Applications of Herbal Excipients and Polymers in Wound Healing

Sachin Kumar Jain
Oriental University, India

Ravikant Gupta
Oriental University, India

Sudha Vengurlekar
Oriental University, India

IGI Global
Scientific Publishing
Publishing Tomorrow's Research Today

Vice President of Editorial	Melissa Wagner
Director of Acquisitions	Mikaela Felty
Director of Book Development	Jocelynn Hessler
Production Manager	Mike Brehm
Cover Design	Jose Rosado

Published in the United States of America by
IGI Global Scientific Publishing
701 East Chocolate Avenue
Hershey, PA, 17033, USA
Tel: 717-533-8845 | Fax: 717-533-7115
Website: https://www.igi-global.com E-mail: cust@igi-global.com

Library of Congress Cataloging-in-Publication Data

LCCN: 2025024574 (CIP Data Pending)
ISBN13: 9798337339771
Isbn13Softcover: 9798337339788
EISBN13: 9798337339795
British Cataloguing in Publication Data
A Cataloguing in Publication record for this book is available from the British Library.

Table of Contents

Detailed Table of Contents

A wound could be defined as a violation of the integrity of living tissue. Wound healing is a complex, tightly controlled process which is vital for protecting the barrier function of skin as well as maintain all other skin functions. Several modifiable and unmodifiable variables could affect this process. Lifestyle habits (smoking, alcohol abuse), oncology treatments (radiation, chemotherapy), medications (steroids, non-steroidal anti-inflammatory drugs, anti-rejection medications) and co-morbidities (diabetes, obesity, protein energy malnutrition) all contribute to this. Diabetes affects nearly all of these healing mechanisms by causing a number of pathological alterations. Increased inflammation and decreased angiogenesis are common features of diabetic wounds. Patients with diabetes have an increased risk of problems related to wound healing following surgery because of these alterations. .

Wound healing is a fundamental physiological process that is critical to the restoration of tissue integrity and function following injury, surgery, or disease. In the realm of healthcare, the significance of effective wound healing cannot be overstated, as it directly influences patient outcomes, healthcare costs, and overall quality of life. Whether wounds are acute, such as surgical incisions and traumatic injuries, or chronic, such as diabetic foot ulcers, pressure ulcers,Wound healing is a fundamental physiological process that is critical to the restoration of tissue integrity and function following injury, surgery, or disease. In the realm of healthcare, the significance of effective wound healing cannot be overstated, as it directly influences patient outcomes, healthcare costs, and overall quality of life. Whether wounds are acute, such as surgical incisions and traumatic injuries, or chronic, such as diabetic foot

Polymers based on polysaccharides have become essential elements in modern wound healing techniques because of their inherent biocompatibility, biodegradability, and functional adaptability. These naturally occurring biopolymers—which include cellulose, dextran, hyaluronic acid, alginate, and chitosan—form the basis for the creation of sophisticated wound dressings. New developments have concentrated on improving these materials' medicinal effectiveness through a variety of changes. For example, by adding stimuli-responsive components, hydrogels that can react dynamically to changes in temperature, pH, and ionic strength have been developed. This allows for the regulated release of bioactive substances and speeds up wound closure. Furthermore, hybrid hydrogel systems that include the beneficial qualities of both components—such as increased mechanical strength and biological activity—have been produced by integrating polysaccharides with synthetic proteins.

Wound healing is a complex biological process involving a cascade of cellular and molecular mechanisms. Recently, natural polymers and herbal excipients have gained attention due to their biocompatibility, therapeutic properties, and low toxicity. This chapter explores the potential of plant-derived gums, natural resins, and herbal oils in wound care. Oils like neem, tea tree, coconut, and calendula exhibit strong antibacterial, anti-inflammatory, and antioxidant actions, aiding in cleansing, infection control, and tissue repair. They also enhance collagen synthesis and hydration. Plant gums such as acacia, guar, and tragacanth support drug delivery, moisture retention, and film formation. Natural resins like myrrh, frankincense, and benzoin offer antimicrobial, astringent, and wound-sealing benefits. Their pharmacological properties, formulation roles, and potential in modern wound care systems are discussed. These agents represent a promising bridge between traditional herbal wisdom and scientific advancement in wound healing.

This chapter explains the role and development of herbal-infused hydrogels in wound healing. This discussion starts with wounds; the wound healing mechanism and factors affecting wound healing and then focuses on the development of wound dressing from the ancient period. It also covers the evolution, and specialized characteristics. Hydrogels are classified based on composition, cross-linking, and functions. This chapter also explains the incorporation of herbal compounds into hydrogels. This chapter shows hydrogel development over the years in wound healing, even though it has challenges that will reduce by future innovation such as development of smart hydrogels in wound management.

This chapter explores the transformative potential of integrating nanotechnology with herbal medicine to advance wound care, addressing challenges like chronic wounds and antimicrobial resistance. It examines how nanoscale systems enhance the delivery, stability, and bioavailability of herbal constituents overcoming limitations like poor solubility and low bioavailability. The discussion covers mechanisms of action, including targeted drug delivery and controlled release, and their applications. Safety concerns, including nanomaterial toxicity and variability in herbal extracts, are analyzed alongside clinical evidence gaps. Future directions, such as green nanotechnology and personalized nanotherapies, are highlighted for their eco-friendly and precision medicine potential. By bridging traditional herbal wisdom with modern nanotechnology, the chapter aims to inspire researchers and clinicians to develop sustainable, effective wound healing therapies, improving patient outcomes while aligning with global healthcare trends.

Wound care stands as a fundamental pillar in the healthcare system, playing a critical role in patient recovery, the prevention of complications, and the enhancement of overall quality of life. Whether resulting from surgical procedures, traumatic injuries, burns, pressure ulcers, or chronic conditions like diabetes, wounds represent a significant medical concern that requires meticulous attention, timely intervention, and specialized careThe impact of inadequate wound management extends beyond individual suffering; it places a substantia. l burden on healthcare systems worldwide in terms of prolonged hospital stays, increased readmission rates, and rising treatment costs. Consequently, effective wound care is not merely a supportive measure but a central component of comprehensive healthcare delivery.At its core, wound care aims to promote healing, reduce the risk of infection, alleviate pain, and restore functionality. It encompasses a wide range of practices, from basic first aid and dressing changes to advanced therapies such.

The process of wound healing involves a number of biochemical processes. Utilizing herbal remedies for wound healing serves to preserve the knowledge of traditional medicine, given its immune-regulating and anti-inflammatory properties, while also aligning with advancements in contemporary biopharmaceutical technology, including the development of innovative biomaterials like hydrogels. Initially, this article presents the innate structural features of healthy skin and the physiological traits associated with chronic wounds in individuals suffering from diabetes and burns. The article goes on to explore the most recent progress in both clinical and experimental research regarding the effects of active constituents in herbal medicine on wound tissue regeneration. It also summarizes current studies investigating the mechanisms of different herbal medicines in healing diabetic and burn wounds. Disruptions in skin integrity contribute to its disorientation, while tissue annihilations lead to the formation of acute or chronic wounds.

Preface

In recent years, the landscape of wound care has undergone a transformative shift—one that is increasingly shaped by a growing awareness of the limitations of conventional synthetic materials and the corresponding rise in demand for sustainable, biocompatible, and patient-friendly alternatives. Among the most promising frontiers in this evolution is the application of herbal excipients and natural polymers. This edited volume, *Applications of Herbal Excipients and Polymers in Wound Healing*, was conceived as a timely and necessary response to this emerging need within the fields of pharmaceutical sciences and biomedical research.

Our aim as editors was to bring together a diverse body of work that captures both the depth and breadth of current research, development, and application of herbal-based materials in wound healing. The chapters included in this book provide a holistic yet technically rigorous overview—ranging from fundamental concepts of natural polymer chemistry and phytochemistry to advanced formulation strategies such as hydrogels, films, dressings, bioadhesives, and nanoformulations.

The book highlights not only the therapeutic potential of herbal excipients and polymers but also their biocompatibility, toxicological safety, and regulatory pathways—critical aspects often overlooked in the enthusiasm surrounding natural materials. We have also taken care to include practical insights from real-world case studies and formulation examples, making this volume especially useful for pharmaceutical scientists, formulation experts, clinicians, and natural product developers alike.

A particular strength of this work lies in its interdisciplinary approach. It bridges traditional knowledge systems and modern pharmaceutical innovation, recognizing the value of both and offering a path forward for their integration. The contributors to this volume—leading researchers, academicians, and professionals from various domains—have lent their expertise to ensure that each chapter is both scientifically sound and practically relevant.

We envision this book as a reference not only for researchers and students in pharmaceutical sciences but also for a broader audience including clinicians, regulatory professionals, and practitioners of traditional medicine. By providing comprehensive knowledge, practical guidelines, and future perspectives, this book aims to inspire new thinking and foster innovation in the design and development of herbal-based wound care therapies.

We would like to extend our heartfelt thanks to all the contributors, reviewers, and support teams whose efforts and commitment made this publication possible. It is our hope that this book serves as a catalyst for further exploration, collaboration, and innovation in this vital area of healthcare.

ORGANIZATION OF THE BOOK

Chapter 1: Introduction to Wound Healing and Its Challenges

This foundational chapter sets the stage by defining wounds and unpacking the multifaceted biological process of wound healing. It delves into the systemic and local factors—ranging from comorbidities like diabetes and obesity to external influences such as medications and lifestyle choices—that impede healing. Special attention is given to the pathophysiology of diabetic wounds, where inflammation and impaired angiogenesis complicate recovery. This chapter provides essential context for understanding why innovative, biocompatible solutions are needed in modern wound care.

Chapter 2: The Role of Herbal Constituents in Wound Healing

Here, the reader is introduced to the therapeutic promise of herbal constituents in wound management. The chapter reviews the biology of acute and chronic wounds and connects it to the use of plant-based actives with antimicrobial, anti-inflammatory, and regenerative properties. Herbal constituents are positioned not merely as alternatives but as functional agents with measurable impacts on healing outcomes, bridging the gap between clinical needs and nature-derived therapies.

Chapter 3: The Role of Some Herbal Constituents in Wound Healing

Expanding on Chapter 2, this chapter offers a detailed analysis of the wound healing process and its stages—hemostasis, inflammation, proliferation, and remodeling—through the lens of herbal intervention. The authors explore how plant-based compounds interact with biological mechanisms such as platelet aggregation, vasoconstriction, and cytokine signaling. Different types of wound healing intentions (primary, secondary, and tertiary) are described, providing a clinical framework to assess the application of herbal actives in diverse wound scenarios.

Chapter 4: Herbal Excipients and Polymers: An Overview

This chapter introduces the core materials that underpin the book: herbal excipients and bioactive polymers. It provides a comprehensive overview of the structural types (gums, mucilages, resins, essential oils) and their functional properties in formulations. Readers will find insights into their roles in controlled release, bioadhesion, film formation, and transdermal systems. Cutting-edge areas such as AI-guided formulation design and standardization efforts are also discussed, illustrating the growing convergence between traditional materials and modern pharmaceutical technology.

Chapter 5: Polysaccharide-Based Polymers

Focused on naturally occurring biopolymers like chitosan, alginate, cellulose, and hyaluronic acid, this chapter explores how polysaccharide-based polymers support wound healing through biodegradability, moisture retention, and bioactivity. Special emphasis is placed on recent innovations such as stimuli-responsive hydrogels and hybrid polymer systems that combine mechanical strength with therapeutic efficacy. These developments signal an exciting future for intelligent wound dressings that adapt to the wound environment.

Chapter 6: Application of Herbal Excipients and Polymers in Wound Healing: Herbal Oils, Gums, and Resins

Here, the focus shifts to specific herbal materials—particularly oils (e.g., neem, tea tree), plant gums (e.g., acacia, guar), and resins (e.g., myrrh, benzoin)—that have long been used in traditional medicine. The chapter evaluates their pharmacological activities, formulation potential, and therapeutic relevance in wound healing. These agents are shown to not only assist in infection control and inflammation reduction but also enhance tissue regeneration and moisture retention, making them invaluable for integrated care approaches.

Chapter 7: Ointments, Creams, and Topical Formulations

This practical chapter examines the formulation and function of semi-solid and topical dosage forms. It outlines the critical considerations in designing herbal-based ointments, creams, and lotions, including ingredient compatibility, skin permeability, and stability. Readers are guided through the advantages of topical delivery—such as localized action and minimal systemic side effects—highlighting the importance of such formulations in both dermatological and systemic applications.

Chapter 8: Bioadhesive Films and Bandages

The final chapter discusses the evolution and promise of bioadhesive wound dressings that combine herbal polymers with advanced drug delivery technologies. Natural biopolymers are explored for their ability to form films and patches that adhere gently to the skin, deliver active agents efficiently, and degrade safely. Examples like pectin-mucilage films and silk fibroin-chitosan combinations illustrate current progress. The chapter also addresses the need for regulatory alignment, standardization, and enhanced clinical validation to facilitate broader adoption of these novel systems.

Chapter 9: Herbal Polymer-Infused Hydrogel Dressings for Enhanced Wound Healing

This chapter examines the unique role of hydrogels as versatile and moisture-retentive dressings and how their therapeutic utility is significantly enhanced when infused with herbal constituents. It traces the historical evolution of wound dressings from ancient remedies to modern hydrogels, emphasizing key characteristics such as biocompatibility, structural integrity, and functionality. The classification of hydrogels—by composition, cross-linking mechanism, and intended function—sets the stage for exploring how plant-based bioactives can be integrated into these systems. The chapter concludes with a discussion on the challenges faced in hydrogel formulation and a look ahead to "smart" hydrogels designed for responsive, targeted, and efficient wound care.

Chapter 10: Nanotechnology in Herbal-Based Wound Care

In this forward-leaning chapter, the convergence of herbal medicine and nanotechnology is explored as a groundbreaking strategy for overcoming common limitations in wound management, including poor drug solubility, low bioavailability, and increasing antimicrobial resistance. Nanoformulations offer controlled release, targeted delivery, and enhanced penetration of herbal actives—amplifying their therapeutic impact. The chapter also addresses critical concerns such as nanotoxicity and batch variability of herbal extracts, highlighting the need for more robust clinical validation. The discussion positions green nanotechnology and personalized nano-therapeutics as promising future directions, presenting a compelling argument for integrative, sustainable wound care solutions.

Chapter 11: Advanced Concepts in Wound Care

Serving as an expansion of Chapter 11, this chapter emphasizes wound care as a central healthcare priority with direct implications on patient outcomes, healthcare costs, and system burden. The narrative contextualizes the broader impact of inadequate wound management, from prolonged hospital stays to increased morbidity. It outlines the clinical imperatives of modern wound care—preventing infection, managing pain, promoting healing—and connects these goals with advanced therapeutic modalities, including herbal nanotechnology. The chapter reinforces the importance of innovative, accessible, and evidence-based wound care as an integral part of modern medical practice.

Chapter 12: Case Studies of Successful Herbal-Based Wound Formulations

This chapter grounds the theoretical discussions in real-world application by presenting clinical and experimental case studies of effective herbal-based wound therapies. Chronic wounds, particularly in patients with diabetes and burns, are used as focal points to demonstrate the impact of specific phytochemicals on tissue regeneration. Through detailed examples, the chapter highlights the role of hydrogels, herbal oils, and natural biomaterials in addressing pathophysiological disruptions such as inflammation and impaired collagen synthesis. The integration of traditional medicinal knowledge with contemporary biomedical innovations is emphasized, offering readers a nuanced understanding of translational potential.

Chapter 13: Precautions in the Use of Herbal Polymers

While the benefits of herbal polymers are numerous, this chapter introduces a critical counterbalance: the need for rigorous safety, standardization, and regulatory oversight. The assumption that "natural" equates to "safe" is challenged, and the authors delve into potential toxicities, allergens, and formulation inconsistencies. Regulatory guidelines, including those from the WHO and regional pharmacopeias, are examined to illustrate the fragmented and evolving governance landscape. The chapter advocates for a cautious yet progressive approach—combining ethnobotanical knowledge with modern toxicology and pharmacovigilance to ensure the responsible use of herbal polymers in wound care.

Chapter 14: Regulatory and Ethical Perspective on Herbal Polymers and Excipients

This chapter provides a deeper dive into the regulatory frameworks shaping the development of herbal-based wound care products. It addresses the lack of standardized procedures for assessing quality, safety, and efficacy—compounded by variability in botanical sources and extraction processes. Ethical considerations, including informed consent and sustainability of sourcing, are also examined. The regulatory stances of major global bodies such as the FDA, EMA, and WHO are compared, and the chapter concludes with a call for harmonized, product-specific guidelines to facilitate the wider adoption of herbal excipients in clinical settings.

Chapter 15: Wound Healing with Herbal Excipients: Navigating Regulatory and Ethical Landscapes

Complementing the previous chapter, this section explores how regulatory fragmentation and ethical dilemmas hinder the integration of herbo-polymeric technologies in mainstream medicine. By analyzing the interdisciplinary science behind herbal excipients and synthetic/natural polymers, the authors present a holistic view of wound dressing innovation. The emphasis is on mimicking the extracellular matrix and creating controlled-release systems that leverage herbal actives. Ethical concerns—such as the cultural appropriation of traditional knowledge and equitable benefit-sharing—are thoughtfully discussed, providing a roadmap for developing responsible and inclusive herbal wound care solutions.

Chapter 16: Challenges and Opportunities in Herbal Wound Care

Focusing on the limitations of current treatment strategies, this chapter outlines the persistent gaps in evidence-based management of chronic wounds, especially those unresponsive to standard therapies. It critically evaluates the role of herbal and natural products as promising yet underutilized alternatives. With the rise of complementary and alternative medicines (CAMs), the chapter identifies research, formulation, and clinical validation as areas ripe for development. The authors encourage interdisciplinary collaboration to overcome the scientific, regulatory, and clinical barriers that currently limit the broader use of herbal therapies in chronic wound management.

CONCLUSION

As editors of *Applications of Herbal Excipients and Polymers in Wound Healing*, it is our distinct pleasure to conclude this volume by reflecting on the journey this book represents—not only in content, but in purpose. This reference work stands at the intersection of tradition and technology, drawing from centuries-old herbal wisdom and aligning it with the rigor and precision of modern pharmaceutical science.

Throughout the chapters, contributors from diverse scientific and clinical backgrounds have explored the multifaceted potential of herbal excipients and polymers in wound care. From foundational principles and material science to advanced delivery systems and regulatory frameworks, each section builds toward a more holistic understanding of how plant-derived materials can reshape wound healing paradigms. Together, these insights point toward a future where sustainable, biocompatible, and evidence-based solutions become integral to both mainstream and alternative medicine.

We have also sought to acknowledge the critical challenges that remain—variability in natural sources, regulatory ambiguities, formulation complexities, and the need for clinical validation. Addressing these issues will require collaborative efforts across disciplines, sectors, and borders. But within these challenges lie equally powerful opportunities: to innovate, to personalize, and to reconnect medicine with nature in responsible and scientifically robust ways.

This book is intended not as a conclusion, but as a beginning—a foundation for further exploration, experimentation, and translation. We hope it serves as a valuable resource for researchers, formulators, clinicians, and students seeking to advance the science and application of herbal materials in wound healing. Most importantly, we hope it inspires continued inquiry into how the natural world can inform and enrich human health in meaningful, measurable ways.

Chapter 1

Introduction to Wound Healing and Its Challenges

Raman Kumari
https://orcid.org/0009-0007-0569-4258
M.M. College of Pharmacy, India

ABSTRACT

A wound could be defined as a violation of the integrity of living tissue. Wound healing is a complex, tightly controlled process which is vital for protecting the barrier function of skin as well as maintain all other skin functions. Several modifiable and unmodifiable variables could affect this process. Lifestyle habits (smoking, alcohol abuse), oncology treatments (radiation, chemotherapy), medications (steroids, non-steroidal anti-inflammatory drugs, anti-rejection medications) and co-morbidities (diabetes, obesity, protein energy malnutrition) all contribute to this. Diabetes affects nearly all of these healing mechanisms by causing a number of pathological alterations. Increased inflammation and decreased angiogenesis are common features of diabetic wounds. Patients with diabetes have an increased risk of problems related to wound healing following surgery because of these alterations. .

INTRODUCTION

Wounds are injuries that happen when the skin's integrity is compromised by abrupt, rash, and typically unanticipated occurrences. The injury can be caused by a variety of things, including cuts, crushes, thermal or radiation burns, or surgical procedures. It can range from superficial damage, which only affects the outer layers of the skin, to the destruction of deep tissues, including muscles, nerves, and blood

DOI: 10.4018/979-8-3373-3977-1.ch001

arteries. The primary issue with wound care is the significant chance of chronicity (Tatarusanu et al., 2023). There are two main categories of wounds: acute wounds and chronic wounds. Acute wounds heal on their own in a very systematic and effective way. Four separate but overlapping phases—haemostasis, inflammation, proliferation, and remodeling—define them. These wounds go through the typical phases of wound healing, including remodelling, proliferation, and inflammation, and within two to four weeks, they exhibit clear indications of healing. On the other hand, chronic wounds do not heal in the same order and frequently become "stalled" in one phase and fail to demonstrate any evidence of healing within 4 weeks (Monika et al., 2022).

Acute Wounds

Tissue damage that "usually results in a sustained restoration of anatomic and functional integrity through an orderly and timely reparative process". There are six types of acute wounds:

1. Abrasions: superficial wounds when the epidermis, the skin's outermost layer, is scraped off. A sliding fall onto a rough surface, such concrete, asphalt, or tree bark, frequently results in abrasions.
2. Avulsions: injuries that result from a body part being violently removed from its natural location. This kind of amputation involves pulling the extremity off instead of cutting it off.
3. Lacerations: A wound brought on by tearing or crushing pressure. Incisions and lacerations can have a stellate (irregular) or linear (regular) appearance.
4. Crush or Cut Wounds: When a heavy object falls on a person, it might crush a portion of the body or cut the body structures with a sharp object, causing wounds. This category includes injuries occurred at home, on the road, and during surgery. Using blades or nails to puncture skin falls under this category as well. These wounds can affect the body's internal structures (dermis and portion of hypoderm) or the epidermis, causing superficial or profound damage, respectively.
5. Velocity or Missile Wounds: When a bullet or other high-speed object penetrates the body, it causes wounds. Velocity wounds include those caused by gunshots or ballistic trauma.
6. Wounds brought on by the acute or long-term effects of ionizing radiation are known as radiation wounds or ulcers. The skin, underlying soft tissues, and even deep structures like bone may be affected (Irfan-Maqsood, 2016).

Chronic Wounds

Chronic wounds are those brought on by metabolic diseases. These wounds require a long time to heal, whereas acute wounds heal in a balanced and brief amount of time. In chronic wounds, the synthesis and breakdown of cells and extracellular matrix, such as collagen, are out of equilibrium. These wounds are often divided into three groups: pressure ulcers, diabetic ulcers, and venous/vascular ulcers. Ischemic wounds are another subtype of chronic wounds. Table 1 describes the etiology of several chronic wounds, including causes, infection risk, dysregulation types, and common treatment options (Ahmad, 2023).

Table 1. Etiology of different types of chronic wounds underlying cause, dysregulation, infection risk and standard of care

Type of Ulcer	Causes	Dysregulation	Infection Risk	Standard of Care
Arterial ulcers	Peripheral artery disease, atherosclerosis/occlusion, critical limb ischemia, dyslipidaemia	Predominance of M1 macrophages, inflammation, oxidative stress, necrosis, nutrient deficiency	High	Restoration of blood flow
Venous ulcers	Endothelial dysfunction, ischemia, increase in intraluminal pressure, venous insufficiency	Inflammation, leakage of fibrin, elevated MMPs levels, oxidative stress, iron overload, tissue metabolites accumulation	High	Restoration of venous hydrostatic pressure
Pressure ulcers	Deep tissue oedema, traumatic injury, pressure, ischemia-reperfusion injury	Inflammation, oxidative stress	High	Relieve of pressure
Diabetic foot ulcers	Impaired angiogenesis, neuropathy, endothelial dysfunction, micro-vascular disease, dysregulated cytokines levels	Inflammation, elevated MMPs levels, hyperglycaemia, hyperlipidaemia, advanced glycation end (AGE) products accumulation	High	Multifactorial counteract of pathogenesis for microenvironment restoration

The Wound Healing Process

The dynamic and complex process of wound healing is made up of four overlapping phases: hemostasis, inflammation, proliferation, and remodeling. Hemostasis starts with blood coagulation, which includes growth factor release, platelet accumulation, degranulation, and fibrin clot formation. Consequently, endothelial cells, macrophages, and fibroblasts participate in wound healing. During the inflammatory stage, neutrophils clear the wound of cellular debris and guard against harmful infections, promoting quickly healing conditions. The symptoms of inflammation, including redness, warmth, erythema, and swelling of the injured skin, are brought on by exudates. Damaged skin causes dead cells to be replaced by new epithelial cells that invade the wound area. The length of the hemostasis and inflammatory phases is determined by the extent of the injury. In the third stage which is proliferative stage, cell proliferation and formation of connective tissue occurs. Further the extracellular matrix (ECM) components like glycosaminoglycan and hyaluronic acid contribute in the granulation tissue production so as to replace the development of primary clot. After an injury, this phase may last for a few days to a few weeks. The last step, which can span anywhere from a few weeks to several months, is a remodeling or maturation phase. At finally, fibroblast cells with scar formation completely restore the surface of the injured tissue (Yasin et al., 2023). The stages of wound healing are shown in Table 2 and Figure 1.

Figure 1. Phases of wound healing

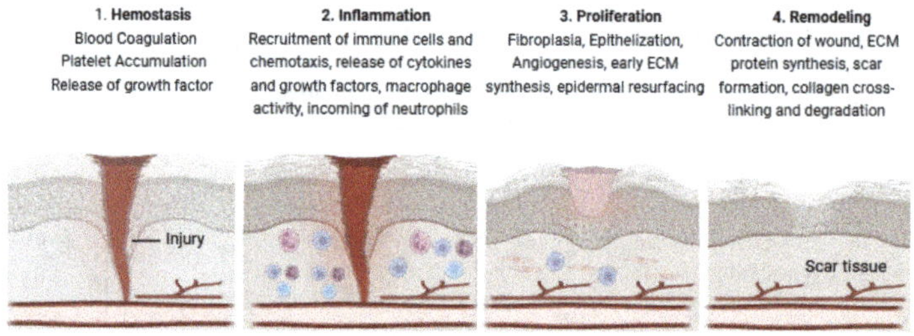

Table 2. Stages of wound healing

Stage	Days	Pathophysiology	Outcomes
Hemostasis	Up to hours	Clotting, Vasoconstriction	Bleeding stops
Inflammation (body prepares itself to fight off infection and repair the injury)	2-5 days	Growth factors and cytokines released, phagocytosis, vasodilation, neutrophils release reactive oxygen species and protease	Redness, swelling, warmth and pain
Proliferation (Promotes new cellular growth to help with healing of the injury)	Up to 3 weeks	Synthesis of collagen (type III), granulation formation, epithelization, angiogenesis, contraction	New blood vessel growth, wound closure
Remodeling (cells are woven together to strengthen the newly healed site)	Up to 2 years	Scar remodeling (type III to I collagen)	Scar strength increases to approximately 80% of original tissue

Hemostasis

Immediately after injury, damaged blood vessels rapid contract and a blood clot form preventing exsanguination from vascular damage (Velnar et al., 2009). Platelets, which are essential for coagulation and hemostasis, get activated when they come into contact with the vascular subendothelial matrix. Glycoprotein VI and other platelet receptors interact with extracellular matrix (ECM) proteins, such as collagen, fibronectin, and von Willebrand factor, to increase adhesion to the blood vessel wall. Thrombin then causes platelets to activate, changing their shape and releasing dense granules and alpha particles that contain bioactive compounds that strengthen coagulation (Golebiewska & Poole, 2015). Fibrin, fibronectin, vitronectin, and thrombospondin combine to create an insoluble clot (eschar), which mainly plugs the site and stops the bleeding. In addition, the eschar serves a variety of secondary purposes, including as protecting against bacterial invasion, acting as a scaffold for incoming immune cells, and housing a reservoir of growth factors and cytokines that direct the behavior of wound cells during the early stages of repair (Zaidi & Green, 2019). In order to attract immune cells to the site of damage, platelets are essential because they can either directly capture immune cells in the eschar or, upon degranulation, release a secretome of chemokine attractants. Indeed, the growth factors found in the platelet secretome also activate fibroblasts and keratinocytes, two types of resident skin cells (Scully et al., 2020). Early suppression of bacterial infection is facilitated by platelets, the most prevalent cell type during early healing. Toll-like receptors (TLRs), which control the synthesis of antimicrobial peptides, are expressed by them in various amounts. By stopping the coagulation process when a sufficient-sized clot has formed, excessive thrombosis is avoided. In this instance, prostacylin inhibits platelet aggregation, antithrombin III inhibits thrombin, and activated protein C degrades coagulation components V through VII. Smooth muscle and endothelial cells, which multiply in response to released platelet-derived growth factor (PDGF), simultaneously heal the damaged vessel wall. To facilitate this process, endothelial progenitors are also enlisted because mature endothelial cells have a restricted ability for proliferation (Wilkinson & Hardman, 2020).

Inflammation

A complex coordination of immune system cells and molecular interactions, including macrophages, neutrophils, lymphocytes, and signaling molecules, is involved in inflammation during wound healing. It starts after hemostasis, when complement cascades and coagulation cause blood vessels to widen. Bradykinin and anaphylatoxins are important players in this process (Nami et al., 2016). By increasing blood artery permeability, anaphylatoxins make it possible for neutrophils and monocytes to get to damage sites. Additionally, they increase the inflammatory response by inducing mast cells to produce histamine and leukotrienes. Inflammatory cell migration at wound sites is facilitated by this increase in EC permeability, which also breaks down cell-to-cell contacts (Petreaca et al., 2007). Neutrophils are the main leukocytes seen in wounds, and they use a variety of strategies to fight infection, including reactive oxygen species (ROS), proteases, and antimicrobial peptides. Through processes involving caspases and cathepsin D, these entities undergo programmed cell death and have a brief lifespan (Schraufstatter et al., 2001). Although neutrophils may not impede wound healing, chronic nonhealing wounds may result from their extended absence. The chemotactic process, which is aided by other immune cells such as neutrophils and keratinocytes, allows monocytes, the predominant inflammatory cells at wound sites, to migrate towards the site of injury. Monocyte migration is guided by CCL2 chemokines, but keratinocytes and neutrophils are also involved (Nathan, 2006). The migration of monocytes to wound sites and their subsequent differentiation into macrophages is essential for wound healing. Macrophages generate cytokines and growth hormones, present antigens, and destroy apoptotic neutrophils. They also offer antigens and eradicate sick cells (Conus et al., 2008). Growth factors that activate and recruit cells, such as TGF-a, TGF-b, bFGF, PDGF, and VEGF, facilitate wound healing by boosting angiogenesis, ECM formation, and proliferation. Additionally, VEGF stimulates angiogenesis by inducing macrophages to produce LIGHT, a cytokine belonging to the TNF-a family, which may result in apoptosis (Simpson & Ross et al., 1972). Coordination between immune system cells and signaling molecules is essential for the systematic progression of wound healing, encompassing both the early inflammatory response and subsequent tissue repair and remodeling phases. The function of macrophages is essential to the healing process because their absence or malfunction significantly hinders wound closure. According to research, the loss of macrophages during the healing phase of skin wounds may lead to inadequate tissue removal, a reduction in fibroblast counts, and a postponement of the healing process. It is crucial to remember, however, that inflammation is not a necessary precondition for the skin's ability to heal wounds (Daley et al., 2005). In wound healing, studies indicate that regulating the inflammatory response can aid in minimizing the production of scars. However, decreased macrophage activity at the site of the lesion can make it more difficult to resolve inflammation, particularly in wounds caused by diabetes. This persistent inflammatory state can hinder wound closure and exacerbate the development of scars, particularly in diabetes wounds where the persistent inflammatory state precludes a resolving phenotype. Lipid mediators that influence inflammation and wound healing include protectins, resolvins, lipoxins, and maresins. In order to resolve and combat inflammation, they trigger actions. Since B and T cells start focused immune responses against infections and foreign substances, they are essential for wound healing. Due to their ability to initiate inflammation and resolve it by apoptosis, which is aided by interferon-c and TNF-a, mast cells are essential for wound healing. They also affect the fibrosis and wound-healing processes.

As long as it is necessary, the inflammatory phase of wound healing will continue, making sure that the wound is free of excess pathogens and debris. However, prolonged inflammation can cause delayed proliferation, significant tissue damage, and the development of a chronic wound. It is believed that a number of substances, including as lipoxins and byproducts of arachidonic acid metabolism, have anti-inflammatory qualities that suppress the immune system and promote the emergence of the subsequent stage of wound healing. The different types of cells involved in inflammation along with their functions is shown in Table 3 (Mamun et al., 2024).

Table 3. Functions of different cell types in wound healing

Cell Type	Functions
Keratinocytes	Forms the outer layer of the skin (epidermis), migrate and proliferate to cover the surface of the wound (re-epithelization), to promote healing secretes growth factors and cytokines
Fibroblasts	For tissue repair – produce collagen, elastin and ECM components, reduces the wound size and is responsible for contraction of the wound
Inflammatory cells	Neutrophils: clears pathogens and debris through phagocytosis and are first responders to the injury. Macrophages: clean up the cellular debris, help release growth factors and regulate inflammation Mast cells: to initiate inflammatory response release histamine along with other inflammatory mediators.
Endothelial cells	Angiogenesis (new blood vessel formation), secrete growth factors to stimulate other cells.
Platelets	Form blood clot in hemostasis stage of wound healing, release growth factors such as platelet-derived growth factor (PDGF) and transforming growth factor ß
Mesenchymal stem cells	Promotes tissue regeneration and secrete factors which modulate inflammation, enhance collagen deposition and angiogenesis

PROLIFERATION

The proliferative stage of the healing cascade can start to fix the defect if the damaging stimulus has stopped, hemostasis has been reached, the inflammatory response is in balance, and the wound is clear of debris. This intricate process includes the simultaneous occurrence of angiogenesis, granulation tissue formation, collagen deposition, epithelialization, and wound retraction.

Angiogenesis

As platelets release TGF-b, PDGF, and FGF, angiogenesis begins as soon as the haemostatic plug forms. In reaction to hypoxia, VEGF is released, which causes endothelial cells to initiate neovascularization and blood vessel repair when combined with other cytokines. When neutrophils invade hypoxic tissue, they activate a family of enzymes known as mixed metalloproteinases (MMP). They stimulate angiogenesis by remodeling the extracellular matrix (ECM) and releasing VEGF. Since the wound's center depends only on diffusion from the healthy capillaries at the wound's periphery, it is initially comparatively avascular. With the progression of angiogenesis, healthy artery offshoots develop a rich vascular network of capillaries throughout the wound. The capillaries are initially brittle and porous, which exacerbates tissue oedema and gives the impression of granulation tissue that is healing (Siefert & Sarkar, 2012).

Fibroblast Migration

Following the wound insult, growth factors produced from the hemostatic clot induce fibroblasts to multiply before migrating to the wound (mostly TGF-b and PDGF). The wound becomes filled with fibroblasts by the third day, which deposit extracellular matrix proteins (fibronectins, hyaluronan, and proteoglycans) and proceed on to generate collagen and fibronectin. Granulation tissue is the pink, fibrous, vascular tissue that forms in the wound site when a clot breaks. In contrast to unwounded tissue, this is made up of a different kind of collagens, with a larger percentage of type 3 collagen. Fibroblasts transform into myofibroblasts and produce pseudopodia after a suitable matrix has been established. This makes it possible for them to attach to the collagen and fibronectin proteins in the surrounding area and support wound contraction. Additionally, myofibroblasts stimulate angiogenesis by mediating MMP activity (Mayrand et al., 2012). Fibroblasts produce collagens, which are essential for giving tissues strength. Collagen deposition reaches its maximum in primary purpose wounds by day five, and this is frequently palpable as a "wound ridge" beneath the skin. An indication that a wound is at risk of dehiscence is when a ridge cannot be felt. A hypertrophic scar may form as a result of excessive collagen production. Hypertrophic scars stay inside the original wound's boundaries but continue to be elevated and erythematous. Wound infections and environments with high levels of stress are risk factors for their development.

Epithelization

Soon after the first injury, epithelial cells begin to migrate from the wound's edges until the entire cell sheet covers the lesion and adheres to the matrix underneath. The epithelial-mesenchymal transition (EMT) is an embryological process that gives epithelial cells the ability to move and cover the surface of wounds (Yang & Weinberg, 2008). This stage can be finished in a day for wounds that are mostly closed. To repopulate epithelial cell levels and finish wound repair, epithelial cells change from a motile to a proliferative phenotype in response to changes in cytokine concentration (De Donatis et al., 2010). The region devoid of epithelial cells in secondary intention wounds may be sizable, and the wound must shrink considerably before epithelialization is finished. Sometimes this won't happen, and the defect can be covered via skin grafting (Hinz, 2006).

Wound Retraction

Seven days after damage, wounds start to constrict, primarily because to myofibroblasts. By drawing the cell bodies closer together, actin and myosin interactions reduce the area of tissue that needs to repair. The rate of contraction might be 0.75 mm each day, resulting in shorter scars. Wound shape is one of several elements that affect this; circular wounds contract the slowest, whereas linear wounds contract the fastest. Contractures and deformities may result from disorders during this healing phase (Hunt, 1988).

REMODELLING

As granulation tissue develops, the extracellular matrix begins to be synthesized and remodeled, a process that lasts for a long time. As the extracellular matrix is continuously remodeled, collagen is continuously synthesized and broken down, reaching a stable state approximately 21 days after injury. The interactions between fibroblasts and the extracellular matrix around them cause wound contraction, which is impacted by several cytokines such as basic fibroblast growth factor, platelet-derived growth factor, and transforming growth factor-β. At the wound site, fibroblasts, neutrophils, and macrophages create particular metalloproteinases that break down collagen. Growth factors, cytokines, and phagocytic stimuli all influence the synthesis and secretion of metalloproteinases. Metalloproteinases include:

- Interstitial collagenases are among the metalloproteinases that cleave fibrillar collagen types I, II, and III.

- Gelatinases, also known as type-IV collagenases, break down fibronectin and amorphous collagen.
- Stromelysins, which catabolize a range of extracellular matrix components, including as amorphous collagen, laminin, fibronectin, and proteoglycans (Enoch & Leaper, 2008).

Different from neutrophil elastase, cathepsin G, plasmin, and other serine proteases that can also break down the extracellular matrix but are not metalloenzymes, metalloproteinases rely on zinc ions to function. Due to their ability to break down vital collagen and impede healing, metalloproteinases' activity is strictly controlled. Usually developed as inactive (zymogen) precursors that need to be activated first, they are carried out by specific proteases (like plasmin), which are probably only found at injury sites. Most mesenchymal cells generate tissue inhibitors of metalloproteinases, which can also quickly stop activated collagenases. Additional wound remodeling results in:

- decreased metalloproteinase activity and increased tissue inhibitory metalloproteinase activity;
- decreased macrophage and fibroblast density;
- haulted capillary outgrowth;
- decreased blood flow and metabolic activity;
- decreased size of the underlying contractile connective tissue (which brings the wound margins close together).

The granulation tissue scaffolding eventually transforms into an avascular scar made up of extracellular matrix components, thick collagen, pieces of elastic tissue, and mostly dormant fibroblasts. As the scar ages, collagen bundles enlarge and fibronectin and hyaluronan are broken down, which correlates with the wound's growing tensile strength. A maximum of 80% of the strength of unwounded skin can be attained, however these collagen fibers never restore the original strength of unwounded skin (Broughton et al., 2006).

Factors That Impair Wound Healing

Impaired wound healing can be caused by a variety of reasons. The factors that affect repair can generally be divided into two categories: systemic and local. Whereas systemic factors are those that impact an individual's ability to heal due to their general health or illness, local factors are those that directly affect the characteristics of the wound itself (Table 4). The systemic factors influence wound healing through local effects, and many of these aspects are interrelated.

Table 4. Factors that impair wound healing

Local Factors	Systemic Factors
Oxygenation	Advanced age and gender
Infection	Obesity
Presence of foreign body	Malnutrition
Inadequate blood supply	Stress
Increased skin tension	Diseases: diabetes mellitus, rheumatoid arthritis, jaundice, uremia, metabolic diseases
Poor venous drainage	Ischemia
Presence of slough and/or non-viable tissue	Life style habits: alcohol and smoking
Continued presence of micro-organisms	Chemotherapy and radiotherapy
Excess local mobility	Immunosuppressant drugs, anticoagulants, corticosteroids
Underlying osteomyelitis	Impaired macrophage activity

Local Factors

Oxygen. In order for cells to manufacture energy by producing ATP, oxygen is crucial for cell metabolism. Additionally, oxygen is required for the healing process of wounds. In addition to preventing infection, oxygen is required to stimulate wound contraction, boost fibroblast cell proliferation, collagen synthesis, keratinocyte differentiation, migration, and re-epithelialization, and induce angiogenesis. Moreover, polymorphonuclear leukocytes' generation of superoxide, which is essential for the oxidative destruction of pathogens, is heavily reliant on oxygen. Due to hypoxia, increased metabolism, and the microenvironment in oxygen-deficient wounds, blood vessels may be damaged and high oxygen consumption may result (Bishop, 2008). Poor tissue oxygenation can be caused by vascular abnormalities brought on by a number of systemic diseases, such as diabetes and senior age. Poor perfusion during the healing process might result in hypoxia in the wound. Poor oxygenation will impede the healing process of wounds. While chronic and sustained hypoxia might impair wound healing, temporary hypoxia brought on by injury can accelerate it. Hypoxia in acute wounds can act as a signal to promote the healing process. Macrophages, keratinocytes, and fibroblast cells can all produce cytokines and growth factors in response to hypoxia. PDGF, TGF-β, VEGF, TNF-, and endothelin-1 are among the cytokines that are generated in response to hypoxia, along with promoter cells that are crucial for angiogenesis, chemotaxis, migration, and cell proliferation in wound healing. Sufficient oxygen concentrations are necessary for the best possible wound healing. As hypoxia can trigger the production of growth factors and angiogenesis, for which oxygen is necessary to sustain the wound healing process, it promotes wound healing (Rodriguez et al., 2008).

Infection. Injuries to the skin may result in a local bacterial infection, which delays the healing process. The majority of pathogenic bacteria are Streptococcal species, Pseudomonas aeruginosa, and Staphylococcus aureus. The human body starts inflammatory processes in reaction to infection, including cytokine release and leukocyte migration (Edwards & Harding et al., 2004). Nevertheless, phagocytic leukocytes trigger the release of endotoxins by bacteria, which leads to localized inflammation and necrosis because of elevated pro-inflammatory cytokines, high metalloproteinase activity, and reduced growth factor release. The first physiological process of healing is the inflammatory response. Chronic inflammation can delay wound retraction and tissue remodeling, interfere with re-epithelialization, and impede the healing process (Rosyid, 2022).

Systemic Factors

Advanced Age and Gender. One of the main risk factors for poor wound healing is aging. The epidermal layer thins with age, and metabolic and systemic changes might result from becoming older. The inflammatory response of the aged is altered in a number of ways, including delayed leukocyte recruitment to the region, reduced growth factor/cytokine release, and diminished macrophage activity as phagocytosis. Decreased fibroblast activity, collagen remodeling, delayed angiogenesis, and re-epithelialization are other effects of aging (Beyene et al., 2020).

Obesity. Chronic obesity contributes to a number of issues with wound healing. Obese wounds frequently include pressure and venous ulcers linked to hematoma, edema, seroma development, and local infection. Reduced skin micro-perfusion, increased production of pro-inflammatory cytokines, and a weakened immune response are cellular and molecular factors linked to poor wound healing in obesity (Sen, 2021).

Stress. Through the dysregulation of endocrine hormones, stress can impede the healing of wounds and a number of systemic disorders. Because stress affects the hypothalamus and neurological system, it can cause an increase in the release of cortisol, glucocorticoids, norepinephrine, and adrenaline. These substances have the ability to reduce leukocyte immunological response and cytokine release, which can interfere with inflammatory processes and slow the healing of wounds (Takahashi et al., 2018).

Nutrition. DNA and protein synthesis are crucial components of the healing process. Any reduction in the cofactors or building blocks (such as amino acids and nucleic acids) required for these processes may be harmful to the wound. Due to the significant quantity of collagen production that occurs, protein deprivation has a substantial effect, but malnutrition of any kind can have serious deleterious effects. Reduced collagen and proteoglycan synthesis, decreased angiogenesis, decreased fibroblast proliferation, and reduced collagen remodeling are all consequences of a depleted protein status (Otranto et al., 2009). When albumin levels are below 1.5 mg/dL, collagen synthesis and wound healing are both negatively impacted. Protein catabolism brought on by inadequate carbohydrate intake or reserve causes the depletion of proteins necessary for repair. Weeks before and after an injury, when acute malnutrition is present, these consequences are most noticeable. Poor healing can also result from vitamin deficits, particularly in zinc, thiamine, and vitamins C and A. Collagen creation requires vitamin C and thiamine (B1), and shortages result in reduced crosslinking and, eventually, wound strength. Although vitamin A plays a crucial role in inflammation, its exact function is unknown. Another essential component for wound healing is zinc, which ought to be added during the perioperative phase, particularly in high-risk groups (such as those with head and neck cancer). Many patients with head and neck cancer who need reconstruction have significant malnutrition, which is generally defined as a weight reduction of 10% or more. Repletive enteral nourishment with a nasogastric tube, even for a little duration, will greatly accelerate the healing process following surgery (Payne et al., 2008).

Life Style Habits

Alcohol. Impaired wound healing is a result of both acute and chronic alcohol consumption. Suppression of host immunity and increased vulnerability to infection are two of the processes involved. Research shows that alcohol reduces the recruitment and activity of neutrophils and pro-inflammatory cytokines at the onset of inflammation, while at a later stage of healing, it increases cytokines and leukocytes. Furthermore, alcohol consumption affects the proliferative phase by reducing angiogenesis in the wound area by VEGF receptor expression. Consequently, oxidative stress molecules and free radicals are formed in the wound region, creating a hypoxic environment. Additionally, drinking alcohol affects extracellular matrix metalloproteinase concentrations, reduces collagen synthesis, and interferes with remodeling processes (Avishai et al., 2017).

Smoking. Smoking has been linked to a higher risk of a number of ailments, including delayed wound healing. Additionally, research indicates that the substances found in tobacco cigarettes—nicotine, carbon monoxide, and hydrogen cyanide—have the potential to influence the processes involved in wound healing. Smoking can hinder wound healing and reduce erythrocyte proliferation, oxygenation, blood flow, and angiogenesis in wounded tissues since hypoxia is one of the primary processes linked to smoking. Additionally, smoking raises blood viscosity, platelet aggregation and adhesiveness, and the risk of embolism and thrombosis. Additionally, cigarette chemicals may reduce collagen remodeling, fibroblast migration, and proliferation. Smoking affects the immune system by decreasing the function of neutrophils, macrophages, and lymphocytes, which increases the risk of infection (Beahrs et al., 2019).

Chemotherapy and Radiotherapy

Chemotherapy. The goal of these therapeutic medicines is to modify cellular replication on several levels. The cells with the highest turnover are the most impacted. There is also a reduction in monocytes and megakaryocytes, which leads to a decrease in circulating platelets and macrophages due to bone marrow inhibition of cells directly involved in the healing process. There are noticeable healing delays.

Radiotherapy. Short-term and long-term impacts are two categories of the various ways that radiation affects wound healing. Radiation changes cellular replication and causes microvascular obliteration and fibrosis in the short term. The impacts on blood vessels are responsible for long-term alterations, which include vessel wall degradation and constriction of all vessel dimensions. The best time to perform surgery on radiation patients is after the acute phase of injury but before the chronic phase has established itself. After radiation therapy, this time frame corresponds to three weeks to three months (Horn et al., 1995).

Sex Hormones in Aged Individuals. It has been demonstrated that older males recover acute wounds more slowly than older females. This can be partially explained by the fact that the wound-healing process seems to be significantly impacted by the male androgens testosterone and 5α-dihydrotestosterone, DHT, and the female estrogens estrogen and 17β-estradiol, as well as their steroid precursor dehydroepiandrosterone (DHEA). It was recently discovered that the majority of the gene expression variations between young and old male human wounds are controlled by estrogen. By controlling several genes linked to regeneration, matrix synthesis, protease inhibition, epidermal function, and the genes mostly linked to inflammation, estrogen influences wound healing. Research shows that while androgens adversely affect the healing of cutaneous wounds, estrogen can help both men and women with age-related healing impairment (Hardman & Ashcroft, 2008).

Drugs. A number of medications can prevent wound healing by interfering with the coagulation cascade, inflammatory mechanisms, or cell proliferation. Corticosteroids, which are commonly used as anti-inflammatory agents and to modulate the immune response, may cause a decrease in growth factors and cytokines, which may modulate wound healing mechanisms and decrease fibroblast proliferation (Franz et al., 2007). Non-steroidal anti-inflammatory drugs (NSAIDs), which are used systemically to treat inflammation and pain, have also been shown to have a negative effect on wound healing by slowing down angiogenesis and fibroblast proliferation. When applied topically, NSAID formulations may promote wound healing and lessen local pain (Krischak et al., 2007). Chemotherapy medications can also impede wound healing because of their potential to lower metabolism and cell proliferation. As a result, wound retraction is delayed and angiogenesis, collagen synthesis, and re-epithelialization are all reduced. Insulin has been shown to enhance the healing of diabetic ulcers by promoting angiogenesis and accelerating re-epithelialization. In rat diabetic ulcer models, metformin can speed up epithelialization, enhance vascular function, and lower the risk of vascular complications. In diabetic ulcer model mice, glibenclamide can stimulate angiogenesis, encourage the production of granulation tissue, and speed up epithelialization (Lee et al., 2014).

Hypertrophic Scarring and Keloids. Excessive immature collagen (type III) and particularly ECM (water and glycoprotein) deposits lead to decreased collagen lysis and an increased proliferative phase of healing, which in turn causes hypertrophic scars and keloids. Although keloids spread outside the bounds of the initial lesion, hypertrophic scars remain inside them. Although they can be found in people of all ethnicities, darker-pigmented people are more likely to be affected. Notably, there haven't been any reports of keloids in albinos yet. Keloid development is most common in African Americans (6–16%). The earlobe, angle of the mandible, upper back and shoulders, upper arms, and anterior chest are the body parts most vulnerable to this aberrant scarring, yet they can appear anywhere. Hormonal aspects are important since they are typically only noticeable in women throughout their reproductive years, which span from puberty to menopause.

It is important to emphasize the necessity of tension-free closures since increased areas of wound tension are also vulnerable. Keloid growth is a concern during the third week, when the proliferative process seems to be continuing unchecked. Determining whether keloid or hypertrophic scarring will occur at this stage is challenging, and despite much investigation, the cause of the change from one to the other remains unknown. Given the increased mRNA expression of TGF-b1 in keloid tissue, TGF-b appears to be a major factor in keloid development (Abdou et al., 2011).

Diabetes. For a variety of reasons, diabetics experience poor wound healing. Diabetes increases the risk of infection in diabetic people due to decreased perfusion brought on by accelerated atherosclerosis and neuropathy. In addition to weakened immunity, this creates the conditions for protracted and aberrant healing. In addition to the evident immunological dysfunction, diabetics also exhibit reduced angiogenesis, slower collagen production and accumulation, and weaker wound tensile strength, all of which contribute to a higher rate of dehiscence. In the diabetic healing wound, strict control of hyperglycemia is crucial; in certain cases, this may even require hospitalization and endocrine advice (Gantwerker & Hom, 2011).

Nanotechnology in Wound Healing

Nanotechnology is an emerging field with numerous applications in skin regeneration. Due to their structural resemblance to the extracellular matrix, nanofibers have drawn particular attention in the field of skin regeneration. Many different types of polymeric nanofibers with unique characteristics have been created and evaluated as skin regeneration scaffolds. Nanofibrous materials can be used as delivery systems for medications, proteins, growth factors, and other compounds in addition to supporting tissue repair. Additionally, nanofibrous materials' shape, biodegradability, and other properties can be manipulated to promote particular wound healing circumstances. Several nanostructured drug delivery methods have been employed to enhance wound healing at various phases, including liposomes, nanoparticles, nanoemulsions, and micelles. The administration of poorly water-soluble medications, enhanced skin penetration, controlled release characteristics, antimicrobial activity, protection of medications from light, heat, enzymes, or pH degradation, stimulation of fibroblast proliferation, and decreased inflammation are just a few advantages that these nanoscale delivery systems have shown to aid in the wound healing process (Alberti et al., 2017).

Metal and Metal Oxide Nanoparticles

Metal-based nanoparticles (NPs) are widely used in biomedicine because of their many advantages, including their better physicochemical qualities, rapid synthesis with predetermined shapes and sizes, easy surface functionalization, and increased biocompatibility. In the biomedical field, gold and silver are the most widely used NPs. Gold nanoparticles are widely used in biosensing because of their optical characteristics and as nanocarriers for medication delivery. Antimicrobial and anticancer properties are the main applications for silver nanoparticles (Rajendran et al., 2018). Three potential mechanisms for their antibacterial activity have been shown: (i) NP accumulation on the microbial membrane will change the microbes' resistance, resulting in the release of membrane proteins, lipopolysaccharides, and intracellular biomolecules; (ii) NPs will generate reactive oxygen species (ROS), causing oxidative damage to cells; and (iii) NPs will be metabolized by the microbes, reducing intracellular ATP and disrupting DNA replication. Nanoparticles of metal and metal oxide exhibit a positive bactericidal effect on drug-resistant types of bacteria. Future research should examine this area, though, as it has also been claimed that when employed on a small size, bacteria might improve their ability to escape these NPs.

Liposomes

A hydrophilic inner core and hydrophobic outer shell make up liposomes. Their capacity to encapsulate hydrophobic and hydrophilic therapeutic substances, including antibiotics and bactericidal ions, has led to extensive research into them as wound healing carriers. By facilitating the passage of medicinal drugs into bacterial cells, liposomes can increase intracellular medication concentrations, hence preventing bacterial growth and biofilm formation. The composition of liposomes can be specifically altered to improve sorption and absorption across the bacterial cell membrane. Various liposomes loaded with antibiotics and exhibiting different surface modifications have been investigated thus far for their ability to control bacterial infections. Liposomes are negatively charged and bind more effectively to the positive-charged bacterial cell membrane than to the neutral or negative-charged membrane. For example, methicillin-resistant *S. aureus* or *S. epidermidis* were successfully combatted by cationic liposomes loaded with vancomycin. The lipid bilayer's shape can be altered, making liposome-based carriers incredibly biocompatible and somewhat immunogenic. In addition, liposomes can be modified and inserted into bandages to continuously and effectively supply therapeutic chemicals to the injured area, inhibiting microorganisms (Kushwaha et al., 2022).

Nanofibers

Nanofibers are filaments with diameters within the nanoscale. Due of its simplicity and low cost, the electrospinning technique is typically used to create them. This method spins polymeric solutions to create fiber meshes by applying a strong electric force between a collector and a needle capillary tip. Because of their organization and random alignment, nanofiber meshes can partially replicate the extracellular matrix (ECM), making them a promising tool in the treatment of chronic wounds. Indeed, its tunable porous shape and high surface area-to-volume ratio can facilitate gas/nutrient exchange and support wound homeostasis. Moreover, nanofibers meshes should also provide moisture to avoid the wound dehydration and bacteria contamination. Additionally, they have the ability to encapsulate biological molecules, medications, or nanocarriers, which enables topical delivery of those substances with the following benefits (lower dose and less side effects). Nanofiber meshes, on the other hand, have been investigated as artificial skin. In order to initiate the wound-healing process, MSCs can either release growth factors or develop into endothelial cells (Blanco-Fernandez et al., 2021).

Hydrogels

In recent years, hydrogels have been investigated as a potential material for wound dressings. Both incisional and excisional wounds can benefit from the use of hydrogel dressings. Since hydrogels can retain a lot of water while maintaining their structural integrity after expanding, they meet the requirements for a 3D cross-linked polymeric network structure. The hydrogels are made up of a number of hydrophilic groups that interact with one another to form a three-dimensional matrix that can hold liquids, such as wound exudates. Biomimetic hydrogels are among the materials for tissue regeneration that resemble natural 3D structures. They can absorb wound exudates, provide a moist environment, and have the same elasticity as native tissue. These hydrogels facilitate gas exchange, which inhibits the growth of anaerobic bacteria, improves cell migration and epithelization into wound hydrogels, and acts as a barrier to bacterial growth. Another possibility is

injectable hydrogels. The ability to fill wounds with irregular spaces, adhesion to wounds, and the capacity to retain bioactive materials and cells in situ are only a few benefits of using injectable hydrogels for skin regeneration. The development of synthetic chemistry and materials science has made it feasible to generate hydrogel in situ after delivery using conventional needles. This guarantees minimal invasion when administering therapeutic payloads and may aid in promoting the body's healing process in the injured area (Dimatteo et al., 2018).

Smart Dressings

Typically, actives are delivered to the wound bead using dressings based on nanotechnology. The physicochemical properties of materials alter when their size is reduced to nanoscales. This is also beneficial in influencing and quickening the healing progression. Healthy skin has a pH of 4.0 to 6.0. It has also also reviewed that the importance of pH in both acute and chronic wound healing, providing additional evidence that the pH of the wound environment shifts from alkaline to neutral and finally acidic as a wound heals. However, this is a generally acknowledged notion. No matter what the pH is, the wound site has a lower pH than the surrounding skin. Because of this pH difference, pH-responsive dressings have been used to treat chronic and infected wounds (Chopra et al., 2023).

CONCLUSION

Wound healing is a complex biological mechanism necessary to restore the integrity of injured tissues. To achieve efficient healing, the passage through hemostasis, inflammation, proliferation, and remodeling stages must happen in a rigorously controlled order. However, a number of local and systemic factors—including oxygenation, infection, age, dietary status, comorbidities, and lifestyle practices—may interfere with this process, therefore resulting in chronic wounds. Particularly in the context of diabetes, obesity, and growing antibiotic resistance, these non-healing wounds present major clinical issues. Though fundamental, conventional wound care techniques are sometimes insufficient for handling challenging wounds. This has brought about a paradigm shift toward creative, technologically driven solutions. Promoting quicker, safer and more effective wound healing, nanotechnology, smart biomaterials and targeted drug distribution systems have created fresh possibilities. More investigation might help these new strategies not just improve healing results but also lower socioeconomic burden of chronic wounds. Overcoming current problems and moving wound management ahead depends on continuous research on the molecular mechanisms of wound healing and the use of cutting- edge therapeutic approaches.

REFERENCES

Abdou, A. G., Maraee, A. H., Al-Bara, A. M., & Diab, W. M. (2011). Immunohistochemical expression of TGF-β1 in keloids and hypertrophic scars. *The American Journal of Dermatopathology*, *33*(1), 84–91. DOI: 10.1097/DAD.0b013e3181d0c3ad PMID: 20559120

Ahmad, N. (2023). In vitro and in vivo characterization methods for evaluation of modern wound dressings. *Pharmaceutics*, *15*(1), 42. DOI: 10.3390/pharmaceutics15010042 PMID: 36678671

Alberti, T., & Coelho, S, D., Voytena, A., Pitz, H., de Pra, M., Mazzarino, L., ... & Veleirinho, B. (2017). Nanotechnology: A promising tool towards wound healing. *Current Pharmaceutical Design*, *23*(24), 3515–3535. PMID: 28472915

Avishai, E., Yeghiazaryan, K., & Golubnitschaja, O. (2017). Impaired wound healing: Facts and hypotheses for multi-professional considerations in predictive, preventive and personalised medicine. *The EPMA Journal*, *8*, 23–33. DOI: 10.1007/s13167-017-0081-y PMID: 28620441

Beahrs, T. R., Reagan, J., Bettin, C. C., Grear, B. J., Murphy, G. A., & Richardson, D. R. (2019). Smoking effects in foot and ankle surgery: An evidence-based review. *Foot & Ankle International*, *40*(10), 1226–1232. DOI: 10.1177/1071100719867942 PMID: 31423824

Beyene, R. T., Derryberry, S. L., & Barbul, A. (2020). The effect of comorbidities on wound healing. *Surgical Clinics*, *100*(4), 695–705. DOI: 10.1016/j.suc.2020.05.002 PMID: 32681870

Bishop, A. (2008). Role of oxygen in wound healing. *Journal of Wound Care*, *17*(9), 399–402. DOI: 10.12968/jowc.2008.17.9.30937 PMID: 18833899

Blanco-Fernandez, B., Castano, O., Mateos-Timoneda, M. Á., Engel, E., & Pérez-Amodio, S. (2021). Nanotechnology approaches in chronic wound healing. *Advances in Wound Care*, *10*(5), 234–256. DOI: 10.1089/wound.2019.1094 PMID: 32320364

Chopra, H., Mohanta, Y. K., Mahanta, S., Mohanta, T. K., Singh, I., Avula, S. K., & Dhama, K. (2023). Recent updates in nanotechnological advances for wound healing: A narrative review. *Nanotechnology Reviews*, *12*(1), 20230129. DOI: 10.1515/ntrev-2023-0129

Conus, S., Perozzo, R., Reinheckel, T., Peters, C., Scapozza, L., Yousefi, S., & Simon, H. U. (2008). Caspase-8 is activated by cathepsin D initiating neutrophil apoptosis during the resolution of inflammation. *The Journal of Experimental Medicine, 205*(3), 685–698. DOI: 10.1084/jem.20072152 PMID: 18299403

Daley, J. M., Reichner, J. S., Mahoney, E. J., Manfield, L., Henry, W. L., Mastrofrancesco, B., & Albina, J. E. (2005). Modulation of macrophage phenotype by soluble product (s) released from neutrophils. *The Journal of Immunology: Official Journal of the American Association of Immunologists, 174*(4), 2265–2272. DOI: 10.4049/jimmunol.174.4.2265 PMID: 15699161

De Donatis, A., Ranaldi, F., & Cirri, P. (2010). Reciprocal control of cell proliferation and migration. *Cell Communication and Signaling: CCS, 8*, 1–4. DOI: 10.1186/1478-811X-8-20 PMID: 20822514

Dimatteo, R., Darling, N. J., & Segura, T. (2018). In situ forming injectable hydrogels for drug delivery and wound repair. *Advanced Drug Delivery Reviews, 127*, 167–184. DOI: 10.1016/j.addr.2018.03.007 PMID: 29567395

Edwards, R., & Harding, K. G. (2004). Bacteria and wound healing. *Current Opinion in Infectious Diseases, 17*(2), 91–96. DOI: 10.1097/00001432-200404000-00004 PMID: 15021046

Enoch, S., & Leaper, D. J. (2008). Basic science of wound healing. *Surgery (Oxford), 26*(2), 31–37. DOI: 10.1016/j.mpsur.2007.11.005

Franz, M. G., Steed, D. L., & Robson, M. C. (2007). Optimizing healing of the acute wound by minimizing complications. *Current Problems in Surgery, 44*(11), 691–763. DOI: 10.1067/j.cpsurg.2007.07.001 PMID: 18036992

Gantwerker, E. A., & Hom, D. B. (2011). Skin: Histology and physiology of wound healing. *Facial Plastic Surgery Clinics of North America, 19*(3), 441. DOI: 10.1016/j.fsc.2011.06.009 PMID: 21856533

George Broughton, I. I., Janis, J. E., & Attinger, C. E. (2006). The basic science of wound healing. *Plastic and Reconstructive Surgery, 117*(7S), 12S–34S. DOI: 10.1097/01.prs.0000225430.42531.c2 PMID: 16799372

Golebiewska, E. M., & Poole, A. W. (2015). Platelet secretion: From haemostasis to wound healing and beyond. *Blood Reviews, 29*(3), 153–162. DOI: 10.1016/j.blre.2014.10.003 PMID: 25468720

Hardman, M. J., & Ashcroft, G. S. (2008). Estrogen, not intrinsic aging, is the major regulator of delayed human wound healing in the elderly. *Genome Biology, 9*, 1–17. DOI: 10.1186/gb-2008-9-5-r80 PMID: 18477406

Hinz, B. (2006). Masters and servants of the force: The role of matrix adhesions in myofibroblast force perception and transmission. *European Journal of Cell Biology*, *85*(3-4), 175–181. DOI: 10.1016/j.ejcb.2005.09.004 PMID: 16546559

Horn, D. B., Adams, G. L., & Monyak, D. (1995). Irradiated soft tissue and its management. *Otolaryngologic Clinics of North America*, *28*(5), 1003–1019. DOI: 10.1016/S0030-6665(20)30472-2 PMID: 8559569

Irfan-Maqsood, M. (2016). Classification of wounds: Know before research and clinical practice. *Journal of Genes and Cells*, *4*(1), 1–4. DOI: 10.15562/gnc.61

Krischak, G. D., Augat, P., Claes, L., Kinzl, L., & Beck, A. (2007). The effects of non-steroidal anti-inflammatory drug application on incisional wound healing in rats. *Journal of Wound Care*, *16*(2), 76–78. DOI: 10.12968/jowc.2007.16.2.27001 PMID: 17319622

Kushwaha, A., Goswami, L., & Kim, B. S. (2022). Nanomaterial-based therapy for wound healing. *Nanomaterials (Basel, Switzerland)*, *12*(4), 618. DOI: 10.3390/nano12040618 PMID: 35214947

Lee, C. H., Hsieh, M. J., Chang, S. H., Lin, Y. H., Liu, S. J., Lin, T. Y., & Juang, J. H. (2014). Enhancement of diabetic wound repair using biodegradable nanofibrous metformin-eluting membranes: In vitro and in vivo. *ACS Applied Materials & Interfaces*, *6*(6), 3979–3986. DOI: 10.1021/am405329g PMID: 24568239

Mamun, A. A., Shao, C., Geng, P., Wang, S., & Xiao, J. (2024). Recent advances in molecular mechanisms of skin wound healing and its treatments. *Frontiers in Immunology*, *15*, 1395479. DOI: 10.3389/fimmu.2024.1395479 PMID: 38835782

Mayrand, D., Laforce-Lavoie, A., Larochelle, S., Langlois, A., Genest, H., Roy, M., & Moulin, V. J. (2012). Angiogenic properties of myofibroblasts isolated from normal human skin wounds. *Angiogenesis*, *15*, 199–212. DOI: 10.1007/s10456-012-9253-5 PMID: 22350743

Monika, P., Chandraprabha, M. N., Rangarajan, A., Waiker, P. V., & Chidambara Murthy, K. N. (2022). Challenges in healing wound: Role of complementary and alternative medicine. *Frontiers in Nutrition*, *8*, 791899. DOI: 10.3389/fnut.2021.791899 PMID: 35127787

Nami, N., Feci, L., Napoliello, L., Giordano, A., Lorenzini, S., Galeazzi, M., & Fimiani, M. (2016). Crosstalk between platelets and PBMC: New evidence in wound healing. *Platelets*, *27*(2), 143–148. DOI: 10.3109/09537104.2015.1048216 PMID: 26030799

Nathan, C. (2006). Neutrophils and immunity: Challenges and opportunities. *Nature Reviews. Immunology*, *6*(3), 173–182. DOI: 10.1038/nri1785 PMID: 16498448

Otranto, M., Souza-Netto, I., Aguila, M. B., & Monte-Alto-Costa, A. (2009). Male and female rats with severe protein restriction present delayed wound healing. *Applied Physiology, Nutrition, and Metabolism*, *34*(6), 1023–1031. DOI: 10.1139/H09-100 PMID: 20029510

Payne, W. G., Naidu, D. K., Wheeler, C. K., Barkoe, D., Mentis, M., Salas, R. E., & Robson, M. C. (2008). Wound healing in PatientsWith cancer. *Eplasty*, *8*, e9. PMID: 18264518

Petreaca, M. L., Yao, M., Liu, Y., DeFea, K., & Martins-Green, M. (2007). Transactivation of vascular endothelial growth factor receptor-2 by interleukin-8 (IL-8/CXCL8) is required for IL-8/CXCL8-induced endothelial permeability. *Molecular Biology of the Cell*, *18*(12), 5014–5023. DOI: 10.1091/mbc.e07-01-0004 PMID: 17928406

Rajendran, N. K., Kumar, S. S. D., Houreld, N. N., & Abrahamse, H. (2018). A review on nanoparticle based treatment for wound healing. *Journal of Drug Delivery Science and Technology*, *44*, 421–430. DOI: 10.1016/j.jddst.2018.01.009

Rodriguez, P. G., Felix, F. N., Woodley, D. T., & Shim, E. K. (2008). The role of oxygen in wound healing: A review of the literature. *Dermatologic Surgery*, *34*(9), 1159–1169. DOI: 10.1111/j.1524-4725.2008.34254.x PMID: 18513296

Rosyid, F. N. (2022). Wounds: Physiological mechanisms and factors affecting healing. *International Journal of Research in Medical Sciences*, *10*(4), 1001–1006. DOI: 10.18203/2320-6012.ijrms20221000

Schraufstatter, I. U., Chung, J., & Burger, M. (2001). IL-8 activates endothelial cell CXCR1 and CXCR2 through Rho and Rac signaling pathways. *American Journal of Physiology. Lung Cellular and Molecular Physiology*, *280*(6), L1094–L1103. DOI: 10.1152/ajplung.2001.280.6.L1094 PMID: 11350788

Scully, D., Sfyri, P., Wilkinson, H. N., Acebes-Huerta, A., Verpoorten, S., Muñoz-Turrillas, M. C., & Matsakas, A. (2020). Optimising platelet secretomes to deliver robust tissue-specific regeneration. *Journal of Tissue Engineering and Regenerative Medicine*, *14*(1), 82–98. DOI: 10.1002/term.2965 PMID: 31603629

Sen, C. K. (2021). Human wounds and its burden: An updated compendium of estimates. *Advances in Wound Care*, *8*(2), 39–48. DOI: 10.1089/wound.2021.0026 PMID: 30809421

Siefert, S. A., & Sarkar, R. (2012). Matrix metalloproteinases in vascular physiology and disease. *Vascular*, *20*(4), 210–216. DOI: 10.1258/vasc.2011.201202 PMID: 22896663

Simpson, D. M., & Ross, R. U. S. S. E. L. L. (1972). The neutrophilic leukocyte in wound repair: A study with antineutrophil serum. *The Journal of Clinical Investigation*, *51*(8), 2009–2023. DOI: 10.1172/JCI107007 PMID: 5054460

Takahashi, A., Flanigan, M. E., McEwen, B. S., & Russo, S. J. (2018). Aggression, social stress, and the immune system in humans and animal models. *Frontiers in Behavioral Neuroscience*, *12*, 56. DOI: 10.3389/fnbeh.2018.00056 PMID: 29623033

Tatarusanu, S. M., Lupascu, F. G., Profire, B. S., Szilagyi, A., Gardikiotis, I., Iacob, A. T., & Profire, L. (2023). Modern approaches in wounds management. *Polymers*, *15*(17), 3648. DOI: 10.3390/polym15173648 PMID: 37688274

Velnar, T., Bailey, T., & Smrkolj, V. (2009). The wound healing process: An overview of the cellular and molecular mechanisms. *The Journal of International Medical Research*, *37*(5), 1528–1542. DOI: 10.1177/147323000903700531 PMID: 19930861

Wilkinson, H. N., & Hardman, M. J. (2020). Wound healing: Cellular mechanisms and pathological outcomes. *Open Biology*, *10*(9), 200223. DOI: 10.1098/rsob.200223 PMID: 32993416

Yang, J., & Weinberg, R. A. (2008). Epithelial-mesenchymal transition: At the crossroads of development and tumor metastasis. *Developmental Cell*, *14*(6), 818–829. DOI: 10.1016/j.devcel.2008.05.009 PMID: 18539112

Yasin, S. N. N., Said, Z., Halib, N., Rahman, Z. A., & Mokhzani, N. I. (2023). Polymer-based hydrogel loaded with honey in drug delivery system for wound healing applications. *Polymers*, *15*(14), 3085. DOI: 10.3390/polym15143085 PMID: 37514474

Young, A., & McNaught, C. E. (2011). The physiology of wound healing. *Surgery (Oxford)*, *29*(10), 475–479. DOI: 10.1016/s0196-0644(88)80351-2

Zaidi, A., & Green, L. (2019). Physiology of haemostasis. *Anaesthesia and Intensive Care Medicine*, *20*(3), 152–158. DOI: 10.1016/j.mpaic.2019.01.005

Chapter 2

The Role of Herbal Constituents in Wound Healing

P. Selvakumar
https://orcid.org/0000-0002-3650-4548
Department of Science and Humanities, Nehru Institute of Technology, Coimbatore, India

T. C. Manjunath
https://orcid.org/0000-0003-2545-9160
Rajarajeswari College of Engineering, India

Jyothsna Devi Kuchipudi
https://orcid.org/0009-0002-6500-6721
School of Allied Healthcare and Sciences, Jain University, India

ABSTRACT

Wound healing is a fundamental physiological process that is critical to the restoration of tissue integrity and function following injury, surgery, or disease. In the realm of healthcare, the significance of effective wound healing cannot be overstated, as it directly influences patient outcomes, healthcare costs, and overall quality of life. Whether wounds are acute, such as surgical incisions and traumatic injuries, or chronic, such as diabetic foot ulcers, pressure ulcers,Wound healing is a fundamental physiological process that is critical to the restoration of tissue integrity and function following injury, surgery, or disease. In the realm of healthcare, the significance of effective wound healing cannot be overstated, as it directly influences patient outcomes, healthcare costs, and overall quality of life. Whether wounds are

DOI: 10.4018/979-8-3373-3977-1.ch002

acute, such as surgical incisions and traumatic injuries, or chronic, such as diabetic foot ulcers, pressure ulcers, and venous leg ulcers, the healing process is central to patient recovery and long-term well-being.

THE IMPORTANCE OF WOUND HEALING IN HEALTHCARE

Wound healing is a fundamental physiological process that is critical to the restoration of tissue integrity and function following injury, surgery, or disease. In the realm of healthcare, the significance of effective wound healing cannot be overstated, as it directly influences patient outcomes, healthcare costs, and overall quality of life. Whether wounds are acute, such as surgical incisions and traumatic injuries, or chronic, such as diabetic foot ulcers, pressure ulcers, wound healing is a fundamental physiological process that is critical to the restoration of tissue integrity and function following injury, surgery, or disease. In the realm of healthcare, the significance of effective wound healing cannot be overstated, as it directly influences patient outcomes, healthcare costs, and overall quality of life. Whether wounds are acute, such as surgical incisions and traumatic injuries, or chronic, such as diabetic foot ulcers, pressure ulcers, and venous leg ulcers, the healing process is central to patient recovery and long-term well-being. Delayed or impaired wound healing not only increases the risk of complications—including infection, prolonged hospitalization, and even amputation—but also contributes to emotional distress, loss of mobility, and decreased social participation for patients. From a clinical perspective, efficient wound healing reduces morbidity and mortality, expedites patient recovery, and enhances the efficacy of medical and surgical interventions. This is especially critical in populations with underlying comorbidities such as diabetes, vascular diseases, and immunosuppression, where wounds tend to heal more slowly and are more prone to complications, (Aburjai et al., 2019) In such cases, advanced wound care interventions and multidisciplinary approaches are often required to manage the healing process effectively. Furthermore, the burden of chronic wounds on healthcare systems worldwide is immense, with billions of dollars spent annually on treatment, management, and associated complications.

As populations age and the prevalence of chronic diseases rises, the demand for effective wound care is expected to increase significantly, placing even greater emphasis on the need for optimized wound healing strategies. In addition to its clinical and economic implications, wound healing has a profound psychosocial impact on patients. Chronic wounds, in particular, are often accompanied by pain, odor, and visible disfigurement, which can lead to psychological issues such as depression, anxiety, and social isolation. The inability to participate in everyday activities or maintain employment due to a non-healing wound further exacerbates these challenges, reducing overall quality of life. Therefore, promoting wound healing is not merely a biological or medical concern but a holistic healthcare priority that intersects with mental health, social support, and patient-centered careHealthcare providers play a crucial role in facilitating wound healing through accurate assessment, timely diagnosis, appropriate intervention, and patient education. Advancements in wound care technologies, including bioengineered skin substitutes, negative pressure wound therapy, antimicrobial dressings, and growth factor treatments, have significantly improved outcomes for many patients. Nevertheless, successful wound management relies heavily on a collaborative approach involving physicians, nurses, wound care specialists, nutritionists, and physical therapists. Equally important is the engagement of patients themselves, who must adhere to treatment protocols, maintain proper hygiene, and manage underlying health conditions to support healing, (Aderibigbe et al., 2018).

THE HISTORY OF HERBAL MEDICINE IN WOUND HEALING

Herbal medicine, rooted in centuries of traditional use, has increasingly gained recognition in modern healthcare as a valuable source of bioactive compounds with significant therapeutic potential. Among its many applications, one of the most promising is the use of herbal constituents in promoting wound healing. Herbal-based treatments have been traditionally employed across cultures to manage cuts, burns, ulcers, and other skin injuries. Today, scientific research is progressively validating these traditional practices, highlighting the remarkable anti-inflammatory, antimicrobial, and antioxidant properties of various plant-derived compounds that are crucial for enhancing wound repair, (Ahmed et al., 2018). These constituents offer a natural, cost-effective, and often safer alternative or complementary option to synthetic pharmaceuticals, especially in settings where access to conventional medicine is limited or where concerns about drug resistance and side effects prevail. The process of wound healing is intricate and involves a tightly regulated sequence of biological events: hemostasis, inflammation, proliferation, and remodeling. Disruption at any of these phases, whether due to infection, oxidative stress, or chronic inflammation, can delay healing and lead to chronic wounds. Herbal constituents intervene at multiple stages of this process, facilitating faster and more complete wound closure. While inflammation is a necessary part of the healing cascade, excessive or prolonged inflammation can be detrimental. Phytochemicals such as curcumin (from *Curcuma longa*), boswellic acids (from *Boswellia serrata*), and glycyrrhizin (from

Glycyrrhiza glabra) have been shown to inhibit key pro-inflammatory cytokines like TNF-α, IL-1β, and IL-6.

These actions not only reduce inflammation but also limit collateral tissue damage and accelerate transition to the proliferative phase. Furthermore, herbal anti-inflammatories are generally associated with fewer side effects compared to corticosteroids or NSAIDs, making them attractive for long-term wound management, (Bihani & Mhaske, 2020). Antimicrobial activity is another critical attribute of many herbal compounds, especially in the context of wound infection—a major impediment to healing. Compounds like asiaticoside (from *Centella asiatica*), aloe-emodin (from *Aloe vera*), and shikonin (from *Lithospermum erythrorhizon*) stimulate fibroblast activity, collagen synthesis, and re-epithelialization. Increased collagen production strengthens the wound bed and supports structural integrity, while enhanced angiogenesis ensures adequate oxygen and nutrient delivery to the regenerating tissue. Some herbs also possess analgesic properties that alleviate pain associated with wounds, improving patient comfort and adherence to treatment. The integration of herbal constituents into wound care products has led to the development of various formulations such as ointments, gels, sprays, and dressings enriched with plant extracts or isolated bioactives. Clinical studies have reported favorable outcomes with such formulations, often showing faster healing times, improved scar appearance, and reduced infection rates. For instance, topical applications of honey—a complex natural product rich in phenolics, enzymes, and sugars—have demonstrated significant efficacy in wound debridement, infection control, and tissue repair. Similarly, hydrogel dressings infused with herbal extracts like turmeric or neem are increasingly being used in both clinical and community settings. Despite these promising attributes, challenges remain in standardizing and validating herbal therapies, (Binsuwaidan et al., 2022). As research continues to bridge the gap between traditional practices and modern science, the integration of herbal medicine into contemporary wound management holds promise for improving outcomes, especially in resource-limited or chronic care settings. (Carvalho et al., 2021). A future where herbal-based interventions complement or even replace synthetic pharmaceuticals in wound healing appears not only plausible but increasingly probable, given the pressing need for effective, sustainable, and accessible healthcare solutions.

FLAVONOIDS AND WOUND HEALING

The use of herbal medicine in wound healing has a rich and deeply rooted history that spans thousands of years, encompassing ancient civilizations, indigenous knowledge systems, and folk remedies passed down through generations. Long before the advent of modern pharmaceuticals and synthetic wound care products, (Chen et al., 2021) humans relied heavily on the natural world—particularly plants—to treat injuries, infections, and chronic wounds. This traditional reliance on herbs was not merely anecdotal but often based on empirical observation and cumulative experiential knowledge. Across continents and cultures, a vast pharmacopeia of medicinal plants emerged, each with unique properties suited to specific types of wounds, from simple cuts and abrasions to complex ulcers and burns. The global historical narrative of herbal wound care is a testament to human ingenuity and the enduring relationship between people and their natural environment. In ancient Egypt, medical papyri such as the Ebers Papyrus (circa 1550 BCE) provide detailed records of herbal remedies used for wound healing. Egyptian physicians employed honey, resins, and various plant extracts like aloe vera and frankincense to disinfect wounds, reduce inflammation, and promote tissue regeneration. Honey, in particular, was renowned for its antibacterial properties and hygroscopic action, drawing moisture from wounds and creating an environment inhospitable to microbial growth. Likewise, aloe vera was valued for its soothing, cooling, and healing effects on burns and open wounds—a use still widely recognized today, (Du et al., 2021). In ancient India, the Ayurvedic system of medicine flourished, offering a sophisticated understanding of wound care known as *Vrana Ropana*. Texts such as the *Sushruta Samhita* (circa 600 BCE) describe over 100 medicinal plants for wound management, including turmeric (*Curcuma longa*), neem (*Azadirachta indica*), and ashwagandha (*Withania somnifera*).

TCM wound healing theory is deeply intertwined with its broader medical philosophy, focusing on balancing internal energies (Qi), enhancing circulation, and removing toxins or "heat" from the body. These treatments often combined herbal knowledge with techniques like acupuncture and moxibustion to support comprehensive healing, (Dunn et al., 2013). In the Greco-Roman world, renowned physicians such as Hippocrates, Dioscorides, and Galen advanced the use of herbs in wound treatment. The Greek physician Dioscorides, in his seminal work *De Materia Medica* (1st century CE), documented hundreds of plant-based remedies for wounds, burns, and ulcers, many of which were adopted across Europe and the Middle East. Ingredients like myrrh, wine, vinegar, thyme, and comfrey were commonly used to cleanse and dress wounds. Galen further emphasized the role of plant-based ointments in post-surgical care, contributing to the development of compound herbal preparations that remained standard practice throughout the Middle, (El-ezz et al., 2022) Ages. Medieval Europe continued the herbal tradition through monastic medicine and folk practices. Monks in monastic infirmaries cultivated medicinal gardens and preserved herbal knowledge through texts such as the *Herbarium* of Apuleius and Hildegard von Bingen's *Physica*. Wound care in this era often involved herbal poultices, salves, and compresses made from calendula, plantain, yarrow, and St. John's wort. Folk medicine, largely practiced by women and local healers, also played a critical role in preserving herbal wound care traditions during times when access to trained physicians or formal medical care was limited. These community-based approaches were rooted in both empirical knowledge and cultural rituals, oft blending healing with spiritual or religious beliefs. Indigenous cultures worldwide developed their own herbal wound healing systems, tailored to the plants available in their specific ecosystems. Native American tribes used poultices of crushed leaves and bark from plants like witch hazel, goldenrod, and slippery elm to soothe wounds and prevent infection. In Africa, traditional healers employed medicinal plants such as *Vernonia amygdalina*, *Aspilia africana*, and *Securidaca longipedunculata* for wound cleansing and tissue repair. Modern formulations—such as herbal-infused dressings, bioactive gels, and sprays—seek to combine traditional efficacy with contemporary biomedical standards. In conclusion, (Elloumi et al., 2022) the history of herbal medicine in wound healing is both expansive and enduring, reflecting the deep-seated human connection to the healing power of nature.

ALKALOIDS AND WOUND HEALING

Flavonoids, a diverse group of naturally occurring polyphenolic compounds found abundantly in fruits, vegetables, herbs, and plant-derived beverages such as tea and wine, have garnered significant scientific interest due to their extensive pharmacological properties, particularly in the context of wound healing. Structurally characterized by a common phenylchroman backbone, flavonoids are subdivided into several classes, (Fathi et al., 2020) including flavonols, flavones, flavanones, isoflavones, anthocyanidins, and catechins, each with distinct chemical properties and biological activities. Flavonoids exert modulatory effects in each of these stages, contributing to faster and more efficient wound closure. In the initial inflammatory phase, flavonoids help regulate the immune response by inhibiting the production of pro-inflammatory cytokines such as tumor necrosis factor-alpha (TNF-α), interleukins (IL-1β, IL-6), and prostaglandins. By dampening the excessive inflammatory response, flavonoids prevent further tissue damage and facilitate the transition to the proliferative phase. For instance, quercetin, one of the most studied flavonols, has demonstrated potent anti-inflammatory effects by modulating the NF-κB signaling pathway and reducing oxidative stress, (Frykberg, 2015) which is commonly elevated in chronic wounds. Oxidative stress, primarily caused by an imbalance between reactive oxygen species (ROS) and antioxidant defenses, is a major factor in delayed wound healing. Excessive ROS can impair fibroblast function, damage extracellular matrix proteins, and delay angiogenesis and re-epithelialization. Flavonoids serve as powerful antioxidants, neutralizing free radicals and enhancing the activity of endogenous antioxidant enzymes like superoxide dismutase (SOD), catalase, and glutathione peroxidase, (Gebremeskel et al., 2018).

Additionally, flavonoids such as kaempferol and naringenin have demonstrated efficacy in improving epithelial regeneration and tensile strength of healed tissue, indicating their role in both functional and aesthetic aspects of wound recovery. The final remodeling phase involves the reorganization of collagen fibers and restoration of tissue architecture. Here, flavonoids continue to exert beneficial effects by modulating the activity of matrix metalloproteinases (MMPs), enzymes that degrade extracellular matrix components. Overactivity of MMPs, particularly in chronic wounds such as diabetic ulcers, leads to extracellular matrix breakdown and impairs tissue integrity. Their antimicrobial mechanisms include disrupting microbial membranes, inhibiting nucleic acid synthesis, and blocking enzyme function. For instance, quercetin and rutin are known to inhibit the growth of *Staphylococcus aureus* and *Pseudomonas aeruginosa*, two of the most common pathogens in infected wounds. The antimicrobial activity of flavonoids, coupled with their low toxicity, positions them as attractive alternatives or adjuncts to conventional antibiotics, particularly in an era of rising antimicrobial resistance. The historical use of flavonoid-rich plants in traditional medicine underscores their longstanding role in wound healing. Plants like *Calendula officinalis* (marigold), *Chamomilla recutita* (chamomile), *Glycyrrhiza glabra* (licorice), and *Hypericum perforatum* (St. John's wort) have been employed in various cultural contexts for treating wounds, burns, and ulcers, (Haq et al., 2020) Modern phytochemical analyses have confirmed that these plants are rich in flavonoids, which account for many of their healing properties. Drawing from both traditional uses and modern scientific validation, flavonoids offer a bridge between herbal medicine and evidence-based clinical practice. As research continues to uncover their molecular mechanisms and optimize their delivery, flavonoids are poised to play an increasingly, (Hou et al., 2021) prominent role in the management of acute and chronic wounds, offering safe, effective, and holistic alternatives in the evolving landscape of regenerative medicine.

TERPENES AND WOUND HEALING

Alkaloids, a broad class of naturally occurring nitrogen-containing compounds primarily found in plants, represent one of the most pharmacologically active groups of secondary metabolites with profound therapeutic potential. Known for their complex chemical structures and potent biological effects, alkaloids have been used in traditional and modern medicine to treat a wide range of conditions, including pain, infections, and inflammation, (Ibrahim et al., 2020). In the realm of wound healing, alkaloids are gaining increasing attention for their multifaceted role in promoting tissue repair, modulating inflammatory responses, and combating microbial infections. These bioactive compounds exhibit diverse pharmacodynamic properties, including anti-inflammatory, antimicrobial, antioxidant, analgesic, and angiogenic effects—all of which are crucial in enhancing the wound healing process. Alkaloids have been shown to modulate inflammatory pathways by inhibiting the production of pro-inflammatory cytokines, reducing leukocyte infiltration, and downregulating enzymes such as cyclooxygenase (COX) and lipoxygenase (LOX), which are involved in the synthesis of inflammatory mediators. For instance, berberine—an isoquinoline alkaloid found in *Berberis vulgaris* and *Coptis chinensis*—has demonstrated potent anti-inflammatory activity by suppressing nuclear factor-kappa B (NF-κB) signaling, a key regulator of inflammation, (Ivanková & Belovičová, 2020). In animal wound models, berberine has been observed to reduce edema, accelerate epithelialization, and enhance tissue granulation, making it a strong candidate for wound therapy.

The integration of alkaloid-rich extracts into topical formulations, such as ointments and dressings, can help reduce microbial load at the wound site, control local infections, and improve the overall healing outcome. Another crucial aspect of wound healing is oxidative stress management. During the inflammatory phase, activated neutrophils and macrophages produce large amounts of reactive oxygen species (ROS) to kill invading pathogens. However, excessive ROS can damage host tissues, impair fibroblast and keratinocyte function, and disrupt the extracellular matrix. Many alkaloids act as natural antioxidants, scavenging ROS and enhancing the activity of endogenous antioxidant enzymes like glutathione peroxidase, catalase, and superoxide dismutase. (Jangde et al., 2018). For instance, matrine and oxymatrine—alkaloids derived from *Sophora flavescens*—have demonstrated angiogenic properties in vitro and in vivo, contributing to enhanced wound vascularization and granulation tissue formation, (Jee et al., 2019) This improved perfusion accelerates the healing process and reduces the risk of wound necrosis, especially in ischemic or diabetic wounds where blood supply is compromised. Traditional medicine systems have long recognized the wound healing properties of alkaloid-containing plants. In Ayurveda, Unani, and Traditional Chinese Medicine (TCM), herbs such as *Argemone mexicana*, *Papaver somniferum*, *Chelidonium majus*, and *Tinospora cordifolia* have been employed for treating wounds, burns, and ulcers. These plants are rich in alkaloids and are often prepared as poultices, decoctions, or infused oils for topical use. Indigenous knowledge, backed by generations of empirical evidence, highlights the value of these natural compounds in promoting healing and preventing infection, (Jones, 2015). Moreover, the pharmacokinetics and bioavailability of alkaloids can vary depending on their chemical structure and formulation. Some alkaloids may exhibit toxicity at higher concentrations, necessitating careful dosage optimization and delivery method refinement. (Kalalinia et al., 2021).

ANTI-INFLAMMATORY EFFECTS OF HERBAL CONSTITUENTS

Terpenes, one of the largest and most diverse classes of naturally occurring organic compounds, are widespread in the plant kingdom and are known for their aromatic properties and potent biological activities. Structurally composed of repeating isoprene units (C5H8), terpenes are categorized based on the number of isoprene units into monoterpenes, sesquiterpenes, diterpenes, triterpenes, and so on. These compounds are synthesized by plants not only for ecological functions—such as attracting pollinators and deterring herbivores—but also for self-defense, especially against microbial invasion and oxidative stress. In the field of phytomedicine, terpenes have attracted considerable attention due to their wide-ranging pharmacological properties, including anti-inflammatory, antimicrobial, antioxidant, analgesic, and regenerative activities. (Kant et al., 2020a). Disruption at any stage can lead to impaired or chronic wounds, particularly in individuals with comorbidities like diabetes or vascular disease, (Kumar et al., 2022) Terpenes can intervene at multiple points in the healing cascade, offering therapeutic effects that complement or even surpass conventional pharmacological agents. One of the primary benefits of terpenes in wound healing is their anti-inflammatory activity, which is crucial in the early stages of wound repair. Excessive or prolonged inflammation can damage tissues, delay healing, and lead to chronic wounds. By preserving the cellular integrity of fibroblasts and keratinocytes, terpenes promote effective tissue regeneration and epithelialization. and accelerates re-epithelialization, making it a key active ingredient in many herbal wound healing formulations.

Clinical studies have confirmed its efficacy in treating burns, surgical wounds, and diabetic ulcers. Its derivatives are now used in standardized creams and topical agents widely available in both traditional and modern healthcare systems, (Lee et al., 2022) Their inclusion in wound dressings or gels has shown to result in more organized and durable scar tissue with fewer complications. Terpenes have been utilized for wound care in traditional medicine for centuries. Indigenous cultures across Asia, Africa, and the Americas have long applied essential oils and terpene-rich plant extracts for wound disinfection, inflammation control, and scar reduction. For instance, the essential oil of lavender (*Lavandula angustifolia*), rich in linalool and linalyl acetate, has traditionally been used for its antiseptic and calming effects. Scientific studies have since supported its use by demonstrating accelerated wound contraction, enhanced collagen synthesis, and reduced inflammation. Similarly, tea tree oil (*Melaleuca alternifolia*), rich in terpinen-4-ol, has been shown to possess antimicrobial and anti-inflammatory effects that significantly enhance wound healing outcomes. These traditional uses have laid the groundwork for the integration of terpenes into modern evidence-based wound care. Despite their many benefits, challenges in standardization, formulation, and delivery of terpene-based therapies remain. (Lüer et al., 2012). Terpenes are volatile and hydrophobic, which can limit their stability and bioavailability when applied topically.

ANTIMICROBIAL EFFECTS OF HERBAL CONSTITUENTS

Inflammation is an essential biological response to tissue injury or infection and is a critical component of the wound healing process. While acute inflammation facilitates immune defense, debris clearance, and tissue repair, chronic or excessive inflammation can be detrimental, resulting in delayed healing, tissue destruction, and the development of non-healing or chronic wounds. In this context, the anti-inflammatory properties of herbal constituents have garnered substantial interest in both traditional and modern medicine due to their capacity to modulate inflammatory responses naturally, safely, and effectively. A growing body of research now supports the use of various plant-derived compounds—including flavonoids, alkaloids, terpenes, saponins, and polyphenols—not only for their anti-inflammatory effects but also for their ability to support and accelerate wound healing processes. These herbal constituents, many of which have been utilized for centuries in traditional medical systems such as Ayurveda, Traditional Chinese Medicine (TCM), and Unani, offer a multi-targeted approach to inflammation management, making them valuable candidates for wound care and tissue regeneration. signaling pathways, including nuclear factor-kappa B (NF-κB), cyclooxygenase-2 (COX-2), and inducible nitric oxide synthase (iNOS). By inhibiting these pathways, curcumin reduces the production of inflammatory mediators such as tumor necrosis factor-alpha (TNF-α), interleukins (IL-1β, IL-6), and prostaglandins. By blocking leukotriene pathways, boswellic acid reduces inflammatory signaling without the gastrointestinal side effects associated with non-steroidal anti-inflammatory drugs (NSAIDs). Studies have demonstrated that boswellic acid reduces edema, leukocyte infiltration, and capillary permeability in inflammatory wound models. Its inclusion in wound ointments and creams has shown to accelerate healing by promoting the resolution of inflammation and facilitating the transition to the proliferative phase of wound healing.y group box 1 (HMGB1) protein, a late-phase mediator of inflammation, (Majtan & Jesenak, 2018).

Apigenin, a flavonoid commonly found in parsley, celery, chamomile, and other herbs, has demonstrated remarkable anti-inflammatory activity. Apigenin inhibits pro-inflammatory enzymes such as COX-2 and iNOS and modulates cytokine production by interfering with mitogen-activated protein kinase (MAPK) and NF-κB pathways. In experimental wound healing models, apigenin has been shown to reduce the infiltration of neutrophils and macrophages at the wound site while promoting keratinocyte and fibroblast proliferation. It also contributes to angiogenesis and matrix remodeling, essential for complete wound recovery. Chamomile-based formulations rich in apigenin are widely used in Europe and Asia for treating minor wounds, insect bites, and dermatitis. Resveratrol, a stilbene-type polyphenol found in grapes, berries, and peanuts, is another herbal constituent with significant anti-inflammatory effects. Resveratrol inhibits (Madgule et al., 2023). TNF-α and interleukin production by modulating NF-κB signaling and activating sirtuins (SIRT1), which are involved in cellular stress responses. In wound healing, resveratrol has been observed to reduce inflammation, enhance angiogenesis, and stimulate fibroblast activity. Its antioxidant properties also mitigate oxidative stress, creating a more favorable environment for healing. Topical applications of resveratrol in diabetic wound models have demonstrated improved re-epithelialization, increased collagen content, and faster wound contraction. The anti-inflammatory effects of quercetin, a flavonol found in onions, apples, and green tea, are well documented. Quercetin modulates immune responses by inhibiting lipopolysaccharide (LPS)-induced cytokine production, suppressing COX-2 expression, and downregulating histamine release. In vitro and in vivo studies have shown that quercetin promotes fibroblast proliferation, enhances collagen synthesis, and accelerates wound closure. Its dual antioxidant and anti-inflammatory effects contribute to its wide applicability in treating inflammatory wounds and skin disorders.

ANTIOXIDANT EFFECTS OF HERBAL CONSTITUENTS.

The antimicrobial properties of herbal constituents play a pivotal role in wound healing, particularly in preventing or managing infections that compromise tissue regeneration and prolong healing time. Infection is one of the primary factors that impairs the normal progression of wound healing by exacerbating inflammation, increasing tissue damage, and facilitating the development of chronic wounds. The overuse and misuse of synthetic antibiotics have led to the alarming rise of multidrug-resistant pathogens, creating an urgent need for alternative antimicrobial agents that are effective, safe, and less likely to cause resistance. Herbal medicine, long used in traditional systems of healthcare across the globe, offers a rich source of natural compounds with potent antimicrobial activity, (Parveen et al., 2018) These plant-derived phytochemicals—including alkaloids, flavonoids, terpenes, saponins, phenolics, and essential oils—exert their effects through diverse mechanisms that disrupt microbial survival and biofilm formation. Increasing scientific interest and research have demonstrated that these constituents not only combat infections but also synergistically support other aspects of the wound healing process, such as inflammation resolution, tissue regeneration, and collagen synthesis.*pylori*—as well as fungi and protozoa. It disrupts microbial membranes, interferes with nucleic acid synthesis, and inhibits bacterial quorum sensing. In wound healing applications, berberine has been incorporated into gels and ointments to prevent infections and accelerate tissue repair, (Pazyar et al., 2014). Its anti-inflammatory and antioxidant properties further support wound closure by reducing oxidative damage and modulating immune responses.

Biofilms provide a protective environment for microorganisms, making them resistant to antibiotics and host immune responses. Flavonoids such as quercetin and catechins help penetrate and disrupt these biofilms, enhancing the susceptibility of pathogens to other antimicrobial agents. creating a favorable environment for tissue repair. In addition, tannins can modulate wound pH and moisture, both of which are critical for maintaining microbial balance and optimizing the healing milieuNeem (*Azadirachta indica*) has been a staple in Ayurvedic medicine for centuries and is valued for its antimicrobial and wound-healing properties. Neem leaves and oil contain compounds like nimbidin, nimbin, and azadirachtin, which have shown activity against a wide range of bacteria and fungi. Neem's antimicrobial efficacy, along with its ability to reduce inflammation, promote collagen formation, and aid tissue regeneration, has led to its use in wound creams, soaps, and antiseptic preparations. In experimental models, neem-based preparations have shown improved wound contraction, faster epithelialization, and reduced bacterial load makes them less likely to induce resistance compared to conventional antibiotics, (Rathod et al., 2022) Moreover, many herbal compounds exert synergistic effects when used in combination, either with each other or with standard antibiotics, enhancing the overall. However, advances in extraction technology, formulation science, and pharmacokinetics are helping to address these barriers. Encapsulation techniques, such as nanoemulsions and liposomal carriers, have been employed to enhance the bioavailability, stability, and controlled release of these compounds in wound environments. The development of herbal-based wound dressings, which integrate antimicrobial constituents into biocompatible scaffolds, is also a promising avenue for creating effective and affordable wound care products. In conclusion, (Yaseen et al., 2020) the antimicrobial effects of herbal constituents represent a vital and multidimensional approach to wound healing.

HERBAL CONSTITUENTS IN WOUND HEALING

Oxidative stress is a critical factor in wound pathology, especially in chronic and non-healing wounds. It refers to the imbalance between the production of reactive oxygen species (ROS) and the body's antioxidant defenses. While ROS play essential roles in cell signaling and microbial killing during the early inflammatory phase of wound healing, excessive and persistent ROS generation can damage cellular components—lipids, proteins, and DNA—ultimately impairing wound healing. This is particularly problematic in patients with underlying conditions such as diabetes, peripheral vascular disease, or prolonged inflammation. Quercetin also stabilizes and protects cell membranes, especially in endothelial cells and fibroblasts, thus preventing oxidative damage in the wound environment. In diabetic wound models, topical application of quercetin has resulted in decreased oxidative markers, increased fibroblast activity, and enhanced angiogenesis, all contributing to faster and more complete wound healing, (Yin et al., 2018) Furthermore, quercetin modulates intracellular signaling pathways such as the Nrf2/Keap1 axis, which is crucial for the activation of cytoprotective genes under oxidative stress conditions. Green tea extracts rich in EGCG have been incorporated into bioactive wound dressings and hydrogels to create a protective antioxidant barrier over wounds. Topical application of resveratrol-based formulations has shown promise in(Zahedi et al., 2010) both acute and chronic wound settings, particularly in ischemic and diabetic wounds where oxidative stress is a major concern. tensile strength of newly formed tissue and reduce exudation in wounds, thus improving the healing process.

Their astringent properties also help in wound contraction and the formation of protective barriers that prevent microbial invasion. ROS and regenerates other antioxidants like vitamin E and glutathione. Vitamin C also supports immune function and endothelial integrity, both of which are crucial during wound healing. Clinical studies have demonstrated that topical and systemic vitamin C accelerates the healing of pressure ulcers, burns, and surgical wounds. Aloe vera gel has been shown to reduce oxidative stress markers and facilitate faster healing with minimal scarring. Aloe vera also contains enzymes such as bradykinase, which help reduce excessive inflammation that can further worsen oxidative damage. promote collagen synthesis, increase tensile strength, and protect dermal fibroblasts from oxidative stress. Centella-based products are commonly used in the management of chronic wounds, including diabetic ulcers and pressure sores, due to their dual antioxidant and regenerative actions. pathways to reduce oxidative load and support cell viability in wound environments., where oxidative stress and microbial colonization coexist and reinforce each other's deleterious effects. In traditional medicine systems such as Ayurveda and Traditional Chinese Medicine (TCM), herbs rich in antioxidants have been used for centuries to treat wounds, burns, and skin ulcers. Ayurvedic formulations like Triphala (a combination of *Emblica officinalis*, *Terminalia chebula*, and *Terminalia bellirica*) and TCM herbs like *Astragalus membranaceus* and *Panax ginseng* are recognized for their rejuvenating and antioxidant effects. These time-tested remedies are increasingly being validated by modern pharmacological research and are being integrated into modern clinical practice. In conclusion, the antioxidant effects of herbal constituents offer a vital and multifaceted contribution to wound healing.

HERBAL CONSTITUENTS AND WOUND HEALING: CASE STUDIES AND SUCCESS STORIES

The role of herbal constituents in wound healing has become an increasingly important area of focus in both ethnopharmacology and modern clinical research. Historically rooted in traditional medicine systems across diverse cultures—such as Ayurveda, Traditional Chinese Medicine (TCM), African traditional medicine, and Unani—herbal remedies have long been utilized for the treatment of skin injuries, ulcers, burns, and surgical wounds. With the growing global interest in natural therapies and the urgent need for alternatives to synthetic drugs, especially antibiotics and corticosteroids, the scientific community has turned its attention to evaluating the efficacy of herbal constituents in promoting wound healing. A robust and expanding body of literature supports the claim that phytochemicals found in medicinal plants—such as flavonoids, alkaloids, terpenoids, saponins, polyphenols, and essential oils—possess properties that aid in each phase of wound healing, including hemostasis, inflammation, proliferation, and remodeling. These compounds exhibit a range of bioactivities such as antimicrobial, anti-inflammatory, antioxidant, and angiogenic effects, which are critical in promoting tissue repair and regeneration, (Zindle et al., 2021). One of the most extensively studied herbal constituents is curcumin, the principal curcuminoid found in *Curcuma longa* (turmeric). Several in vitro and in vivo studies have demonstrated curcumin's ability to enhance wound contraction, stimulate fibroblast proliferation, increase collagen synthesis, and modulate various growth factors like TGF-β and VEGF. Its potent anti-inflammatory and antioxidant effects—primarily through the inhibition of the NF-κB pathway and activation of Nrf2—make curcumin especially useful in treating chronic wounds where oxidative stress and prolonged inflammation are predominant. Clinical studies have supported these findings, with curcumin-loaded hydrogels, nanofibers, and films showing improved healing in surgical wounds, burns, and diabetic foot ulcers. However, its low bioavailability and rapid degradation remain limitations, leading researchers to develop nanoformulations and encapsulated systems to enhance its stability and therapeutic impact. The mucilaginous gel of *Aloe barbadensis* contains compounds such as acemannan, aloin, and vitamins A, C, and E—all of which contribute to its anti-inflammatory, moisturizing, and antioxidant effects.

Aloe vera has been shown to enhance collagen deposition, stimulate fibroblast activity, and reduce the duration of the inflammatory phase. A meta-analysis published in *Journal of Wound Care* (2020) concluded that Aloe vera significantly reduces healing time in burn injuries compared to standard treatments. However, variability in Aloe product quality, source, and processing methods can affect outcomes, emphasizing the need for standardization and quality control in commercial formulations, (Xu et al., 2018). Centella asiatica (Gotu kola), rich in triterpenoids like asiaticoside and madecassoside, has also been the subject of extensive research. Studies have shown that Centella extracts promote fibroblast proliferation, increase collagen synthesis, and improve angiogenesis. Clinical trials in patients with venous ulcers and diabetic wounds have demonstrated faster healing and reduced scar formation when treated with Centella-based ointments or dressings. The World Health Organization has recognized *Centella asiatica* as a medicinal plant with scientifically proven wound-healing properties, (Wayal & Gurav, 2021). However, berberine's bitter taste, poor gastrointestinal absorption, and potential cytotoxicity at high doses have limited its systemic use, though topical formulations have shown promising safety and efficacy profiles. Another widely cited herbal constituent is epigallocatechin-3-gallate (EGCG), a catechin found in green tea (*Camellia sinensis*). EGCG offers antioxidant, antimicrobial, and anti-inflammatory actions. It has been shown to inhibit matrix metalloproteinases (MMPs), which degrade extracellular matrix components and delay wound closure, especially in chronic wounds. In animal studies, topical EGCG reduced wound size and increased collagen fiber alignment and tensile strength. Its incorporation into hydrogels and polymeric scaffolds for wound dressings is a growing area of interest. Despite the compelling evidence for the benefits of herbal constituents in wound healing, the literature also highlights important limitations and challenges. One key concern is the variability in phytochemical content due to differences in plant species, geographic origin, harvesting time, and extraction method. (Wang et al., 2022). This inconsistency can affect the reproducibility and efficacy of herbal treatments. Additionally, many studies rely on in vitro or animal models, and while these provide valuable mechanistic insights, there remains a need for more robust, large-scale, and well-controlled clinical trials in humans.

HERBAL CONSTITUENTS AND WOUND HEALING: FUTURE DIRECTIONS

Herbal medicine has long played a central role in the treatment of wounds, cuts, ulcers, and burns across various cultures worldwide. As modern medicine continues to seek alternatives to synthetic drugs and antibiotic resistance, herbal constituents have gained renewed attention for their potential to enhance wound healing. The literature surrounding herbal constituents and their applications in wound healing includes not only laboratory and preclinical studies but also real-world case studies and clinical trials that underscore the effectiveness of plant-derived substances. Numerous success stories, ranging from the use of individual herbal compounds like curcumin and aloe vera to combinations of traditional herbs, illustrate the promising therapeutic potential of herbal medicine in promoting tissue repair, preventing infection, and reducing scar formation (Vijayakumar et al., 2024). The combination of its anti-inflammatory, antioxidant, and antimicrobial properties has made curcumin a staple in modern wound care protocols, particularly for chronic and non-healing wounds. Similarly, (Tessema & Molla, 2021) is the application of *Aloe vera* gel in second-degree burns. A clinical trial published in *Phytotherapy Research* (2020) demonstrated that topical application of Aloe vera gel led to a 50% reduction in healing time for patients with burn injuries compared to those treated with standard burn creams. The gel's ability to maintain a moist wound environment, reduce inflammation, and promote collagen synthesis is well-documented, and the trial also noted a significant reduction in pain and scarring. This success story aligns with numerous other studies that have explored Aloe vera's benefits for wound healing, including chronic wounds like diabetic ulcers. Notably, Aloe vera's bioactive compounds, including acemannan, polysaccharides, and vitamins A, C, and E, contribute to its ability to stimulate fibroblast activity, increase collagen production, and reduce excessive inflammation at the wound site. **Centella Asiatica** (Gotu kola) is another herb that has gained recognition for its wound-healing properties. A clinical trial conducted in India, published in the *International Journal of Pharmaceutical Sciences and Research* (2021), highlighted the use of Centella asiatica extracts in the treatment of venous leg ulcers. The trial revealed that patients receiving topical Centella extract showed faster wound closure and reduced edema compared to those treated with conventional saline dressings. (Tekleyes et al., 2021).

Centella's active triterpenoid compounds, particularly asiaticoside and madecassoside, have been shown to stimulate fibroblast proliferation, collagen formation, and angiogenesis. The study found that the wound healing process was significantly accelerated, with reduced risk of secondary infection and scarring. The anti-inflammatory and antioxidant properties of Centella asiatica were further demonstrated by a reduction in pro-inflammatory cytokines and oxidative stress markers in the treated group, underscoring the herb's multifaceted role in promoting tissue repaiith complete tissue regeneration and no signs of infection. This success story is consistent with research showing that honey possesses antimicrobial, anti-inflammatory, and debridement properties that are vital in treating chronic wounds and preventing infection. The natural composition of honey—rich in hydrogen peroxide, methylglyoxal, and phenolic compounds—contributes to its powerful ability to fight pathogens and promote healing. Its hygroscopic nature helps in maintaining a moist environment conducive to cell migration and tissue regeneration, making it a valuable tool in wound healing. Another case study worth mentioning in wound healing. A study published in *Wound Medicine* (2021) focused on the application of green tea catechins in diabetic foot ulcers. The study included 30 patients with chronic diabetic wounds who were treated with a gel containing epigallocatechin gallate (EGCG), the main antioxidant component in green tea.

THE CHALLENGES OF USING HERBAL CONSTITUENTS IN WOUND HEALING

Herbal medicine has long played a vital role in the treatment of wounds, injuries, and burns, particularly in traditional healing systems across the world. As modern medicine grapples with issues such as antibiotic resistance, prolonged inflammation, and the limitations of synthetic drugs, herbal constituents have garnered increasing attention, (Sugumaran et al., 2024) for their potential to enhance wound healing. The future of herbal constituents in wound healing holds tremendous promise, particularly with advances in pharmaceutical technologies, biotechnological innovation, and growing interest in integrative medicine. The following discussion explores the future directions for research and development in this field, focusing on improving the efficacy, bioavailability, and application of herbal-based therapies in wound management. One of the primary challenges associated with the use of herbal constituents in wound healing is their bioavailability and stability when applied topically. Many bioactive compounds in plants, such as flavonoids, alkaloids, and terpenoids, exhibit poor solubility, limited skin penetration, and rapid degradation, which significantly hampers their therapeutic potential. To address these limitations, the future of herbal medicine in wound healing will rely heavily on nanotechnology to enhance the delivery of herbal constituents to the wound site. Another promising direction for future research in herbal wound healing involves combination therapies. While individual herbal constituents, such as turmeric (curcumin), honey, and aloe vera, have shown effectiveness in wound healing, emerging evidence suggests that the synergistic effects of combining multiple herbal agents may offer enhanced therapeutic outcomes. Researchers are exploring various herbal combinations for their potential to address multiple aspects of the wound healing process, such as inflammation, infection, and tissue regeneration, simultaneously. A promising area of research is the combination of antimicrobial herbs like Manuka honey, Garlic (*Allium sativum*), and Berberine with anti-inflammatory agents like Turmeric and Gotu Kola (*Centella Asiatica*). Manuka honey's proven antimicrobial properties are enhanced when combined with flavonoids from plants like green tea and chamomile to target infection while promoting tissue repair. The combined anti-inflammatory, antimicrobial, and regenerative properties of these combinations have shown remarkable potential in animal models of chronic wounds, where both infection and excessive inflammation hinder the healing process.

The future will likely see a growing trend of multifunctional herbal formulations that combine multiple herbs, enhancing the efficiency of wound care and offering broader therapeutic benefits. regulatory conditions, the quality and consistency of herbal products can vary significantly due to differences in plant sources, extraction methods, and geographic location. The future of herbal medicine in wound healing will depend on rigorous quality control measures to ensure that herbal preparations are potent, safe, and reproducible. critical step in this process will involve developing standardized herbal extracts that contain consistent levels of active compounds, ensuring therapeutic efficacy.(Sreenivasulu et al., 2022) The use of Good Manufacturing Practices (GMP), phytochemical profiling, and analytical testing techniques, such as high-performance liquid chromatography (HPLC) and mass spectrometry, will become the norm in the production of herbal wound-healing products. Furthermore, collaborations between herbalists, pharmacologists, and regulatory bodies will play an essential role in ensuring the safety and efficacy of herbal-based therapies, making them more acceptable and trusted in clinical settings. Additionally, integrative medicine is expected to gain further traction in wound care. Herbal remedies will likely be integrated into conventional wound care protocols, combining the best of both worlds: the natural healing properties of herbs with the advanced technologies of modern medicine. This could include combining herbal constituents with advanced wound dressings, biomaterial scaffolds, and growth factor therapies to create a more comprehensive and holistic approach to wound management. The combination of evidence-based herbal treatments with cutting-edge technologies offers significant promise for improving outcomes in chronic, difficult-to-heal wounds. ulcers, pressure sores, and post-surgical wounds. Moreover, the development of regulatory frameworks for herbal medicines, particularly in wound healing, will be crucial for their widespread acceptance in the medical community.

THE OPPORTUNITIES OF HERBAL CONSTITUENTS IN WOUND HEALING

The use of herbal constituents in wound healing has gained significant attention in recent years, driven by the increasing need for alternative therapies in the face of rising concerns over antibiotic resistance, chronic wound management, and the limitations of synthetic drugs. Despite the promising results in both laboratory studies and clinical applications, the widespread integration of herbal constituents into wound healing practices faces numerous challenges. These hurdles span regulatory concerns, scientific and technological barriers, scalability issues, quality control, and the integration of herbal treatments with conventional medicine. Overcoming these challenges is crucial to the acceptance, efficacy, and safe use of herbal treatments in mainstream healthcare. efficacy, herbal products are often treated with less scrutiny in many parts of the world. Contamination with heavy metals, pesticides, or microbial pathogens can pose significant health risks, particularly when used in wound care, where the skin's integrity is compromised, and there is a direct route for pathogens to enter the body. Moreover, there is a risk of adulteration—the deliberate substitution or addition of cheaper or ineffective ingredients to herbal products. (Sivamani et al., 2012). This is especially prevalent in areas where herbal medicine is not subject to strict regulations. For example, the use of substandard or contaminated herbal ingredients could lead to wound infections or delayed healing, ultimately harming patients and undermining trust in herbal treatments. To mitigate these risks, stringent Good Manufacturing Practices (GMP), phytochemical analysis, and quality testing protocols must be implemented. Adopting modern analytical techniques such as high-performance liquid chromatography (HPLC) and mass spectrometry can aid in ensuring the consistency and purity of herbal products, thereby enhancing their reliability and safety in clinical use. By investing in advanced formulation technologies, clinical research, and standardized manufacturing processes, these challenges can be mitigated. As research advances and regulatory frameworks evolve, the potential of herbal constituents in wound healing will likely be realized, providing new, safe, and natural alternatives to conventional wound care treatments.

THE FUTURE OF HERBAL CONSTITUENTS IN WOUND HEALING

Herbal constituents have long been valued for their therapeutic properties, with many plants offering potent biological activities that can support various aspects of human health. In the field of wound healing, the potential of herbal ingredients is increasingly recognized due to their multifaceted effects, which include anti-inflammatory, antimicrobial, antioxidant, and regenerative properties. As the limitations of conventional wound healing therapies, such as the overuse of antibiotics and the growing incidence of chronic wounds, become more apparent, the demand for alternative or complementary treatments is on the rise. This increasing interest in natural remedies opens up significant opportunities for herbal constituents to play a pivotal role in improving patient outcomes and enhancing the healing process of wounds. The following analysis explores the key opportunities of herbal constituents in wound healing, from the molecular mechanisms involved to the broader implications for clinical practice. Healing lies in their ability to address chronic wounds, which represent a major burden on healthcare systems globally. Chronic wounds, such as diabetic ulcers, venous leg ulcers, pressure ulcers, and surgical wounds, often fail to heal due to prolonged inflammation, infection, poor tissue regeneration, and impaired blood flow. These wounds can take months or even years to heal, leading to prolonged patient suffering, reduced quality of life, and high treatment costs. Herbal constituents offer a natural alternative to traditional therapies, with many plants known for their antimicrobial properties. This is particularly relevant in the context of antimicrobial resistance (AMR), which is increasingly undermining the effectiveness of conventional antibiotics. (Ramakrishnan et al., 2022). Wound infections caused by multidrug-resistant organisms, such as Methicillin-resistant Staphylococcus aureus (MRSA) and Pseudomonas aeruginosa, are common and can complicate the healing process.

Several herbs, including Manuka honey, Garlic (Allium sativum), and Echinacea, have demonstrated significant antimicrobial activity against a broad spectrum of pathogens. For instance, Manuka honey contains methylglyoxal, a compound with potent antimicrobial properties, making it highly effective in managing wound infections, promoting faster healing, and reducing the need for antibiotics. The use of these herbal remedies can not only help prevent infection but also reduce the dependence on synthetic antibiotics, thereby playing a crucial role in combating the growing issue of antimicrobial resistance. The opportunity here is vast—herbal products with antimicrobial properties can complement existing wound care treatments, helping to mitigate the risk of infection while supporting the body's natural healing processesing, where tissue regeneration occurs. Furthermore, certain herbs such as Centella Asiatica (commonly known as Gotu Kola) have been shown to stimulate collagen synthesis, a crucial aspect of wound healing. Collagen, the primary structural protein in connective tissue, plays a vital role in the formation of new skin and the closure of wounds. Gotu Kola's ability to stimulate collagen production has made it a key ingredient in many wound healing products. Similarly, Aloe Vera has long been used for its ability to promote wound healing, thanks to its polysaccharides, which can enhance tissue regeneration and reduce scarring. The opportunity in this area is significant: By incorporating herbal constituents into wound healing regimens, healthcare providers can potentially accelerate the healing process, leading to faster recovery times, less scarring, and improved outcomes for patients. These effects can be especially beneficial for individuals with chronic wounds, where conventional therapies often fail to deliver quick results.

RECOMMENDATIONS FOR FUTURE RESEARCH AND DEVELOPMENT

The exploration of herbal constituents in wound healing has illuminated a powerful potential for natural remedies to complement and enhance modern wound care practices. Throughout this discourse, we have examined the multifaceted role that herbal constituents play in promoting faster and more effective wound healing. Moreover, compounds like curcumin, found in turmeric, and epigallocatechin gallate (EGCG), found in green tea, show promise in reducing oxidative stress and protecting cellular integrity, which is essential for optimal wound healing. These bioactive molecules contribute to wound healing by promoting cell proliferation, collagen formation, and the revascularization of the wound bed, which are all crucial steps in tissue repair. (Centella Asiatica) and Aloe Vera offer substantial benefits in stimulating tissue regeneration, promoting collagen synthesis, and reducing scarring. Rigorous scientific research is needed to identify and isolate the most effective compounds and ensure their efficacy in clinical applications. Another challenge is the regulatory landscape surrounding herbal medicines, which is often less stringent than that for pharmaceuticals. As the demand for herbal remedies increases, it will be essential for regulatory bodies to establish clear guidelines for the safety, efficacy, and quality control of herbal products used in wound care. This would help ensure that patients and healthcare providers can trust the products they use and that herbal remedies are safe for widespread clinical application. Furthermore, the scalability of herbal medicine can be an issue, especially for herbs that require extensive cultivation or specific growing conditions. To meet the growing demand for herbal-based wound care products, sustainable sourcing and ethical farming practices must be prioritized to prevent overharvesting and ensure that these products are available for long-term use, health condition, and their response to previous treatments, ensuring that the most effective combination of therapies is used for optimal healing, alternative. Many herbal constituents can be sourced from widely available and renewable plant resources, which can be cultivated using sustainable farming practices.

CONCLUSION

One of the most significant drivers of the future of herbal constituents in wound healing is the increasing body of research surrounding their bioactive properties. Over the last few decades, there has been a surge in scientific studies investigating the mechanisms by which herbal constituents promote wound healing. Research has revealed that compounds from a variety of plants—ranging from flavonoids and alkaloids to terpenes and polyphenols—exhibit anti-inflammatory, antimicrobial, antioxidant, and regenerative properties that are crucial for wound repair and tissue regeneration. As the scientific community continues to explore the molecular mechanisms behind these healing processes, the future of herbal constituents in wound healing will likely benefit from targeted research efforts focused on identifying novel plant compounds with superior efficacy in promoting wound closure, tissue regeneration, and scar minimization. For instance, flavonoids like quercetin and luteolin, which have demonstrated anti-inflammatory effects, could potentially be optimized in future formulations to reduce chronic inflammation in wounds. Similarly, the antioxidant properties of compounds found in green tea or pomegranate could be enhanced to better protect cells from oxidative damage and support faster tissue healing. Moreover, the biochemical profiling of herbal constituents will help identify the specific active compounds responsible for wound-healing effects. This knowledge will provide opportunities for creating more potent, standardized formulations, ensuring that herbal treatments are not only effective but also safe and consistent. As research continues, new plant species with novel bioactive compounds may emerge, potentially expanding the range of available treatments for chronic and difficult-to-heal wounds overcome this barrier, future formulations will likely focus on novel drug delivery technologies that can enhance the penetration and sustained release of herbal compounds into the wound site. Nanotechnology is one promising approach for improving the bioavailability of herbal constituents. The use of nanoemulsions, nanoparticles, and liposomes can enhance the topical delivery of active ingredients directly to the wound site. For example, nanoencapsulation of curcumin or Aloe Vera compounds could improve their stability and bioavailability, increasing their potential to reduce inflammation, promote tissue regeneration, and accelerate wound healing. Moreover, these nanoformulations could be designed to release herbal compounds in a controlled manner over time, providing prolonged therapeutic effects and reducing the need for frequent applications. Similarly, hydrogels and bioactive wound dressings incorporating herbal constituents are gaining attention as highly effective, sustained-release platforms for wound care. These formulations not only enhance the therapeutic effects of the herbs but also maintain a moist wound environment, which has been shown to promote optimal healing. The development of smart wound dressings that release herbal constituents in response to changes in the wound environment (e.g., pH or temperature) will further enhance the precision and personalization of wound healing therapies, ortunity to complement conventional treatments, offering a more holistic and patient-centered approach to wound management. Integrative wound care strategies could involve the combination of topical herbal treatments with conventional therapies, such as antibiotic ointments, surgical debridement, or negative pressure wound therapy (NPWT). For example, Aloe Vera or Manuka honey could be applied in conjunction with more standard medical interventions to improve healing, reduce scarring, and prevent infection. Gotu Kola (Centella Asiatica), with its collagen-promoting effects, could be used in combination with conventional treatments for burns and surgical wounds to accelerate tissue repair and reduce the formation of hypertrophic scars. Moreover, as the field of personalized medicine advances, herbal constituents may be tailored to meet the specific needs of individual patients. Genetic, environmental, and lifestyle factors can affect how a patient's body responds to various treatments. The future of wound healing will likely see the development of personalized wound care regimens that include custom formulations of herbal remedies, optimizing the efficacy of healing based on the patient's unique characteristics. By considering factors like genetic predisposition to scarring, immune response, and the type of wound, practitioners could recommend a targeted combination of herbal and conventional therapies that align with the patient's specific healing requirements.ng practices, ensuring that medicinal plants are cultivated responsibly and that their use does not lead to environmental degradation. Sustainably cultivated herbal products and fair-trade practices will become increasingly important as consumers and healthcare professionals alike seek environmentally friendly, ethical solutions.

REFERENCES

Aburjai, T., Al-Janabi, R., Al-Mamoori, F., & Azzam, H. (2019). In vivo wound healing and antimicrobial activity of Alkanna strigose. *Wound Med*, *25*(1), 100152.

Aderibigbe, B. A., & Buyana, B. (2018). Alginate in wound dressings. *Pharmaceutics*, *10*(2), 42. PMID: 29614804

Ahmed, O. M., Mohamed, T., Moustafa, H., Hamdy, H., Ahmed, R. R., & Aboud, E. (2018). Quercetin and low level laser therapy promote wound healing process in diabetic rats via structural reorganization and modulatory effects on inflammation and oxidative stress. *Biomedicine and Pharmacotherapy*, *101*, 58–73. PMID: 29477473

Bihani, T., & Mhaske, N. (2020). Evaluation of in vivo wound healing activity of Plumeria obtusa L. (Champa) spray in rats. *Wound Med.*, *28*, 100176.

Binsuwaidan, R., Elekhnawy, E., Elseady, W. S., Keshk, W. A., Shoeib, N. A., Attallah, N. G., Mokhtar, F. A., Abd El Hadi, S. R., Ahmed, E., & Magdeldin, S. (2022). Anti-bacterial activity and wound healing potential of Cycas thouarsii R. Br n-butanol fraction in diabetic rats supported with phytochemical profiling. *Biomedicine and Pharmacotherapy*, *155*, 113763. PMID: 36182739

Carvalho, M. T. B., Araújo-Filho, H. G., Barreto, A. S., Quintans-Júnior, L. J., Quintans, J. S. S., & Barreto, R. S. S. (2021). Wound healing properties of flavonoids: A systematic review highlighting the mechanisms of action. *Phytomedicine*, *90*, 153636. PMID: 34333340

Chen, L.-Y., Cheng, H.-L., Kuan, Y.-H., Liang, T.-J., Chao, Y.-Y., & Lin, H.-C. (2021). Therapeutic potential of luteolin on impaired wound healing in streptozotocin-induced rats. *Biomedicines*, *9*(7), 761. PMID: 34209369

Du, X., Wu, L., Yan, H., Jiang, Z., Li, S., Li, W., Bai, Y., Wang, H., Cheng, Z., & Kong, D.. (2021). Microchannelled alkylated chitosan sponge to treat noncompressible hemorrhages and facilitate wound healing. *Nature Communications*, *12*(1), 4733. PMID: 34354068

Dunn, L., Prosser, H. C., Tan, J. T., Vanags, L. Z., Ng, M. K., & Bursill, C. A. (2013). Murine model of wound healing. [j Visual Exp]. *Journal of Visualized Experiments*, *75*, e50265. PMID: 23748713

El-ezz, A., Abdel-Rahman, L. H., Al-Farhan, B. S., Mostafa, D. A., Ayad, E. G., Basha, M. T., Abdelaziz, M., & Abdalla, E. M. (2022). Enhanced in vivo wound healing efficacy of a novel hydrogel loaded with copper (II) schiff base quinoline complex (CuSQ) solid lipid nanoparticles. *Pharmaceuticals*, *15*(8), 978. PMID: 36015126

Elloumi, W., Mahmoudi, A., Ortiz, S., Boutefnouchet, S., Chamkha, M., & Sayadi, S. (2022). Wound healing potential of quercetin-3-O-rhamnoside and myricetin-3-O-rhamnoside isolated from Pistacia lentiscus distilled leaves in rats model. *Biomedicine and Pharmacotherapy*, *146*, 112574. PMID: 35062055

Fathi, A. N., Sakhaie, M. H., Babaei, S., Babaei, S., Slimabad, F., & Babaei, S. (2020). Use of bromelain in cutaneous wound healing in streptozocin-induced diabetic rats: An experimental model. *Journal of Wound Care*, *29*(9), 488–495. PMID: 32924815

Frykberg Robert, G. (2015). Challenges in the treatment of chronic wounds. *Advances in Wound Care (New Rochelle, N.Y.)*, *4*(9), 560–582. PMID: 26339534

Gebremeskel, L., Bhoumik, D., Sibhat, G. G., & Tuem, K. B. (2018). In vivo wound healing and anti-inflammatory activities of leaf latex of aloe megalacantha baker (Xanthorrhoeaceae). *Evidence-Based Complementary and Alternative Medicine: eCAM*, *2018*, 1–7. PMID: 30057643

Haq, A., Kumar, S., Mao, Y., Berthiaume, F., & Michniak-Kohn, B. (2020). Thymoquinone-loaded polymeric films and hydrogels for bacterial disinfection and wound healing. *Biomedicines*, *8*(10), 386. PMID: 32998437

Hou, Y., Xin, M., Li, Q., & Wu, X. (2021). Glycyrrhizin micelle as a genistein nanocarrier: Synergistically promoting corneal epithelial wound healing through blockage of the HMGB1 signaling pathway in diabetic mice. *Experimental Eye Research*, *204*, 108454. PMID: 33497689

Ibrahim, A. A. E., Bagherani, N., Smoller, B. R., Reyes-Baron, C., & Bagherani, N. (2020). Functions of the Skin. In Smoller, B., & Bagherani, N. (Eds.), *Atlas of Dermatology, Dermatopathology and Venereology* (pp. 1–11). Springer International Publishing.

Ivanková V, Belovičová M 2020 Consequences of chronic wounds on patient's lif. Україна Здоров'я нації. 2(3).

Jangde, R., Srivastava, S., Singh, M. R., & Singh, D. (2018). In vitro and In vivo characterization of quercetin loaded multiphase hydrogel for wound healing application. *International Journal of Biological Macromolecules*, *115*, 1211–1217. PMID: 29730004

Jee, J.-P., Pangeni, R., Jha, S. K., Byun, Y., & Park, J. W. (2019). Preparation and in vivo evaluation of a topical hydrogel system incorporating highly skin-permeable growth factors, quercetin, and oxygen carriers for enhanced diabetic wound-healing therapy. *International Journal of Nanomedicine*, *14*, 5449. PMID: 31409998

Jones, M. L. (2015). A short history of the development of wound care dressings. *British Journal of Healthcare Assistants*, *9*(10), 482–485.

Kalalinia, F., Aamiri, N., Bayat, S., Movaffagh, J., & Hahsemi, M. (2021). (20211 burn wound healing effect of bromelain-loaded chitosan nanofibers. *Journal of Burn Care & Research; Official Publication of the American Burn Association*, *42*(1), S192–S192.

Kant, V., Jangir, B. L., Kumar, V., Nigam, A., & Sharma, V. (2020a). Quercetin accelerated cutaneous wound healing in rats by modulation of different cytokines and growth factors. *Growth Factors (Chur, Switzerland)*, *38*(2), 105–119. PMID: 32957814

Kumar, S., Kumar, A., Kumar, N., Singh, P., Singh, T. U., Singh, B. R., Gupta, P. K., & Thakur, V. K. (2022). In vivo therapeutic efficacy of Curcuma longa extract loaded ethosomes on wound healing. *Veterinary Research Communications*, *46*(4), 1033–1049. PMID: 35796857

Lee, G., Ko, Y.-G., Bae, K. H., Kurisawa, M., Kwon, O. K., & Kwon, O. H. (2022). Green tea catechin-grafted silk fibroin hydrogels with reactive oxygen species scavenging activity for wound healing applications. *Biomaterials Research*, *26*(1), 1–6. PMID: 36352485

Lüer, S., Troller, R., & Aebi, C. (2012). Anti-bacterial and antiinflammatory kinetics of curcumin as a potential antimucositis agent in cancer patients. *Nutrition and Cancer*, *64*(7), 975–981. PMID: 22973975

Madgule, M., Vinayaka, N., Sonkhaskar, Y. M., Patel, D. R., Karthikeyan, R., & Selvakumar, P. (2023). Mechanical properties and microstructure of activated TIG welded similar joints of Inconel alloys by desirability approaches. *Materials Today: Proceedings*, *77*, 528–533.

Majtan, J., & Jesenak, M. (2018). β-Glucans: Multi-functional modulator of wound healing. *Molecules (Basel, Switzerland)*, *23*(4), 80. PMID: 29614757

Parveen, A., Kulkarni, N., Yalagatti, M., Abbaraju, V., & Deshpande, R. (2018). In vivo efficacy of biocompatible silver nanoparticles cream for empirical wound healing. *Journal of Tissue Viability*, *27*(4), 257–261. PMID: 30190175

Pazyar, N., Yaghoobi, R., Rafiee, E., Mehrabian, A., & Feily, A. (2014). Skin wound healing and phytomedicine: A review. *Skin Pharmacology and Physiology*, *27*(6), 303–310. PMID: 24993834

Ramakrishnan, T., Mohan Gift, M. D., Chitradevi, S., Jegan, R., & Subha Hency Jose, P. Nagaraja, Rajneesh Sharma H.N., Selvakumar P., Sintayehu Mekuria Hailegiorgis, (2022). "Study of Numerous Resins Used in Polymer Matrix Composite Materials", Advances in Materials Science and Engineering, vol. 2022, Article ID 1088926, 8 pages, 2022. https://doi.org/DOI: 10.1155/2022/1088926

Rathod, L., Bhowmick, S., Patel, P., & Sawant, K. (2022). Calendula flower extract loaded collagen film exhibits superior wound healing potential: Preparation, evaluation, in-vitro & in-vivo wound healing study. *Journal of Drug Delivery Science and Technology*, *72*, 103363.

Sivamani, R. K., Ma, B. R., Wehrli, L. N., & Maverakis, E. (2012). Phytochemicals and naturally derived substances for wound healing. *Advances in Wound Care (New Rochelle, N.Y.)*, *1*(5), 213–217. PMID: 24527308

Sreenivasulu, A., & Manimozhi, T. Satheesh kumar P., Selvakumar P. and Singh P.,(2022). "The Model of Smart Sensing Device For Sensitive Nanoclusters Modification in Sensing Properties," 2022 2nd International Conference on Advance Computing and Innovative Technologies in Engineering (ICACITE), Greater Noida, India, 2022, pp. 1043-1047, doi: DOI: 10.1109/ICACITE53722.2022.9823846

Sugumaran, K. M. D., Pandiyarajan V., Y. B S, Selvakumar P. and M. S, (2024). "Analysis of Electromyography Signals for Control of Mechanical Prosthesis using Machine Learning Techniques," 2024 2nd International Conference on Intelligent Data Communication Technologies and Internet of Things (IDCIoT), Bengaluru, India, 2024, pp. 1059-1067, doi: DOI: 10.1109/IDCIoT59759.2024.10467707

Tekleyes, B., Huluka, S. A., Wondu, K., & Wondmkun, Y. T. (2021). Wound healing activity of 80% methanol leaf extract of zehneria scabra (lf) sond (cucurbitaceae) in mice. *Journal of Experimental Pharmacology*, *13*, 537. PMID: 34104005

Tessema, Z., & Molla, Y. (2021). Evaluation of the wound healing activity of the crude extract of root bark of Brucea antidysentrica, the leaves of Dodonaea angustifolia and Rhamnus prinoides in mice. *Heliyon*, *7*(1), e05901. PMID: 33521349

Vijayakumar, G. (2024). Muniyandi Rajkumar, Rajiv Chandar N, Selvakumar P and Ramesh Duraisamy, (2024). Environmentally friendly TDS removal from waste water by electrochemical ion exchange batch-type recirculation (EIR) technique. *Environmental Science. Water Research & Technology*, *10*, 826–835. DOI: 10.1039/D3EW00793F

Wang, L., Hu, L., Peng, Z., Cao, H., Cao, D., Long, Y., & Zou, Z. (2022). Luteolin is an effective component of platycodon grandiflorus in promoting wound healing in rats with cutaneous scald injury. *Clinical, Cosmetic and Investigational Dermatology*, *15*, 1715–1727. PMID: 36032411

Wayal, S. R., & Gurav, S. S. (2021). Evaluation of wound healing potential of Bhallatakadi Ghrita–cow ghee based polyherbal formulation: In-vivo excision and incision wound model. *Journal of Complementary & Integrative Medicine*, *18*(3), 507–515. PMID: 33691354

Xu, N., Wang, L., Guan, J., Tang, C., He, N., Zhang, W., & Fu, S. (2018). Wound healing effects of a Curcuma zedoaria polysaccharide with platelet-rich plasma exosomes assembled on chitosan/silk hydrogel sponge in a diabetic rat model. *International Journal of Biological Macromolecules*, *117*, 102–107. PMID: 29772339

Yaseen, H. S., Asif, M., Saadullah, M., Asghar, S., Shams, M. U., Bazmi, R. R., Saleem, M., Yousaf, H. M., & Yaseen, M. (2020). Methanolic extract of Ephedra ciliata promotes wound healing and arrests inflammatory cascade in vivo through downregulation of TNF-α. *Inflammopharmacology*, *28*(6), 1691–1704. PMID: 32385747

Yin, G., Wang, Z., Wang, Z., & Wang, X. (2018). Topical application of quercetin improves wound healing in pressure ulcer lesions. *Experimental Dermatology*, *27*(7), 779–786. PMID: 29733461

Zahedi, P., Rezaeian, I., Ranaei-Siadat, S. O., Jafari, S. H., & Supaphol, P. (2010). A review on wound dressings with an emphasis on electrospun nanofibrous polymeric bandages. *Polymers for Advanced Technologies*, *21*(2), 77–95.

Zindle, J. K., Wolinsky, E., & Bogie, K. M. (2021). A review of animal models from 2015 to 2020 for preclinical chronic wounds relevant to human health. *Journal of Tissue Viability*, *30*(3), 291–300. PMID: 34103213

Chapter 3
The Role of Some Herbal Constituents in Wound Healing

Sandipan Babasaheb Jige
S.R. College, India

Shubhangi Hemant Fulamarkar
Independent Researcher, USA

ABSTRACT

The wound healing is natural physiological reaction to tissue injury, but it is not simple phenomenon and involves a complex interplay between numerous cell types, cytokines, mediators and vascular system. The wound healing activity reviews evaluation and treatment of wounds and discuss different wound healing phases. The injury occurs initial phase an outpouring of lymphatic fluid and blood, during process adequate hemostasis is achieved. The extrinsic and intrinsic coagulation pathway is activated and play role in stopping blood loss. The aggregation of platelets follows arterial vasoconstriction to damaged endothelial lining. The wound healing is process of skin recovering from significant damage, it has three general parts like primary, secondary and tertiary it also referred as intentions.

INTRODUCTION

In the plants healing power is ancient idea, the people on all continents long applied poultices and imbibed infusions of hundreds. In the history therapeutic result been mixed quite often cure or relive symptoms. In the Bible about 30 healing plants described, it indeed frankincense and myrrh probably enjoyed their status of great

DOI: 10.4018/979-8-3373-3977-1.ch003

worth due to their medicinal properties. The Indian medicinal system like Ayurveda describes many herbal plants for the wound healing. For the utilize impressive array of knowledge assembled by indigenous peoples about plant and animal products used to maintain health is scientific branch known as ethnobotany. The herbal plants like basil, onion, garlic, turmeric, cinnamon and aloe are wound healer herbs. They show properties like anti-inflammation, ant-bacterial, anti-fungal, anti-biotic and anti-oxidant (Upadhaya et. al. 2009).

In the history in Mediterranean region the Greek surgeon Discorides published 600 plants in De Materia Medica in 77 A.D. The De Materia Medica contains medicinal importance and herbal collection information. In India collection of plants studied in the Rig-Veda and its classification into Vruksha means tree. In China herb has concoctions for pharmaceutical purpose in 481 B.C. In 1542 the De Historia published by herbalists Leonheart Fuchs, The species plantrum published by Carl Linnaeus in 1753. The Hippocrates in the period 460-380 B. C. discuss about 400 plant species and develops system of diagnosis and prognosis with herb help. In India in 25,000 B. C. first medicine text Ayurveda known for theory of illness occur in term imbalance with herb and dietary control for restore equilibrium use. The Arabic botanist Abdullah Ben Al Bitar in the period 1021-1080 written book 'Explanation of Dioscorides' on herb. This books glossary contains about 1,400 drugs names which are listed alphabetic order in Arabic, Persian or Spanish and Greek languages. In the Bible about 30 plants describes as healing plants, indeed frankincense and myrrh probably enjoy their start of great worth due to medicinal properties. In 1803 the German scientist Frederich Sertumer extracted first plant drug morphine (Badri & Renu, 2011). He extracted white crystal from of crude opium poppy plant then aconitine from monkshood, emetine from ipecacuanha, quinine from Peruvian bark and atropine from deadly nightshade plant. In the recent period in 2015 two natural products discovered one is avermectin a macrocyclic lactone isolates from soil microorganism Streptomyces avermitilis and other artemisinin a sesquiterpene lactone contain peroxide bridge from plant Artemisia annuna astraceae family member. This discovery wins Nobel Prize in physiology and medicine.

The medicine is increasingly respected to use of antimicrobial and other drugs which are derived from plants. The plant has limitless ability to synthesize aromatic substance most are phenols or their oxygen substituted derivatives. The secondary metabolism which has at least 12,000 isolate from number estimate to less than 10% of total. Many substances serve as plant defense mechanism against predation by microorganisms, insects and herbivores (Baron, 2020). Some terpenoids produce odors, other for flavor like capsaicin and some herb used as seasonal food and produce useful medicinal compounds.

Objectives

- To study the importance of herbal constituents in wound healing
- To focus on role of herbal constituents in wound healing
- To study the future of constituents
- To aware young generation about the herbal importance

ANALYSIS AND RESULTS

The herbal medicine widely used around the world, in rural area local traditional medicine includes herbalism is only source of health care to people. In developing area alternative medicine include use of dietary supplement is marketed aggressively use claims of traditional medicine. The traditional Chinese medicine makes use wide variety of plants among other material and techniques (De Guzman Ladion, 2002). The drugs derived from plants include opiates, cocaine and cannabis both medical and recreational uses. The different countries various times made use of illegal drugs, partly on basis of risks involved in taking psychoactive drugs. The herbal medicines are important for wound healing and other different illness of body.

History of Herbal Use as Medicine

The written record of the medicinal plant use comes from the Sumerians in Mesopotamia date back over 5,000 years. In which about 250 plants herbal recipes documented, around 1550 BC. Ebers Papyrus described more than 700 plant based remedies. In the China around 2500 BC Shen Nung creates with compiling text on medicinal plants known as 'Pen T'Sao'. In the India Vedas like Rig-Veda and Athava-Veda maintain information about medicinal plants and their uses. In Greek the physician like Hippocrates and Galan documented herbal uses, with developing system of diagnosis and treatment based on herbal properties. About 60,000 years ago in Paleolithic era medicinal plants used evidence occur in archaeology. In medieval period the Monasteries plays important role in preserving and dissemination knowledge of herbal medicine. The modern medicine system depends on traditional knowledge and many modern drugs derived from the natural plant resources. The herbal medicine widely continues practiced for its potential treating chronic condition and complementary approach to the conventional medicine (Ghosh & Gaba, 2013). The great physician Hippocrates known as father of medicine for his work like classification of herbs, development of diagnostic and therapeutic system based on their properties. The Chinese emperor legendary credited with compiling first pharmacopoeia 'Pen T'Sao'. The herbal medicine plays vital role in cultural tradition of many societies with knowledge often passed from one generation to another generation. In some culture herbalism means of cultural resistance and survival to marginalized communities (Singh et al., 2024). The herbal medicines used for general health problems like digestive issues, respiratory ailments, skin problems and menstrual disorders. It also used for stress management, as complementary theory for chronic diseases.

Types of Wounds

The wounds have general five types like abrasion, laceration, avulsion, puncture and incision.

Abrasion

When the skin rubs or slides against rough surface then this type of wounds occurs. In abrasion examples includes scarped knee, rod rash, it produces little blood then wound sanitize is important and removal of any debris for prevention of infection is necessary (Guetner, 2008).

Laceration

It is deep opening or tear of skin, the laceration occurs due to accidents or incidents usually. It involves knives, machinery or other sharp tools, in this wound significant bleeding occurs.

Avulsion

It involves forcefully tearing away the underlying tissues and skin, it is result of violent incidents like animal attacks, explosions or motor vehicles accidents.

Puncture

It is show small hole in the soft tissues splinters and needles cause an acute puncture wound that affects only outer layers of tissue. The knife or gunshot wounds damage deep muscles and internal organs which results significant bleeding (Haalboom, 2018).

Incision

It is clean straight cut of skin, many surgical procedure use incisions. The accidents involve knives, broken glass, razor blades and other sharp objects cause incisions. The incisions cause heavy rapid bleeding, the deep incisions damage muscles or nerve and likely require starches.

Types of Wounds Healing

The skin recovering from the significant damage process known as wound healing it also known as intentions. The wound healing has three types primary, secondary and tertiary wound healing.

Primary Wound Healing

The primary wound healing involves stiches, staples or glue to close a wound. It is method which helps body focus on healing a smaller area of injury.

Secondary Wound Healing

The wound is very large then secondary wound healing recommended. After cleaning wound is allow for heal naturally, it take long time for healing. It also higher risk of infection and contamination so that consistent care and attention is required.

Tertiary Wound Healing

It refers as healing delayed primary closure, the treatment involves prolonged time based method of closing of wound. The doctor fears that trap infectious germ or tissue in wound by closing it soon. It allows some natural healing or other treatment therapies before closing it with sutures.

The Properties for Wound Healing Herbal

The herbal remedies for wound healing shows some their properties as follows.

Anti-Inflammatory Properties

The herbs are possess anti-inflammatory compounds which help to reduce the swelling, redness and pain related with wounds. For the example the extract of turmeric and chamomile plants helps modulate inflammatory response.

Anti-Bacterial and Antiseptic Properties

The herbs possess antioxidant properties which helps combat or prevent wound infections by inhibiting the growth of bacteria. For example honey, garlic and tea tree oil is known for their good antibacterial properties.

Antioxidant Properties

The antioxidant properties of herb help to protect cells from damage caused by free radicals which hinder the healing process. The fruits and vegetables the herbs like turmeric and a green tree has rich with antioxidants properties which is important in wound healing.

Regenerative and Tissue Repair Properties

Some herbs promote the formation of new tissue and accelerate healing process by cell growth and collagen synthesis stimulation. For example aloe Vera herb known for the skin regeneration promotes and green tea enhances collagen production. The herbal remedies increase angiogenesis by forming new blood vessels it is essential for delivering nutrients and oxygen to the wound site.

Other Properties

Some herbs help in cleaning and removing dead tissues from wound facilitating the heal process commonly known as debridement. Some herbs known for moist environment they create this environment for conducive to wound healing. Some herbs help in minimize scarring that heals wounds. For example aloe vera has soothing regenerative and moisturizing properties,

Wound Healing Herbals

The plants has riches different phytochemicals like polyphenols, alkaloids, carotenoids, terpenes, sulfur contain groups and terpenoids which possess enormous antibacterial and antioxidant properties. In antioxidant, antibacterial, anti-inflammation, anticancer and antiviral activity this natural products occur especially polyphenols. The antibiotic medicine has fight with infection which is caused by bacteria in human and animals. It works either killing bacteria or grows and multiplies. In wound healing there are many herbal plants which is used, the different phytochemicals of that herbal plant work on it for cure (Arie B. and et. al 2015). The body's first line of defense is skin which guard against mechanical, chemical and thermal damage to interior organs. The highly developed immune response also serves as barrier against pathogenic infections. The wound healing is dynamic process occurs with numerous cellular activities like inflammation, proliferation, homeostasis and remodeling it require harmonious integration proper, for repair effectively damage tissues. The microorganism quickly enters after damage beneath skin which results in chronic wounds and fatal infections. The pharmacological properties occur in natural phyto-medicines so it widely and effectively employed on wound treatment and infection prevention. For the treatment of cutaneous wounds since ancient time phytotherapy used, it reduce onset of infection and minimize usage of antibiotic that causes critical antibiotic resistance. In Northern hemisphere number of botanicals that used in wound healing like Achiella millefolium, Aloe vera, Calendula officinals, Athaea officinals, Matricaria chmomilla, Curcuma long, Jojoba (Simmondsia chinensis), Eucalyptus (Eucalyptus globulus), Pine, pomegranate and green tea. The herbal medicines known as complementary and alternative medicine it used over decades to treat medical ailments and promote wellness by their bioactive ingredients. The herbal medicine also called as complementary and alternative medicines which used over decades to treat medical ailments and promote wellness by their bioactive ingredients (Dede Cumings and et. al. 2024). The human discover many plant species over time which is effective as treatments for specific illness. In Chinese medicine, Unani, Ayurveda and Russian herbalism the herbal medicine used as standard practice. The medicine systems apply botanicals to treat wounds and other dermatological problems. Some following herbal plants has plays important role in wound healing.

Tea Tree Oil

The plant is known for the antiseptic and antimicrobial properties, botanically plant known as Melaeuca alternifolia, which is member of family myrtaceae. The tree oil has antimicrobial and anti-inflammatory properties it prevent infection in wounds and combine with traditional methods encourage healing. The research on the tree oil shows reduce inflammation and stimulate white blood cell activity, which is important in healing process. The tree oil demonstrates effectiveness against range of bacteria like staphylococcus aureus it infects wounds generally. The antimicrobial properties of the tree oil prevent or reduce risk of infection in cuts, abrasions and other wounds. In body natural healing processes take place by inhibiting bacterial growth by tea oil. The inflammation is natural part of wound healing but excessive inflammation hinders healing. The tree oil balance healing environment it is traditionally also used due to antibacterial and anti-inflammatory property.

Aloe Vera

It is botanically known as Aloe barbadensis which is member of family lilaceae, the aloe means 'alloeh' which means bitter in Arabic language. In new food products aloe used due to its medicinal and functional qualities (Goetz, 2019). The early Egyptians called for aloe vera as 'plant of immorality' and it used in traditional medicine more than 2000 years in Arab, Greek, Egyptian, Japanese and Korean. The diseases like external and internal ulcers, skin issues, constipation, hyperlipidemia and diabetes treats. The aloe vera used in laxative medications, cosmetic products, cleaners, lotions, shampoos and hair tonics. It also used in preparation for makeup and fragrances, shaving creams and bath products (Antherton, 1998). In biological activities like detoxification, digestion aloe is related; the plant has bioactive because of antibacterial, anti-inflammatory, anti-rheumatoid, anti-arthritis and antimicrobial activities. The leaf skin, green pulp, flower and gel has demonstrates antioxidant activities. From ancient time it is used as wounds cure; it also treats chronic wounds like pressure ulcers, burn wounds, cracked nipples, surgical wounds, psoriasis and genital herpes. In the swelling, wound contraction and angiogenesis aloe vera hydrogel used, it results 29% reduction in overall healing time and complete wound closure within fifteen days (Sonawane et. al., 2021). Aloe vera can be applied topically as a cream or gel, or can be impregnated into a dressing and applied to the wound. The Aloe vera plant has been used in a large number of cultures due to its therapeutic properties. The gel from the pulp of its leaves is used in both cosmetics and alternative therapies, helping in rejuvenation, wound healing, and the treatment of dermatological diseases.

Calendula

It is commonly known as pot marigold and botanically Calendula officinalis which is member of family asteraceae. It is used from long time in ethano-pharmacology, traditional medicine for skin inflammation and healing wounds includes lipophilic and aqueous calendula alcoholic extract. It is import for anti-inflammatory, antioxidant, antibacterial, antifungal, anti-edematous and immune stimulant properties (Raina R. and et. al. 2008). The plant contains flavonoids, terpenoids, phenolic acids, carotenoids, quinones, coumarins, amino acids, volatile oils, and lipid. The plant is used in breast cancer treatment, acne treatment, gastric ulcer treatment and in wound healing. The calendula ointment used for accelerate cesarean recovery, it significantly speed up healing of cesarean wounds.

Eucalyptus

It is botanically known as Eucalyptus globulus which is member of family myrtaceae. It is quick growing, high quality woody biomass and excellent adaptability plant. It shows many species the essential oil extracted from plants leaves used as antiseptic worldwide (Alam et. Al., 2018). It is used in symptoms of cold, cough, sore throats and other illness, the pure essential oil and gentamycin optimized nano emulsion. It is used in wound healing research, collagen estimation and histological evaluation (Grattapaglia & Kirst, 2008). The dried leaves extracted in ethanol also show optimal wound healing results with more cell proliferation.

Jojoba

It is botanically known as Simmondsia chinensis which is member of family simmondsiaceae or buxaceae. The plant is dioecious desert shrub produces seeds that given liquid wax esters as valuable ingredient in lubricants used in cosmetics and industries. The oil is naturally occur light yellow capable for healing wounds and rebuilding skin barriers (Sen, 2019). The oil contains bioactive substance like polyphenols, alkaloids and flavonoids with addition of 97% linear long chain esters. The jojoba oil dry nano emulsion powder reduced bleeding and inflammatory cell infiltration in acute long injury. The oil emphasizes its efficiency anti-inflammatory and radical scavengers used in treatment of wounds. The fibroblasts and keratinocytes wound closure is notable accelerated by jojoba liquid wax. The jojoba liquid wax promotes collagen production of fibroblast, its pharmacological characters suggest employed in in clinical setts to treat wounds due to its effect on skin cell.

Curcumin

It is botanically known as Curcuma longa commonly called turmeric it is member of family zingiberaceae. The curcumin contain chief constituent is curcumin which is discovered by Vogel and Pelletier 200 years ago. The traditional medicine of curcumin used in treatment of weight loss, digestive problems and gastrointestinal and skin inflammation (Dosoky & Setzer, 2018). The curcumin contains bisdemethoxycurcumin, demethoxycurcumin and curcumin the bioactive cucurminoids is anti-inflammatory, anticancer anti-aging properties. The curcumin is important in the healing of wounds it formed granulation tissue that predominantly composed deposition collagen and regenerate epithelium (Gupta, Patchva, & Aggarwal, 2013). The curcumin reduce matrix metallopeptidase-9 and necrosis factor alpha and speed up healing wounds with controlling different cytokines (Kocaadam & Sanlier, 2017).

Plantago

It is botanically known as Plantago major commonly called Chitrak it is member of family plantaginaceae. It is herb having rosette shaped leaves which is used in folk medicine. The seeds and leaves in folk medicine used variety of ailments problems and respiratory issues. It has anti-inflammatory, antimicrobial and anti-tumor properties which is important in wounds treatment (Kizi, 2022). The plant contains caffeic acid, terpenoids, lipids, flavonoids and derivatives of polysaccharides. It is used for burn wounds its ointments not contains qualities for wound healing but also function as analgesic and antibacterial agent. The extract of freeze dried leaves made from water and ethanol stimulate effect that might useful source of many bioactive compounds which has wound healing potential. The Plantago is traditional medicinal plants used in management of diarrhea.

Pomegranate

It is botanically known as Punica granantum commonly called as pomegranate it is member of family lythraceae having sub family punicoideae. The old fruit is full of bioactive components like phenols, flavonoids, hydrolysable, proteins, vitamins, tannins and minerals (Lukiswanto et. al., 2019). The fruit has different parts like peel which consists 49-555 of total fruit size, arils it is about 45-52% in which 18-20% seeds and 26-30% juices. The seeds of fruit riches phytochemicals with high antioxidant activity, the peel extract are significant effect on burn wounds. The pomegranate is medicinal plant recover burn wounds, the research shows 10% standard pomegranate extract heals serious second burn wounds which characterized by angiogenesis, the mature and complete epithelium has low number inflammatory cells and high collagen density with good organization (Magangana T. P and et. al. 2020). The cream of pomegranate flower extract help faster wound healing, the pomegranate peel ointment also improve wound contraction and time of epithelialization.

Neem

It is botanically known as Azadirachata indica commonly called as neem it is member of family meliaceae. The leaf extract and essential oil extracted from seeds is known for antimicrobial effect which is important for infected wounds. It maintains wound and lesion free secondary infection by reducing bacterial population. The neem extract prevents inflammation and subsequent increase wound healing. The leaf extract of neem and oil of seeds has antimicrobial effect which mainly attributes its compound like margosic acid, glycerides of fatty acids, butyric acid and trace valeric acid. The stem bark after burning the ash mixed with coconut oil used for wound healing. The neem plant has play antimicrobial role by inhibitory effect on microbial growth. It also play role as free radical scavenging properties due to presence of antioxidant azadirachtin and nimbolide. It also show anti-inflammatory regulation of proinflammatory enzyme activities including cyclooxygenase and lipoxygenase.

Cinnamon

It is botanically known as Cinnamomum verum commonly called as cinnamon it is member of family lauraceae. It is traditionally used as medicine the bark used spice, condiment and flouring agent. It has antioxidant, antiulcer, antimicrobial, anti-diabetic, hypoglycemic, hypolipidemic and anti-inflammatory properties. The cinnamon is beneficial in all types of wounds like diabetic and infected wounds (Vaibhavi, Rakesh, & Pankaj, 2010) The cinnamon has significant level of phenols it enhance glucose uptake in animals. The extract accelerates wound healing by their antioxidant properties. The cinnamaldhyde is main component of cinnamon bark oil and it is key contributor of its flavor and aroma and it has antibacterial properties. The Eugenol is another chemical constituent found in its bark and leaf oil it is antioxidant and anti-inflammatory properties. The cumarin is important constituent it is potential liver toxicity.

Chmomilla

It is botanically known as Matricaria chamomilla commonly called as chmomilla it is member of family astraceae. The plant is important in dysmenorrhea, digestive disorders, conjunctivitis, cough, cold, eye infection, kidney stones, insomnia and headaches. The plant is sedative, antispasmodic, antiseptic and antiemetic its tea is reduce symptoms of minor gastrointestinal complains like bloating and spams. The anti-inflammatory properties potentially help for condition like skin inflammation, gingivitis and inflammatory bowel disease. In traditional medicine chmomilla used different infection like respiratory and gastrointestinal it also used in skin irritation, hemorrhoids and wounds. It also treats neuropsychiatric, respiratory, gastrointestinal and liver disorder like diseases (Quave, 2018). The chmomilla is sedative, antiseptic, antispasmodic and antiemetic the phytochemistry shows about 120 constituents. The essential oils contain terpenoids like α- bisabodol and its oxides, A and B bisabolone oxide, a chamazulene and β- farnesene. The plant inhibits growth of bacteria and microorganisms by preventing infection and promoting cleaning produce healing environment. It also protects wound area damage from free radicals, aids in tissue repair. The increase production of collagen which help wound strength and structure, encourage migration and proliferation of fibroblast cells which play important role in wound healing. The chmomilla promote faster wound closure stimulate collagen production with increased number of fibroblast to fast tissue regeneration.

Garlic

It is botanically known as Allium sativum commonly called as garlic it is member of family amaryllidaceae. The herb contains active component 'allicin' it is important in wounds healing due to antimicrobial and anti-inflammatory properties. It also stimulates fibroblast activity which crucial for tissue repairs. The allicin inhibit growth of bacteria and fungi it prevent or reduce wound infection due to antimicrobial and antifungal properties (Pazyar et. Al., 2014). The garlic modulates inflammatory response in wound with promoting more efficient healing process. In collagen production, tissue repair and faster wound closure allicin plays important role. In the animals research indicate the garlic extracts or ointments accelerate wound healing. The raw garlic causes skin irritation, redness or even burn in some individuals. The natural remedy garlic cause multitude of dermatoses includes limited to irritant contact dermatitis.

Table 1. Showing plants constituent and wound healing properties

Sr. No	Plant name	Botanical name	Family	Active constituents	Wound healing properties
01	Tea tree oil	Melaeuca alternifolia	Myrtaceae	Terpien-4-ol	Antiseptic and Antimicrobial
02	Aloe vera	Aloe barbadensis	Lilaceae	Acemannan, Aloin	Anti-inflammatory, Anti-microbial
03	Marigold	Calendula officinalis	Asteraceae	Triterpenoids	Anti-inflammatory, Antimicrobial
04	Eucalyptus	Eucalyptus globulus	Myrtaceae	Eucalyptol	Antiseptic
05	Jojoba	Simmondsia chinensis	Buxaceae	Eicosanoid	Anti-inflammatory
06	Plantago	Plantago major	Plantaginaceae	Caffeic acid	Anti-inflammatory, Antimicrobial
07	Garlic	Allium sativum	Amaryllidaceae	Allicin	Antimicrobial Anti-inflammatory
08	Pomegranate	Punica granantum	Lythraceae	Ellagitannins	Antioxidant
09	Neem	Azadirachata indica	Meliaceae	Azadirachata	Wound healing, Anti-inflammatory,
10	Chamomilla	Matricaria chamomilla	Asteraceae	Terpenoids α-bisabodol	Antispasmodic, Antiseptic

continued on following page

Table 1. Continued

Sr. No	Plant name	Botanical name	Family	Active constituents	Wound healing properties
11	Cinnamon	Cinnamomum verum	Lauraceae	Coumarin	Antioxidant, Antiulcer,
12	Turmeric	Curcuma longa	Zingiberaceae	Curcumin	Anti-inflammatory, Antioxidant

The traditional medicine is sum of knowledge, skill and practices based on theories, beliefs and experiences indigenous to different culture used for prevention and diagnosis, improvement or physical treatment and mental illness also health maintenance. The different parts of plants or whole plant has used in formulation of decoctions, tincture, ointments, plaster, paste and different part of medicine in external administration. The herbal remedies like herb, herbal ingredients, herbal formulation and herbal products have significant potential in treating wounds of microbial infection. The herbal medicines obtained naturally from plants root, stem, leaves, flower and seeds which improve health and health illness. The changing lifestyle has impact on consumer's health and cause major shift of medical needs. The individual consume processed food and suffer from health complains.

HERBAL PRODUCTS MARKET

The report of World Health Organization around 80% world's population consult traditional health practitioner for plant based medicine. The cosmetic industry offer promising prospects for exports of natural ingredients from developing countries into developed nation. The wound healing ointments used for superficial wound healing like abrasions, cuts, burns and scars. These also control inflammation and infection so its demand increasing due to rising prevalence of chronic injuries and number of surgical procedures. The chronic wound has major challenge for physician it projected problem for more than 1.5% world's population. The increase in natural remedies awareness has rising prevalence chronic wounds. The market project USD 216.59 billion by 2032. The compound annual growth rate of 6.83% from 2025 to 2032, the market projected growth from USD 251.25 billion in 2025 to USD 437 billion by 2032. The Europe dominates herbal medicine market with market share of 44.55% in 2024. The Asian and Pacific regions countries like China and India has rich history of herbal medicine and has key market of wound healing products.

CONCLUSION

The wound healing has two stages include inflammation process, tissue formation and tissue remodeling. The inflammatory phase involves different stages like platelet accumulation, leukocyte migration and coagulation. The tissue formation has different stages like re-epithelialization, angiogenesis, and fibroplasia and wound contracts. The remodeling phase lasted for one month and dermis respond to injury with production of collagen and matrix protein and return pre-injury phenotype. The herbal medicine is play important role in wound healing due to different properties like antimicrobial, antioxidant and antimicrobial effect. It also promotes collagen synthesis and encourages cell proliferation. The wound healing phenomenon is co-ordinated with cellular and biochemical phases collaborate synergistically promote restoration of injured tissues. The wound healing process entails different group of cells, mix outside cells and influence soluble signaling molecule like stimulatory factor and cell signaling proteins. The medicinal plants increasingly recognize their wound healing. The medicinal plants increasingly recognized for their potential with their lower side effects infected or open wounds. The implementation of improved quality assurance methods identify assessment and quantified plant based constituents coupled with planned preclinical and clinical research. The medicine is increasingly respected to use of antimicrobial and other drugs which are derived from plants. The plant has limitless ability to synthesize aromatic substance most are phenols or their oxygen substituted derivatives. The wound healing is done by the bioactive compounds of plants.

REFERENCES

Alam, P., Shakeel, F., Anwer, M. K., Foudah, A. I., & Alqarni, M. H. (2018). Wound healing study of eucalyptus oil containing nanoemulsion in rat model. *Journal of Oleo Science*, *67*(8), 957–968. DOI: 10.5650/jos.ess18005 PMID: 30012898

Badri, P. N., & Renu, S. (2011). Role of medicinal plants in wound healing. *Research Journal of Medicinal Plant*, *5*(4), 392–405. DOI: 10.3923/rjmp.2011.392.405

Baron, J. M., Glatz, M., & Proksch, E. (2020). Optimal support of wound healing: New insights. *Dermatology (Basel, Switzerland)*, *236*(6), 593–600. DOI: 10.1159/000505291 PMID: 31955162

Cumings, D., Holmes, A., & Fahs, B. (2024). *Healing herbals: How to grow, store and maximize their medicinal power*. Good Books.

De Guzman Ladion, H. (2002). *Healing wonders of herbs: Guide to the effective use of medicinal plants*. Inter-American Division Publishing Association.

Dosoky, N. S., & Setzer, W. N. (2018). Chemical composition and biological activities of essential oils of Curcuma species. *Nutrients*, *10*(9), 1196. Advance online publication. DOI: 10.3390/nu10091196 PMID: 30200410

Ghosh, P. K., & Gaba, A. (2013). Phyto-extracts in wound healing. *Journal of Pharmacy & Pharmaceutical Sciences*, *16*(5), 760–820. PMID: 24393557

Goetz, P. (2019). Aloe vera. *Phytothérapie*, *17*(6), 352–356. DOI: 10.3166/phyto-2019-0213

Grattapaglia, D., & Kirst, M. (2008). Eucalyptus applied genomics: From gene sequences to breeding tools. *The New Phytologist*, *179*(4), 911–929. DOI: 10.1111/j.1469-8137.2008.02503.x PMID: 18537893

Gupta, S. C., Patchva, S., & Aggarwal, B. B. (2013). Therapeutic roles of curcumin: Lessons learned from clinical trials. *The AAPS Journal*, *15*(1), 195–218. DOI: 10.1208/s12248-012-9432-8 PMID: 23143785

Haalboom, M. (2018). Chronic wounds: Innovations in diagnostics and therapeutics. *Current Medicinal Chemistry*, *25*(42), 5772–5781. DOI: 10.2174/0929867324666170710120556 PMID: 28699502

Kizi, K. S. A. (2022). Pharmacological properties of Plantago major L. and its active constituents. *International Journal of Medical Science and Public Health Research*, *3*(4), 9–12. DOI: 10.37547/ijmsphr/volume03issue04-03

Kocaadam, B., & Şanlier, N. (2017). Curcumin, an active component of turmeric (Curcuma longa), and its effects on health. *Critical Reviews in Food Science and Nutrition*, *57*(13), 2889–2895. DOI: 10.1080/10408398.2015.1077195 PMID: 26528921

Lukiswanto, B. S., Miranti, A., Sudjarwo, S. A., Primarizky, H., & Yuniarti, W. M. (2019). Evaluation of wound healing potential of pomegranate (Punica granatum) whole fruit extract on skin burn wound in rats (Rattus norvegicus). *Journal of Advanced Veterinary and Animal Research*, *6*(2), 202–207. DOI: 10.5455/javar.2019.f333 PMID: 31453192

Magangana, T. P., Makunga, N. P., Fawole, O. A., & Opara, U. L. (2020). Processing factors affecting the phytochemical and nutritional properties of pomegranate (Punica granatum L.) peel waste: A review. *Molecules (Basel, Switzerland)*, *25*(20), 4690. Advance online publication. DOI: 10.3390/molecules25204690 PMID: 33066412

Pazyar, N., Yaghoobi, R., Rafiee, E., Mehrabian, A., & Feily, A. (2014). Skin wound healing and phytomedicine: A review. *Skin Pharmacology and Physiology*, *27*(6), 303–310. DOI: 10.1159/000357477 PMID: 24993834

Quave, C. L. (2018). Wound healing with botanicals: A review and future perspectives. *Current Dermatology Reports*, *7*(4), 287–295. DOI: 10.1007/s13671-018-0247-4 PMID: 31106027

Raina, R., Prawez, S., Verma, P. K., & Pankaj, N. K. (2008). Medicinal plants and their role in wound healing. *Vet Scan*, *3*(1), 24.

Sen, C. K. (2019). Human wounds and its burden: An updated compendium of estimates. *Advances in Wound Care*, *8*(2), 39–48. DOI: 10.1089/wound.2019.0946 PMID: 30809421

Singh, M. A., Wahi, A., Teotia, A., Thota, P., Varshney, R., & Gupta, M. (2024). *Novel phyto-pharmaceuticals used for wound healing*. CRC Press.

Sonawane, S. R., Gokhale, J. S., Mulla, M. Z., Kandu, V. R., & Patil, S. A. (2021). A comprehensive overview of functional and rheological properties of Aloe vera and its application in foods. *Journal of Food Science and Technology*, *58*(4), 1217–1226. DOI: 10.1007/s13197-020-04661-6 PMID: 33746250

Upadhaya, A.. (2009). *Healing herbs of India*. Satish Serial Publishing House.

Vaibhavi, J., Rakesh, R., & Pankaj, K. (2010). Cinnamon: A pharmacological review. *Journal of Advanced Scientific and Engineering Research*, *1*(2), 19–23.

KEY TERMS AND DEFINIITONS

Ayurveda: it is commonly known as science of life, it is traditional Indian system of medicine which practiced for over 5000 years. The Ayurveda focus on holistic healing, balance in body, mind and sprit by natural approaches like diet, lifestyle and herbal remedies.

Coagulation: It is commonly called as clotting in this process where blood changes from liquid to gel like state from clot. It is crucial process help in stop bleeding from damaged blood vessels and key part of the body.

Ethnobotany: It is study of relationship between people and plants focus on how different cultures interact with and utilize plants in their daily lives. It encompasses traditional knowledge of how plants used for food, medicine, shelter and various other purposes. In this study how people and region make use indigenous plants, it provides food, shelter, medicines, dyes, oils, gums, resins, latex, waxes, tannins and also contribute air for breathe.

Indigenous people: It is communities that live historical continuity with pre-invasion and pre-colonial societies that develop on their territories and consider distinct themselves from other societies now prevailing in those territories. They are original inhabitants of region with strong link to their ancestral lands and unique cultures, languages and traditions.

Wound: It is an injury to body by violence, accident or surgery typically involves laceration or breaking of skin membrane and damage underlying tissues. It also known as break in tissue epithelial integrity, which occur due to physical trauma like tearing, cutting or puncturing skin or from blunt force trauma cause contusion.

Chapter 4

Herbal Excipients and Polymers: An Overview

Rupayan Roy
https://orcid.org/0000-0002-8118-431X
Department of Fashion Technology, National Institute of Fashion Technology, Kannur, India

Ayona Padhi
Department of Fashion Technology, National Institute of Fashion Technology, Kannur, India

Arya Rajesh Nambiar
Department of Fashion Technology, National Institute of Fashion Technology, Kannur, India

Vaibhavi Sanjay Bhosale
Department of Fashion Technology, National Institute of Fashion Technology, Kannur, India

ABSTRACT

Complex drug delivery systems and therapeutic applications may use natural chemicals and polymeric materials. Herbal excipients—plant-derived gums, mucilages, resins, and essential oils—are used with bioactive polymers to build multifunctional pharmaceutical platforms in this chapter. Current formulations benefit from anti-inflammatory, antibacterial, antioxidant, and wound-healing herbal excipients. Film-forming, bioadhesive, and controlled-release natural and synthetic polymers such chitosan, alginate, gelatin, and PVA are useful carriers. Herbal actives and polymers form hydrogels, films, nanofibers, and transdermal systems for wound

DOI: 10.4018/979-8-3373-3977-1.ch004

healing, dermatological treatment, and chronic illness management. This chapter covers herbal excipients and polymers' taxonomy, physicochemical properties, functional roles, and formulation methods. It discusses new research, standardization, scalability, and AI-guided formulation design. Traditional herbal and polymer sciences can inform current biomedicine.

INTRODUCTION

Excipients are pharmacologically inactive chemicals that are crucial in the formulation and development of pharmaceutical dosage forms. Traditionally viewed as inactive additives, contemporary formulation sciences acknowledge excipients as crucial enhancers in drug administration, improving solubility, stability, bioavailability, and patient adherence (Chaudhari & Patil, 2012). Their functions encompass not only bulking agents but also binders, diluents, disintegrants, suspending agents, and preservatives. As pharmacological formulations increase in complexity—particularly in controlled and targeted delivery systems—the choice and efficacy of excipients have become essential factors in formulation science (Usman et al., 2019; Dave et al., 2015).

The worldwide shift towards safer, ecological, and biocompatible pharmaceutical ingredients has stimulated interest in herbal excipients. These originate from botanical sources such as gums, mucilages, oils, and resins, exhibiting advantageous properties such as non-toxicity, biodegradability, and environmental sustainability (Pawar et al., 2025). Beyond their structural or functional roles in formulations, some herbal excipients possess intrinsic pharmacological characteristics, including anti-inflammatory, antibacterial, and antioxidant actions, thereby serving as bioactive excipients (Singh et al., 2021; Feng et al., 2023). Their extensive historical application in traditional medical systems confers credibility and consumer acceptance, particularly in areas where herbal medicine is intricately woven into cultural healthcare practices. Furthermore, regulatory bodies are increasingly endorsing plant-derived compounds with established safety records, hence facilitating their integration into contemporary pharmaceutical formulations (Nagarajan et al., 2025). Herbal excipients play crucial roles in the formulation of herbal and conventional pharmaceuticals. They can be categorized based on their functional contributions such as binding, diluting, disintegrating, thickening, emulsifying, and stabilizing the active ingredients as shown in Table 1.

Table 1. Classification of herbal excipients based on their functional roles

Type	Function	Examples of Herbal Excipients
Binders	Help bind ingredients together in tablets or granules	Acacia gum, Tragacanth, Guar gum
Diluents	Add bulk to formulations to aid in accurate dosing	Cellulose, Starch, Kaolin
Disintegrants	Facilitate the breakup of tablets for better absorption	Plantago ovata (Isabgol), Alginates, Starch
Thickeners	Increase viscosity in liquid formulations	Xanthan gum, Pectin, Carrageenan
Emulsifiers	Stabilize emulsions by reducing surface tension	Lecithin (Soy), Acacia gum, Quillaja saponins
Stabilizers	Maintain the physical and chemical integrity of formulations	Aloe vera gel, Gelatin (from plant sources), Gums

Notwithstanding the potential of herbal excipients, obstacles including batch-to-batch variability, inadequate mechanical strength, and stability concerns remain. These constraints need their incorporation with natural and synthetic polymers, which can enhance their functional efficacy in medicinal systems. Biopolymers, including chitosan, alginate, gelatin, and pectin, present benefits such as film-forming capacity, mucoadhesiveness, and biodegradability, whilst synthetic alternatives like polyvinyl alcohol (PVA) and polylactic acid (PLA) deliver enhanced mechanical strength and structural integrity. The integration of herbal bioactives with polymer matrices has proven effective in creating sophisticated drug delivery systems, including hydrogels, films, microspheres, and nanoparticles (Chavda et al., 2022). These hybrid systems improve drug stability, facilitate regulated release, and support focused therapeutic efficacy. Chitosan-based systems infused with neem extract demonstrate potential in wound healing, whereas curcumin-alginate films have been noted for their prolonged anti-inflammatory and antibacterial properties (Sharma et al., 2021; Tamilarasi et al., 2022).

This chapter seeks to deliver a thorough examination of herbal excipients and their synergistic incorporation with both natural and synthetic polymers in pharmaceutical formulations. It aims to clarify the physicochemical and biological properties that render herbal excipients and polymers appropriate for contemporary drug delivery systems. Emphasis is placed on the formulation science of polymer-herbal hybrids, their therapeutic potential, and the problems that must be resolved for broader clinical and commercial implementation. This chapter aims to provide insights into contemporary trends, research deficiencies, and prospective developments in this swiftly advancing domain by examining emerging research, applications, and case studies.

CLASSIFICATION OF HERBAL EXCIPIENTS

In the progression of formulation science, excipients have transcended their traditional function as inert transporters. Currently, they actively contribute to stability, bioavailability, patient adherence, and regulated medication release. The increasing interest in herbal excipients arises from their environmental sustainability, biocompatibility, biodegradability, and low toxicity. Their incorporation into pharmaceutical compositions signifies a synthesis of traditional wisdom and contemporary science. Herbal excipients are categorized based on their functional role or botanical origin, each providing distinct benefits in medication administration and formulation design. The classification of herbal excipients is often based on their functional contributions to formulations. As illustrated in Figure 1.

Types: Binders, Diluents, Disintegrants, Thickeners, etc.

Herbal excipients can be classified according to their functional roles in medicinal formulations. These encompass binders, diluents, disintegrants, thickeners, emulsifiers, and stabilizers—each essential to the formulation's efficacy.

Binders augment the mechanical integrity of tablets by consolidating the powdered components. Examples encompass Acacia arabica (gum acacia), Tragacanth, and Aegle marmelos, which offer efficient binding properties, commendable compressibility, and biodegradability (Aklilu, 2002; Arshi, 2011).

Diluents, or fillers, are employed when active substances are present in minimal quantities and necessitate volumetric modification. Herbal powders, including maize starch, Glycyrrhiza glabra (licorice) root, and microcrystalline cellulose sourced from plant fibers, are frequently utilized.

Disintegrants are essential for the disintegration of solid dose forms within the gastrointestinal tract. Natural disintegrants, including Plantago ovata mucilage, Hibiscus esculentus extract, and Lepidium sativum seeds, enhance water absorption and swelling properties, facilitating pill disintegration.

Thickeners facilitate the attainment of the necessary viscosity in semi-solid or liquid compositions. Gums such as Sterculia urens (karaya), Boswellia serrata (frankincense), and Cassia tora are utilized to stabilize emulsions and suspensions (Prasad et al., 2023).

Figure 1. Classification of herbal excipients based on functional roles

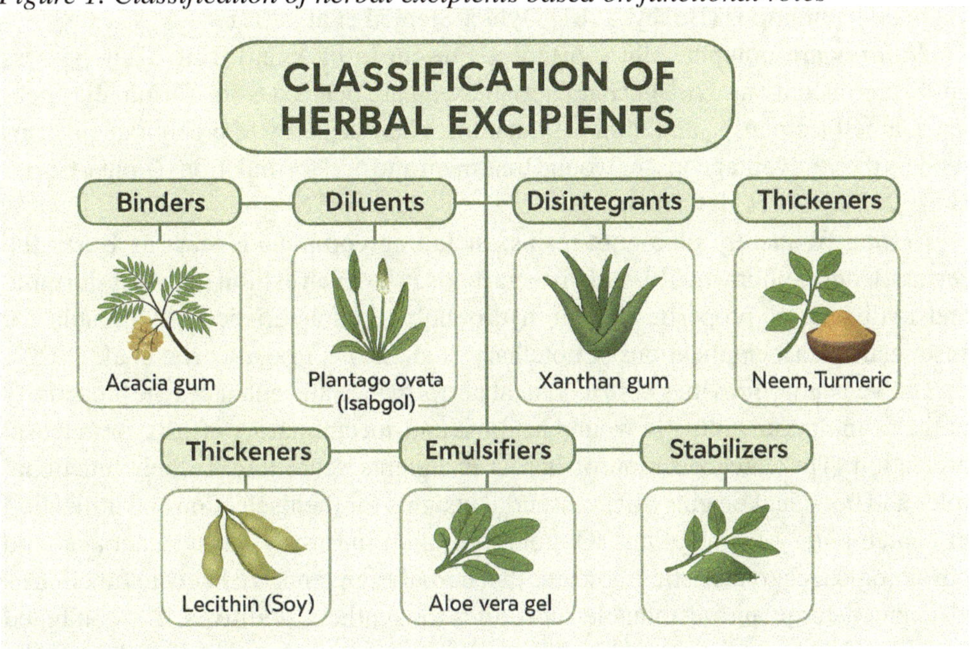

Emulsifiers such saponins derived from Quillaja saponaria maintain oil-water interfaces in topical and cosmetic formulations, providing a natural substitute for synthetic surfactants (Oleszek & Hamed, 2010).

By substituting synthetic additives, these functional herbal compounds provide therapeutic and biopharmaceutical advantages, hence improving the overall acceptability of herbal-based drug delivery systems.

Source-Based Classification: Gums, Mucilages, Tannins, Resins

Herbal excipients can be classified according to their origin or composition, encompassing gums, mucilages, tannins, and resins.

Gums are exudates rich in polysaccharides that are released in response to damage and exhibit high hydrophilicity. Acacia senegal (gum acacia), Astragalus gummifer (tragacanth), and Sterculia urens are frequently included in oral and topical preparations due to their swelling, emulsifying, and suspending characteristics (Mirhosseini & Amid, 2012; Hamman et al., 2015a).

Mucilages, generated intracellularly, expand upon exposure to water, resulting in gel formation. Mucilages from Plantago ovata, Hibiscus esculentus, and Cydonia oblonga (quince seeds) improve mucoadhesive characteristics in buccal, nasal, and vaginal formulations (Boney, 1981; Dybka-Stępień et al., 2021).

Tannins are polyphenolic substances present in bark and fruit. They possess antibacterial and antioxidant characteristics and are derived from Terminalia chebula, Camellia sinensis, and Punica granatum. Their capacity to precipitate proteins renders them advantageous for wound treatment and oral formulations (Fraga-Corral et al., 2021; Jain et al., 2014).

Resins, frequently oleo-gum-resins, including compounds such as Boswellia serrata, Commiphora mukul, and Pistacia lentiscus, which exhibit both film-forming and antibacterial properties. Their hydrophobic characteristics are suitable for sustained-release applications (Choudhary et al., 2014; Fraga-Corral et al., 2020).

Each category provides both technical performance and enhances the bioactivity of the formulation, aiding in wound healing, anti-inflammatory effects, or mucosal protection. The categorization of herbal excipients according to their functional roles and botanical origins offers essential insights for their selection and utilization in contemporary formulations. Ongoing research into their physicochemical and physiological characteristics indicates that herbal excipients are likely to function as efficient, natural, and sustainable substitutes for synthetic additives. The combined benefits of therapeutic synergy and formulation improvement position them at the leading edge of green pharmaceuticals and customized drug delivery systems.

ADVANTAGES OF HERBAL EXCIPIENTS

The rising desire for green and sustainable options in pharmaceutical formulation has positioned herbal excipients as formidable prospects, owing to their distinctive blend of functional, medicinal, and ecological advantages. These organically produced compounds, obtained from diverse plant components including seeds, bark, leaves, and roots, are progressively supplanting or augmenting synthetic excipients in contemporary drug delivery methods. Their benefits encompass various areas—extending from physiological compatibility to economic and environmental sustainability—rendering them a favored option for formulators and researchers.

Biocompatibility and Biodegradability

A notable advantage of herbal excipients is their superior biocompatibility, which denotes their capacity to cohabit with living tissues without provoking adverse immunological reactions or discomfort. These botanical materials exhibit chemical similarities to human biological molecules, facilitating enhanced absorption and integration with bodily systems (Mu et al., 2014). Mucilages from Plantago ovata and gums such as Acacia senegal exhibit enhanced compatibility in topical, oral, and parenteral drug delivery formulations (Biswas et al., 2020).

Moreover, these materials exhibit compatibility and are biodegradable, indicating they decompose through enzymatic or microbial processes into non-toxic byproducts. This characteristic guarantees that leftover excipients do not accumulate in the body or the environment, hence minimizing long-term negative effects and ecological consequences (Pifferi & Restani, 2003). Tragacanth and Guar gum undergo complete degradation under physiological conditions, rendering them especially advantageous for controlled-release systems for mucoadhesive drug delivery (Bayer, 2023).

This dual attribute—biocompatibility and biodegradability—corresponds effectively with global efforts in green pharmacy and sustainability-oriented research in pharmaceutics.

Cost-Effectiveness and Local Availability

Herbal excipients are typically more economical than synthetic counterparts because of their natural availability and simplicity of production, especially in agricultural economies such as India, China, and many African countries. These materials frequently necessitate minimal chemical processing, thereby substantially decreasing production and purifying expenses (*Nazemi et al., 2023*). Cassia tora, Tamarind seed polysaccharides, and Aloe vera gel are extensively cultivated and collected economically in tropical and subtropical climates.

Furthermore, the local availability of these excipients diminishes the necessity for extensive transportation and importation of synthetic agents, hence enhancing cost efficiency and supply chain stability. The dependence on indigenous herbal excipients fosters rural employment and the development of local herbal economies, hence enhancing economic upliftment and self-sufficiency (Karkare et al., 2022). Formulators in resource-constrained environments have particularly profited from utilizing locally sourced gums, mucilages, and resins, which satisfy functional needs such as binding, emulsifying, and thickening at a significantly lower cost than synthetic alternatives (Prasad et al., 2022).

Low Toxicity and Minimal Side Effects

Herbal excipients typically have low toxicity, a characteristic that has been substantiated throughout centuries of traditional application in diverse herbal and Ayurvedic formulations. In contrast to certain synthetic excipients that can induce hypersensitivity, irritation, or organ-specific toxicity with prolonged use, the majority of herbal compounds remain non-toxic at therapeutic dosages (Rousseaux, 2023).

For example, Boswellia resin, Neem gum, and Okra mucilage have exhibited safety in both topical and oral uses (Malabadi et al., 2021).

These drugs typically exhibit low adverse effects, rendering them appropriate for sensitive demographics, including children, elderly individuals, and people with impaired immune systems (Davies & O'mahony, 2015). Natural excipients frequently exhibit supplementary pharmacological properties, including antibacterial, anti-inflammatory, or antioxidant actions, hence diminishing the necessity for additional additions in formulations (Braithwaite et al., 2014).

Furthermore, herbal excipients typically demonstrate reduced systemic absorption, thereby diminishing the risk of toxicity associated with buildup. For instance, gums such as Acacia arabica and mucilages from Hibiscus esculentus predominantly function locally inside the gastrointestinal system and are excreted without metabolic alteration (Alamgir & Alamgir, 2018).

Their multifunctionality—as both excipients and therapeutic agents—improves formulation efficiency and diminishes the likelihood of unpleasant reactions typically associated with synthetic additions like sodium lauryl sulphate, polyethylene glycol, or parabens (Pockle et al., 2023).

Herbal excipients provide multiple benefits that correspond with the fundamental tenets of sustainable, safe, and patient-focused pharmaceuticals. Their biocompatibility enhances patient tolerance, but biodegradability reduces environmental impact. They are economically feasible because to local availability and reduced processing requirements, particularly in underdeveloped nations. Most importantly, they provide a high safety profile, characterized by low toxicity and little side effects, hence facilitating their broad acceptance in both traditional and alternative medical systems.

As research advances into the structural, functional, and therapeutic properties of these plant-derived materials, herbal excipients are set to transform pharmaceutical formulation science. The incorporation of these natural components satisfies technological specifications and corresponds with global trends in green pharmacy, personalized medicine, and sustainable healthcare solutions.

BIOACTIVE POLYMERS: PROPERTIES AND APPLICATIONS

Bioactive polymers, whether sourced from natural origins or synthesized with biocompatible characteristics, are essential in contemporary pharmaceutical and biomedical sciences. These polymers function as structural elements and actively contribute to therapeutic results by interacting with biological tissues, assisting in regulated medication release, enhancing healing, and promoting tissue regeneration. Bioactive polymers are appealing due to their multifunctionality, tunability, and capacity to combine with diverse delivery systems. Due to the growing interest in biomaterials and natural treatments, bioactive polymers, particularly those derived from herbal or semi-synthetic sources, are being thoroughly investigated for their use in drug delivery, wound healing, and tissue engineering (Bhatia & Bhatia, 2016).

Characteristics of Ideal Bioactive Polymers

An efficient bioactive polymer must exhibit a synthesis of mechanical, chemical, and biological properties to guarantee its efficacy in various biomedical applications.

Mucoadhesion

Mucoadhesive polymers prolong the retention of medicines at mucosal locations, resulting in enhanced bioavailability and targeted pharmacological action. This attribute is particularly advantageous in oral, buccal, nasal, and vaginal drug delivery systems (Shaikh et al., 2011). Polymers like chitosan, carbopol, and sodium alginate have significant mucoadhesion owing to their ionic and hydrogen-bonding capabilities, facilitating extended interaction with mucin layers (Cazorla-Luna et al., 2021).

Mechanical Integrity and Elasticity

Mechanical robustness is essential for the structural integrity of dosage forms, including films, patches, and scaffolds. Polymers such as polyvinyl alcohol (PVA) and gelatin offer superior flexibility and tensile strength, essential for patient adherence and application to dynamic anatomical regions (Zulkiflee & Fauzi, 2021). Combining various polymers enables the tailoring of mechanical properties for particular purposes; for example, the integration of gelatin with PVA enhances elasticity while preserving biocompatibility (Mushtaq et al., 2022).

Film-Forming Capability

The capacity to form a film is essential for topical medication delivery systems, particularly in wound dressings and transdermal patches. Polymers like cellulose derivatives (e.g., hydroxypropyl methylcellulose or HPMC), pectin, and gelatin provide translucent, permeable, and consistent films capable of encapsulating active medicinal components (*Boateng et al., 2008*). These films serve as physical barriers, safeguarding wounds from microbial invasion and regulating moisture loss, so expediting wound healing.

Role in Drug Delivery, Wound Healing, and Tissue Engineering

Drug Delivery

Bioactive polymers have revolutionized medicine delivery by facilitating continuous release, precise targeting, and safeguarding of sensitive pharmaceuticals. Polymers such as alginate and chitosan create hydrogels that encapsulate medicines and facilitate their regulated release over time, enhancing therapeutic efficacy and minimizing dose frequency (El-Tanani et al., 2025). In oral formulations, these polymers can evade enzymatic breakdown and regulate gastrointestinal transit time, facilitating site-specific administration (Brown et al., 2020).

Nanoparticles composed of PLGA (poly lactic-co-glycolic acid), PCL (polycaprolactone), or chitosan are progressively utilized for targeted cancer therapy, as they can be engineered with ligands that attach to tumor-specific receptors (Al-Sahlawi et al., 2024). The mucoadhesive properties of many herbal polymers improve the administration of poorly soluble or unstable medicines by concentrating them at the absorption site. Figure 2 highlights major application areas of herbal-polymer composites

Figure 2. Applications of herbal-polymer composite systems in wound healing, transdermal delivery, and tissue engineering

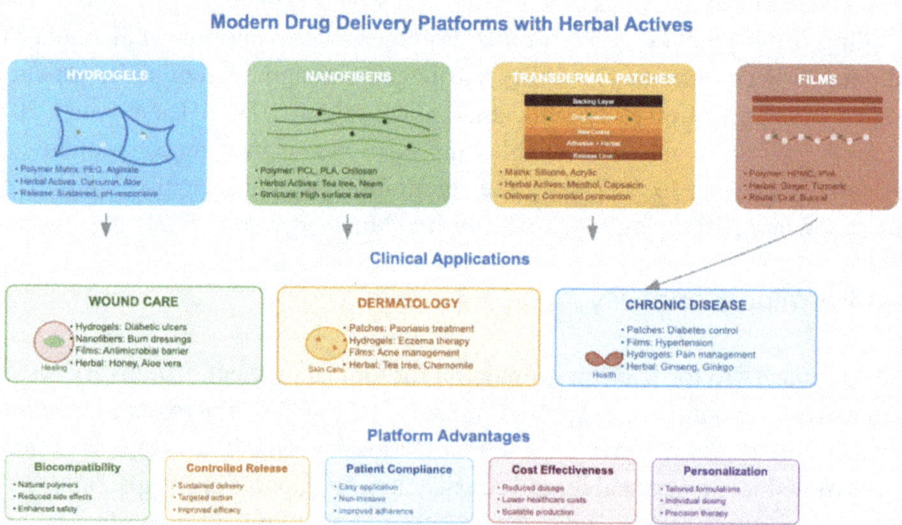

Wound Healing

In wound care, bioactive polymers function as hemostatic agents, moisture regulators, and medicament transporters. Chitosan-based dressings enhance wound healing by facilitating macrophage activation, collagen deposition, and exhibiting antibacterial properties (Liu et al., 2018). Alginate, extracted from brown seaweed, absorbs exudate and creates a gel that preserves a moist wound environment, essential for epithelialization (Alrata et al., 2024).

Gelatin and collagen scaffolds infused with herbal extracts (such as curcumin, neem, or aloe vera) provide synergistic therapeutic effects, merging the regeneration qualities of biopolymers with the anti-inflammatory and antioxidant attributes of phytochemicals (Soni et al., 2023). These formulations exemplify the integration of natural and synthetic components for sophisticated wound care.

Tissue Engineering

In regenerative medicine, bioactive polymers are constructed into three-dimensional scaffolds that replicate the extracellular matrix, facilitating cell adhesion, proliferation, and differentiation. Gelatin, collagen, cellulose acetate, and polycaprolactone are extensively utilized in the engineering of skin, bone, cartilage, and neural tissues (Iovene et al., 2021).

Recent advancements entail the integration of herbal bioactives with polymers to build composite scaffolds that administer growth hormones, regulate inflammation, and expedite tissue regeneration. Chitosan-collagen scaffolds infused with turmeric or neem extracts have exhibited enhanced cell viability and accelerated wound closure in animal models (Pramanik et al., 2024).

Key Examples of Bioactive Polymers

Chitosan

Chitosan, derived from chitin (found in crustacean shells), is a biodegradable, mucoadhesive polymer with intrinsic antimicrobial and hemostatic properties. It has been employed in drug-loaded films, hydrogels, and nanoparticles for diverse applications, including wound dressings and gene delivery (Sharma et al., 2022).

Alginate

Alginate is an anionic polysaccharide obtained from brown algae, notable for its gel-forming ability in the presence of divalent cations like calcium. It is widely used in controlled release, wound care, and encapsulation technologies due to its mild gelling conditions and high biocompatibility (Abka-Khajouei et al., 2022).

Polyvinyl Alcohol (PVA)

A synthetic polymer with excellent mechanical strength and film-forming capacity, PVA is often blended with natural polymers to improve elasticity and hydration properties. Its non-toxic and flexible nature makes it suitable for hydrogels, contact lenses, and drug patches (*Teodorescu et al., 2018*).

Gelatin

It is extensively used in tissue engineering and as a carrier for herbal and synthetic drugs in hydrogels and microparticles (Gorgieva & Kokol, 2011).

Cellulose Derivatives

Hydroxypropyl methylcellulose (HPMC), methylcellulose, and carboxymethyl cellulose are widely used due to their viscosity-modifying, emulsifying, and stabilizing properties. These polymers are central to oral and topical dosage forms, offering hydration control and film integrity (*Yin et al., 2023*).

Bioactive polymers have become indispensable in pharmaceutical formulation, offering a versatile platform for designing advanced drug delivery systems, wound dressings, and tissue engineering scaffolds. Their properties—mucoadhesion, mechanical resilience, and film-forming ability—enable targeted, controlled, and effective therapy. Polymers such as chitosan, alginate, PVA, and gelatin exemplify the bridge between functional excipients and therapeutic agents, especially when integrated with herbal actives. As interdisciplinary innovations grow, the fusion of polymer science with herbal pharmaceutics offers immense promise in creating smart, biocompatible, and eco-friendly healthcare solutions.

SYNERGISTIC ROLE OF HERBAL EXCIPIENTS AND POLYMERS

The combined collection of herbal excipients with natural and synthetic polymers has unveiled new possibilities in pharmaceutical composition. Herbal excipients such gums, mucilages, and tannins possess bioactive characteristics and biocompatibility, whereas polymers, particularly biodegradable and bioactive types, ensure structural integrity and controlled drug release. Their amalgamation yields synergistic effects that augment the stability, bioavailability, and therapeutic efficacy of medicinal dosage forms. This combination enhances pharmacological advantages and facilitates the development of regulated drug delivery systems, thereby minimizing toxicity and enhancing patient adherence (Veerapandian et al., 2023). The integration of herbal excipients with bioactive polymers like chitosan, alginate, and PVA is paving the way for multifunctional drug delivery systems, as conceptually represented in Figure 3.

Improved Drug Stability and Bioavailability

A major difficulty in formulation science is maintaining the stability of labile pharmaceuticals and improving the bioavailability of poorly soluble substances. Herbal excipients such mucilage from Plantago ovata, guar gum, and acacia possess intrinsic stabilizing qualities attributed to their polysaccharide composition, which creates protective colloidal structures (Bhosale et al., 2014). When combined with polymers like chitosan, polyvinyl alcohol (PVA), or HPMC, the resulting matrix protects the medication from environmental degradation, including pH fluctuations, enzymatic activity, or oxidative stress (Ciolacu et al., 2020).

Furthermore, the improvement of bioavailability has been noted when mucoadhesive polymers, such as chitosan, are utilized in conjunction with herbal stabilizers. The mucoadhesion extends residence time at absorption sites, while herbal gums create protective coatings that inhibit early drug breakdown (Mansuri et al., 2016). Combining chitosan with okra mucilage has demonstrated improved absorption for anti-inflammatory medications due to increased mucosal permeability (Noreen et al., 2022).

Sustained and Controlled Release Systems

Regulated and prolonged medication release is crucial for decreasing dose frequency, mitigating side effects, and ensuring stable therapeutic concentrations. The utilization of herbal excipients as rate-controlling agents in polymeric matrices is attracting interest because of their swelling, gelling, and erosion properties. Xanthan gum, a microbial gum derived from plants, is frequently utilized in conjunction with carbopol or HPMC to formulate dual-phase release profiles—characterized by an initial burst release followed by sustained delivery. (Zhou et al., 2022).

Research indicates that resin-based herbal excipients, such as boswellic acid resin, can be integrated with biodegradable polymers to make microspheres or nanoparticles exhibiting sustained release properties. These methods provide targeted administration, particularly in colon-specific formulations, by withstanding degradation in the upper gastrointestinal tract and releasing active components exclusively upon arrival in the colon (Yadav et al., 2016). Furthermore, polysaccharides such as pectin and guar gum, when integrated with polymers like Eudragit, create pH-sensitive delivery systems that guarantee drug release exclusively in designated settings. This method is especially advantageous for colon-targeted therapies and anti-inflammatory compositions (Singh & Nayak, 2023a).

Figure 3. Integration of herbal excipients and bioactive polymers for advanced drug delivery systems

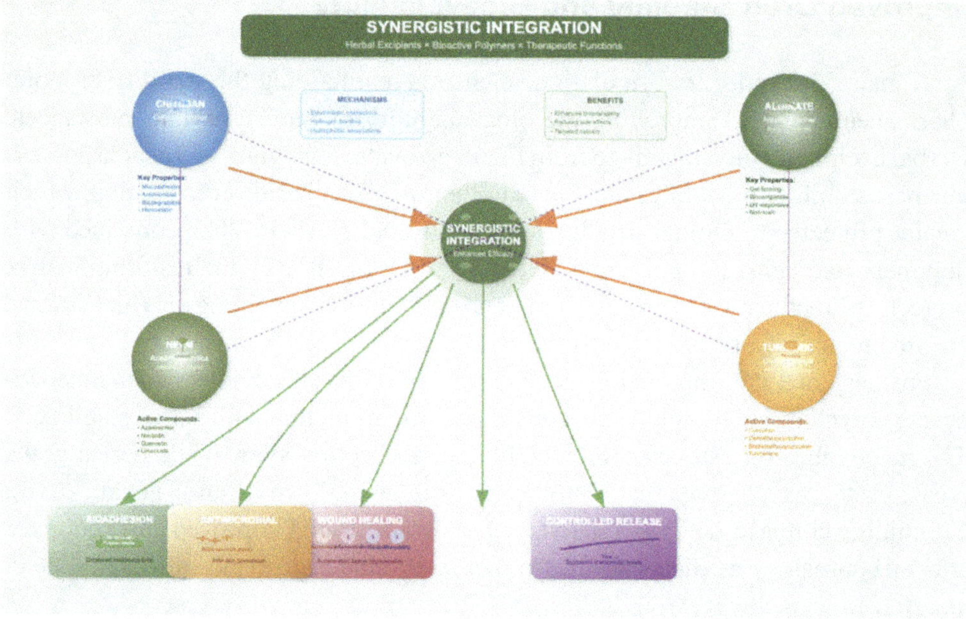

Enhanced Antimicrobial and Antioxidant Activities

The use of herbal excipients into polymeric systems might augment the antibacterial and antioxidant properties of formulations, particularly beneficial in wound dressings, ophthalmic solutions, and topical gels. Numerous herbal excipients, such as neem gum, turmeric extract, and acacia, exhibit inherent antibacterial properties. When encapsulated or combined with biocompatible polymers, their efficacy is augmented by sustained release and improved penetration (Muruganantham et al., 2022). Chitosan, recognized for its antimicrobial and film-forming characteristics, when integrated with curcumin-loaded herbal excipients, can provide an antibacterial wound dressing with significant therapeutic potential (Vinchhi et al., 2024). This combination facilitates extended efficacy against microbial biofilms and establishes a physical barrier to infection.

Gelatin-alginate films infused with green tea polyphenols or tannins exhibit notable free radical scavenging ability and antibacterial properties. These films are particularly advantageous in biomedical applications that need the simultaneous reduction of oxidative stress and infection risk (Vilchez et al., 2020). Furthermore, nanofibrous scaffolds using plant extracts and polymeric carriers are being engineered for tissue regeneration, leveraging their dual functions of antioxidant properties and structural support (Do et al., 2022).

Mechanistic Insight: Why the Synergy Works

The synergistic interaction between herbal excipients and polymers results from their complimentary characteristics:

- The hydrophilic characteristics of numerous herbal excipients promote polymer swelling and diffusion-mediated release.
- The presence of chemical functionalities (hydroxyl, carboxyl, and amino groups) in both components facilitates robust hydrogen bonding, leading to enhanced encapsulation efficiency.
- The bioactivity of herbal compounds provides pharmacological effects, whereas polymers give mechanical and physicochemical regulation (Srivastava & Misra, 2018).

These combinations result in multifunctional delivery systems that provide physical support, modulate medication release, and enhance therapy through intrinsic bioactivity.

The synergistic integration of herbal excipients with natural or synthetic polymers represents a novel and promising approach in contemporary pharmaceutics. Collectively, they provide a robust arsenal for the creation of stable, bioavailable, and versatile drug delivery systems. Their integration facilitates advancements in sustained-release platforms, bioadhesive formulations, and therapeutic scaffolds, rendering them essential in both traditional and innovative dosage forms. Future study must investigate standardized methodologies, mechanistic modeling, and clinical trials to fully harness the promise of these synergistic systems and integrate traditional herbal knowledge with advanced pharmaceutical technologies.

CHALLENGES AND REGULATORY ASPECTS

The integration of herbal excipients and polymers in pharmaceutical formulations offers many therapeutic benefits. This integration presents obstacles. Challenges concerning standardization, quality assurance, polymer compatibility, and regulatory frameworks frequently obstruct the extensive development and acceptance of these systems. Comprehending these issues is crucial for converting laboratory-scale ideas into clinically and economically viable solutions.

Standardization and Quality Control of Herbal Raw Materials

A primary hurdle in developing herbal-polymer drug delivery systems is the standardization of herbal raw materials. Herbal excipients, like natural compounds, demonstrate batch-to-batch variability attributable to variations in plant species, geographical origin, harvesting time, drying methods, and storage conditions (Steinhoff, 2021). This heterogeneity might affect essential physicochemical parameters such as viscosity, swelling index, solubility, and bioactivity, which are vital for formulation efficacy.

In contrast to synthetic excipients produced under regulated settings with clearly defined chemical profiles, herbal excipients are susceptible to adulteration, contamination, and variable phytochemical composition (Alengebawy et al., 2021). Gum acacia obtained from various regions may exhibit varying molecular weights and gelling properties, influencing medication release profiles in matrix tablets.

Standardization necessitates the application of rigorous analytical methodologies, including HPLC, FTIR, and NMR, in conjunction with approved pharmacognostic criteria. Furthermore, microbiological load testing, pesticide residue analysis, and heavy metal evaluation are essential to guarantee safety and efficacy (Alves et al., 2020). The absence of globally recognized pharmacopoeial standards for the majority of herbal excipients intensifies the problem, necessitating global regulatory harmonization.

Compatibility with Synthetic Polymers

A further technological barrier in the development of hybrid formulations is the physicochemical compatibility between herbal excipients and synthetic or semi-synthetic polymers. Incompatibility can present as precipitation, phase separation, diminished bioactivity, or instability during processing or storage (Ćirić et al., 2020).

Polymers such as polyvinyl alcohol (PVA), carbopol, or Eudragit may adversely interact with herbal constituents because to variations in pH sensitivity, solubility, or ionic characteristics. Tannin-rich herbal excipients may create insoluble complexes with basic polymers, influencing drug release dynamics and formulation stability (Bagade & Doke, 2023). To resolve compatibility difficulties, researchers must perform preformulation experiments utilizing Fourier Transform Infrared Spectroscopy (FTIR), Differential Scanning Calorimetry (DSC), and X-ray diffraction (XRD) to evaluate probable chemical interactions. The inclusion of plasticizers, co-polymers, or surface modifiers may alleviate incompatibility; however, this complicates the formulation and elevates costs.

Moreover, thermal and mechanical processing methods (such as hot-melt extrusion and freeze-drying) may compromise heat-sensitive herbal constituents unless meticulously calibrated. Achieving a balance between the mechanical properties of polymers and thermolabile phytochemicals is a significant formulation challenge (Thakkar et al., 2020).

Regulatory Hurdles in Herbal-Polymer Formulations

The regulatory framework for herbal-polymer combinations is intricate due to the dual classification of these formulations as pharmaceuticals, nutraceuticals, or herbal medicines, contingent upon their constituents, intended use, and jurisdiction (Vandghanooni et al., 2025). Regulatory bodies such as the FDA (USA), EMA (Europe), and AYUSH (India) possess divergent criteria for herbal products and excipients, frequently lacking comprehensive frameworks for their amalgamation with synthetic polymers.

For example, although synthetic polymers such as HPMC or PEG are designated as GRAS (Generally Recognized as Safe), the incorporation of a non-standardized herbal excipient may modify the regulatory classification and need toxicological data, clinical safety investigations, and new drug applications (NDAs) (Jangid & Sharma, 2025). This incurs substantial expenses and delays in product development. Moreover, the labeling standards, product claims, and evidence of efficacy for herbal-polymer medication systems are often inadequately delineated, resulting in ambiguity and regulatory opposition. The absence of monographs for numerous herbal excipients in official compendia further restricts their acceptability.

Intellectual Property (IP) concerns further complicate the situation. Synthetic polymer compositions can be patented based on their structure and technique; however, herbal-based inventions may encounter obstacles due to the conventional knowledge clause in patent law, unless uniqueness and inventiveness are clearly demonstrated (Volenzo & Odiyo, 2020).

Sustainability, Ethics, and Consumer Perception

A developing concern is the ethical procurement and sustainability of herbal raw resources. Overharvesting, habitat degradation, and inadequate fair-trade standards can compromise the perceived ecological sustainability of herbal compositions (Ogaji et al., 2012). Furthermore, consumer distrust regarding the scientific validity of herbal formulations endures, particularly in controlled markets. Herbal excipients sourced from endangered or unsustainable origins may also face regulatory examination. Certification in accordance with WHO-GACP (Good Agricultural and Collection Practices) or organic labels is increasingly vital for market acceptance and customer confidence.

The collaboration between herbal excipients and polymers presents significant potential in medication delivery, although numerous scientific and regulatory obstacles must be addressed. The standardization of herbal ingredients, establishing compatibility with synthetic polymers, and navigating intricate regulatory frameworks are essential elements for successful formulation and commercialization. Confronting these difficulties necessitates interdisciplinary collaboration among pharmaceutical scientists, herbal specialists, regulatory authorities, and industrial stakeholders. With the rising global demand for natural and sustainable therapies, it is essential to establish cohesive norms and evidence-based frameworks that promote innovation while guaranteeing safety, efficacy, and quality.

RECENT ADVANCES AND EMERGING TRENDS

The amalgamation of herbal excipients with sophisticated polymeric systems has precipitated considerable advancements in medication delivery. Recent advancements include intelligent polymeric systems that respond to phytochemical stimuli, 3D-printed drug delivery systems employing herbal matrices, and the use of artificial intelligence (AI) to forecast polymer-herb interactions. These developments seek to improve therapeutic efficacy, customization, and safety in pharmaceutical formulations (Zhang et al., 2019).

Smart Polymeric Systems with Phytochemical Triggers

Smart polymers, or stimulus-responsive polymers, can undergo physical or chemical transformations in reaction to certain environmental stimuli, like pH, temperature, or the presence of particular biomolecules (Brazel, 2009). Utilizing phytochemicals as activators in these systems presents an innovative method for targeted and regulated medication release.

pH-responsive polymers can be engineered to release pharmaceuticals in the acidic milieu of tumor tissues or inflamed regions. Phytochemicals such as tannic acid, recognized for their pH-sensitive characteristics, can be included into polymer matrices to facilitate site-specific drug delivery (Ofridam et al., 2021). Likewise, temperature-sensitive polymers integrated with thermogenic herbal extracts can provide regulated medication release in reaction to localized hyperthermia (Su et al., 2022).

Furthermore, enzymatically sensitive polymers that decompose in the presence of specific enzymes can be customized utilizing botanical constituents that influence enzymatic activity. This technique guarantees that the medicine is released exclusively under specific biological conditions, hence improving treatment accuracy and reducing systemic adverse effects (Fatimi et al., 2022).

3D-Printed Drug Delivery Systems Using Herbal Matrices

Three-dimensional (3D) printing technology has transformed the production of customized medicine delivery devices. The use of herbal matrices in 3D printing provides biocompatibility, biodegradability, and the integration of therapeutic characteristics intrinsic to natural products (Latos-Brozio et al., 2022).

Natural polymers, including alginate, gelatin, and cellulose derivatives obtained from botanical sources, function as superior bioinks for 3D printing. These materials can be designed to form intricate structures with regulated porosity and mechanical strength, appropriate for diverse drug delivery applications (Metwally et al., 2023).

For instance, 3D-printed scaffolds infused with herbal extracts have been created for wound healing purposes, offering both structural reinforcement and antibacterial properties (Serrano et al., 2023a). Moreover, customized oral dosage forms using herbal excipients can be developed to address specific patient requirements, enhancing adherence and therapeutic results.

The adaptability of 3D printing facilitates the incorporation of many medications and excipients into a singular dosage form, permitting combination therapies and intricate release profiles. This methodology corresponds with the increasing demand for individualized therapy and the application of natural goods in healthcare (Vaz & Kumar, 2021).

AI-Based Prediction of Polymer-Herb Interaction

The intricate interactions between polymers and herbal excipients require sophisticated technologies for prediction and optimization. Artificial intelligence (AI) and machine learning (ML) algorithms have become formidable instruments in modeling and forecasting these interactions, enabling the development of efficient and secure medication delivery systems (*Ali et al., 2024*). AI models can examine extensive datasets to discern patterns and forecast the physicochemical compatibility of particular polymers and herbal constituents. This predictive ability facilitates the selection of suitable combinations that guarantee stability, efficacy, and controlled drug release.

Moreover, AI-driven simulations can predict the behavior of polymer-herb systems across many physiological circumstances, thereby diminishing the dependence on large experimental trials (Gholap et al., 2024). This expedites the development process and improves the accuracy of formulation design. The incorporation of AI in this field facilitates the detection of any harmful interactions, hence enhancing the safety evaluation of new formulations. As AI technologies advance, their utilization in forecasting polymer-herb interactions will become more refined, fostering innovation in pharmaceutical creation.

The integration of herbal excipients with sophisticated polymeric technologies, such as smart polymers, 3D printing, and AI-driven modeling, signifies a substantial advancement in drug delivery systems. These developing trends have the promise for highly individualized, efficient, and secure treatment solutions. Ongoing multidisciplinary research and collaboration are crucial to fully harness the advantages of these advances and to tackle the problems related to their deployment in clinical environments.

CONCLUSION

Together and separately, herbal excipients and polymers alter pharmaceutical and biomedical formulation creation. Herbal excipients help create safer, more effective healthcare products due to their biodegradability, healing properties, and natural origin. Natural and manmade polymers provide structural integrity, controlled release, and site-specific delivery. Combining these two materials allows scientists to create practical, eco-friendly, and patient-compliant hybrid systems. These combinations are promising in wound healing, medication delivery, and tissue engineering. Lack of standardization, compatibility limitations, and regulatory concerns prevent large-scale deployment despite the benefits. Herbal active molecular characterisation, polymer-herb compatibility studies, AI-guided formulation design, and industry-academia translational research should be prioritized. Innovation in herbal wisdom and polymer technology could change therapeutic delivery systems, providing tailored, sustainable, and high-performance solutions in modern medicine.

REFERENCES

Abka-Khajouei, R., Tounsi, L., Shahabi, N., Patel, A. K., Abdelkafi, S., & Michaud, P. (2022). Structures, properties and applications of alginates. *Marine Drugs*, *20*(6), 364. PMID: 35736167

Aklilu, T. E. G. E. G. N. E. (2002). *Evaluation of Local Gum of Acacia Polyacantha as a Binder in Tablet Formulations*. AAU Institutional Repository.

. Al-Sahlawi, F., Alabdali, A. Y. M., Chinnappan, S., Al-Samydai, A., & Maki, M. A. A. (2024). Polymer-based nanoparticles in targeted cancer therapy: a review. *Journal of Applied Pharmaceutical Science, 14*(9), 057-068.

. Alamgir, A. N. M., & Alamgir, A. N. M. (2018). Secondary metabolites: Secondary metabolic products consisting of C and H; C, H, and O; N, S, and P elements; and O/N heterocycles. *Therapeutic use of medicinal plants and their extracts: volume 2: phytochemistry and bioactive compounds*, 165-309.

Alengebawy, A., Abdelkhalek, S. T., Qureshi, S. R., & Wang, M. Q. (2021). Heavy metals and pesticides toxicity in agricultural soil and plants: Ecological risks and human health implications. *Toxics*, *9*(3), 42. PMID: 33668829

Ali, K. A., Mohin, S. K., Mondal, P., Goswami, S., Ghosh, S., & Choudhuri, S. (2024). Influence of artificial intelligence in modern pharmaceutical formulation and drug development. *Future Journal of Pharmaceutical Sciences*, *10*(1), 53.

Alrata, L., Abdulsattar, D., Madrigal, S., Pyeatte, S. R., Zaghloul, M., Abu-Amer, W., & Zayed, M. A. (2024). Alginate Formulation for Wound Healing Applications. *Advances in Wound Care*. PMID: 39531216

Alves, T. F., Morsink, M., Batain, F., Chaud, M. V., Almeida, T., Fernandes, D. A., & Severino, P. (2020). Applications of natural, semi-synthetic, and synthetic polymers in cosmetic formulations. *Cosmetics*, *7*(4), 75.

Arshi, A. (2011). *Formulation and evaluation of tablets using natural gum as a binder* (Master's thesis, Rajiv Gandhi University of Health Sciences (India)).

Bagade, O., & Doke, P. (2023). Lipid and Polymer Based Nano-Phytotherapeutics. *Nanofabrication*, *8*(1), 1–33.

Bayer, I. S. (2023). Controlled drug release from nanoengineered polysaccharides. *Pharmaceutics*, *15*(5), 1364. PMID: 37242606

. Bhatia, S., & Bhatia, S. (2016). Natural polymers vs synthetic polymer. *Natural polymer drug delivery systems: nanoparticles, plants, and algae*, 95-118.

Bhosale, R. R., Osmani, R. A. M., & Moin, A. (2014). Natural gums and mucilages: A review on multifaceted excipients in pharmaceutical science and research. *International Journal of Pharmacognosy and Phytochemical Research*, *15*(6), 4.

. Biswas, D., Das, S., MOHANTO, S., & MANTRY, S. (2020). Extraction, modification, and characterization of natural polymers used in transdermal drug delivery system: an updated review. *EXTRACTION, 13*(7).

Boateng, J. S., Matthews, K. H., Stevens, H. N., & Eccleston, G. M. (2008). Wound healing dressings and drug delivery systems: A review. *Journal of Pharmaceutical Sciences*, *97*(8), 2892–2923. PMID: 17963217

Boney, A. D. (1981). Mucilage: The ubiquitous algal attribute. *British Phycological Journal*, *16*(2), 115–132.

Braithwaite, M. C., Tyagi, C., Tomar, L. K., Kumar, P., Choonara, Y. E., & Pillay, V. (2014). Nutraceutical-based therapeutics and formulation strategies augmenting their efficiency to complement modern medicine: An overview. *Journal of Functional Foods*, *6*, 82–99.

Brazel, C. S. (2009). Magnetothermally-responsive nanomaterials: Combining magnetic nanostructures and thermally-sensitive polymers for triggered drug release. *Pharmaceutical Research*, *26*, 644–656. PMID: 19005741

Brown, T. D., Whitehead, K. A., & Mitragotri, S. (2020). Materials for oral delivery of proteins and peptides. *Nature Reviews. Materials*, *5*(2), 127–148.

Cazorla-Luna, R., Martín-Illana, A., Notario-Pérez, F., Ruiz-Caro, R., & Veiga, M. D. (2021). Naturally occurring polyelectrolytes and their use for the development of complex-based mucoadhesive drug delivery systems: An overview. *Polymers*, *13*(14), 2241. PMID: 34301004

Chaudhari, S. P., & Patil, P. S. (2012). Pharmaceutical excipients: A review. *Int J Adv Pharm Biol Chem*, *1*(1), 21–34.

Chavda, V. P., Patel, A. B., Mistry, K. J., Suthar, S. F., Wu, Z. X., Chen, Z. S., & Hou, K. (2022). Nano-drug delivery systems entrapping natural bioactive compounds for cancer: Recent progress and future challenges. *Frontiers in Oncology*, *12*, 867655. PMID: 35425710

Choudhary, P. D., & Pawar, H. A. (2014). Recently investigated natural gums and mucilages as pharmaceutical excipients: An overview. *Journal of Pharmaceutics*, *2014*(1), 204849. PMID: 26556189

Ciolacu, D. E., Nicu, R., & Ciolacu, F. (2020). Cellulose-based hydrogels as sustained drug-delivery systems. *Materials (Basel), 13*(22), 5270. PMID: 33233413

Ćirić, A., Krajišnik, D., Čalija, B., & Đekić, L. (2020). Biocompatible non-covalent complexes of chitosan and different polymers: Characteristics and application in drug delivery. *Arhiv za Farmaciju, 70*(4), 173–197.

Dave, V. S., Saoji, S. D., Raut, N. A., & Haware, R. V. (2015). Excipient variability and its impact on dosage form functionality. *Journal of Pharmaceutical Sciences, 104*(3), 906–915. PMID: 25561249

Davies, E. A., & O'mahony, M. S. (2015). Adverse drug reactions in special populations–the elderly. *British Journal of Clinical Pharmacology, 80*(4), 796–807. PMID: 25619317

Do, N. H., Truong, Q. T., Le, P. K., & Ha, A. C. (2022). Recent developments in chitosan hydrogels carrying natural bioactive compounds. *Carbohydrate Polymers, 294*, 119726. PMID: 35868739

Dybka-Stępień, K., Otlewska, A., Góźdź, P., & Piotrowska, M. (2021). The renaissance of plant mucilage in health promotion and industrial applications: A review. *Nutrients, 13*(10), 3354. PMID: 34684354

El-Tanani, M., Satyam, S. M., Rabbani, S. A., El-Tanani, Y., Aljabali, A. A., Al Faouri, I., & Rehman, A. (2025). Revolutionizing Drug Delivery: The Impact of Advanced Materials Science and Technology on Precision Medicine. *Pharmaceutics, 17*(3), 375. PMID: 40143038

Fatimi, A., Okoro, O. V., Podstawczyk, D., Siminska-Stanny, J., & Shavandi, A. (2022). Natural hydrogel-based bio-inks for 3D bioprinting in tissue engineering: A review. *Gels (Basel, Switzerland), 8*(3), 179. PMID: 35323292

Feng, M., Dai, X., Yang, C., Zhang, Y., Tian, Y., Qu, Q., & Shi, X. (2023). Unification of medicines and excipients: The roles of natural excipients for promoting drug delivery. *Expert Opinion on Drug Delivery, 20*(5), 597–620. PMID: 37150753

Fraga-Corral, M., García-Oliveira, P., Pereira, A. G., Lourenço-Lopes, C., Jimenez-Lopez, C., Prieto, M. A., & Simal-Gandara, J. (2020). Technological application of tannin-based extracts. *Molecules (Basel, Switzerland), 25*(3), 614. PMID: 32019231

Fraga-Corral, M., Otero, P., Cassani, L., Echave, J., Garcia-Oliveira, P., Carpena, M., & Simal-Gandara, J. (2021). Traditional applications of tannin rich extracts supported by scientific data: Chemical composition, bioavailability and bioaccessibility. *Foods, 10*(2), 251. PMID: 33530516

Gholap, A. D., Uddin, M. J., Faiyazuddin, M., Omri, A., Gowri, S., & Khalid, M. (2024). Advances in artificial intelligence in drug delivery and development: A comprehensive review. *Computers in Biology and Medicine*, •••, 108702. PMID: 38878397

. Gorgieva, S., & Kokol, V. (2011). Collagen-vs. gelatine-based biomaterials and their biocompatibility: review and perspectives. *Biomaterials applications for nanomedicine, 2*(2011), 17-52.

Hamman, H., Steenekamp, J., & Hamman, J. (2015). Use of natural gums and mucilages as pharmaceutical excipients. *Current Pharmaceutical Design*, *21*(33), 4775–4797. PMID: 26290212

Iovene, A., Zhao, Y., Wang, S., & Amoako, K. (2021). Bioactive polymeric materials for the advancement of regenerative medicine. *Journal of Functional Biomaterials*, *12*(1), 14. PMID: 33672492

Jain, A., Radiya, P., Wadekar, R., Limaye, S., & Pawar, C. (2014). Natural excipients-an alternative to synthetic excipients: A comprehensive review. *International Journal of Pharmaceutical and Medicinal Research*, 2(4), 123–127.

Jangid, A. K., & Sharma, S. (2025). Overview of Herbal Nanoparticles: A Patent Review. *Current Nanomedicine*.

Karkare, P., Odijie, M. E., Ukaoha, K., & van Seters, J. (2022). Inconsistent policies or political realities. *Nigeria's trade and industrial policy imperatives (No. Discussion Paper No. 31)*.

Latos-Brozio, M., Masek, A., & Piotrowska, M. (2022). Polymeric forms of plant flavonoids obtained by enzymatic reactions. *Molecules (Basel, Switzerland)*, *27*(12), 3702. PMID: 35744827

Liu, H., Wang, C., Li, C., Qin, Y., Wang, Z., Yang, F., & Wang, J. (2018). A functional chitosan-based hydrogel as a wound dressing and drug delivery system in the treatment of wound healing. *RSC Advances*, *8*(14), 7533–7549. PMID: 35539132

Malabadi, R. B., Kolkar, K. P., & Chalannavar, R. K. (2021). Natural plant gum exudates and mucilage: Pharmaceutical updates. *Int J Innov Sci Res Rev*, *3*(10), 1897–1912.

Mansuri, S., Kesharwani, P., Jain, K., Tekade, R. K., & Jain, N. K. (2016). Mucoadhesion: A promising approach in drug delivery system. *Reactive & Functional Polymers*, *100*, 151–172.

Metwally, W. M., El-Habashy, S. E., El-Hosseiny, L. S., Essawy, M. M., Eltaher, H. M., & El-Khordagui, L. K. (2023). Bioinspired 3D-printed scaffold embedding DDAB-nano ZnO/nanofibrous microspheres for regenerative diabetic wound healing. *Biofabrication, 16*(1), 015001. PMID: 37751750

Mirhosseini, H., & Amid, B. T. (2012). A review study on chemical composition and molecular structure of newly plant gum exudates and seed gums. *Food Research International, 46*(1), 387–398.

Mu, Q., Jiang, G., Chen, L., Zhou, H., Fourches, D., Tropsha, A., & Yan, B. (2014). Chemical basis of interactions between engineered nanoparticles and biological systems. *Chemical Reviews, 114*(15), 7740–7781. PMID: 24927254

. Muruganantham, S., Krishnaswami, V., Anitha Manikandan, D., Aravindaraj, N., Suresh, J., Murugesan, M., & Kandasamy, R. (2022). Gums as Pharmaceutical Excipients: An Overview. *Gums, Resins and Latexes of Plant Origin: Chemistry, Biological Activities and Uses*, 145-189.

Mushtaq, F., Raza, Z. A., Batool, S. R., Zahid, M., Onder, O. C., Rafique, A., & Nazeer, M. A. (2022). Preparation, properties, and applications of gelatin-based hydrogels (GHs) in the environmental, technological, and biomedical sectors. *International Journal of Biological Macromolecules, 218*, 601–633. PMID: 35902015

. Nagarajan, P., Kannan, S., Raj, A., Louis, L. R. P., Bazeer, A. B., Kaliaperumal, R., ... & Patil, S. J. (2025). Future Prospects in Medicinal Plant-Derived Drug Development: Unveiling Opportunities and Challenges. *Biotechnology and Phytochemical Prospects in Drug Discovery*, 241-266.

Nazemi, Z., Sahraro, M., Janmohammadi, M., Nourbakhsh, M. S., & Savoji, H. (2023). A review on tragacanth gum: A promising natural polysaccharide in drug delivery and cell therapy. *International Journal of Biological Macromolecules, 241*, 124343. PMID: 37054856

Noreen, S., Hasan, S., Ghumman, S. A., Bukhari, S. N. A., Ijaz, B., Hameed, H., & Ejaz, H. (2022). pH responsive Abelmoschus esculentus mucilage and administration of methotrexate: In-vitro antitumor and in-vivo toxicity evaluation. *International Journal of Molecular Sciences, 23*(5), 2725. PMID: 35269867

Ofridam, F., Tarhini, M., Lebaz, N., Gagnière, É., Mangin, D., & Elaissari, A. (2021). pH-sensitive polymers: Classification and some fine potential applications. *Polymers for Advanced Technologies, 32*(4), 1455–1484.

Ogaji, I. J., Nep, E. I., & Audu-Peter, J. D. (2012). Advances in natural polymers as pharmaceutical excipients. *Pharmaceutica Analytica Acta, 3*(1), 1–16.

. Oleszek, W., & Hamed, A. (2010). Saponin-based surfactants. *Surfactants from renewable resources*, 239-249.

Pawar, S. R., Patel, P., & Jain, K. (2025). Herbal Formulations: Development, Challenges, Testing, Stability, and Regulatory Guidelines. In *Advances in Pharmaceutical Product Development* (pp. 379–397). Springer Nature Singapore.

Pifferi, G., & Restani, P. (2003). The safety of pharmaceutical excipients. *Il Farmaco*, *58*(8), 541–550. PMID: 12875883

Pockle, R. D., Masareddy, R. S., Patil, A. S., & Patil, P. D. (2023). A comprehensive review on pharmaceutical excipients. *Therapeutic Delivery*, *14*(7), 443–458. PMID: 37464784

Pramanik, S., Aggarwal, A., Kadi, A., Alhomrani, M., Alamri, A. S., Alsanie, W. F., & Bellucci, S. (2024). Chitosan alchemy: Transforming tissue engineering and wound healing. *RSC Advances*, *14*(27), 19219–19256. PMID: 38887635

Prasad, N., Thombare, N., Sharma, S. C., & Kumar, S. (2022). Gum arabic–A versatile natural gum: A review on production, processing, properties and applications. *Industrial Crops and Products*, *187*, 115304.

Prasad, N., Thombare, N., Sharma, S. C., & Kumar, S. (2023). Recent development in the medical and industrial applications of gum karaya: A review. *Polymer Bulletin*, *80*(4), 3425–3447.

Rousseaux, C. G. (2023). Herbal remedies. In *Haschek and Rousseaux's handbook of toxicologic pathology* (pp. 183–303). Academic Press.

Serrano, D. R., Kara, A., Yuste, I., Luciano, F. C., Ongoren, B., Anaya, B. J., & Lalatsa, A. (2023). 3D printing technologies in personalized medicine, nanomedicines, and biopharmaceuticals. *Pharmaceutics*, *15*(2), 313. PMID: 36839636

Shaikh, R., Singh, T. R. R., Garland, M. J., Woolfson, A. D., & Donnelly, R. F. (2011). Mucoadhesive drug delivery systems. *Journal of Pharmacy & Bioallied Sciences*, *3*(1), 89–100. PMID: 21430958

Sharma, A., Puri, V., Bakshi, I. S., & Kumar, P. (2022). Herbal bioactive-incorporated scaffolds for wound healing applications. In *Herbal Bioactive-Based Drug Delivery Systems* (pp. 311–330). Academic Press.

Sharma, S., Sudhakara, P., Singh, J., Ilyas, R. A., Asyraf, M. R. M., & Razman, M. R. (2021). Critical review of biodegradable and bioactive polymer composites for bone tissue engineering and drug delivery applications. *Polymers*, *13*(16), 2623. PMID: 34451161

Singh, J., & Nayak, P. (2023). pH-responsive polymers for drug delivery: Trends and opportunities. *Journal of polymer science, 61*(22), 2828–2850.

. Singh, P., Mishra, G., & Dinda, S. C. (2021). Natural excipients in pharmaceutical formulations. *Evidence Based Validation of Traditional Medicines: A comprehensive Approach*, 829-869.

Soni, S., Namdeo, S., Agrawal, P., Haider, T., & Soni, V. (2023). Novel modalities of delivering herbal medicines for wound healing: A review. *Dermatological Reviews, 4*(5), 194–210.

. Srivastava, S., & Misra, A. (2018). Quality control of herbal drugs: Advancements and challenges. *New Age Herbals: Resource, Quality and Pharmacognosy*, 189-209.

Steinhoff, B. (2021). Challenges in the quality of herbal medicinal products with a specific focus on contaminants. *Phytochemical Analysis, 32*(2), 117–123. PMID: 31402494

Su, C., Chen, Y., Tian, S., Lu, C., & Lv, Q. (2022). Natural materials for 3D printing and their applications. *Gels (Basel, Switzerland), 8*(11), 748. PMID: 36421570

Tamilarasi, G. P., Krishnan, M., Sabarees, G., Gouthaman, S., Alagarsamy, V., & Solomon, V. R. (2022). Emerging trends in curcumin embedded electrospun nanofibers for impaired diabetic wound healing. *Applied Nanoscience, 3*(4), 202–232.

Teodorescu, M., Bercea, M., & Morariu, S. (2018). Biomaterials of poly (vinyl alcohol) and natural polymers. *Polymer Reviews (Philadelphia, Pa.), 58*(2), 247–287.

Thakkar, S., Anklam, E., Xu, A., Ulberth, F., Li, J., Li, B., & Tong, W. (2020). Regulatory landscape of dietary supplements and herbal medicines from a global perspective. *Regulatory Toxicology and Pharmacology, 114*, 104647. PMID: 32305367

Usman, S., Fawzy, K. A., Beevi, R., & Usman, A. (2019). Basis of Pharmaceutical Formulation. In *Nanoscale Networking and Communications Handbook* (pp. 281–319). CRC Press.

. Vandghanooni, S., Jaymand, M., & Eskandani, M. (2025). The use of nanomedicines in the healthcare systems: A policy brief. *Drug Development and Industrial Pharmacy*, (just-accepted), 1-17.

Vaz, V. M., & Kumar, L. (2021). 3D printing as a promising tool in personalized medicine. *AAPS PharmSciTech, 22*, 1–20. PMID: 33458797

Veerapandian, M., Ramasundaram, S., Jerome, P., Chellasamy, G., Govindaraju, S., Yun, K., & Oh, T. H. (2023). Drug delivery application of functional nanomaterials synthesized using natural sources. *Journal of Functional Biomaterials*, *14*(8), 426. PMID: 37623670

Vilchez, A., Acevedo, F., Cea, M., Seeger, M., & Navia, R. (2020). Applications of electrospun nanofibers with antioxidant properties: A review. *Nanomaterials (Basel, Switzerland)*, *10*(1), 175. PMID: 31968539

Vinchhi, P., Wui, W. T., & Patel, M. M. (2024). Healing with herbs: An alliance with 'nano'for wound management. *Expert Opinion on Drug Delivery*, *21*(7), 1115–1141. PMID: 39095934

Volenzo, T., & Odiyo, J. (2020). Integrating endemic medicinal plants into the global value chains: The ecological degradation challenges and opportunities. *Heliyon*, *6*(9). PMID: 32995638

Yadav, B. K., Gidwani, B., & Vyas, A. (2016). Rosin: Recent advances and potential applications in novel drug delivery system. *Journal of Bioactive and Compatible Polymers*, *31*(2), 111–126.

Yin, Y., Huang, J., Wang, T., Yang, R., Hu, H., Manuka, M., & Ma, B. (2023). Effect of Hydroxypropyl methyl cellulose (HPMC) on rheology and printability of the first printed layer of cement activated slag-based 3D printing concrete. *Construction & Building Materials*, *405*, 133347.

Zhang, J., Jiang, X., Wen, X., Xu, Q., Zeng, H., Zhao, Y., & Wang, Y. (2019). Bio-responsive smart polymers and biomedical applications. *JPhys Materials*, *2*(3), 032004.

Zhou, Y., Wang, M., Yan, C., Liu, H., & Yu, D. G. (2022). Advances in the application of electrospun drug-loaded nanofibers in the treatment of oral ulcers. *Biomolecules*, *12*(9), 1254. PMID: 36139093

Zulkiflee, I., & Fauzi, M. B. (2021). Gelatin-polyvinyl alcohol film for tissue engineering: A concise review. *Biomedicines*, *9*(8), 979. PMID: 34440183

Chapter 5
Polysaccharide-Based Polymers

Neha Raghuwanshi
https://orcid.org/0009-0003-9096-0362
Amity Institute of Pharmacy, Amity University, Mumbai, India

ABSTRACT

Polymers based on polysaccharides have become essential elements in modern wound healing techniques because of their inherent biocompatibility, biodegradability, and functional adaptability. These naturally occurring biopolymers—which include cellulose, dextran, hyaluronic acid, alginate, and chitosan—form the basis for the creation of sophisticated wound dressings. New developments have concentrated on improving these materials' medicinal effectiveness through a variety of changes. For example, by adding stimuli-responsive components, hydrogels that can react dynamically to changes in temperature, pH, and ionic strength have been developed. This allows for the regulated release of bioactive substances and speeds up wound closure. Furthermore, hybrid hydrogel systems that include the beneficial qualities of both components—such as increased mechanical strength and biological activity—have been produced by integrating polysaccharides with synthetic proteins.

INTRODUCTION TO POLYSACCHARIDE BIOMATERIALS

Polysaccharide-based biomaterials are a class of naturally occurring polymers composed of long chains of monosaccharide units linked by glycosidic bonds. These biopolymers are derived from various natural sources, including terrestrial plants (e.g., cellulose and starch), marine organisms (e.g., alginate from brown algae and chitosan from crustacean shells), and microbial fermentation products (e.g., dextran and xanthan gum) (Liu et al., 2024; Wang et al., 2025). Their molecular

DOI: 10.4018/979-8-3373-3977-1.ch005

structures typically include abundant functional groups such as hydroxyl (-OH), amino ($-NH_2$), and carboxyl (-COOH), which contribute to their hydrophilicity and reactivity. These reactive groups also allow extensive chemical modification, enabling tailoring of mechanical strength, biodegradability, and biological activity for specific biomedical applications.

Structurally, polysaccharides range from linear to highly branched architectures, and their physicochemical properties—such as viscosity, solubility, gelation behavior, and thermal stability—can be finely tuned through structural modifications. This tunability facilitates the design of advanced wound dressings in the form of hydrogels, films, foams, sponges, scaffolds, and electrospun nanofibers (Zhang et al., 2020; Liu et al., 2024). Such versatility makes polysaccharide-based materials especially suitable for dynamic and complex wound healing environments, where materials must adapt to moisture levels, microbial presence, and varying tissue regeneration phases.

Figure 1. A detailed microscopic illustration depicting the molecular structure of various polysaccharide biomaterials

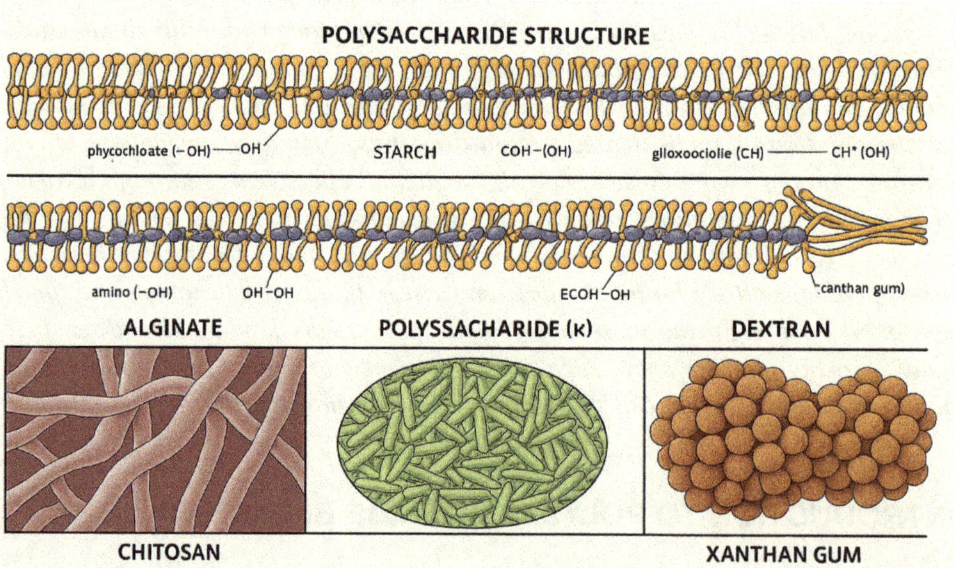

KEY ADVANTAGES OVER SYNTHETIC POLYMERS IN WOUND CARE

One of the foremost advantages of polysaccharide-based polymers over synthetic counterparts lies in their biocompatibility and biodegradability. Unlike synthetic materials, which may elicit immune reactions or leave behind harmful residues, polysaccharides degrade into non-toxic byproducts that are often metabolized or excreted naturally by the body (Wang et al., 2025). This makes them highly suitable for temporary implants or wound dressings that do not require surgical removal.

Additionally, polysaccharides can mimic components of the extracellular matrix (ECM), creating a biologically relevant microenvironment that enhances cellular activities such as adhesion, migration, and proliferation. For example, chitosan's structural similarity to glycosaminoglycans—a key ECM component—facilitates its interaction with skin cells, promoting rapid tissue regeneration (Zhang et al., 2020).

Polysaccharide-based materials also possess intrinsic biological functionalities that contribute directly to wound healing. Chitosan, for instance, is known for its antimicrobial, hemostatic, and mucoadhesive properties, making it particularly effective in infected or bleeding wounds (Liu et al., 2024). Alginate forms ionically crosslinked hydrogels in the presence of calcium ions, which not only absorb exudates but also maintain a moist healing environment and support ionic balance—factors essential for fibroblast function and re-epithelialization (Wang et al., 2025).

Furthermore, many polysaccharides serve as excellent carriers for therapeutic agents, such as antibiotics, antioxidants, anti-inflammatory drugs, and growth factors. Their porous structure and chemical modifiability enable controlled release mechanisms, thereby providing sustained therapeutic effects and minimizing systemic toxicity (Zhang et al., 2020).

From a fabrication standpoint, polysaccharides are easy to process using green chemistry techniques, such as aqueous-based formulations and low-temperature drying, which help preserve bioactivity and reduce environmental impact (Liu et al., 2024). The sustainability and renewability of their sources also enhance their appeal in the context of eco-friendly biomedical product development.

In summary, the inherent biocompatibility, tunable physicochemical properties, biological functionality, and sustainable sourcing of polysaccharide-based polymers render them superior to many synthetic alternatives in wound care. Their continued development is expected to play a crucial role in next-generation wound management systems that emphasize not only healing efficacy but also patient comfort, environmental sustainability, and cost-effectiveness.

Figure 2. Polysaccharide based bymecr polymers over polymers in wound care

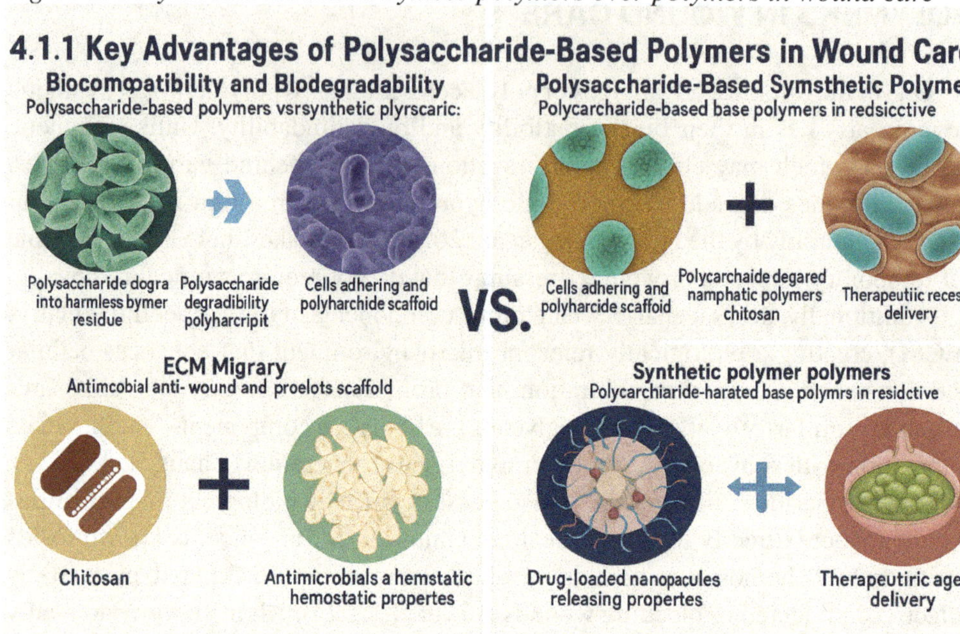

MAJOR POLYSACCHARIDES IN WOUND HEALING

Polysaccharides have become prominent candidates in wound care due to their biocompatibility, tunable physicochemical properties, and functional roles in tissue repair. The most widely used polysaccharides in this context include chitosan, alginate, hyaluronic acid, cellulose derivatives, and dextran. These materials contribute to wound healing by offering antimicrobial protection, maintaining a moist wound environment, promoting tissue regeneration, and serving as structural scaffolds.

Chitosan

Chitosan, a cationic polysaccharide obtained by deacetylation of chitin, exhibits a unique combination of wound healing properties. It possesses strong antibacterial activity due to its polycationic nature, which disrupts microbial cell membranes, making it effective against both Gram-positive and Gram-negative bacteria (Wang et al., 2021). Its moisture retention ability helps maintain a hydrated wound environment that accelerates epithelialization. Additionally, chitosan facilitates tissue regeneration by enhancing fibroblast proliferation and collagen deposition (Liu et al., 2023). It can also be processed into hydrogels, films, and sponges, making it an excellent scaffold for tissue repair.

Alginate

Alginate is a naturally occurring anionic polysaccharide derived from brown seaweed, composed mainly of guluronic and mannuronic acid blocks. In wound healing, alginate forms hydrogels upon contact with wound exudate, thereby providing moisture retention and absorbing excess fluids (Ranjbar-Mohammadi & Bahrami, 2018). Calcium alginate dressings also release calcium ions that aid in hemostasis and can form a gel matrix that promotes cell migration and granulation tissue formation (Zhang et al., 2020). Additionally, alginate can be combined with antimicrobial agents to enhance antibacterial activity, and its gelling nature makes it a suitable scaffold for cellular growth.

Hyaluronic Acid

Hyaluronic acid (HA) is a non-sulfated glycosaminoglycan found in the extracellular matrix of connective tissues. It plays a crucial role in all phases of wound healing. Its moisture-retaining property is due to its strong water-binding ability, which maintains a hydrated environment that supports angiogenesis and cell proliferation (Chen et al., 2022). HA also contributes to tissue regeneration by stimulating keratinocyte migration and fibroblast activity while modulating inflammatory responses (Fang et al., 2021). HA-based hydrogels are widely used as injectable matrices and scaffolds in tissue engineering, offering a bioactive interface for skin regeneration.

Cellulose Derivatives

Cellulose derivatives such as carboxymethyl cellulose (CMC) and hydroxypropyl cellulose (HPC) are commonly used in wound dressings due to their excellent moisture retention and swelling capabilities. These semi-synthetic polysaccharides are structurally robust and can be blended with antimicrobial agents to provide antibacterial protection (Patel et al., 2020). CMC, in particular, promotes tissue regeneration by facilitating cell attachment and migration. Furthermore, cellulose derivatives can be fabricated into fibrous mats or hydrogels, serving as effective scaffolds for skin tissue repair.

Dextran

Dextran is a branched polysaccharide produced by certain bacterial strains. It is especially useful in drug delivery systems for wound healing due to its hydrophilicity and biocompatibility. Dextran-based hydrogels retain moisture, offer antimicrobial potential when conjugated with agents like silver nanoparticles, and enable controlled release of growth factors (Hajimiri et al., 2020). Their viscoelastic and porous structure supports tissue regeneration and provides a scaffold that mimics the extracellular matrix.

Figure 3. Major polysaccharides in wound healing

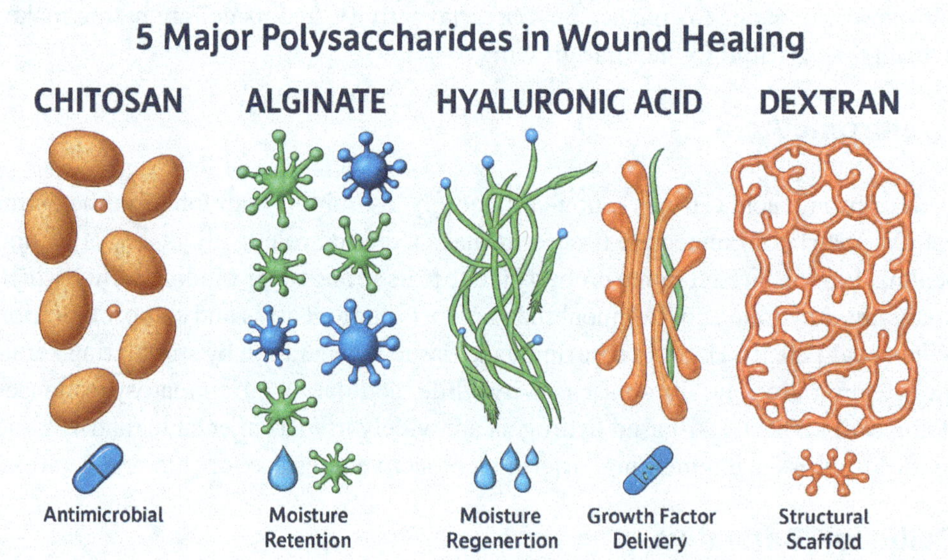

FUNCTIONALIZATION AND MODIFICATION

Crosslinking and Stimuli-Responsive Modifications

Polysaccharide-based hydrogels have shown immense promise in wound healing due to their innate biocompatibility and degradability. However, native forms often lack mechanical robustness and dynamic functionality. To address this, functionalization via crosslinking and incorporation of stimuli-responsive features has gained substantial attention.

Crosslinking improves hydrogel integrity and modulates degradation kinetics. Covalent (chemical) crosslinking, such as using genipin or glutaraldehyde, has been used to enhance the structural stability of chitosan and alginate hydrogels (Feng et al., 2019). On the other hand, physical crosslinking, through ionic bonding (e.g., calcium ions with alginate) or hydrogen bonding, enables milder processing and improved biocompatibility (Tao et al., 2023). Dynamic covalent crosslinking approaches using Schiff base reactions or boronate esters impart reversible, self-healing capabilities to hydrogels (Qian et al., 2022).

Stimuli-responsive modifications allow hydrogels to react to environmental triggers like pH, temperature, or redox state. For instance, pH-responsive hydrogels can swell in acidic conditions, which is relevant in chronic wounds (He et al., 2021). Similarly, thermosensitive systems like methylcellulose or chitosan-glycerophosphate solutions form gels at body temperature, facilitating in situ application (Jiang et al., 2023). Redox-sensitive hydrogels that degrade in response to elevated reactive oxygen species (ROS) are also being explored for controlled drug release in inflamed wounds (Yang et al., 2021).

Together, crosslinking and responsiveness enhance hydrogel mechanical integrity, drug-release kinetics, and adaptability to wound microenvironments, aligning well with clinical needs.

Incorporation of Bioactive Agents

Another important strategy in polysaccharide modification is the incorporation of bioactive agents, such as growth factors, antimicrobial compounds, and antioxidants, to accelerate healing and prevent complications like infection or chronic inflammation.

Growth factors, including epidermal growth factor (EGF), basic fibroblast growth factor (bFGF), and vascular endothelial growth factor (VEGF), are pivotal in promoting cell proliferation, angiogenesis, and extracellular matrix remodeling. Encapsulating these within hydrogels allows for controlled and localized delivery. For instance, hyaluronic acid hydrogels loaded with VEGF significantly enhanced granulation tissue formation in diabetic wounds (Wang et al., 2021).

Antimicrobial agents such as silver nanoparticles, zinc oxide, or antibiotics can be incorporated into chitosan or cellulose matrices to combat infections. For example, a carboxymethyl cellulose hydrogel loaded with silver nanoparticles demonstrated excellent antibacterial efficacy and promoted wound closure in infected models (Ali et al., 2022).

Antioxidants, like quercetin, curcumin, or tannic acid, neutralize ROS that hinder the healing process. Recent research shows that dextran-based hydrogels incorporating quercetin improved wound healing outcomes by reducing oxidative stress and inflammation (Liu et al., 2020).

By combining structural polysaccharides with therapeutic agents, functionalized hydrogels can address complex wound pathophysiology, offering a multifactorial approach to healing.

Figure 4. Crosslinking and stimuli responsive modifications in polysaccharide hydrogel for wound healing

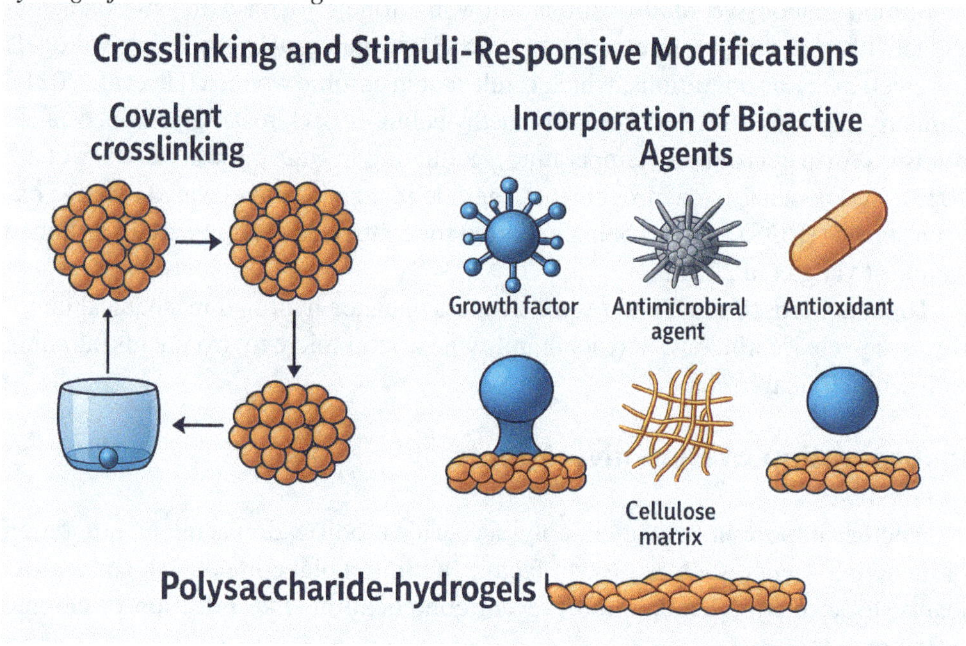

FABRICATION TECHNIQUES

The development of advanced fabrication techniques has significantly enhanced the application of polysaccharide-based polymers in wound healing. These techniques, including electrospinning for nanofiber mats, 3D bioprinting, and the creation of injectable hydrogels, have enabled the production of materials that closely mimic the natural extracellular matrix (ECM), providing structural support and promoting cellular activities essential for tissue regeneration.

Electrospun Nanofiber Mats

Electrospinning is a versatile technique that produces nanofibers with diameters ranging from tens to hundreds of nanometers, offering a high surface-area-to-volume ratio ideal for wound healing applications. Polysaccharide-based nanofibers, such as those derived from chitosan, alginate, and hyaluronic acid, have been extensively studied due to their biocompatibility, biodegradability, and inherent bioactivity. These nanofibers can be fabricated using electrospinning to create mats that serve as scaffolds for cell attachment, proliferation, and differentiation. For instance, chitosan-based nanofiber mats have demonstrated antimicrobial properties and enhanced cell migration, making them suitable for treating infected wounds (Tan et al., 2022).

The electrospinning process parameters, such as solution concentration, voltage, and collector distance, play a crucial role in determining the morphology and properties of the nanofibers. By optimizing these parameters, researchers can tailor the mechanical strength, porosity, and degradation rate of the nanofiber mats to meet specific clinical needs. Additionally, the incorporation of bioactive agents, such as growth factors or antimicrobial peptides, into the electrospun nanofibers has been explored to further enhance their therapeutic efficacy **(Tan et al., 2022).**

3D Bioprinting

3D bioprinting has emerged as a groundbreaking technology in tissue engineering, allowing for the precise deposition of bioinks to create complex, three-dimensional structures that mimic native tissues. Polysaccharide-based hydrogels, such as those derived from alginate, chitosan, and hyaluronic acid, serve as excellent bioinks due to their tunable rheological properties, biocompatibility, and ability to support cell viability and function. These hydrogels can be crosslinked post-printing to stabilize the printed structures.

Recent advancements have focused on enhancing the mechanical properties and printability of polysaccharide-based bioinks. For example, the incorporation of gelatin methacrylate (GelMA) into alginate-based bioinks has improved their printability and mechanical strength, facilitating the fabrication of more robust and functional tissue constructs (Wang et al., 2024). Moreover, the use of 3D bioprinting allows for the creation of scaffolds with complex architectures, such as multi-layered structures and vascular networks, which are essential for the regeneration of large tissue defects (Wang et al., 2024).

Injectable Hydrogels

Injectable hydrogels offer a minimally invasive approach to wound treatment, allowing for the delivery of therapeutic agents directly to the site of injury. Polysaccharide-based injectable hydrogels, such as those derived from carboxymethyl chitosan (CMCS) and sodium alginate, can undergo gelation in situ through various mechanisms, including ionic crosslinking and Schiff base reactions. These hydrogels can encapsulate bioactive molecules, such as growth factors or antimicrobial agents, and release them in a controlled manner to promote wound healing. (Fang et al.,2023)

The injectability and self-healing properties of these hydrogels are crucial for their application in wound healing. For instance, CMCS-based hydrogels have been shown to exhibit good injectability and self-healing abilities, facilitating their application in irregularly shaped wounds (Xuan et al., 2021). Furthermore, the incorporation of nanofillers, such as polymethyl methacrylate (PMA) nanofibers, into the hydrogels has been explored to enhance their mechanical properties and promote cell adhesion and proliferation (Xuan et al., 2021).

Figure 5. Polysaccharide fabricaride based polymer wound healing application

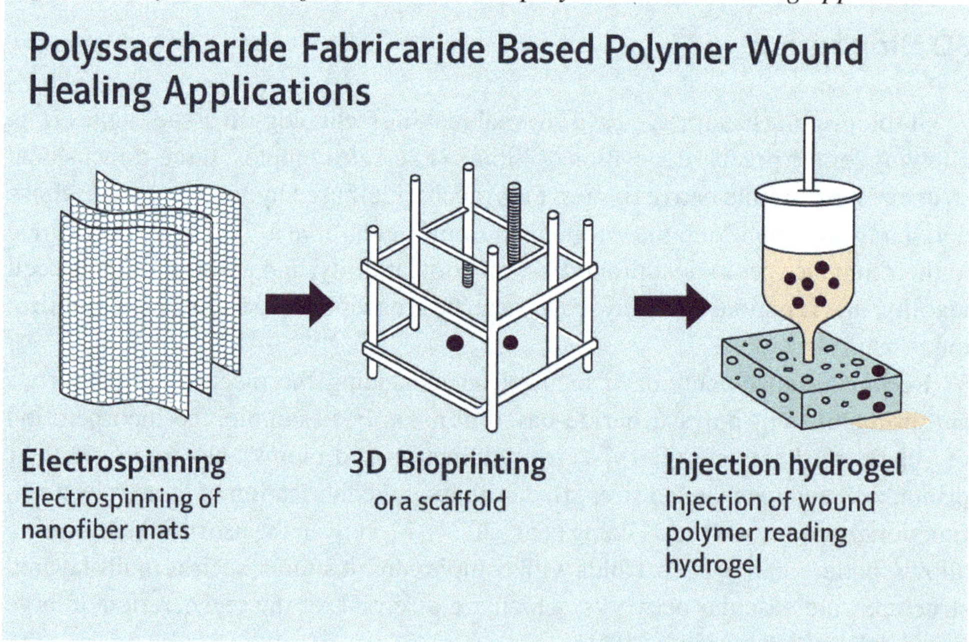

These fabrication techniques have significantly advanced the field of wound healing by providing versatile and effective materials that promote tissue regeneration. The continuous development and optimization of these methods hold great promise for the future of regenerative medicine.

COMPOSITE AND HYBRID SYSTEMS

Polysaccharide Blends with Synthetic Polymers or Proteins

Polysaccharides are naturally abundant and biocompatible, making them an ideal candidate for use in biomedical applications, particularly in wound healing. However, their mechanical properties, such as strength and elasticity, can be limiting in some applications. Therefore, blending polysaccharides with synthetic polymers or proteins enhances their physical properties while maintaining their biocompatibility and biodegradability.

The incorporation of synthetic polymers like poly(lactic acid) (PLA), poly(ethylene glycol) (PEG), or proteins such as collagen into polysaccharides like chitosan, hyaluronic acid, and alginate improves the mechanical stability, processability, and functional properties of the composite systems (Salmaso & Caliceti, 2021). For example, the combination of chitosan with PLA has been shown to produce composite scaffolds that offer improved mechanical strength compared to chitosan alone, making them more suitable for load-bearing applications in wound healing (Zhang, Zhang, & Zhang, 2023).

Moreover, polysaccharide-based composites can mimic the natural extracellular matrix (ECM), which is crucial for cellular adhesion, proliferation, and differentiation during tissue regeneration. Gelatin, a natural protein, is often blended with polysaccharides to form hydrogels that provide a three-dimensional structure for cell growth. Hyaluronic acid combined with gelatin, for example, forms hydrogels with enhanced mechanical properties that promote cell attachment and growth, making them ideal for soft tissue regeneration **(Zhou, Zhang, & Zhang, 2024).**

Example

In a recent study, a chitosan-based composite hydrogel was created by blending chitosan with PEG. This composite exhibited enhanced mechanical properties and controlled biodegradability, which facilitated its use in the treatment of chronic wounds. The incorporation of PEG into the chitosan matrix improved its elasticity and moisture retention, which are essential for promoting wound healing **(Wang, Zhang, & Wei, 2024).** This example highlights the flexibility and adaptability of polysaccharide-based hybrid systems in wound care applications.

Dual Drug Delivery Applications

Composite and hybrid systems can also be designed for dual drug delivery applications, a strategy that enhances therapeutic efficacy by delivering multiple therapeutic agents simultaneously or sequentially. This approach has significant potential in the treatment of complex conditions such as chronic wounds, infections, and cancer, where a combination of drugs may be needed to address multiple aspects of the disease simultaneously.

One of the primary advantages of using polysaccharide-based composite systems in dual drug delivery is their ability to encapsulate and release two or more drugs in a controlled manner. For instance, a composite hydrogel made from chitosan and PEG was designed to release both an anti-inflammatory agent and an antimicrobial drug in response to changes in pH and temperature, providing a synergistic effect for wound healing (Zhang et al., 2023). This system helps combat both infection and inflammation, which are two common challenges in chronic wound healing.

Another example of dual drug delivery involves the combination of hyaluronic acid with polylactic-co-glycolic acid (PLGA), a synthetic polymer. In this case, hyaluronic acid served as a carrier for hydrophobic anticancer drugs, while PLGA encapsulated hydrophilic drugs like growth factors. This combination allowed for the sequential release of the anticancer drug followed by the release of growth factors, thereby promoting both the reduction of cancer cells and the regeneration of healthy tissue (Salmaso & Caliceti, 2021).

The controlled release properties of these systems are critical, as they allow for precise modulation of drug concentrations over time, improving the overall efficacy and reducing the side effects of individual drugs. The release kinetics of dual drug systems can be controlled by adjusting factors such as the polysaccharide-to-synthetic polymer ratio, the degree of crosslinking, and the type of bioactive agent incorporated.

Example

A recent study on dual-drug delivery systems used chitosan-based nanoparticles to deliver both antibiotics and growth factors. These nanoparticles were designed to release the antibiotics first to fight bacterial infection, followed by the release of growth factors to promote tissue regeneration. The system was tested on infected wound models in rats and showed improved healing and reduced infection rates compared to single-drug treatments (Nguyen Le et al., 2022). This example demonstrates the practical application of dual-drug delivery systems in treating complex wounds.

Figure 6. Composite and hybrid system of polysaccharide blends with symthetic polymers

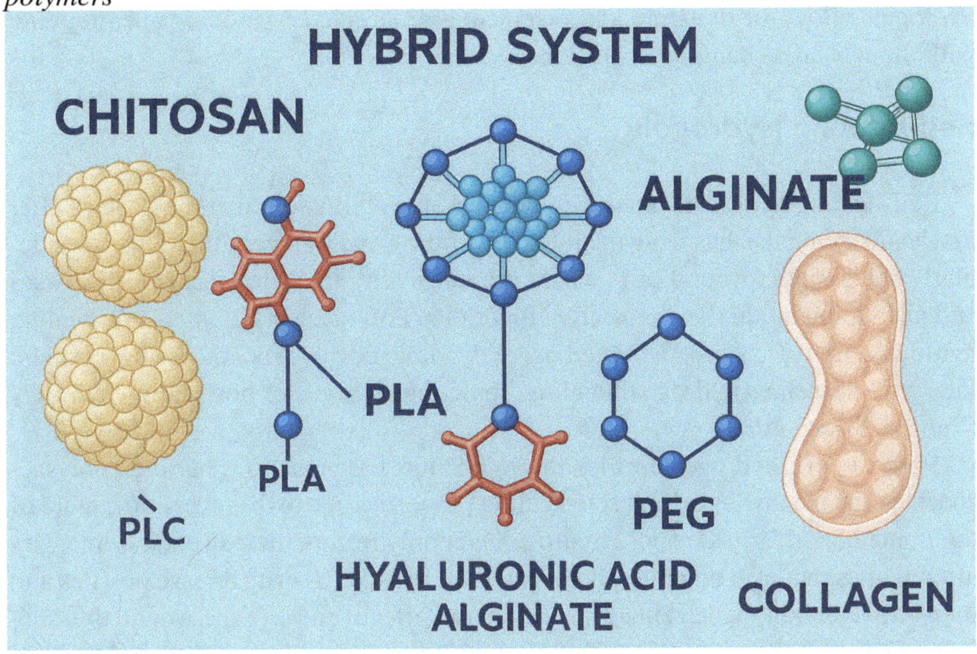

SMART AND RESPONSIVE DRESSINGS

Stimuli-Responsive Hydrogels

Stimuli-responsive hydrogels are engineered to undergo reversible changes in their physical or chemical properties in response to specific environmental triggers, such as pH, temperature, ionic strength, or the presence of reactive oxygen species (ROS). Polysaccharides like chitosan, hyaluronic acid, and alginate are often used to fabricate these hydrogels due to their natural abundance and ability to undergo modification with functional groups that facilitate crosslinking and stimuli-response (Damiri, Fatimi, Santos, Varma, & Berrada, 2023).

For instance, chitosan-based hydrogels have been developed to respond to variations in pH and temperature, enabling controlled release of therapeutic agents at the wound site. These hydrogels swell or contract in response to the acidic environment of chronic wounds, modulating drug release rates and enhancing healing efficacy (Damiri et al., 2023). Similarly, hyaluronic acid-based hydrogels have been designed to respond to ROS, which are elevated in chronic wounds, inducing the degradation of the hydrogel matrix and facilitating the sustained release of growth factors to promote tissue regeneration (Gao, Golland, Tronci, & Thornton, 2021). These hydrogels allow for dynamic and responsive drug delivery in real-time, aligning with the wound's changing conditions.

Self-Healing Hydrogels

Self-healing hydrogels possess the remarkable ability to repair themselves after mechanical damage, ensuring the integrity of the dressing over time. This is particularly beneficial in wound care, where dressings are subject to mechanical stresses and need to maintain their protective functions. Polysaccharide-based self-healing hydrogels are typically constructed using dynamic covalent bonds or non-covalent interactions such as hydrogen bonding, ionic interactions, or host-guest chemistry (Yang & Wang, 2023).

For example, hydrogels formed through Schiff base reactions between polysaccharides and aldehydes exhibit self-healing properties due to the reversible nature of the imine bonds formed. These hydrogels not only restore their structural integrity after damage but also maintain their functionality, such as drug release profiles and moisture retention, which enhances the overall effectiveness of the wound dressing (Mo, Zhang, & Zhang, 2021). Self-healing polysaccharide-based materials have thus proven to be highly beneficial in maintaining the dressing's performance during prolonged application.

Biosensor-Integrated Dressings

Integrating biosensors into polysaccharide-based dressings enables real-time monitoring of the wound environment, providing valuable information for personalized wound management. These biosensor-integrated dressings can detect biomarkers such as glucose, pH, temperature, and ROS, all of which are indicative of the wound's healing status (Khalid et al., 2020). For example, a redox-responsive hyaluronic acid-based hydrogel has been developed to detect variations in glutathione levels, a marker of wound healing. The hydrogel's properties change in response to glutathione concentration, allowing for non-invasive monitoring of the wound's healing progress (Gao et al., 2021).

In addition, electrospun nanodiamond-silk fibroin membranes have been explored as multifunctional platforms for biosensing and wound healing. These membranes detect temperature changes associated with infection and inflammation, providing real-time feedback on the wound's condition without the need to remove the dressing (Khalid et al., 2020). This integration of biosensing technology with polysaccharide-based materials ensures more efficient and dynamic monitoring, which is crucial for improving patient care in chronic wound treatment.

Clinical Applications and Future Directions

The clinical application of smart polysaccharide-based dressings is advancing rapidly. Several formulations are undergoing preclinical and clinical evaluations due to their ability to respond to dynamic wound conditions, deliver therapeutic agents in a controlled manner, and provide real-time monitoring of wound status. The next steps in research include enhancing the functionality of these dressings by incorporating multiple stimuli-responsive elements, improving biosensor integration, and scaling production for clinical use (Yang & Wang, 2023).

Moreover, standardizing protocols for evaluating the safety and performance of these dressings will be crucial for their clinical adoption. Future research will likely focus on the integration of artificial intelligence (AI) to better predict wound healing responses based on real-time data provided by these smart materials (Gao et al., 2021).

CASE STUDIES AND APPLICATIONS

Real-World Uses of Chitosan, Alginate, and Hyaluronic Acid

Polysaccharide-based materials such as chitosan, alginate, and hyaluronic acid (HA) are widely used in clinical applications for their beneficial properties in wound healing, tissue regeneration, and drug delivery systems. These polysaccharides are highly biocompatible and have shown promising results in both preclinical and clinical settings.

Chitosan-Based Applications

Wound Healing

Chitosan has been widely studied for its wound healing potential due to its antimicrobial properties, biocompatibility, and ability to promote tissue regeneration. A study by **Soni et al. (2021)** developed a chitosan-based wound dressing for the treatment of chronic diabetic ulcers. The dressing was found to enhance healing by improving collagen deposition and epithelialization, as well as by providing a protective barrier against bacterial infection. This study showed that chitosan dressings promoted faster tissue regeneration compared to traditional dressings.

Drug Delivery

Chitosan is also used in controlled drug delivery applications due to its ability to form gels and nanoparticles. In a clinical study, chitosan nanoparticles were used to deliver antibiotics to infected wounds, showing that they improved drug stability, prolonged the release of antibiotics, and minimized side effects, making them an effective delivery vehicle in wound care (Moghadam et al., 2020).

Alginate-Based Applications

Wound Dressings

Alginate, derived from brown seaweed, is a hydrophilic polysaccharide that forms gels when in contact with wound exudate. Alginate-based dressings are commonly used in the management of exudative wounds, such as diabetic ulcers and burns. A clinical study by Tottoli et al. (2020) showed that alginate dressings effectively managed exudate and maintained a moist environment, which accelerated the healing process and reduced infection rates in chronic wounds.

Tissue Engineering

Alginate has also been incorporated into tissue engineering applications. **Wu et al. (2020)** explored the use of alginate-based scaffolds to support mesenchymal stem cells (MSCs) for cartilage repair. When combined with other biomaterials like hyaluronic acid and collagen, the alginate scaffold enhanced cell viability and promoted cartilage regeneration in animal models, showcasing its potential in regenerative medicine.

Hyaluronic Acid-Based Applications

Wound Healing and Regeneration

Hyaluronic acid (HA), a naturally occurring glycosaminoglycan, plays a critical role in wound healing by promoting cell migration, collagen formation, and tissue repair. A clinical trial by Yamaguchi et al. (2019) evaluated HA-based hydrogel dressings in patients with burns and chronic ulcers. The study demonstrated that HA promoted faster wound closure, enhanced epithelial regeneration, and reduced scarring compared to conventional treatments.

Osteoarthritis and Joint Regeneration

In addition to wound healing, HA is widely used in the treatment of osteoarthritis (OA) due to its ability to lubricate joints and reduce inflammation. A study by Lee et al. (2020) investigated the use of HA injections in OA patients. The results showed significant improvements in joint mobility and pain relief, demonstrating the effectiveness of HA in managing degenerative joint diseases.

Figure 7. Real-world application of chitosan and hyaluronic acid wound healing and drug delivery

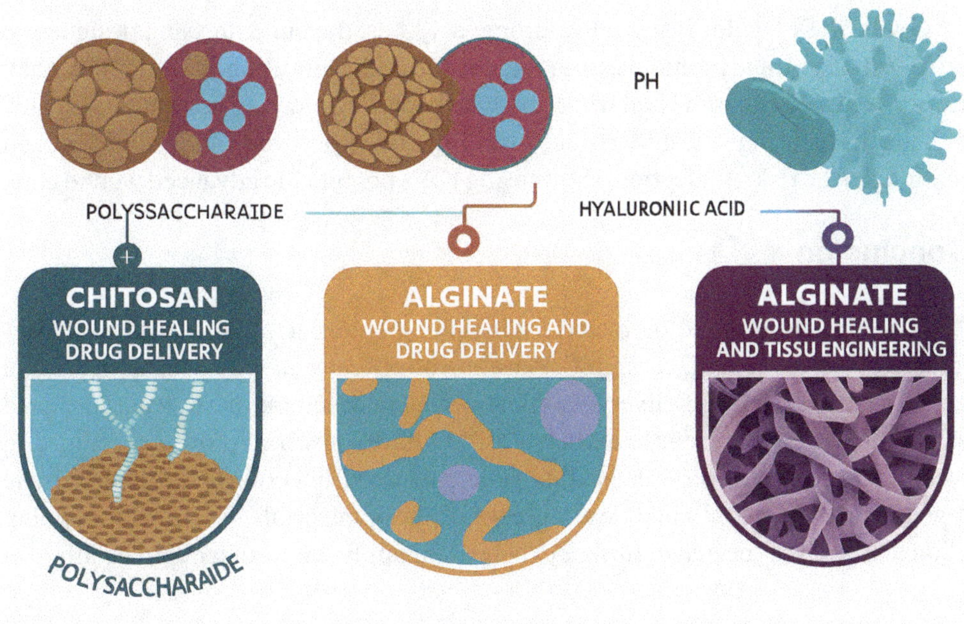

Clinical Products and Trial Outcomes

Chitosan-Based Products

ChitoClear®. This is a chitosan-based wound dressing that has been clinically proven to accelerate wound healing. In a randomized controlled trial, **Ryu et al. (2017)** used ChitoClear® to treat diabetic foot ulcers. The results indicated that the chitosan dressing significantly improved healing rates compared to standard care, reducing infection and promoting faster tissue regeneration.

Alginate-Based Products

Kaltostat®. A widely used alginate dressing in clinical practice, Kaltostat® is indicated for moderate to heavily exuding wounds. In a study by Darouiche et al. (2020), the efficacy of Kaltostat® was evaluated in patients with chronic wounds. The findings suggested that the alginate dressing was superior to conventional dressings in managing exudate, promoting faster healing, and reducing the incidence of infections.

Hyaluronic Acid-Based Products

Hyalofill®. Hyalofill® is a hyaluronic acid-based wound dressing designed to provide moisture and promote tissue regeneration in chronic wounds. In a clinical trial, **López et al. (2021)** used Hyalofill® to treat venous leg ulcers. The results indicated that the dressing significantly reduced healing time, improved patient comfort, and minimized the risk of infection, showcasing HA's potential in advanced wound care.

Conclusion

Polysaccharide-based biomaterials, including chitosan, alginate, and hyaluronic acid, have demonstrated significant clinical efficacy in wound healing, tissue regeneration, and drug delivery. Clinical products based on these materials, such as ChitoClear®, Kaltostat®, and Hyalofill®, have shown improved outcomes in wound care, including faster healing times, reduced infections, and better tissue regeneration. The continued development of these materials, along with ongoing clinical trials, is expected to further expand their applications in modern healthcare.

CHALLENGES AND FUTURE OUTLOOK

Production and Regulatory Issues

Despite the growing interest in polysaccharide-based polymers for biomedical applications, several challenges remain in their large-scale production and regulatory approval. One of the primary hurdles in the production of polysaccharide-based biomaterials is the cost and scalability of manufacturing. Polysaccharides like chitosan, alginate, and hyaluronic acid are typically derived from natural sources such as crustaceans, seaweed, and bacteria, respectively. While these sources are abundant, the extraction and purification processes can be costly and labor-intensive, which limits the scalability of these materials for industrial applications. Furthermore, to meet the requirements of the medical and pharmaceutical industries, polysaccharide-based products must undergo rigorous quality control measures to ensure their consistency and safety. The development of more efficient and cost-effective methods for the extraction and processing of polysaccharides will be key to overcoming this barrier (Mohammad et al., 2021; Karami et al., 2019).

Another significant challenge is regulatory approval. The regulatory process for biomaterials, particularly for medical and wound care applications, can be lengthy and complex. Polysaccharides are naturally occurring and biocompatible, which supports their safety profiles; however, their clinical use still requires thorough preclinical testing, toxicological assessments, and clinical trials to ensure that they meet the standards set by regulatory agencies such as the FDA and the European Medicines Agency (EMA). Variations in production methods, such as the use of synthetic modifications or additives in polysaccharide formulations, may also require additional regulatory scrutiny (Zhao et al., 2020). Regulatory hurdles, along with concerns related to product standardization, can slow the time-to-market for novel polysaccharide-based biomaterials.

Emerging Trends: AI-Based Design and Biodegradable Electronics

The future of polysaccharide-based polymers is poised to be shaped by several emerging trends that could enhance their performance and applicability in medical and technological fields. One such trend is the application of artificial intelligence (AI) in the design and optimization of polysaccharide-based materials. AI-driven algorithms and machine learning techniques have the potential to revolutionize the development of biomaterials by enabling the design of new materials with tailored properties. Through AI-based modeling and simulations, researchers can predict how different polysaccharide compositions will behave under various conditions, allowing for the rapid development of optimized materials for specific applications, such as controlled drug delivery or tissue regeneration (Gao et al., 2021).

AI also has the potential to enhance the sustainability of polysaccharide production. By using machine learning to optimize extraction processes or develop more efficient biosynthetic pathways, AI could contribute to the reduction of costs and environmental impact associated with polysaccharide manufacturing (Singh et al., 2022). For instance, AI models could identify more sustainable raw materials, such as plant-based polysaccharides, and improve processes for converting biomass into commercially viable products. The combination of AI with green chemistry principles could lead to the development of highly efficient and eco-friendly polysaccharide-based materials for various biomedical and environmental applications.

Another exciting area of development is biodegradable electronics, a field that intersects with polysaccharide-based polymers in the design of environmentally friendly electronic devices. Polysaccharides like chitosan, alginate, and cellulose derivatives have been explored as components in biodegradable electronic materials due to their natural abundance, biocompatibility, and ability to degrade without leaving toxic residues. Recent studies have demonstrated that polysaccharide-based films and hydrogels can be used as substrates, flexible conductors, or insulators in biodegradable electronics, making them suitable for applications such as disposable medical sensors, bioelectronics, and environmentally friendly packaging (Liu et al., 2020; Lee et al., 2021).

Biodegradable electronics are particularly promising in the medical field, where electronic devices are often used for monitoring, diagnostic, or therapeutic purposes. Bioelectronics made from polysaccharides could eliminate the need for traditional electronic waste disposal methods, which often result in pollution. The future of this field involves designing fully biodegradable, high-performance electronic systems that can dissolve or degrade safely after use, reducing environmental impact (Patel et al., 2022).

Conclusion and Future Outlook

While polysaccharide-based biomaterials show immense promise in various biomedical applications, they still face significant challenges in terms of production scalability, regulatory approval, and cost-effectiveness. The ongoing advancement of AI-based design methods and biodegradable electronics presents exciting opportunities to overcome some of these challenges. The integration of AI into the development of polysaccharide materials will enhance their customization and efficiency, while biodegradable electronics could pave the way for more sustainable medical and technological innovations. As research continues and novel solutions emerge, the future of polysaccharide-based polymers holds great potential in improving patient care and advancing medical technologies.

SUMMARY

Polysaccharide-based polymers, such as chitosan, alginate, hyaluronic acid, and cellulose derivatives, are revolutionizing the world of wound healing and biomedical applications. These natural wonders offer a range of benefits over synthetic polymers, from superior tissue regeneration and moisture retention to impressive antibacterial action. With their unique ability to promote healing, polysaccharides are becoming go-to materials for advanced wound care solutions. Cutting-edge modifications, like crosslinking for added strength and stimuli-responsive properties, are elevating these materials to new heights, while the incorporation of bioactive agents, such as growth factors, makes them even more effective and adaptable. Additionally, advanced fabrication techniques, including nanofiber mats, 3D bioprinting, and injectable hydrogels, are setting the stage for custom-tailored, next-generation wound dressings.

While the future is bright for polysaccharide-based biomaterials, challenges such as scalable production, regulatory complexities, and cost-efficiency remain. However, the emerging trend of AI-driven design is unlocking new possibilities for optimizing these materials, helping to overcome barriers and accelerate innovation. Looking ahead, the potential of biodegradable electronics, integrated with polysaccharides, offers exciting new avenues for sustainable medical solutions. With the addition of smart features like self-healing properties and biosensors, the next generation of polysaccharide-based wound care products promises to be more efficient, responsive, and environmentally friendly. As research continues to push boundaries, these biomaterials will undoubtedly become key players in advancing healthcare and shaping the future of medical technology.

REFERENCES

Ali, R., Ali, M., Nisar, S., Ahmad, T., & Mahmood, A. (2022). Fabrication of carboxymethyl cellulose-silver nanoparticle composite hydrogel for infected wound healing applications. *International Journal of Biological Macromolecules, 201*, 408–417. DOI: 10.1016/j.ijbiomac.2022.03.045

Chen, G., Yu, Y., Wu, Y., Zeng, Y., & Liu, J. (2022). Applications of hyaluronic acid-based hydrogels for skin wound healing: A comprehensive review. *International Journal of Biological Macromolecules, 208*, 518–529. DOI: 10.1016/j.ijbiomac.2022.03.029

Damiri, F., Fatimi, A., Santos, A. C. P., Varma, R. S., & Berrada, M. (2023). Smart stimuli-responsive chitosan hydrogel for drug delivery: A review. *Journal of Materials Chemistry. B, 11*(1), 10538–10565. DOI: 10.1039/D3TB01712E PMID: 37909361

Darouiche, R. O.. (2020). Alginate-based wound dressings: A randomized controlled trial in chronic wound management. *Journal of Wound Care, 29*(6), 353–362. DOI: 10.12968/jowc.2020.29.6.353

Fang, Y., Egorov, M., Behnisch, J., & Yang, F. (2021). Hyaluronic acid in skin wound healing. *Polymers, 13*(12), 2104. DOI: 10.3390/polym13122104

Fang, Z., Lin, T., Fan, S., Qiu, X., Zhong, Z., Yang, G., Yang, J., Zhang, G., Feng, Y., Ai, F., Shi, Q., & Wan, W. (2023). Antibacterial, injectable, and adhesive hydrogel promotes skin healing. *Frontiers in Bioengineering and Biotechnology, 11*, 1180073. DOI: 10.3389/fbioe.2023.1180073 PMID: 37334269

Feng, Q., Li, Y., Yang, Y., Zhang, Z., & Xiao, B. (2019). Injectable and self-healing polysaccharide-based hydrogels for hemostasis and wound healing. *Frontiers in Bioengineering and Biotechnology, 7*, 288. DOI: 10.3389/fbioe.2019.00288

Gao, J.. (2021). Artificial intelligence in the design and optimization of biomaterials for medical applications. *Materials Science and Engineering R Reports, 145*, 100426. DOI: 10.1016/j.mser.2020.100426

Gao, Z., Golland, B., Tronci, G., & Thornton, P. D. (2021). A redox-responsive hyaluronic acid-based hydrogel for chronic wound management. *arXiv*. https://arxiv.org/abs/2101.01638

Hajimiri, M., Shahverdi, A., Oryan, A., Mohammadi, A. A., & Bandegi, A. R. (2020). A review on dextran hydrogels: Synthesis, properties, and biomedical applications. *Carbohydrate Polymers, 232*, 115800. DOI: 10.1016/j.carbpol.2019.115800

He, W., Ma, Z., Wang, Z., Zheng, Y., Sun, Y., & Wang, Y. (2021). A multifunctional hydrogel dressing with pH-responsive drug release, antioxidant and antibacterial activities for chronic wound healing. *Materials Science and Engineering C, 124*, 112019. DOI: 10.1016/j.msec.2021.112019

Jiang, Y., Liu, Z., Guo, S., Zhang, Y., & Huang, Y. (2023). Thermosensitive chitosan-based hydrogels for controlled drug delivery and wound healing. *Carbohydrate Polymers, 301*, 120347. DOI: 10.1016/j.carbpol.2022.120347

Karami, Z.. (2019). Polysaccharide-based biomaterials: Challenges in commercial production. *Biomaterials Science*, *7*(12), 3856–3869. DOI: 10.1039/C9BM01194F

Khalid, A., Bai, D., & Abraham, A.. (2020). Electrospun nanodiamond-silk fibroin membranes: A multifunctional platform for biosensing and wound healing applications. *arXiv*. https://arxiv.org/abs/2006.00614

Lee, J. H.. (2020). Efficacy of hyaluronic acid in the treatment of osteoarthritis: A systematic review and meta-analysis. *Journal of Clinical Medicine*, *9*(8), 2480. DOI: 10.3390/jcm9082480 PMID: 32748835

Lee, K. Y.. (2021). Biodegradable electronics based on polysaccharide-based materials for medical applications. *Nature Communications*, *12*, 1459. DOI: 10.1038/s41467-021-21606-0

Liu, M., Jin, J., Zhong, X., Liu, L., Tang, C., & Cai, L. (2023). Polysaccharide hydrogels for skin wound healing. *Heliyon*, *9*(3), e12999. DOI: 10.1016/j.heliyon.2023.e12999 PMID: 39144923

Liu, M., Jin, J., Zhong, X., Liu, L., Tang, C., & Cai, L. (2024). Polysaccharide hydrogels for skin wound healing. *Heliyon*, *10*(15), e35014. DOI: 10.1016/j.heliyon.2024.e35014 PMID: 39144923

Liu, M., Zhang, X., Yang, H., Yang, Q., & Wei, X. (2020). Dextran-based injectable hydrogels embedded with quercetin for promoting chronic wound healing. *ACS Omega*, *5*(17), 9642–9649. DOI: 10.1021/acsomega.0c00374

Liu, S.. (2020). Polysaccharide-based materials for biodegradable bioelectronics: Progress and prospects. *Biomaterials*, *237*, 119822. DOI: 10.1016/j.biomaterials.2020.119822

López, J. A.. (2021). Clinical trial of Hyalofill® in the treatment of venous leg ulcers: A prospective randomized study. *The Journal of Dermatological Treatment*, *32*(2), 173–181. DOI: 10.1080/09546634.2021.1870736

Mo, X., Zhang, L., & Zhang, Y. (2021). Polysaccharide-based hydrogels: New insights and futuristic prospects in wound healing. *PubMed.* https://pubmed.ncbi.nlm.nih.gov/36395945/

Moghadam, A. M.. (2020). Chitosan nanoparticles for controlled delivery of antibiotics in wound infections: A clinical approach. *Pharmaceutical Development and Technology*, *25*(5), 543–552. DOI: 10.1080/10837450.2020.1751294

Mohammad, M.. (2021). Biocompatibility and production of polysaccharide-based biomaterials for wound healing applications. *Journal of Biomaterials Science. Polymer Edition*, *32*(10), 1335–1346. DOI: 10.1080/09205063.2021.1923181

Nguyen Le, N.-M., Le-Vinh, B., Friedl, J. D., Jalil, A., & Kali, G. (2022). Polyaminated pullulan, a new biodegradable and cationic pullulan derivative for mucosal drug delivery. *Carbohydrate Polymers*, *277*, 118848. DOI: 10.1016/j.carbpol.2021.118848

Patel, A.. (2022). Bioelectronics and biodegradable sensors: Future prospects of polysaccharide-based materials. *Journal of Electronic Materials*, *51*(7), 3567–3584. DOI: 10.1007/s11664-022-09409-1

Patel, M., Gade, S., & Jadhav, P. (2020). Cellulose-based dressings for wound healing applications: A review. *Materials Today: Proceedings*, *33*, 2987–2993. DOI: 10.1016/j.matpr.2020.02.604

Qian, Y., Lin, X., Sun, Y., Wang, J., & Zhao, Y. (2022). Self-healing hydrogels with antibacterial and antioxidant activities based on dynamic Schiff base linkages for wound healing. *International Journal of Biological Macromolecules*, *213*, 321–331. DOI: 10.1016/j.ijbiomac.2022.07.153

Ranjbar-Mohammadi, M., & Bahrami, S. H. (2018). Alginate-based wound dressings: Recent advances and future perspectives. *Carbohydrate Polymers*, *206*, 473–488. DOI: 10.1016/j.carbpol.2018.11.035

Ryu, W. H.. (2017). Clinical evaluation of chitosan-based wound dressing in diabetic foot ulcers: A randomized controlled trial. *Diabetes Research and Clinical Practice*, *126*, 117–123. DOI: 10.1016/j.diabres.2017.01.027

Salmaso, S., & Caliceti, P. (2021). Pullulan-based bioconjugates for ocular drug delivery. *European Journal of Pharmaceutical Sciences*, *158*, 105667. DOI: 10.1016/j.ejps.2021.105667

Singh, S.. (2022). Artificial intelligence in green chemistry: Designing sustainable polysaccharides for biomedical applications. *Green Chemistry*, *24*(2), 512–523. DOI: 10.1039/D1GC03982A

Soni, N. S.. (2021). Chitosan-based hydrogels in the treatment of chronic diabetic ulcers: A clinical trial. *Biomaterials Science*, *9*(4), 633–644. DOI: 10.1039/D0BM02180D

Tan, G., Wang, L., Pan, W., & Chen, K. (2022). Polysaccharide electrospun nanofibers for wound healing applications. *International Journal of Nanomedicine*, *17*, 3913–3931. DOI: 10.2147/IJN.S371900 PMID: 36097445

Tao, Y., Li, J., Hu, W., & Zhou, X. (2023). Advances in ionically crosslinked polysaccharide hydrogels for biomedical applications. *Gels (Basel, Switzerland)*, *9*(3), 206. DOI: 10.3390/gels9030206 PMID: 36975655

Tottoli, E. M.. (2020). Alginate-based dressings in chronic wound care: A review of their properties and clinical applications. *Journal of Applied Biomaterials & Functional Materials*, *18*(1), 1–10. DOI: 10.1177/2280800019900693

Wang, J., Wang, X., Yuan, X., & Zhang, W. (2021). Bioactive hyaluronic acid-based hydrogel loaded with VEGF for promoting diabetic wound healing. *Materials Science and Engineering C*, *120*, 111719. DOI: 10.1016/j.msec.2020.111719

Wang, J., Wang, X., Yuan, X., & Zhang, W. (2024). Recent advances in 3D bioprinted polysaccharide hydrogels for biomedical applications: A comprehensive review. *International Wound Journal*. Advance online publication. DOI: 10.1111/iwj.14533 PMID: 38069620

Wang, L., Mu, Y., Xu, M., & Gao, J. (2021). Recent advances of chitosan-based injectable hydrogels for wound healing. *Journal of Materials Chemistry. B*, *9*(15), 3279–3291. DOI: 10.1039/D0TB02785B

Wang, R., Chen, M., Pan, W., Chu, Y., & Chen, F. (2025). The design principle of natural polysaccharide hydrogels for promoting wound healing: A prospective review. *Journal of Materials Chemistry. B*. Advance online publication. DOI: 10.1039/D4TB02576H PMID: 40145143

Wang, Y., Zhang, X., & Wei, X. (2024). Recent advances in polysaccharide-based hydrogels for controlled delivery of therapeutic biomolecules. *ACS Biomaterials Science & Engineering*, *10*(1), 1–15. DOI: 10.1021/acsbiomaterials.0c01784 PMID: 38186359

Wu, Y.. (2020). 3D printing of alginate-based scaffolds for cartilage tissue engineering. *Materials Science and Engineering C*, *116*, 111198. DOI: 10.1016/j.msec.2020.111198

Xuan, H., Wu, S., Fei, S., Li, B., Yang, Y., & Yuan, H. (2021). Injectable nanofiber-polysaccharide self-healing hydrogels for wound healing. *Materials Science and Engineering C, 128*, 112264. DOI: 10.1016/j.msec.2021.112264 PMID: 34474823

Yamaguchi, N.. (2019). Hyaluronic acid-based hydrogel dressings for burn wound healing: A clinical evaluation. *Journal of Burn Care & Research; Official Publication of the American Burn Association, 40*(4), 512–518. DOI: 10.1093/jbcr/iry047

Yang, G., Xiao, Z., Ren, X., Long, H., & Qian, H. (2021). Redox-responsive hydrogels for drug delivery and tissue engineering applications. *Reactive & Functional Polymers, 163*, 104895. DOI: 10.1016/j.reactfunctpolym.2021.104895

Yang, J., & Wang, S. (2023). Polysaccharide-based multifunctional hydrogel bio-adhesives for wound healing: A review. *Gels (Basel, Switzerland), 9*(2), 138. DOI: 10.3390/gels9020138 PMID: 36826308

Zhang, L., Zhang, Y., & Zhang, L. (2023). Exploring the potential of polysaccharide-based hybrid hydrogel systems for their biomedical and therapeutic applications: A review. *International Journal of Biological Macromolecules, 256*, 128348. DOI: 10.1016/j.ijbiomac.2023.128348 PMID: 38007021

Zhang, X., Zhang, Z., & Zhang, L. (2020). Rational design and latest advances of polysaccharide-based hydrogels for wound healing. *Biomaterials Science, 8*(8), 2040–2055. DOI: 10.1039/D0BM00055H PMID: 32118241

Zhao, Y.. (2020). Regulatory hurdles for polysaccharide-based biomaterials in wound care: Challenges and solutions. *Biomaterials, 235*, 119758. DOI: 10.1016/j.biomaterials.2020.119758

Zhou, X., Zhang, X., & Zhang, L. (2024). A review of recent advances of cellulose-based intelligent-responsive hydrogels as vehicles for controllable drug delivery system. *International Journal of Biological Macromolecules, 264*, 130525. DOI: 10.1016/j.ijbiomac.2024.130525 PMID: 38431004

Chapter 6
Application of Herbal Excipients and Polymers in Wound Healing:
Herbal Oil, Gums, and Resins

Yogita Dhurandhar
https://orcid.org/0009-0003-9825-1026
Guru Ghasidas Vishwavidyal, India

Jeevan Lal Prajapati
Guru Ghasidas Vishwavidyalaya, India

Aspee Singh
Guru Ghasidas Vishwavidyalaya, India

Shubham Tomar
Central Drugs Standard Control Organisation, New Delhi, India

Kamta Prasad Namdeo
Guru Ghasidas Vishwavidyalaya, India

ABSTRACT

Wound healing is a complex biological process involving a cascade of cellular and molecular mechanisms. Recently, natural polymers and herbal excipients have gained attention due to their biocompatibility, therapeutic properties, and low toxicity. This chapter explores the potential of plant-derived gums, natural resins, and herbal oils in wound care. Oils like neem, tea tree, coconut, and calendula exhibit strong anti-bacterial, anti-inflammatory, and antioxidant actions, aiding in cleansing, infection control, and tissue repair. They also enhance collagen synthesis and hydration.

DOI: 10.4018/979-8-3373-3977-1.ch006

Plant gums such as acacia, guar, and tragacanth support drug delivery, moisture retention, and film formation. Natural resins like myrrh, frankincense, and benzoin offer antimicrobial, astringent, and wound-sealing benefits. Their pharmacological properties, formulation roles, and potential in modern wound care systems are discussed. These agents represent a promising bridge between traditional herbal wisdom and scientific advancement in wound healing.

INTRODUCTION TO WOUND HEALING AND NATURAL THERAPEUTICS

One essential physiological process that repairs damaged tissues' integrity and functionality is wound healing. Each of the overlapping phases of this dynamic and highly controlled process hemostasis, inflammation, proliferation, and remodeling is influenced by complex cellular and molecular interactions. The skin's protective barrier function, which protects the body from infection, dehydration, and environmental dangers, depends on wound healing that is effective. But this process can be hampered by a number of internal and environmental conditions, including aging, infections, diabetes, and malnutrition, which frequently leads to chronic wounds or delayed healing (Schultz et al., 2011). Natural therapies have gained popularity in recent years as a substitute for or addition to traditional wound care methods. In addition to their long history in traditional medicine, natural products made from plants, minerals, and bees are currently receiving more attention and validation from contemporary science. Because of their accessibility, affordability, and biocompatibility, as well as their multipurpose qualities that can promote wound healing while reducing adverse effects, these agents are frequently preferred. Natural remedies that have demonstrated encouraging wound-healing qualities include honey, Aloe vera, curcumin, Centella asiatica, Calendula officinalis, and tea tree oil (Shedoeva et al., 2019). The antibacterial and anti-inflammatory properties of honey, especially Manuka honey, encourage tissue regeneration and keep wounds moist. Curcumin promotes collagen synthesis and fibroblast activity, whereas aloe vera is calming, moisturizing, and collagen-stimulating. While Calendula officinalis is antibacterial and tissue-regenerative, Centella asiatica promotes collagen production and angiogenesis. In infected wounds, tea tree oil lowers inflammation. The application of these natural remedies in topical formulations and sophisticated wound care systems is growing (Mandal & Mandal, 2011).

MECHANISM OF WOUND HEALING: A BRIEF OVERVIEW

The process of wound healing is a biological process that involves the restoration of the integrity of the skin or tissue after an injury has occurred. This process relies on careful orchestration. Hemostasis, inflammation, proliferation, and remodeling (or maturation) are the four main phases that can be generically separated into this complex process. Additionally, these phases overlap with one another. In each phase, there are particular cellular and molecular events that contribute to the healing and regeneration of the damaged tissue. These events set the stage for the subsequent phases. Hemostasis, which happens right after the damage, is the first step in the process. The body starts vasoconstriction to stop blood loss when blood vessels are injured. Platelets cling to the exposed collagen in the injured vessel walls after rapidly aggregating at the site of injury (Wallace et al., 2023). A fibrin clot forms as a result of the coagulation cascade being triggered by chemical signals released by these platelets. In addition to halting the bleeding, this clot offers incoming cells that are necessary for the healing process a temporary scaffold. The inflammatory phase, which usually lasts a few days to several hours, comes after hemostasis. In this stage, immune cells like neutrophils and monocytes can enter the wound site because the previously narrowed blood arteries enlarge. Through phagocytosis, neutrophils are essential in removing infections and cellular debris from the wound. Monocyte-derived macrophages take over as the predominant cell type in inflammation. By producing cytokines and growth factors that promote the subsequent stage of healing, these macrophages play a crucial role in coordinating the shift from inflammation to tissue repair. Depending on the degree of the wound, the proliferative phase may extend for a few weeks following the injury onset (LaPelusa & Dave, 2023). The extracellular matrix (ECM) and collagen components that make up the structural framework of new tissue are produced by the proliferation of fibroblasts during this stage. To give the healing tissue nutrition and oxygen, angiogenesis the growth of new blood vessels is induced. The process of re-epithelialization occurs when keratinocytes, or epithelial cells, move across the wound bed to repair the epidermis. Granulation tissue a transient matrix full of fibroblasts, endothelial cells, and extracellular matrix proteins starts to form in the wound, promoting tissue regeneration. Last but not least, the remodeling phase, which can last anywhere from a few weeks to many months, aims to restore the tissue's strength and functionality (Diller & Tabor, 2022). The wound's tensile strength is increased during this phase when stronger type I collagen gradually replaces the initially deposited collagen type III. As superfluous capillaries retreat, the area's blood vessel density decreases. Once their functions are completed, fibroblasts and other cells go through apoptosis, which reorganizes the extracellular matrix to resemble the original tissue structure. Depending on the extent of the incision and the effectiveness of the healing process, the result could be either scar formation or full tissue regeneration (Schultz et al., 2011).

ROLE OF EXCIPIENTS AND POLYMERS IN WOUND HEALING

In contemporary wound care, improving the healing process requires the creation of potent topical formulations and sophisticated delivery technologies. The design of these formulations relies heavily on excipients and polymers, which enhance the therapeutic efficacy, stability, and bioavailability of active wound-healing agents. Despite being regarded as inert chemicals in the past, excipients have important roles in wound healing, including promoting drug penetration, creating protective barriers, hydrating, and regulating the release of active drugs (Sheokand et al., 2023). The use of natural and synthetic polymers in drug delivery systems and wound dressings is also common because they offer structural support and functional advantages that promote tissue regeneration. Humectants, such as glycerin and propylene glycol, are frequently used excipients in wound healing formulations because they preserve moisture and prevent wound desiccation; emulsifiers, such as lecithin and polysorbates, ensure the stability of creams and ointments; and preservatives, such as parabens or benzyl alcohol, prevent microbial contamination. Therapeutic compounds can more efficiently reach deeper tissue layers when certain excipients serve as penetration enhancers (Satchanska et al., 2024). Excipients have a little but important role in the healing process by keeping the wound environment wet, hygienic, and favorable for cell migration. Contrarily, polymers are necessary for the production of several wound care products, such as hydrogels, films, foams, sponges, and nanofiber scaffolds. These substances may be designed to assist cell adhesion, regulate the release of medicinal substances, and resemble the extracellular matrix (ECM). The biocompatibility, biodegradability, and inherent biological activity of natural polymers including chitosan, alginate, gelatin, and hyaluronic acid make them popular. For example, seaweed-derived alginate generates hydrogels that absorb wound exudate and encourage granulation, whereas chitosan demonstrates antibacterial and hemostatic qualities. Synthetic polymers with exceptional mechanical strength, such as polyvinyl alcohol (PVA), polyethylene glycol (PEG), and polylactic acid (PLA), can be altered to provide particular release patterns or rates of degradation (Gounden & Singh, 2024). Furthermore, the ability of smart polymers that react to temperature, pH, or enzymes to release pharmaceuticals in a regulated and responsive manner is drawing attention. This could improve focused therapy and reduce systemic adverse effects. These polymers can be coupled with bioactive substances to provide advanced wound dressings that actively aid in healing by supporting tissue regeneration, providing prolonged drug administration, and acting as an antibacterial. These dressings also protect and hydrate the wound (Thang et al., 2023).

OVERVIEW OF HERBAL-BASED EXCIPIENTS AND POLYMERS

Herbal-Based Excipients

Inactive chemicals that are produced from plants are known as herbal-based excipients. These herbal-based excipients are utilized in medicine formulations to assist in the processing, transport, or stability of the active pharmaceutical ingredients (Table 1).

Herbal-Based Polymers

Polymers derived from herbs are macromolecules that bind, thicken, form films, and act as controlled-release agents. These polymers are acquired from natural sources and serve a variety of functional purposes (Kalpana Manivannan et al., 2024).

Table 1. Common examples of herbal-based excipients and polymers

Natural Source	Excipients/Polymers	Pharmaceutical role
Plantago ovata (psyllium)	Mucilage	Binder, disintegrant
Hibiscus esculentus (okra)	Polysaccharides	Sustained-release agent
Tamarindus indica (tamarind)	Tamarind seed polysaccharide	Mucoadhesive, thickener
Trigonella foenum-graecum (fenugreek)	Galactomannan	Gelling agent
Grewia gum	Mucilage	Emulsifier, binder
Aloe vera	Gel polysaccharides	Film-former, moisturizer
Acacia (Gum arabic)	Natural gum	Emulsifying agent, binder
Sterculia urens (karaya gum)	Polysaccharide	Controlled-release matrix

HERBAL OILS IN WOUND HEALING

The high concentration of bioactive chemicals that herbal oils contain, including flavonoids, terpenoids, alkaloids, tannins, and vital fatty acids, makes them an essential component in the process of wound healing. A wide variety of pharmacological actions, such as anti-inflammatory, antibacterial, antioxidant, and analgesic effects, are exhibited by these natural components (table 2). Collectively, these activities contribute to the faster and more effective regeneration of wounds. Herbal oils, when applied topically, form a barrier that protects the wound from getting infected by microorganisms and avoiding the loss of moisture. Additionally, they encourage the regeneration of skin tissues (Cedillo-Cortezano et al., 2024).

Therapeutic Properties & Mechanism of Action of Herbal Oils

Antimicrobial Action

Terpinen-4-ol, azadirachtin, and thymol are among the substances found in many herbal oils, including tea tree, neem, and thyme oils, that cause microbial cell membranes to rupture. By lowering the microbial burden at the wound site, this action stops infection and permits the body's natural healing processes to continue (Mondello et al., 2022).

Anti-Inflammatory Effect

By inhibiting enzymes like COX-2 and modulating pro-inflammatory cytokines like IL-1, IL-6, and TNF-α, herbal oils help to reduce edema and inflammation. Sesquiterpenes and flavonoids found in oils like chamomile, eucalyptus, and lavender help control the inflammatory response and reduce tissue damage (Horváth et al., 2022).

Antioxidant Activity

By harming cells and extracellular matrix constituents, reactive oxygen species (ROS) can impede the healing process. Antioxidants (such as tocopherols and polyphenols) found in herbal oils like calendula and rosemary scavenge ROS, protecting tissues and promoting cellular repair (Ukaegbu et al., 2025).

Promotion of Fibroblast Proliferation and Collagen Synthesis

Oils that promote fibroblast activity and increase the production of type I and III collagen both necessary for wound tensile strength and tissue regeneration include calendula and gotu kola (Centella asiatica). This promotes granulation tissue development and re-epithelialization (Witkowska et al., 2024).

Angiogenesis Stimulation

In order to provide nutrition and oxygen to the healing tissue, several herbal oils promote angiogenesis, the development of new blood vessels. Compounds in oils like frankincense and turmeric boost vascular endothelial growth factor (VEGF), which is one growth factor that is modulated to help achieve this (Johnson & Wilgus, 2014).

Moisture Retention and Barrier Formation

Herbal oils' high lipid content contributes to the preservation of a moist environment, which promotes the migration of epithelial cells and rapid wound healing. They create a semi-occlusive coating that keeps the wound wet while shielding it from outside impurities (Saporito et al., 2017).

Table 2. Commonly used herbal oils

Herbal Oil	Source Plant	Primary Health Benefits
Tea Tree Oil	*Melaleuca alternifolia*	Antibacterial, antifungal, acne treatment, supports wound healing
Lavender Oil	*Lavandula angustifolia*	Calming, promotes sleep, relieves stress and anxiety, soothes burns and insect bites
Peppermint Oil	*Mentha piperita*	Aids digestion, relieves headaches, boosts energy, helps with respiratory issues
Eucalyptus Oil	*Eucalyptus globulus*	Decongestant, relieves coughs, antimicrobial, reduces muscle pain
Rosemary Oil	*Rosmarinus officinalis*	Improves memory and concentration, promotes hair growth, anti-inflammatory
Chamomile Oil	*Matricaria chamomilla / Chamaemelum nobile*	Anti-inflammatory, calming, good for skin irritation and anxiety
Frankincense Oil	*Boswellia serrata*	Reduces stress, boosts immunity, promotes cellular health, anti-aging for skin
Clove Oil	*Syzygium aromaticum*	Pain relief (especially dental), antimicrobial, aids digestion

continued on following page

Table 2. Continued

Herbal Oil	Source Plant	Primary Health Benefits
Lemon Oil	*Citrus limon*	Detoxifying, improves mood, antibacterial, supports digestion
Oregano Oil	*Origanum vulgare*	Antiviral, antifungal, supports immune system, strong antimicrobial properties
Basil Oil	*Ocimum basilicum*	Mental clarity, reduces stress, relieves respiratory problems
Ginger Oil	*Zingiber officinale*	Reduces inflammation, aids digestion, improves circulation
Thyme Oil	*Thymus vulgaris*	Antimicrobial, respiratory support, immune booster
Cinnamon Oil	*Cinnamomum zeylanicum*	Antibacterial, boosts circulation, helps control blood sugar
Neem Oil	*Azadirachta indica*	Skin health, antifungal, anti-inflammatory, insect repellent

Formulation Approaches

Herbal oils have emerged as attractive natural agents in contemporary pharmaceutical and cosmeceutical formulations owing to their diverse therapeutic characteristics. These oils, derived from diverse plant parts, are abundant in bioactive ingredients including terpenes, flavonoids, and phenolic compounds, which have antibacterial, anti-inflammatory, antioxidant, and wound-healing properties (table 3). With customer demand increasingly favoring safer, natural alternatives, herbal oils provide a biocompatible and environmentally sustainable choice for formulation scientists. Herbal oils are useful excipients that improve skin penetration, act as emollients, or act as natural preservatives in topical administration systems in addition to being active agents. Their flexibility in formulation science is demonstrated by their inclusion into a range of dosage forms, including ointments, gels, creams, emulsions, and nanoformulations. In order to create natural and efficient healthcare solutions, this chapter examines novel formulation techniques that make use of herbal oils, emphasising their physicochemical functions, stability issues, and therapeutic contributions.

Table 3. Formulation approaches using herbal oils

S.no	Formulation Type	Description	Common Herbal Oils Used	Therapeutic application
1	Massage Oils	Herbal oils diluted in carrier oils for therapeutic body massage.	Lavender, Peppermint, Rosemary, Eucalyptus	Muscle relaxation, stress relief, pain relief
2	Aromatherapy Blends	Essential oils used in diffusers or inhalers to affect mood or respiratory health	Lavender, Eucalyptus, Lemon, Frankincense	tress, insomnia, respiratory issues
3	Balms & Ointments	Thickened oil-based formulations with beeswax or shea butter for topical application.	Tea Tree, Clove, Chamomile, Neem	Skin infections, burns, wounds, eczema
4	Creams & Lotions	Emulsions of oil and water phases, often including herbal oils for skin therapy.	Calendula, Chamomile, Neem, Lavender	Moisturizing, anti-aging, dermatitis, sunburn relief
5	Hair Oils and Serums	Herbal oils blended with base oils to nourish scalp and promote hair health.	Rosemary, Amla, Brahmi, Tea Tree	Hair growth, dandruff control, scalp nourishment
6	Bath Oils	Oils added to bathwater to enhance relaxation and skin moisturization.	Lavender, Rose, Ylang-Ylang, Chamomile	Stress relief, skin softening, aromatherapy
7	Oral Care Products	Oils incorporated into mouthwashes or toothpaste for antimicrobial benefits.	Clove, Peppermint, Tea Tree	Gum health, fresh breath, oral infections
8	Inhalers & Steam Therapy	Oils used in steam or portable inhalers for sinus relief and respiratory support.	Eucalyptus, Peppermint, Oregano	Congestion, cold relief, asthma
9	Capsules & Softgel	Herbal oils encapsulated for internal use	Oregano, Ginger, Turmeric oil	Immunity boost, inflammation, digestive aid
10	Sprays	Herbal oils diluted in water/ alcohol base for room or body sprays.	Lemon, Lavender, Peppermint	Air purification, deodorizing, mood enhancement

PLANT GUMS IN WOUND HEALING

Natural biopolymers called plant gums have demonstrated encouraging potential in wound healing applications because of their distinct biological and physicochemical characteristics. When a tree or shrub is injured or under stress from the environment, it usually produces exudates. Because of their capacity to create viscous solutions or gels, as well as their biocompatibility and biodegradability, they are perfect for use in biomedical applications, especially in the creation of drug delivery systems and wound dressings (Table 4). These natural materials can help speed up the healing process by keeping the wound site wet, encouraging cell growth, and acting as carriers for antibacterial and therapeutic chemicals (Table 5).

Table 4. Plant gums in wound healing: mechanism of action, benefits, and purposes

S.no	Mechanism of action	Description	Benefits
1	Moisture Retention	Gums are highly hydrophilic, forming gels that retain moisture at the wound site.	Promoting faster epithelial cell migration, preventing scab formation, Enhancing tissue regeneration
2	Barrier Formation	When applied to wounds, plant gums can form a protective physical film or hydrogel layer	Shields the wound from microbial invasion and environmental contaminants, minimizes mechanical trauma, Prevents dehydration of the wound surface
3	Cell Proliferation and Migration	Some gums, due to their polysaccharide nature, can support cell adhesion and stimulate the migration of fibroblasts and keratinocytes, which are crucial for tissue repair and skin regeneration	Tissue repair and skin regeneration
4	Controlled Drug Delivery	Gums can serve as carriers for antibiotics, anti-inflammatory agents, and growth factors, allowing for sustained and targeted release of therapeutic agents at the wound site.	Therapeutic benfits
5	Antioxidant and Anti-inflammatory Effects	Many gums possess intrinsic bioactivity, such as scavenging free radicals and reducing inflammation, which supports the overall healing process	Enhancing tissue regeneration

Characteristics and Sources of Natural Gums

- **Biocompatibility**: They are non-toxic and generally safe for direct application on skin and wounds (Hamdani et al., 2019).
- **Hydrophilicity**: Gums have high water-holding capacity, helping to maintain a moist wound environment, which is critical for optimal healing (Hamdani et al., 2019).
- **Film-Forming Ability**: They can form protective films or gels over wounds, acting as physical barriers to microbial contamination (Hamdani et al., 2019).
- **Biodegradability**: Plant gums naturally degrade over time without causing harm, making them eco-friendly and safe (Hamdani et al., 2019).
- **Bioadhesiveness**: Many plant gums can adhere well to biological tissues, improving their effectiveness in wound dressing applications (Hamdani et al., 2019).

Table 5. Natural gum and its roles

S.no	Natural gum	Sources	Therapeutic role
1	Gum Acacia	*Acacia senegal*	Soothing, film-forming, anti-inflammatory
2	Gum Tragacanth	*Astragalus gummifer*	Thickening, bioadhesive, wound protection
3	Gum Karaya	*Sterculia urens*	Absorbent, swellable, good for burn and exudative wounds
4	Guar Gum	*Cyamopsis tetragonoloba*	Gelling, used as a matrix for drug release in wound dressings
5	Xanthan Gum	*Xanthomonas campestris*	Stabilizing, moisturizing, used in hydrogel formulations
6	Locust Bean Gum	*Ceratonia siliqua*	Moisture retention, supportive in hydrogel dressings

Gum-Based Hydrogels and Films

Innovative biomaterials called gum-based hydrogels and films are made from natural plant or microbial gums and have demonstrated great potential in the treatment of wounds. In addition to being biodegradable and biocompatible, these materials can be developed to have certain physical, chemical, and biological characteristics that make them appropriate for use in wound care (Table 6). Three-dimensional networks of hydrophilic polymers that can hold a lot of water are called hydrogels. Hydrogels are created when gums like xanthan, guar, or gellan gum are crosslinked; these hydrogels can support tissue regeneration and keep wounds moist. Films are sheets of gum-based material that are applied thinly to the wound site. They serve as barriers that keep out germs and stop moisture loss while accelerating the healing process (Kaur et al., 2024).

Table 6. Gum-based hydrogels and its properties

S.no	Types of gum	Properties
1	Xanthan Gum	Offers good viscosity and is often combined with other polymers for mechanical strength
2	Guar Gum	its swelling ability and used in hydrogel formulations.
3	Gellan Gum	Forms stable gels and is used in both hydrogels and films for its flexibility and stability
4	Locust Bean Gum	Enhances film-forming capacity and mechanical strength.
5	Tragacanth Gum and Gum Arabic	Biocompatible and used for their emulsifying and film-forming properties.

Applications in Wound Healing

- **Acute Wounds:** For minor cuts and abrasions, gum-based films provide a protective layer (Abdi et al., 2024).
- **Chronic Wounds:** Such as diabetic ulcers or pressure sores, where sustained drug delivery and a moist environment are crucial (Abdi et al., 2024).
- **Burns:** Hydrogels soothe and cool the skin, maintain hydration, and reduce infection risk.
- **Post-surgical Sites:** Offer controlled healing with minimal scarring (Abdi et al., 2024).

NATURAL RESINS IN WOUND MANAGEMENT

Resins that are naturally occurring are substances that are semi-solid, sticky, and primarily made of terpenoids and phenolic chemicals. When it comes to plants, they provide the function of a protective barrier, preventing infection and closing wounds. They also provide extra therapeutic benefits when applied to human wounds, which allows them to replicate the defensive role that they provide. Natural resins aid in the healing of wounds through a variety of cooperative processes. Their ability to combat bacteria is one of their main functions (Sipponen et al., 2012). Resins like myrrh and propolis have shown broad-spectrum efficacy against fungi and bacteria, assisting in the prevention or management of wound infections. This lowers the possibility of complications and promotes a more hygienic healing environment. Furthermore, numerous resins exhibit significant anti-inflammatory characteristics that aid in reducing swelling, erythema, and discomfort. By diminishing the local inflammatory response, resins facilitate a more pleasant and stable milieu for tissue healing. Resins demonstrate significant antioxidant properties, allowing them to neutralize detrimental free radicals. This safeguards impaired cells from oxidative stress and facilitates accelerated tissue regeneration while minimizing scarring. Barrier formation is an additional benefit. When applied to a wound, resins frequently form a physical barrier that keeps out external pollutants and stops moisture loss, both of which are necessary to keep the healing environment wet and promote the migration of epithelial cells (El-Sakhawy et al., 2023).

Pharmacological Activities of Resins

Many plants, especially trees like conifers, naturally secrete complex mixtures of biologically active substances called resins. Usually, they are made of organic materials such as phenolic compounds, volatile oils, and resin acids. Resins have many pharmacological qualities that have been used in both conventional and modern medicine because of their rich chemical makeup. Antimicrobial activity is a major resin pharmacological activity. Resins have strong antibacterial, antifungal, and antiviral properties. This is due to volatile oils and phenolic chemicals disrupting microbial cell membranes and enzyme systems. Bee propolis has high antibacterial action against Staphylococcus aureus and Candida albicans. As an antiseptic, benzoin resin is commonly used to treat respiratory and skin infections (Dilworth et al., 2023). Resins are anti-inflammatory too. These are mostly due to their capacity to suppress prostaglandins and leukotrienes. Incense, made from Boswellia serrata resin, is a popular example. Boswellic acids inhibit leukotriene-producing 5-lipoxygenase. This makes Boswellia useful for treating arthritis, asthma, and IBD. Many resins are analgesic and anti-inflammatory. Their anti-inflammatory and central pain-modulating properties may explain these effects. Scientific research indicates the analgesic properties of frankincense and myrrh resins for joint and muscular pain.

Resins' antioxidant properties are also essential. Cancer, cardiovascular disease, and neurological diseases are connected to free radicals and oxidative stress (Siddiqui, 2011). Propolis and pine resin include flavonoids and phenolic acids that scavenge ROS and decrease oxidative damage, protecting against many illnesses. Resins exhibit interesting anticancer properties. Certain resin elements can cause apoptosis, prevent angiogenesis, and disrupt cancer cell signaling. Frankincense boswellic acids have been shown to kill glioma and leukemia cells in lab experiments. Propolis has anticancer efficacy in animal and in vitro models. Another area of study is resins' hepatoprotective (liver-protecting) properties. Resins can help shield the liver from oxidative stress and toxin-induced damage by modulating hepatic enzyme activity and exhibiting antioxidant qualities. Research has indicated that frankincense resin may help maintain liver health by protecting against chemically induced liver damage in animal models (Elumalai et al., 2022). Additionally, some resins have antiulcer and gastroprotective qualities. They aid in healing, lowering the production of gastric acid, and creating a protective coating over the stomach mucosa. Pistacia lentiscus is the source of mastic gum, a well-known resin that has long been used to treat Helicobacter pylori infections and peptic ulcers. Clinical settings are now acknowledging its beneficial effects on the gastrointestinal tract as well. Furthermore, because of their expectorant and antitussive (cough-suppressing) qualities, resins have long been used to treat respiratory conditions. They aid in the removal of mucus from the airways and soothe the mucous membranes. Because of their positive benefits on the respiratory system, benzoin and myrrh resins are frequently found in cough syrups and throat lozenges (Soulaidopoulos et al., 2022). Resins applied topically have shown promising results in skin regeneration and wound healing. Their antibacterial, anti-inflammatory, and tissue-regenerative properties are responsible for this. To promote quicker and cleaner wound healing, propolis and dragon's blood resin, for instance, are used in ointments and bandages for wounds, burns, and ulcers (Table 7). Additionally, resins have carminative and antispasmodic qualities that help ease flatulence, cramping, and spasms in the gastrointestinal tract. Because of its capacity to relax smooth muscles and release gas, asafoetida, a resin derived from the Ferula plant, has long been used to treat digestive issues (Table 8) (J. Yang et al., 2022).

Table 7 Examples of resin in wound management

S.no	Resin Type	Origin	Key Properties	Applications in Wound Management
1	Propolis	Resinous substance collected by honeybees from plant buds	Antibacterial, antifungal, anti-inflammatory, antioxidant	Used in creams, gels, sprays, and dressings to prevent infection and enhance tissue regeneration
2	Tolu Balsam	Resin from *Myroxylon balsamum* tree	Antiseptic, healing stimulant	Used in topical preparations for chronic wounds, abrasions, and ulcers
3	Colophony	Solidified resin from pine trees	Antiseptic, film-forming, tackiness	Used in medical adhesive bandages, tapes, and surgical drapes
4	Mastic	Resin from *Pistacia lentiscus* trees	Antimicrobial, antioxidant, anti-inflammatory	Being studied for oral wound care and skin ulcers; incorporated in bioactive dressings
5	Benzoin Resin	Derived from *Styrax* species	Antimicrobial, soothing, forms protective barrier	Used in compound tincture of benzoin for minor wounds, skin protectants, and post-surgical care
6	Myrrh	Resin from *Commiphora* species trees	Antiseptic, anti-inflammatory, analgesic	Traditional wound cleanser; used in modern formulations for chronic ulcers and infected wounds
7	Storax	Resin from *Liquidambar* species	Antiseptic, fragrant, soothing	Used in traditional poultices; under research for biofilm-resistant wound coatings

Table 8. Resin-based formulations and applications

S.no	Resin used	Formulation	Applications
1	Myrrh	Tincture, essential oil, paste	Antiseptic, anti-inflammatory, dental care
2	Asafoetida	Powder, tincture	Antispasmodic, digestive aid, flatulence relief
3	Benzoin	Tincture	Respiratory infections, skin protectant
4	Shellac	Enteric coating, varnish	Pharmaceutical coating, controlled drug release
5	Colophony	Adhesive, topical plasters	Dental cements, bandage adhesives, ointment bases
6	Mastic gum	Chewing gum, capsules	Gastroprotective, anti-H. pylori, oral hygiene

continued on following page

Table 8. Continued

S.no	Resin used	Formulation	Applications
7	Propolis	Tincture, ointment, lozenge	Antimicrobial, wound healing, oral health
8	Boswellia	Capsules, tablets, ointment, resin extract	Anti-inflammatory, arthritis, asthma, inflammatory bowel disease

ADVANTAGES OF HERBAL POLYMERS OVER SYNTHETIC AGENTS

The search for safer, more efficient, and ecologically friendly biomaterials has led to a growing preference for herbal polymers over their synthetic counterparts in the rapidly changing field of wound care. Because of their many uses in wound healing, herbal polymers biopolymers made from natural plant sources like gums, mucilages, resins, and herbal oils present a strong substitute. Although synthetic polymers like polyvinyl alcohol (PVA), polyethylene glycol (PEG), and polylactic acid (PLA) have been widely used in the creation of contemporary wound care systems, their drawbacks such as possible cytotoxicity, environmental persistence, and high processing costs have led to a move toward natural, plant-based substitutes. In the context of wound care and topical drug delivery systems, this section examines the numerous benefits of herbal polymers over synthetic agents (Sheokand et al., 2023).

Biocompatibility and Non-Toxicity

Biocompatibility is a major benefit of herbal polymers. These polymers from edible or medicinal plants are non-toxic and well-tolerated on human tissue. Their low immune response and discomfort make them ideal for chronic wound management that requires sustained skin contact. Gum acacia and aloe vera mucilage are known for their relaxing and non-sensitizing properties. However, some synthetic polymers leach monomers or stabilizers that might cause cytotoxicity, allergies, or irritation. Additionally, some synthetic excipients require considerable purification to meet safety criteria, increasing production complexity and cost (Orive & Desimone, 2024).

Biodegradability and Environmental Safety

Our herbal polymers degrade spontaneously into harmless components through enzymatic and microbiological action. Environment-friendly green chemistry and sustainable healthcare are achieved. Disposing of guar gum, xanthan gum, and mastic gum does not harm soil or aquatic environments. Synthetic polymers biodegrade poorly, causing microplastic contamination and environmental buildup. Even with biodegradable synthetic polymers, their breakdown may need industrial composting facilities, limiting their usefulness and environmental friendliness (George et al., 2019).

Enhanced Moisture Retention and Barrier Formation

Moisture increases epithelial cell movement and prevents scab formation, promoting wound healing. Hydrogels and biofilms made from herbal polymers such tragacanth gum, guar gum, and xanthan gum retain moisture and prevent desiccation.

Bioadhesive barriers from these polymers protect wounds from microbiological and mechanical stress. They cling better to biological tissues than synthetic chemicals, especially in damp environments (W. Yang et al., 2024).

Cost-Effectiveness and Accessibility

Low-resource and rural healthcare settings can save money on synthetic excipients with natural polymers. They are renewable, locally available, and requires little infrastructure for production and extraction. Sustainable harvesting of indigenous plant species can produce herbal ingredients like acacia gum and okra polysaccharides with low environmental impact. Instead, synthetic polymers use petrochemicals or energy-intensive production methods. In certain regions, their global supply networks are less accessible due to economic and geopolitical volatility (Sipponen et al., 2012).

Compatibility with Bioactive Compounds and Natural Oils

Hydrophobic natural oils, plant extracts, and essential oils sometimes work better with herbal polymers. Their amphiphilia allows them to generate stable emulsions, gels, and films that transport lipophilic bioactive substances to wounds. Formulations with xanthan gum and tea tree oil exhibit synergistic antibacterial and healing properties. Surfactants, emulsifiers, or chemical alterations may be needed to make synthetic polymers compatible, which complicates and may be harmful (Iñiguez-moreno et al., 2021).

Support for Traditional and Ethnopharmacological Systems

The concepts of Ayurveda, Traditional Chinese Medicine, Unani, and other traditional medical systems that have long used plant-based medicines to treat wounds are all in line with the usage of herbal polymers. Their use into contemporary wound dressings creates culturally aware and comprehensive healthcare alternatives by bridging the gap between traditional knowledge and scientific innovation. Despite their scientific advancements, synthetic drugs are frequently not culturally accepted in societies that rely on traditional medicine and may be perceived as alien or incompatible with native therapeutic methods (Albahri et al., 2023).

RECENT ADVANCES AND NOVEL DELIVERY SYSTEMS

Wound treatment has seen tremendous progress as a result of the combination of contemporary pharmaceutical technologies with natural herbal excipients. Nanoformulations and smart hydrogels are two of the most promising developments; they are intended to improve bioavailability, targeted distribution, and responsive medication release at the wound site (Awlqadr et al., 2025).

Nanoformulations

The delivery of herbal oils, gums, and resins for wound healing applications has advanced significantly with the use of nanoformulations. Herbal bioactives are encapsulated in nanoscale carriers as liposomes, nanoparticles, or nanoemulsions in these systems. This method overcomes the drawbacks of conventional herbal preparations and provides a number of important advantages. First off, by shielding volatile or chemically sensitive herbal ingredients from environmental deterioration like oxidation or UV light, nanoencapsulation increases their durability. Second, nanoformulations ensure deeper and more effective therapeutic activity at the wound site by improving the penetration of active substances through the epidermal barrier because of their tiny particle size and large surface area. These systems also allow for the controlled and prolonged release of herbal ingredients, which prolongs the duration of therapeutic effects and lessens the frequency of reapplication. This reduces the possibility of adverse consequences while also increasing patient compliance (Kumari et al., 2022).

Types and Examples

a. **Resin-loaded nanoparticles: Propolis-loaded chitosan nanoparticles**: Exhibit sustained antimicrobial activity and enhance wound closure.

Boswellia-loaded polymeric nanoparticles: Used for anti-inflammatory and collagen-stimulating effects.

b. **Herbal oil nanoemulsions**:

Neem oil nanoemulsion: Offers enhanced antimicrobial action and faster epithelialization.

Tea tree oil nanocapsules: Improve stability and reduce skin irritation.

c. **Gum-based nanocarriers**: **Xanthan gum-coated nanoparticles**: Provide mucoadhesion and improved retention at the wound site.
d. **Smart hydrogels responsive to wound pH or enzymes:** Smart hydrogels are sophisticated, stimuli-responsive delivery devices that may release therapeutic drugs precisely and at specified sites by dynamically adapting to the wound microenvironment. The purpose of these hydrogels is to react to a range of physiological cues that are frequently connected to wounds. They can, for example, sense and respond to pH shifts, such as the higher alkaline conditions usually present in infected wounds, to start the release of active ingredients. Furthermore, it is possible to create smart hydrogels that react to particular enzymes, such as matrix metalloproteinases (MMPs), which are frequently overexpressed in chronic wounds. This enables precise and efficient drug delivery. In addition to their responsiveness, these hydrogels are important for sustaining the ideal conditions for wound healing because they maintain moisturebalance and guarantee sufficient oxygen permeability, two factors that are critical for effective tissue regeneration and repair (Bordbar-Khiabani & Gasik, 2022).

Examples

- **pH-sensitive hydrogels:** Gum acacia/alginate hydrogels loaded with herbal extracts (e.g., turmeric or aloe vera) that release actives under elevated pH found in infected wounds.
- **Enzyme-responsive hydrogels:** Collagenase-triggered hydrogels releasing myrrh extract or boswellic acids upon enzymatic activity.
- **Thermo-sensitive hydrogels:** Resins embedded in poloxamer-based hydrogels that gel at body temperature and gradually release active compounds (Jahanbekam et al., 2025).

CHALLENGES AND LIMITATIONS IN HERBAL-BASED WOUND HEALING

Herbal-based wound healing has garnered a lot of interest because of its traditional use, affordability, and natural origin. Nevertheless, in spite of these benefits, a number of obstacles and restrictions prevent its extensive clinical use. Insufficient standardization is one of the main problems. The stability and repeatability of herbal formulations' medicinal benefits are impacted by the compositional variations that frequently occur based on plant species, harvesting seasons, and preparation techniques. Many herbal therapies are also not well supported by clinical data. The majority are supported by laboratory research or anecdotal reports; few extensive, randomized clinical trials have been conducted to confirm their effectiveness in people (Shedoeva et al., 2019b). Poor phytochemical bioavailability is another issue. Herb compounds are often poorly absorbed, weakly soluble, or rapidly metabolized, reducing wound site concentration. Acute or severe wounds that need rapid healing are not suitable for herbal therapies since they work slowly. They're harder to use without regulation. Unlike pharmaceutical pharmaceuticals, herbal products are not strictly regulated, resulting in contamination, mislabeling, and uneven potency. Safety is another issue. While frequently considered safe, some herbal medicines might produce adverse responses or toxicity, especially in sensitive or preexisting diseases (Thangapazham et al., 2016). Modern wound-care incompatibility is another issue. Advanced wound dressings and conventional therapies like antibiotics and skin grafts may not work well with herbal extracts, limiting their use in full treatment schemes. The short shelf life and poor stability of many herbal formulations, especially aqueous ones, make storage and transit difficult, especially in rural or resource-limited places. Scalability and commercial production are issues. Different agricultural and processing methods make it hard to mass-produce herbal items with consistent quality. Finally, herbal ingredient methods of action are poorly understood. These chemicals' evolution into effective therapeutic agents is limited by a lack of molecular understanding of how they promote healing. Complete realization of the potential of herbal-based wound healing in modern healthcare depends on addressing these constraints by research, control, and creativity (Pang et al., 2023).

REGULATORY ASPECTS AND SAFETY CONSIDERATIONS

A robust regulatory and safety framework is required for the use of herbal products in wound healing in order to guarantee patient safety, effectiveness, and quality. Guidelines are provided by a number of national and international organizations for the creation, evaluation, and marketing of herbal medications. In order to evaluate the safety and effectiveness of herbal products, the World Health Organization (WHO) has released extensive guidelines that place a strong emphasis on pharmacovigilance, quality control, and good agriculture and collecting practices (GACP) (Wang et al., 2023). An analogous regulatory framework is offered by the European Medicines Agency (EMA) through its Committee on Herbal Medicinal medicines (HMPC), which assesses herbal ingredients and preparations utilized in conventional and proven pharmaceutical medicines. Although those that make therapeutic claims must go through medication approval procedures, the USFDA mostly regulates herbal products as dietary supplements under the Dietary Supplement Health and Education Act (DSHEA) (Gatt et al., 2024). Ayurveda, Unani, Siddha, and homeopathy are among the traditional medical systems regulated and promoted in India by the Ministry of AYUSH, which has set safety, effectiveness, and quality control criteria. Herbal wound healing products must pass safety tests before being approved. When applied to open or compromised skin, preclinical assessments include dermal irritation, sensitization, and toxicity studies evaluate the risk of allergic reactions, skin damage, or systemic side effects. These investigations determine safe dosage levels and detect dangerous formulation ingredients (Pandey et al., 2013). Laboratory testing, long-term clinical surveillance, and post-market monitoring are needed to track adverse effects in larger populations. To inform consumers and healthcare professionals about herbal wound care products' contents, usage directions, contraindications, and adverse effects, proper labeling is necessary. Labels must also include the botanical source, plant part, preparation process, and active component concentration. Sustainability and sourcing are ethical and ecological issues. For endangered medicinal plant species and environmental conservation, sustainable harvesting and traceable supply chains are essential. Local populations that grow and harvest medicinal herbs benefit from ethical sourcing (Ekor, 2014).

FUTURE PERSPECTIVES AND RESEARCH DIRECTIONS

Standardizing formulations to assure quality and consistency should be the main emphasis of future research on herbal excipients and polymers in wound healing, since natural source variability is still a problem. To learn more about how they promote tissue regeneration and repair, more research into their molecular mechanisms of action is required. These natural substances may have more therapeutic potential if they are added to sophisticated drug delivery systems like hydrogels or nanoparticles (Safta et al., 2025). Investigating synergistic pairings with synthetic materials may also increase efficacy. Preclinical discoveries must be validated by clinical studies, and scalable production techniques and sustainable sourcing ought to be given top priority. In the end, incorporating these organic substances into personalized medical strategies may transform wound care (Joseph et al., 2023).

CONCLUSION

Herbal excipients and polymers, comprising oils, gums, and resins, possess considerable potential in wound healing owing to their natural origin, biocompatibility, and multifunctional therapeutic attributes, including anti-inflammatory, antibacterial, and regenerative activities. Their integration into contemporary wound care formulations offers a possible substitute for synthetic drugs. Nonetheless, obstacles like uniformity, mechanistic comprehension, and clinical validation persist. Ongoing research and technology advancements may enable these natural substances to significantly contribute to the creation of safer, more effective, and sustainable wound healing therapies.

REFERENCES

Abdi, G., Jain, M., Patil, N., Tariq, M., Choudhary, S., Kumar, P., Raj, N. S., Mohsen Ali, S. S., & Uthappa, U. T. (2024). Tragacanth gum-based hydrogels for drug delivery and tissue engineering applications. *Frontiers in Materials*, *11*, 1296399. DOI: 10.3389/FMATS.2024.1296399/XML/NLM

Albahri, G., Badran, A., Hijazi, A., Daou, A., Baydoun, E., Nasser, M., & Merah, O. (2023). The Therapeutic Wound Healing Bioactivities of Various Medicinal Plants. *Life (Chicago, Ill.)*, *13*(2), 317. DOI: 10.3390/LIFE13020317 PMID: 36836674

Awlqadr, F. H., Majeed, K. R., Altemimi, A. B., Hassan, A. M., Qadir, S. A., Saeed, M. N., Faraj, A. M., Salih, T. H., Abd Al-Manhel, A. J., Najm, M. A. A., Tsakali, E., Van Impe, J. F. M., Abd El-Maksoud, A. A., & Abedelmaksoud, T. G. (2025). Nanotechnology-based herbal medicine: Preparation, synthesis, and applications in food and medicine. *Journal of Agriculture and Food Research*, *19*, 101661. DOI: 10.1016/J.JAFR.2025.101661

Bordbar-Khiabani, A., & Gasik, M. (2022). Smart Hydrogels for Advanced Drug Delivery Systems. *International Journal of Molecular Sciences*, *23*(7), 3665. DOI: 10.3390/IJMS23073665 PMID: 35409025

Cedillo-Cortezano, M., Martinez-Cuevas, L. R., López, J. A. M., Barrera López, I. L., Escutia-Perez, S., & Petricevich, V. L. (2024). Use of Medicinal Plants in the Process of Wound Healing: A Literature Review. *Pharmaceuticals*, *17*(3), 303. DOI: 10.3390/PH17030303 PMID: 38543089

Diller, R. B., & Tabor, A. J. (2022). The Role of the Extracellular Matrix (ECM) in Wound Healing: A Review. *Biomimetics*, *7*(3), 87. DOI: 10.3390/BIOMIMETICS7030087 PMID: 35892357

Dilworth, L. L., Riley, C. K., & Stennett, D. K. (2023). *Plant constituents: carbohydrates, oils, resins, balsams, and plant hormones. Pharmacognosy: Fundamentals* (2nd ed.). Applications, and Strategies., DOI: 10.1016/B978-0-443-18657-8.00021-9

Ekor, M. (2014). The growing use of herbal medicines: Issues relating to adverse reactions and challenges in monitoring safety. *Frontiers in Pharmacology*, *4*, 177. DOI: 10.3389/FPHAR.2013.00177 PMID: 24454289

El-Sakhawy, M., Salama, A., & Tohamy, H. A. S. (2023). Applications of propolis-based materials in wound healing. *Archives of Dermatological Research*, *316*(1), 61. DOI: 10.1007/S00403-023-02789-X PMID: 38151671

Elumalai, P., Muninathan, N., Megalatha, S. T., Suresh, A., Kumar, K. S., Jhansi, N., Kalaivani, K., & Krishnamoorthy, G. (2022). An Insight into Anticancer Effect of Propolis and Its Constituents: A Review of Molecular Mechanisms. *Evidence-Based Complementary and Alternative Medicine: eCAM*, *2022*(1), 5901191. DOI: 10.1155/2022/5901191 PMID: 35754701

Gatt, A. R., Vella Bonanno, P., & Zammit, R. (2024). Ethical considerations in the regulation and use of herbal medicines in the European Union. *Frontiers in Medical Technology*, *6*, 1358956. DOI: 10.3389/FMEDT.2024.1358956 PMID: 38948354

George, A., Shah, P. A., & Shrivastav, P. S. (2019). Guar gum: Versatile natural polymer for drug delivery applications. *European Polymer Journal*, *112*, 722–735. DOI: 10.1016/J.EURPOLYMJ.2018.10.042

Gounden, V., & Singh, M. (2024). Hydrogels and Wound Healing: Current and Future Prospects. *Gels (Basel, Switzerland)*, *10*(1), 43. DOI: 10.3390/GELS10010043 PMID: 38247766

Hamdani, A. M., Wani, I. A., & Bhat, N. A. (2019). Sources, structure, properties and health benefits of plant gums: A review. *International Journal of Biological Macromolecules*, *135*, 46–61. DOI: 10.1016/J.IJBIOMAC.2019.05.103 PMID: 31121233

Horváth, A., Pandur, E., Sipos, K., Micalizzi, G., Mondello, L., Böszörményi, A., Birinyi, P., & Horváth, G. (2022). Anti-inflammatory effects of lavender and eucalyptus essential oils on the in vitro cell culture model of bladder pain syndrome using T24 cells. *BMC Complementary Medicine and Therapies*, *22*(1), 119. DOI: 10.1186/S12906-022-03604-2 PMID: 35490236

Iñiguez-moreno, M., Ragazzo-sánchez, J. A., & Calderón-santoyo, M. (2021). An Extensive Review of Natural Polymers Used as Coatings for Postharvest Shelf-Life Extension: Trends and Challenges. *Polymers 2021, Vol. 13, Page 3271*, *13*(19), 3271. DOI: 10.3390/POLYM13193271

Jahanbekam, S., Asare-Addo, K., Alipour, S., & Nokhodchi, A. (2025). Smart hydrogels and the promise of multi-responsive in-situ systems. *Journal of Drug Delivery Science and Technology*, *107*, 106758. DOI: 10.1016/J.JDDST.2025.106758

Johnson, K. E., & Wilgus, T. A. (2014). Vascular Endothelial Growth Factor and Angiogenesis in the Regulation of Cutaneous Wound Repair. *Advances in Wound Care*, *3*(10), 647. DOI: 10.1089/WOUND.2013.0517 PMID: 25302139

Joseph, T. M., Kar Mahapatra, D., Esmaeili, A., Piszczyk, Ł., Hasanin, M. S., Kattali, M., Haponiuk, J., & Thomas, S. (2023). Nanoparticles: Taking a Unique Position in Medicine. *Nanomaterials 2023, Vol. 13, Page 574, 13*(3), 574. DOI: 10.3390/NANO13030574

Kalpana Manivannan, R., Sharma, N., Kumar, V., Jayaraj, I., Vimal, S., & Umesh, M. (2024). A comprehensive review on natural macromolecular biopolymers for biomedical applications: Recent advancements, current challenges, and future outlooks. *Carbohydrate Polymer Technologies and Applications*, *8*, 100536. DOI: 10.1016/J.CARPTA.2024.100536

Kaur, H., Gogoi, B., Sharma, I., Das, D. K., Azad, M. A., Das Pramanik, D., & Pramanik, A. (2024). Hydrogels as a Potential Biomaterial for Multimodal Therapeutic Applications. *Molecular Pharmaceutics*, *21*(10), 4827. DOI: 10.1021/ACS.MOLPHARMACEUT.4C00595 PMID: 39290162

Kumari, S., Goyal, A., Gürer, E. S., Yapar, E. A., Garg, M., Sood, M., & Sindhu, R. K. (2022). Bioactive Loaded Novel Nano-Formulations for Targeted Drug Delivery and Their Therapeutic Potential. *Pharmaceutics*, *14*(5), 1091. DOI: 10.3390/PHARMACEUTICS14051091 PMID: 35631677

LaPelusa, A., & Dave, H. D. (2023). Physiology, Hemostasis. *StatPearls*. https://www.ncbi.nlm.nih.gov/books/NBK545263/

Mandal, M. D., & Mandal, S. (2011). Honey: Its medicinal property and antibacterial activity. *Asian Pacific Journal of Tropical Biomedicine*, *1*(2), 154. DOI: 10.1016/S2221-1691(11)60016-6 PMID: 23569748

Mondello, F., Fontana, S., Scaturro, M., Girolamo, A., Colone, M., Stringaro, A., Di Vito, M., & Ricci, M. L. (2022). Terpinen-4-ol, the Main Bioactive Component of Tea Tree Oil, as an Innovative Antimicrobial Agent against Legionella pneumophila. *Pathogens (Basel, Switzerland)*, *11*(6), 682. DOI: 10.3390/PATHOGENS11060682/S1 PMID: 35745536

Orive, G., & Desimone, M. F. (2024). Biopolymers Take Center Stage in Wound Healing Advancements. *Pharmaceutics*, *16*(6), 755. DOI: 10.3390/PHARMACEUTICS16060755 PMID: 38931877

Pandey, M. M., Rastogi, S., & Rawat, A. K. S. (2013). Indian Traditional Ayurvedic System of Medicine and Nutritional Supplementation. *Evidence-Based Complementary and Alternative Medicine: eCAM*, *376327*. Advance online publication. DOI: 10.1155/2013/376327 PMID: 23864888

Pang, Q., Yang, F., Jiang, Z., Wu, K., Hou, R., & Zhu, Y. (2023). Smart wound dressing for advanced wound management: Real-time monitoring and on-demand treatment. *Materials & Design*, *229*, 111917. DOI: 10.1016/J.MATDES.2023.111917

(PDF) A Review on Herbal Excipients in Pharmaceutical Formulations. (n.d.). Retrieved May 20, 2025, from https://www.researchgate.net/publication/387721347_A_Review_on_Herbal_Excipients_in_Pharmaceutical_Formulations

Safta, D. A., Bogdan, C., Iurian, S., & Moldovan, M.-L. (2025). Optimization of Film-Dressings Containing Herbal Extracts for Wound Care—A Quality by Design Approach. *Gels 2025, Vol. 11, Page 322, 11*(5), 322. DOI: 10.3390/GELS11050322

Saporito, F., Sandri, G., Bonferoni, M. C., Rossi, S., Boselli, C., Cornaglia, A. I., Mannucci, B., Grisoli, P., Vigani, B., & Ferrari, F. (2017). Essential oil-loaded lipid nanoparticles for wound healing. *International Journal of Nanomedicine*, *13*, 175. DOI: 10.2147/IJN.S152529 PMID: 29343956

Satchanska, G., Davidova, S., & Petrov, P. D. (2024). Natural and Synthetic Polymers for Biomedical and Environmental Applications. *Polymers*, *16*(8), 1159. DOI: 10.3390/POLYM16081159 PMID: 38675078

Schultz, G. S., Chin, G. A., Moldawer, L., & Diegelmann, R. F. (2011). Principles of Wound Healing. *Diabetic Foot Problems*, 395–402. DOI: 10.1142/9789812791535_0028

Shedoeva, A., Leavesley, D., Upton, Z., & Fan, C. (2019a). Wound Healing and the Use of Medicinal Plants. *Evidence-Based Complementary and Alternative Medicine: eCAM, 2684108*. Advance online publication. DOI: 10.1155/2019/2684108 PMID: 31662773

Sheokand, B., Vats, M., Kumar, A., Srivastava, C. M., Bahadur, I., & Pathak, S. R. (2023). Natural polymers used in the dressing materials for wound healing: Past, present and future. *Journal of Polymer Science*, *61*(14), 1389–1414. DOI: 10.1002/POL.20220734

Siddiqui, M. Z. (2011). Boswellia Serrata, A Potential Antiinflammatory Agent: An Overview. *Indian Journal of Pharmaceutical Sciences*, *73*(3), 255. DOI: 10.4103/0250-474X.93507 PMID: 22457547

Sipponen, A., Kuokkanen, O., Tiihonen, R., Kauppinen, H., & Jokinen, J. J. (2012). Natural coniferous resin salve used to treat complicated surgical wounds: Pilot clinical trial on healing and costs. *International Journal of Dermatology*, *51*(6), 726–732. DOI: 10.1111/J.1365-4632.2011.05397.X PMID: 22607295

Soulaidopoulos, S., Tsiogka, A., Chrysohoou, C., Lazarou, E., Aznaouridis, K., Doundoulakis, I., Tyrovola, D., Tousoulis, D., Tsioufis, K., Vlachopoulos, C., & Lazaros, G. (2022). Overview of Chios Mastic Gum (Pistacia lentiscus) Effects on Human Health. *Nutrients, 14*(3), 590. DOI: 10.3390/NU14030590 PMID: 35276949

Thang, N. H., Chien, T. B., & Cuong, D. X. (2023). Polymer-Based Hydrogels Applied in Drug Delivery: An Overview. *Gels (Basel, Switzerland), 9*(7), 523. DOI: 10.3390/GELS9070523 PMID: 37504402

Thangapazham, R. L., Sharad, S., & Maheshwari, R. K. (2016). Phytochemicals in Wound Healing. *Advances in Wound Care, 5*(5), 230. DOI: 10.1089/WOUND.2013.0505 PMID: 27134766

Ukaegbu, K., Allen, E., & Svoboda, K. K. H. (2025). Reactive Oxygen Species and Antioxidants in Wound Healing: Mechanisms and Therapeutic Potential. *International Wound Journal, 22*(5), e70330. DOI: 10.1111/IWJ.70330 PMID: 40288766

Wallace, H. A., Basehore, B. M., & Zito, P. M. (2023). Wound Healing Phases. *StatPearls*. https://www.ncbi.nlm.nih.gov/books/NBK470443/

Wang, H., Chen, Y., Wang, L., Liu, Q., Yang, S., & Wang, C. (2023). Advancing herbal medicine: Enhancing product quality and safety through robust quality control practices. *Frontiers in Pharmacology, 14*, 1265178. DOI: 10.3389/FPHAR.2023.1265178 PMID: 37818188

Witkowska, K., Paczkowska-Walendowska, M., Garbiec, E., & Cielecka-Piontek, J. (2024). Topical Application of Centella asiatica in Wound Healing: Recent Insights into Mechanisms and Clinical Efficacy. *Pharmaceutics, 16*(10), 1252. DOI: 10.3390/PHARMACEUTICS16101252 PMID: 39458583

Yang, J., Pi, A., Yan, L., Li, J., Nan, S., Zhang, J., & Hao, Y. (2022). Research Progress on Therapeutic Effect and Mechanism of Propolis on Wound Healing. *Evidence-Based Complementary and Alternative Medicine: eCAM, 5798941*. Advance online publication. DOI: 10.1155/2022/5798941 PMID: 35911156

Yang, W., Zhang, Q., Zhou, J., Li, L., Li, Y., Zhu, L., Narain, R., Nan, K., & Chen, Y. (2024). Self-Healing Guar Gum-Based Nanocomposite Hydrogel Promotes Infected Wound Healing through Photothermal Antibacterial Therapy. *Biomacromolecules, 25*(6), 3432–3448. DOI: 10.1021/ACS.BIOMAC.4C00080 PMID: 38771294

Chapter 7
Ointments, Creams, and Topical Formulations

P. Selvakumar
https://orcid.org/0000-0002-3650-4548
Department of Science and Humanities, Nehru Institute of Technology, Coimbatore, India

T. C. Manjunath
https://orcid.org/0000-0003-2545-9160
Rajarajeswari College of Engineering, Bangalore, India

Maurya Manjunath
https://orcid.org/0000-0001-9563-9269
JSS Academy of Higher Education and Research, Mysuru, India

ABSTRACT

Topical formulations are a class of pharmaceutical and cosmetic products that are applied directly to the skin or mucous membranes. These formulations are designed to deliver active ingredients to specific areas of the body, offering a targeted approach to treatment. The skin, being the largest organ of the human body, serves as both a barrier and a potential pathway for the absorption of various substances. Topical formulations, therefore, utilize this unique characteristic of the skin to deliver therapeutic agents while avoiding the systemic side effects commonly associated with oral or injectable medications. As such, they play a crucial role in the treatment of various dermatological conditions, local pain management, and even certain systemic diseases.The development of topical formulations is an intricate process that takes into account the skin's physiology, the chemical properties of the active ingredients, and the desired therapeutic effect.

DOI: 10.4018/979-8-3373-3977-1.ch007

INTRODUCTION ABOUT THE TOPICAL FORMULATIONS

Topical formulations are a class of pharmaceutical and cosmetic products that are applied directly to the skin or mucous membranes. These formulations are designed to deliver active ingredients to specific areas of the body, offering a targeted approach to treatment. The skin, being the largest organ of the human body, serves as both a barrier and a potential pathway for the absorption of various substances. Topical formulations, therefore, utilize this unique characteristic of the skin to deliver therapeutic agents while avoiding the systemic side effects commonly associated with oral or injectable medications. As such, they play a crucial role in the treatment of various dermatological conditions, local pain management, and even certain systemic diseases. The development of topical formulations is an intricate process that takes into account the skin's physiology, the chemical properties of the active ingredients, and the desired therapeutic effect. These formulations come in various forms, including creams, ointTopical formulations are a class of pharmaceutical and cosmetic products that are applied directly to the skin or mucous membranes, (Anderson & Brown, 2024). These formulations are designed to deliver active ingredients to specific areas of the body, offering a targeted approach to treatment. The skin, being the largest organ of the human body, serves as both a barrier and a potential pathway for the absorption of various substances. Topical formulations, therefore, utilize this unique characteristic of the skin to deliver therapeutic agents while avoiding the systemic side effects commonly associated with oral or injectable medications. As such, they play a crucial role in the treatment of various dermatological conditions, local pain management, and even certain systemic diseases. The development of topical formulations is an intricate process that takes into account the skin's physiology, the chemical properties of the active ingredients, and the desired therapeutic effect. (Tiwari & Ochieng, 2024). The skin consists of three primary layers: the epidermis, the dermis, and the hypodermis. The outermost layer, the epidermis, serves as the primary barrier to external substances. It is composed of keratinocytes, which form a protective layer that limits the permeability of the skin. Beneath the epidermis lies the dermis, a deeper layer that contains blood vessels, hair follicles, sweat glands, and collagen fibers, which provide structural support and enable the skin to perform various functions.

`The process of drug absorption through the skin is known as percutaneous absorption, and it typically involves the crossing of active ingredients through the stratum corneum, the outermost layer of the epidermis. Several factors can influence the absorption of topical medications, including the molecular size, solubility, and concentration of the active ingredients, as well as the formulation type and the condition of the skin itself.: Creams are semiliquid emulsions, typically composed of water and oil, that provide a balanced combination of hydration and lubrication.

They are easy to apply and absorb relatively quickly, making them ideal for use on large areas of skin or in conditions that require hydration and soothing. (Athavale et al., 2025). Due to their occlusive nature, ointments are particularly effective in treating dry or scaly skin conditions as they prevent moisture loss and enhance the absorption of active ingredients. They are commonly used in the treatment of eczema, psoriasis, and other inflammatory skin conditions. They are often used for their non-greasy feel and quick absorption. Gels are preferred for areas of the skin that require a more drying effect or where a greasier formulation may be undesirable. They are commonly used for acne treatment or for localized pain relief to deliver the active ingredient to the target site in an effective manner. Several mechanisms play a role in the absorption and action of topical medications. The active ingredients move from an area of higher concentration (the formulation) to an area of lower concentration (the skin). This process is influenced by factors such as the molecular size of the drug and the integrity of the skin's barrier molecules to penetrate more easily. (Tripathi & Deshmukh, 2025) Common permeation enhancers include alcohols, fatty acids, and surfactants can enhance the absorption of the active ingredients while also providing a moisturizing effect ingredients over an extended period. This controlled release allows for continuous delivery of the medication, maintaining therapeutic levels of the drug in the skin and minimizing fluctuations in drug concentration. Topical formulations are widely used in the treatment of various conditions, ranging from minor skin irritations to chronic diseases. Common applications include: Despite their many advantages, topical formulations face several challenges, particularly concerning drug delivery. (Baker & Sanchez, 2025) The skin's natural barrier function limits the penetration of many drugs, and developing formulations that can overcome this barrier without causing irritation or other side effects is a key area of research. Advances in nanotechnology, such as the use of nanoparticles, liposomes, and microneedles, are showing promise in improving drug delivery to the skin and enhancing the bioavailability of active ingredients. In conclusion, topical formulations remain a vital and evolving area of pharmaceutical and cosmetic science. Their ability to deliver targeted therapies with minimal systemic side effects makes them an invaluable tool for treating a wide range of conditions. As research and technology continue to advance, the future of topical formulations looks promising, offering even more efficient and effective ways to treat and maintain skin health and deliver therapeutic agents.

TYPES OF TOPICAL FORMULATIONS: OINTMENTS, CREAMS, AND MORE

Topical drug delivery has emerged as one of the most significant advancements in both the pharmaceutical and cosmetic industries. This method involves the application of therapeutic agents directly to the skin or mucous membranes, offering numerous advantages over other routes of administration, such as oral or injectable therapies. The skin, being the body's largest organ, is uniquely positioned to act as both a barrier and a potential entry point for active ingredients, making topical formulations an ideal option for treating a variety of conditions and for cosmetic enhancement. The importance of topical delivery is highlighted by its ability to provide localized, controlled, and non-invasive treatment while minimizing the systemic side effects often associated with oral or injectable drugs. As both pharmaceutical and cosmetic industries continue to innovate, the development of effective topical formulations remains at the forefront, transforming the way we approach skin health, therapeutic interventions, and aesthetic treatments plays a crucial role in the absorption and effectiveness of topical formulations. As the body's first line of defense, the skin's primary function is to protect underlying tissues from harmful substances and pathogens. This protective barrier, however, also presents challenges for drug absorption, requiring formulations to be designed with specific mechanisms to enhance the penetration of active ingredients. Understanding the skin's structure is essential to developing effective topical formulations. . (Chakrabarti & Lin, 2023) The outermost layer, the stratum corneum, is composed of dead skin cells that form a strong barrier to foreign substances. Beneath it lies the living layers of the epidermis and dermis, which contain blood vessels, nerve endings, and connective tissue. For topical formulations to be effective, they must penetrate this outer layer and reach the deeper layers where they can exert their therapeutic effects. (Chandel & Ghosh, 2024). Topical delivery offers the distinct advantage of targeting localized areas directly, allowing for higher concentrations of the active ingredient to be delivered precisely where needed. This targeted delivery minimizes the need for systemic absorption, which is a common concern with oral medications. By bypassing the gastrointestinal system and liver metabolism, topical treatments often reduce the risk of systemic side effects or toxicity, making them a safer and more effective alternative for many patients., particularly those affecting the skin and mucous membranes. The ability to apply drugs directly to the site of action allows for faster onset of action, greater precision in targeting, and the potential for sustained-release formulations. Some of the most common therapeutic areas where topical delivery has proven invaluable include and antibiotics. (Uddin & Jensen, 2024) Topical delivery provides targeted therapy to the affected area, reducing the need for systemic treatment that might cause unwanted side effects like gastrointestinal distress, headaches, or systemic immunosuppression. For instance, corticosteroid creams can reduce inflammation and itching without significantly impacting the entire immune system anti-inflammatory drug (NSAID) gels, are increasingly being used for localized pain relief.

These products allow for controlled, sustained release of the active ingredients, delivering pain relief directly to the site of discomfort without the systemic side effects that oral pain medications can cause, such as drowsiness, gastrointestinal irritation, or dependency or progesterone provide an alternative to oral hormone replacement therapy (HRT). These patches allow for steady, controlled delivery of hormones directly into the bloodstream, bypassing the digestive system and avoiding the risks associated with oral hormone therapy, including liver strain and fluctuations in hormone levels are used to treat localized infections, particularly in wound care and surgical settings. Applying these agents directly to the site of infection reduces the likelihood of resistance development and minimizes the need for systemic antibiotics, which can have broader effects on the body's microbiota designed to improve skin appearance, such as anti-aging treatments, moisturizers, and skin brighteners. Retinoids, vitamin C, peptides, and antioxidants are commonly included in topical formulations aimed at reducing the appearance of fine lines, wrinkles, hyperpigmentation, and other signs of aging appearance. Skin care products, such as moisturizers, sunscreens, anti-aging creams, and acne treatments, rely on topical delivery mechanisms to improve skin condition, protect from environmental damage, and address various aesthetic concerns. The key advantages of topical delivery in cosmetic applications include precision, non-invasiveness, and ease of use. Some of the major areas where topical delivery plays a crucial role in cosmetics include hydration to the skin's surface and helping to repair the skin's natural barrier. Ingredients such as hyaluronic acid, glycerin, and ceramides are commonly used in topical formulations to enhance moisture retention and restore the skin's natural barrier function. (Das & Tripathi, 2025). These products are essential in treating dry, flaky, or sensitive skin, especially in conditions like eczema, psoriasis, and atopic dermatitis. (UV) radiation. Topical delivery of sunscreens allows for localized protection by applying ingredients such as zinc oxide or avobenzone directly to the skin, forming a physical or chemical barrier against harmful UV rays. This localized effect ensures targeted protection without the need for systemic absorption of the active ingredients to rise, topical delivery systems have become essential in delivering active ingredients that reduce the visible signs of aging. Retinoids, peptides, growth factors, and antioxidants are commonly used in these formulations to promote collagen production, reduce wrinkles, and improve skin elasticity. These products provide a non-invasive alternative to procedures like Botox or facelifts, offering more gradual and accessible solutions for individuals seeking to maintain youthful skin. Acne treatments are among the most commonly used topical products. Over-the-counter acne medications, such as benzoyl peroxide, salicylic acid, and retinoids, help reduce inflammation, unclog pores, and control excess sebum production. (Valdez & Krishnan, 2023). These products target the root causes of acne by delivering active ingredients directly to the site of inflammation, making them an effective option for both mild and severe acne management advantages, there are still challenges to overcome, particularly with regard to the permeability of the skin's protective barrier. The stratum corneum, as the main barrier to drug absorption, limits the efficacy of many topical formulations. As a result, ongoing research is focused on developing advanced drug delivery systems that can enhance skin penetration and improve drug bioavailability. Techniques such as liposomes, microneedles, nanoparticles, and iontophoresis are being explored to improve drug delivery through the skin. In conclusion, the importance of topical delivery in both pharmaceutical and cosmetic applications cannot be overstated. The ability to provide targeted, localized, and controlled therapy with minimal systemic side effects makes topical formulations an invaluable tool in modern medicine and skin care. As technology continues to evolve, the future of topical drug delivery looks promising, with new innovations set to expand its applications, improve treatment efficacy, and enhance patient outcomes.

OINTMENTS AND ITS CHARACTERISTICS AND APPLICATIONS

Topical formulations have long been integral in the treatment of a wide variety of skin conditions, from minor irritations to chronic diseases. These formulations are designed to deliver active ingredients to the skin or mucous membranes, providing localized effects with minimal systemic absorption. Topical drugs are often preferred due to their non-invasive nature, precise application, and ability to minimize side effects when compared to oral or injectable treatments. As such, a variety of topical formulations have been developed, each with its own unique characteristics and advantages, making them suitable for different therapeutic and cosmetic applications. (Desai & Anand, 2024). This discussion explores the various types of topical formulations, including ointments, creams, gels, lotions, foams, and patches, highlighting their distinct properties, uses, and the underlying factors that influence their formulation. thick, greasy, and oil-based, which makes them highly effective for treating dry, scaly, or cracked skin conditions. The primary ingredients in ointments are oils, waxes, and fatty substances such as petrolatum, which form an occlusive barrier over the skin. This barrier helps to lock in moisture, reduce transepidermal water loss (TEWL), and enhance the absorption of active ingredients into the skin. They are often used for conditions like eczema, psoriasis, Due to their thick consistency and occlusive nature, ointments tend to remain on the skin for extended periods, providing prolonged therapeutic effects. Ointments are commonly used in the treatment of inflammatory skin conditions, including eczema, psoriasis, and atopic dermatitis, where the skin requires both hydration and protection from environmental irritants oils with the refreshing, light feel of water.

This makes creams less greasy than ointments, with a more cosmetically acceptable texture. Creams are versatile and can be formulated for a variety of uses, including both dermatological and cosmetic applications, (Fernandez & Zhao, 2024). Creams are less greasy than ointments and can be applied more comfortably to larger skin areas, such as the face, arms, or legs. The skin compared to ointments, making them suitable for use when a faster onset of action is desiredGels are semi-solid systems in which the active ingredients are dispersed in a water-based or alcohol-based medium that has a jelly-like consistency. Gels are often used for their non-greasy, lightweight texture and fast absorption properties. They provide a cooling effect upon application and are typically clear or translucent, which makes them more aesthetically pleasing than ointments or creams, especially for facial use disorders. Gels are commonly used for acne treatments, as well as for localized pain relief (such as with menthol or lidocaine gels). They are also employed in the cosmetic industry for products aimed at tightening or refreshing the skin that contain a higher percentage of water than creams, making them thinner and more fluid. (Edwards & Patel, 2023). They are typically used for larger areas of the body or areas where a less greasy formulation is needed. Lotions provide quick absorption and are often used for conditions that require hydration but not heavy occlusion, (Wang & Fernandes, 2023). Lotions are typically used in the treatment of mild to moderate skin dryness or irritation. They are commonly found in moisturizers and are used to provide relief from conditions like sunburn or insect bites are created when a foaming agent is incorporated into a liquid formulation, producing a product that is light, airy, and easy to apply. Foams often have a rapid spreadability and absorb quickly into the skin, leaving little to no residue. Its concentration and effectiveness Foams are commonly used for scalp treatments (such as dandruff control), hair loss treatments, and acne products.

CREAMS: FORMULATION AND USE

Ointments have been a cornerstone in the world of topical drug delivery for centuries. Known for their emollient and occlusive properties, ointments are semi-solid formulations that offer a versatile and effective means of administering active ingredients directly to the skin. These formulations are typically oil-based and are designed to be applied to the skin, where they are absorbed or remain on the surface to exert localized effects. Ointments are widely used in both pharmaceutical and cosmetic applications due to their ability to provide hydration, protect the skin, and facilitate the penetration of active ingredients. Despite their greasy nature, ointments continue to be an essential part of therapeutic skin care, particularly for the treatment of various dermatological conditions and lotions. Their composition typically consists of a high proportion of lipophilic (fat-loving) components, such as petrolatum, mineral oil, lanolin, or other oils and waxes. This gives ointments their characteristic greasy texture and a higher viscosity compared to water-based formulations like creams or lotions. The active pharmaceutical ingredients (APIs), and the additives that stabilize the formulation, improve texture, or enhance the effectiveness of the product. (Vijayakumar et al., 2024). The base in an ointment is crucial as it controls the spreadability, consistency, and adherence to the skin. Oil-based bases such as petrolatum or hydrophobic emulsions can hold active ingredients in suspension, allowing for controlled release over time. The high lipid content of ointments also means that they are usually thicker and more viscous than creams or lotions, which are often water-based. This increased viscosity contributes to the barrier-forming properties of ointments, allowing them to trap moisture within the skin, especially in cases of dry, cracked, or inflamed skin. (Ghosh & Pillai, 2025) The occlusive effect of ointments can also makes ointments especially beneficial for treating conditions involving dry, cracked, or inflamed skin. In conditions such as eczema or psoriasis, where the skin barrier is compromised, ointments help seal in moisture, promote skin hydration, and provide a protective shield that reduces further irritation. Ointments also function as emollients, softening and soothing the skin. The emollient properties of ointments are particularly valuable for individuals with dry or rough skin, as they help smooth the skin's surface and restore its natural texture. By moisturizing the outer layers of the skin, ointments can improve skin elasticity and reduce the appearance of scaling or flakiness that often accompanies conditions like dermatitis.to other topical formulations such as gels or creams.

This slow release can be advantageous in certain therapeutic applications, as it prolongs the time during which the active ingredients remain on the skin. For example, ointments are commonly used in the treatment of chronic conditions that require sustained delivery of medication, such as inflammatory skin diseases or localized pain formulations. For individuals with sensitive skin, ointments provide a gentler alternative to creams or lotions, which may contain preservatives, emulsifiers, or other additives that could cause allergic reactions use. The two main types of ointments are:-water-soluble. Hydrocarbon-based ointments are typically thicker, provide excellent occlusion, and are highly effective at retaining moisture. Because they do not contain water, hydrocarbon ointments are less likely to spoil and have a longer shelf life components, allowing them to incorporate small amounts of water into the formulation. These ointments are less greasy than hydrocarbon ointments but still retain their occlusive properties. They are often used when a slightly lighter texture is desired, but the moisturizing and barrier-forming benefits of an ointment are still needed are used extensively in the pharmaceutical field for the treatment of a variety of conditions, particularly those affecting the skin. The following outlines some of the most common therapeutic applications of ointments or damaged skin. They are frequently prescribed for the treatment of provide quick relief by reducing inflammation and locking in moisture. The occlusive effect of ointments helps promote healing by preventing further water loss from the skin, (Wagner & Kumar, 2024). Thick, scaly patches of skin. Ointments containing corticosteroids, coal tar, or vitamin D analogs can help reduce the thickness of the lesions and provide relief from itching and inflammation skin, such as that caused by cold weather, excessive handwashing, or certain medical conditions. Ointments help create a barrier that retains moisture and promotes the repair of the skin's natural barrier and protect the wound from infection. Ointments containing antimicrobial agents such as silver sulfadiazine or honey are commonly applied to burns, abrasions, or surgical wounds. These ointments not only help to maintain a moist environment conducive to healing but also prevent microbial growth, reducing the risk of infectionpain, neuropathic pain, or arthritic pain. The slow absorption of these ointments ensures that the active ingredients provide prolonged relief at the site of application containing ingredients like clotrimazole or terbinafine are commonly prescribed for fungal conditions such as athlete's foot or ringworm. Similarly, antibiotic ointments containing ingredients like bacitracin or mupirocin are used to treat superficial bacterial infections, cuts, and scrapes or menopause. Transdermal hormonal ointments, such as estrogen or testosterone, allow for controlled delivery of the active ingredient directly through the skin. (Gupta & Bhatia, 2024). This avoids the gastrointestinal metabolism of oral hormones and allows for more stable and consistent hormone levels. Ointments are a powerful and versatile form of topical formulation, offering numerous benefits in the treatment of a variety of skin conditions. Their emollient and occlusive properties make them ideal for dry, irritated, or damaged skin, while their slow and prolonged release of active ingredients provides sustained therapeutic effects. Despite their greasy texture, ointments remain a preferred choice for the treatment of dermatological conditions such as eczema, psoriasis, and dry skin, as well as in the management of pain, infections, and wounds. While they may not always be suitable for all users or all areas of the body, ointments continue to play a crucial role in both pharmaceutical and cosmetic applications, delivering effective and localized treatment with minimal systemic side effects.

KEY DIFFERENCES BETWEEN OINTMENTS AND CREAMS

Creams are one of the most commonly used and versatile forms of topical medication. These semi-solid emulsions have gained significant popularity in both pharmaceutical and cosmetic industries due to their balanced texture, ease of application, and efficacy in treating a variety of skin conditions. As emulsions, creams consist of a mixture of both water and oil-based components, which makes them an ideal choice for delivering active ingredients to the skin while maintaining a light, non-greasy texture. (Hansen & Ng, 2025) The formulation, application, and benefits of creams vary depending on the specific use case, ranging from therapeutic purposes such as the treatment of dermatological conditions to cosmetic uses like moisturizing and anti-aging products. This comprehensive discussion will cover the formulation, characteristics, therapeutic applications, cosmetic uses, and the benefits and limitations of creams, providing an in-depth understanding of their role in topical skincare aqueous phase (water) and the oil phase (lipophilic or fat-soluble ingredients). These phases are combined using an emulsifying agent, which stabilizes the mixture and prevents the separation of the oil and water components. Creams are classified based on their oil-to-water ratio, In these formulations, the oil phase is dispersed in water, which makes the cream light and easy to spread. This type of cream typically has a non-greasy feel, and it is well-suited for individuals with oily or combination skin.

The high water content provides a refreshing sensation upon application, which makes these creams ideal for daytime use or for those who prefer a lightweight texture. O/W creams are often used for moisturizing, sunscreen applications, and the treatment of inflammatory skin conditions such as eczema or contact dermatitis the other hand, have water droplets dispersed in an oil phase. These creams are thicker, heavier, and more occlusive, making them suitable for dry or cracked skin that requires a higher level of hydration and protection. W/O creams create a barrier on the skin's surface, which helps lock in moisture and reduce water loss. These creams are often used in products for dry, sensitive, or aging skin and are commonly found in night creams or formulations designed for colder climates where the skin is more prone to dehydration. In both types of emulsions, stabilizing agents such as surfactants, emulsifiers, and preservatives are added to improve the shelf life of the product and prevent microbial contamination. Common emulsifiers include cetyl alcohol, stearic acid, or polysorbates, which help bind the water and oil components together. In addition to the emulsifying agents, creams typically contain several key ingredients that contribute to their intended effect: These ingredients can vary widely depending on the therapeutic or cosmetic goal. Common APIs include corticosteroids (for anti-inflammatory purposes), antifungal agents (for treating infections), antibiotics (for treating bacterial skin infections), and analgesics (for localized pain relief). Other active ingredients may include retinoids (for anti-aging and acne treatment), hyaluronic acid (for hydration), or peptides (for skin rejuvenation).skin cells, creating a smooth surface and preventing moisture loss. Common emollients used in creams include glycerin, lanolin, and various vegetable oils. Humectants, such as glycerin, propylene glycol, or urea, help attract water to the skin and retain moisture, contributing to the skin's hydration and elasticity spoilage or infection. Preservatives like parabens, phenoxyethanol, or ethylhexylglycerin are often added to extend the shelf life of the product and prevent bacterial, fungal, or yeast growth. These preservatives are generally used in small amounts and are carefully selected to ensure they do not irritate or sensitize the skin. (Iqbal & Nair, 2024). However, these ingredients can sometimes cause irritation or allergic reactions, particularly in individuals with sensitive skin. Fragrance-free and hypoallergenic formulations are typically available for those with more sensitive skin or conditions like eczema or rosacea carbomers, or cellulose derivatives. These ingredients ensure that the cream remains stable and consistent in texture, making it easy to apply and spread across the skin. The balanced nature of creams allows them to provide hydration and healing properties while delivering active ingredients to the skin. Some common therapeutic uses of creams include: Topical analgesic creams are often used to provide localized pain relief. These creams typically contain ingredients like lidocaine, menthol, or capsaicin that work by numbing the area or providing a cooling or warming sensation. They are commonly used to treat conditions such as arthritis, muscle strains, back pain, and neuropathic pain soothing ingredients like aloe vera, hydrocortisone, or calamine are often used to reduce inflammation, cool the skin, and accelerate the healing process. These creams provide relief from the burning sensation and promote faster recovery of the skin a protective barrier. Creams containing ingredients like zinc oxide or silver sulfadiazine are frequently used in the treatment of burns, cuts, and other wounds. These creams help keep the wound moist, reduce the risk of infection, and speed up the healing process. They are used in skincare and beauty products to hydrate, nourish, and protect the skin. Some common cosmetic uses of creams include:

FORMULATION CONSIDERATIONS: ACTIVE INGREDIENTS AND EXCIPIENTS

Topical formulations, such as ointments and creams, are integral components of modern medicine and skincare. Both serve as vehicles for delivering active ingredients to the skin, treating a variety of conditions ranging from dermatological issues to cosmetic concerns. Although ointments and creams are often used interchangeably in daily language, they have distinct differences in their formulation, properties, applications, and effectiveness. Understanding these differences is crucial not only for medical professionals prescribing these products but also for consumers choosing the right product for their specific needs. In this comprehensive discussion, we will delve into the key differences between ointments and creams, focusing on their composition, texture, clinical uses, advantages and disadvantages, and the specific contexts in which each formulation is best suited of the primary distinctions between ointments and creams lies in their composition. These differences influence their texture, spreadability, and how they interact with the skin ointment is predominantly composed of petroleum jelly, mineral oil, lanolin, or other waxes and oils. The oil content of ointments often exceeds 80%, which imparts a thick, greasy texture that adheres to the skin. Due to the oil content, ointments are typically hydrophobic, meaning they lack water in their formulation. As a result, ointments do not easily wash off with water, and they are often more occlusive in nature content, with a composition where water constitutes around 50% to 80% of the formula, with the remainder being oils and emulsifiers. (Khan & Rodrigues, 2023) This dual-phase structure allows for better hydration of the skin while maintaining the moisturizing benefits of oils. Emulsifiers such as cetyl alcohol, stearic acid, and polysorbates stabilize the water-oil mixture, ensuring a uniform product that does not separate. The water phase of creams imparts a lighter texture, making them easier to spread and less greasy compared to ointments process, and patient preference more difficult to apply evenly, especially over large areas. When applied to the skin, ointments leave a shiny, oily residue that can be difficult to wash off. While this greasy texture may be undesirable for some users, it is an advantage in specific therapeutic applications where an occlusive effect is necessary to prevent water loss and promote healing. Ointments are often used in cases of severely dry skin, eczema, or psoriasis, where moisture retention is critical small areas and allows for quicker absorption into the skin. Creams typically leave a less greasy finish compared to ointments, and the texture is lighter, making them more pleasant for general skincare and everyday use. They often feel cool upon application and are ideal for individuals who prefer a less heavy product that doesn't leave a noticeable residue the active ingredients is needed. For example, the slow and sustained release of a corticosteroid in an ointment form may be beneficial for treating inflammatory skin conditions such as eczema or psoriasis, where long-lasting effects are desired tend to be more rapidly absorbed compared to ointments, which may make them more suitable for acute conditions or for use on areas of the body where quick relief or faster action is required. (Malhotra & Jain, 2024) For instance, creams containing antifungal or antibacterial agents are often absorbed swiftly to treat infections on the skin's surface highly effective in managing conditions that involve dry, cracked, or inflamed skin, as they help lock in moisture and create a favorable environment for healing. The occlusive nature of ointments is particularly beneficial in conditions.

The higher water content of creams allows for better initial hydration, making them effective in treating conditions that require rapid rehydration of the skin. However, the lack of a thick occlusive barrier means that creams are generally better suited for milder skin conditions where skin hydration is required but the need for a strong protective barrier is less pronounced. creams are used in the treatment of a wide range of skin conditions, but their specific therapeutic applications differ based on their formulation properties provide sustained relief and protect the skin. For instance, ointments containing analgesic agents, such as lidocaine or menthol, are used for localized pain relief in conditions like arthritis or muscle strain. The slower absorption of the active ingredients helps provide prolonged relief. Each formulation offers distinct advantages and disadvantages, which depend on the specific needs of the user and the condition being treated. Creams are lighter and more easily spread over the skin, making them convenient for daily use and suitable for larger application areas. Creams absorb quickly, which is ideal for individuals (Lee & Chen, 2023) who need a quick-acting product or who want to avoid feeling greasy after application. The light texture and non-greasy nature of creams make them a popular choice for facial skincare, especially for individuals with sensitive or acne-prone skin. While ointments and creams both serve the essential role of delivering topical treatments to the skin, their differences in composition, texture, and function make them suited for different purposes. other hand, are lighter, easier to apply, and absorb more quickly, making them preferable for milder conditions, facial skincare, and daily moisturizing needs. Understanding the key differences between these two types of formulations can help consumers make informed choices about which product to use, depending on their skin type, the condition being treated, and the desired effect. Whether it's the long-lasting protection of ointments or the quick absorption and comfort of creams, both have their place in the world of topical treatments and skincare.

EMULSIONS AND STABILITY: CHALLENGES IN TOPICAL FORMULATIONS

In the development of topical formulations, such as ointments, creams, gels, and lotions, several critical factors must be considered to ensure the product is effective, safe, and stable. Among these factors, the choice and balance of active ingredients and excipients are central to the success of the formulation. The active ingredients are responsible for the therapeutic or cosmetic effects of the product, while excipients serve a variety of supportive roles, including improving the formulation's stability, enhancing the skin's absorption of the active ingredients, and providing desirable sensory properties. Both active ingredients and excipients must be carefully selected and optimized to create a product that meets the specific needs of the intended use, whether it’s for pharmaceutical treatment or cosmetic skincare. This analysis will explore the key formulation considerations for both active ingredients and excipients, with a focus on their roles, selection criteria, and interactions effect. In the pharmaceutical context, these ingredients can include drugs, biologically active compounds, and other substances that provide a beneficial effect when applied to the skin. (Mehta et al., 2025). The choice of active ingredient depends on the condition being treated, the mechanism of action required, and the specific patient population. In cosmetic formulations, active ingredients are typically included to target specific skin concerns, such as hydration, anti-aging, acne treatment, or hyperpigmentation effect, such as corticosteroids, antifungals, antibiotics, and analgesics. The choice of API is driven by the clinical objective, for example, the treatment of inflammatory skin conditions (corticosteroids), infections (antibiotics), or localized pain (analgesics). In dermatological formulations, APIs are often delivered to the skin to act locally without systemic absorption, though some formulations may allow for partial systemic delivery, especially in chronic conditions. improve skin health, appearance, and function. Common active ingredients in skincare products include hyaluronic acid (for hydration), retinoids (for anti-aging and acne), vitamin C (for brightening), peptides (for anti-aging and collagen synthesis), and niacinamide (for reducing redness and inflammation).

These ingredients are often chosen based on their specific properties, such as collagen stimulation, antioxidant activity, or barrier repair: The active ingredient must demonstrate the desired therapeutic or cosmetic effect, supported by scientific evidence of its effectiveness. This includes clinical studies, dermatological testing, and regulatory approvals. For pharmaceutical products, efficacy must be proven through clinical trials, while for cosmetic products, marketing claims may be supported by in-vitro or consumer use studies. (Norris & Ahmed, 2024) outermost layer of the skin, presents a significant barrier to the absorption of many substances, and the ability of an active ingredient to cross this barrier is a critical consideration. For this reason, the physicochemical properties of the active ingredient, such as molecular size, polarity, and solubility, are important factors in formulation design. For example, smaller molecules like corticosteroids or retinoids may penetrate the skin more easily, while larger molecules may require penetration enhancers to aid absorption., and some biologics, can degrade over time when exposed to light, heat, or oxygen. Therefore, the formulation must protect these ingredients from degradation, which may include using air-tight packaging, antioxidants, or chelating agents potent ingredients, like retinoids or corticosteroids, may cause irritation, especially when used in high concentrations or on sensitive skin. Formulations must be optimized to minimize irritation while maintaining efficacy., and fragrance. Excipients also contribute to the safety, ease of use, and effectiveness of the final product. There are several categories of excipients, each serving a specific function within the formulation the solubility of the active ingredient but also its release and absorption in the skin. For example, water-based vehicles may be used in lighter formulations like gels and lotions, while oil-based vehicles are often used in ointments for more occlusive effects include cetyl alcohol, stearyl alcohol, polysorbates, and lecithin.

RHEOLOGY AND TEXTURE: IMPORTANCE IN TOPICAL FORMULATIONS

The creation of stable emulsions is crucial for ensuring the efficacy, safety, and aesthetic properties of topical products. However, the process of formulating and maintaining emulsions in a stable form is fraught with challenges, which require careful consideration of ingredients, formulation techniques, and storage conditions. Stability is a key concern in emulsion formulations, as any disruption in the balance of the oil and water phases can lead to separation, phase inversion, or degradation of the active ingredients. This section explores the various aspects of emulsions in topical formulations, the challenges associated with maintaining their stability, and strategies to address these challenges. In O/W emulsions, water is the continuous phase, with oil droplets dispersed throughout, while in W/O emulsions, oil is the continuous phase, with water droplets dispersed within it. The selection of emulsion type plays a critical role in determining the formulation's characteristics, including its texture, feel, absorption rate, and use for specific therapeutic or cosmetic applications. for use in products that require rapid absorption and minimal residue, such as lotions and creams. The predominance of water in these formulations allows for good spreadability and hydration of the skin. (O'Connor & Dubey, 2025) They are commonly used for moisturizing, anti-aging, and sun protection products of oil, making them ideal for dry or dehydrated skin, as they create a barrier to reduce moisture loss. W/O emulsions are used in richer creams and ointments for treating conditions like eczema, psoriasis, or other forms of severe skin dryness change in the appearance or texture of the product. Such issues not only affect the product's efficacy but also its safety, as unstable emulsions can lead to degradation of active ingredients or microbial contamination. Several factors contribute to the instability of emulsions: stability. Emulsifiers work by reducing the surface tension between the oil and water phases, facilitating the formation of a stable dispersion. However, if the emulsifier is not properly chosen or if its concentration is insufficient, the emulsion can break down, leading to phase separation. The stability of an emulsion can also be influenced by the type of emulsifier used, with some being more effective in stabilizing oil-in-water emulsions, while others work better in water-in-oil systems., transforming an oil-in-water emulsion into a water-in-oil emulsion or vice versa.

This phenomenon is often caused by temperature fluctuations, changes in pH, or the introduction of certain ingredients that disrupt the balance between the oil and water phases. For example, an emulsion formulated to be oil-in-water might invert to water-in-oil if exposed to high temperatures during storage. Phase inversion leads to changes in texture, appearance, and performance, often making the product unusable crucial to its stability. Smaller droplets provide a larger surface area, which helps keep the oil and water phases dispersed. If the droplet size increases or if there is aggregation of droplets, the emulsion can become unstable and prone to separation. The use of high-shear mixing or homogenization during formulation can help achieve a fine and uniform droplet size, but over time, the emulsified droplets may coalesce, leading to instability of ingredients, or cause phase separation. For example, exposure to high temperatures can cause the breakdown of emulsifiers and lead to the separation of the oil and water phases. Similarly, freezing temperatures can result in the formation of ice crystals, which disrupt the structure of the emulsion. (Omar & Wang, 2023) Therefore, controlling storage conditions is essential for maintaining the stability of emulsions, and manufacturers often provide specific storage instructions to avoid temperature extremes the charge and behavior of the emulsifiers and other ingredients. For instance, certain emulsifiers may only be effective within a specific pH range. If the pH of the product shifts outside of this range due to the addition of other ingredients or through degradation, the emulsion may break down. Furthermore, the pH of the skin itself, typically ranging from 4.5 to 5.5, should be considered when formulating topical emulsions to ensure compatibility and to prevent irritation or instability with the inclusion of preservatives, emulsions can become contaminated if the formulation is not adequately protected or if preservatives lose their effectiveness over time. Preservative selection must be aligned with the formulation's characteristics, ensuring broad-spectrum antimicrobial activity while minimizing potential irritation or sensitivity chemical, and microbial stability of the product. Some of these strategies include or combination of emulsifiers, formulators can improve the stability of the emulsion. Additionally, ensuring the correct concentration of emulsifiers is critical for maintaining stability without compromising the texture or sensory properties of the product.) is used to improve the stability of the emulsion. Co-emulsifiers work synergistically with the primary emulsifier to enhance the viscosity, stabilize the emulsion, and prevent phase separation. This approach can also improve the feel and sensory attributes of the final product, which is important in cosmetic formulation and help stabilize the formulation. These ingredients help maintain the uniformity of the product, reduce the likelihood of phase separation, and enhance the emulsion's spreadability and texture. However, care must be taken to ensure that the thickening agents do not interfere with the efficacy of active ingredients or the sensory experience of the product., the addition of antioxidants and preservatives is essential. Antioxidants, such as vitamin (Pradeep et al., 2025). E or butylated hydroxytoluene (BHT), help prevent the oxidation of oils and active ingredients, which could otherwise lead to the breakdown of the formulation. Preservatives like phenoxyethanol, ethylhexylglycerin, or parabens are used to inhibit microbial growth and extend shelf life, particularly in emulsions containing water remain stable. A gentle, controlled heating and cooling process can help minimize the risk of phase inversion and prevent ingredient degradation.

During production, emulsions are often created by slowly adding the oil phase to the water phase under controlled mixing to form a stable dispersion the active ingredients. Air-tight containers, such as pumps or tubes, help minimize exposure to oxygen, which can lead to oxidation, and protect the formulation from microbial contamination are essential in the formulation of topical products, offering a versatile means of delivering active ingredients to the skin in a controlled, effective manner. However, maintaining the stability of emulsions is a complex challenge that requires careful attention to formulation parameters, including emulsifier selection, phase stability, temperature control, and preservative management. Instability in emulsions can lead to undesirable product characteristics, such as phase separation, texture changes, or loss of efficacy. By understanding the factors that influence emulsion stability and implementing strategies to mitigate these challenges, formulators can create high-quality, stable emulsion-based products that effectively meet the needs of consumers and patientsv, (Qureshi & Dasgupta, 2024). Products are applied directly to the skin, necessitating rigorous testing to ensure their safety, efficacy, and consistency. Effective QC encompasses a range of activities, from raw material assessment to final product testing, all aimed at maintaining high-quality standards and compliance with regulatory Adherence to Good Manufacturing Practices (GMP) is fundamental in ensuring the quality of topical formulations. GMP guidelines, as outlined by regulatory bodies like the U.S. Food and Drug Administration (FDA) and the Central Drugs Standard Control Organization (CDSCO) in India, provide a framework for maintaining product quality. These practices encompass aspects such as personnel training, equipment calibration, sanitation, and documentation to maintain product integrity and traceability properties of topical formulations. A comprehensive stability study, (Ranjitha et al., 2025) including both long-term and accelerated testing, is essential for determining the appropriate shelf life and storage conditions for topical formulations. For example, nanoparticles such as solid lipid nanoparticles (SLNs) and nanostructured lipid carriers (NLCs) are being increasingly incorporated into cosmetic and pharmaceutical formulations to enhance the delivery of active ingredients like vitamins, antioxidants, and anti-aging compounds. (Sameer Babu et al., 2025) The use of nanocarriers also opens up possibilities for controlled or sustained release formulations, where the active ingredients are gradually released over time, ensuring prolonged therapeutic effects wound healing. the most exciting trends in topical formulations is the integration of wearable technology with skincare products. Sensors embedded in patches, smartwatches, or even clothing can monitor a variety of skin parameters, including hydration, temperature, UV exposure, and pH levels. (Thomas & Farooq, 2023). This real-time data can then be used to personalize topical formulations, adjusting the rich with potential, driven by innovations in nanotechnology, biotechnology, regenerative medicine, sustainability, and digital health. These biologically active ingredients, combined with advances in delivery systems, are likely to become central to the next generation of skincare treatments, offering both therapeutic and anti-aging benefits. Furthermore, gene therapy and RNA-based therapies are starting to make their way into topical formulations. (Tanaka & Velasquez, 2024) Although still in the early stages of development, these therapies hold the potential to treat genetic skin conditions or repair skin damage at the genetic level.

CONCLUSION

The future of topical formulations is poised to undergo significant transformations, driven by technological innovations, enhanced understanding of skin biology, and evolving consumer needs. As the demand for more effective, personalized, and sustainable skincare and therapeutic solutions increases, advancements in material science, drug delivery technologies, and digital health are paving the way for a new generation of topical products. These innovations hold the promise of improving both the efficacy and safety of treatments, while offering consumers more control and customization over their skincare and medical needs. This section will explore several of the key areas where breakthroughs are expected to shape the future of topical formulations skin's natural barrier to the absorption of active ingredients. The skin's outermost layer, the stratum corneum, acts as a protective shield that prevents the easy entry of foreign substances. However, advancements in nanotechnology, including the use of nanoparticles, liposomes, and nanoemulsions, are breaking down these barriers and facilitating deeper, more efficient delivery of active ingredients into the skin. Nanocarriers can significantly improve the solubility and stability of both hydrophilic and lipophilic drugs, enhancing the bioavailability of therapeutic agents. By utilizing nanoparticles that are small enough to penetrate the skin's barrier, these systems can deliver drugs with high precision, minimizing systemic side effects and increasing localized therapeutic effects. Nanomaterials, including silver nanoparticles and nanofibers, are being incorporated into wound dressings to enhance antimicrobial properties and promote faster tissue regeneration. The ability of these nanomaterials to target specific areas of the skin and modulate cellular processes at the molecular level represents a breakthrough in treating chronicmaterials that respond to changes in temperature, pH, light, or other factors to release active ingredients in a controlled, targeted manner. The use of "smart polymers," such as thermo-responsive, pH-sensitive, or photo-responsive materials, enables the design of formulations that release their active ingredients only when needed, thereby enhancing efficacy and reducing side effects. For example, thermo-responsive hydrogels can undergo a phase transition at body temperature, transforming from a gel to a liquid and enabling better distribution and absorption of the active ingredient. Similarly, pH-sensitive formulations can release their payload when they encounter acidic or alkaline conditions, which could be particularly useful in treating conditions such as acne (which often involves an imbalance in skin pH) or eczema (which is associated with an altered skin barrier). Furthermore, these systems can allow for sustained or delayed release, which improves patient compliance by reducing the frequency of applications and ensuring consistent therapeutic levels over time. Additionally, these smart delivery systems can be integrated with wearable technology, such as sensors or patches, to monitor skin conditions and adjust the formulation accordingly. For instance, a wearable patch might release a therapeutic agent when it detects elevated inflammation or when the skin's moisture level drops below a certain threshold. This integration of real-time data with formulation design could revolutionize how we approach the management of skin conditions, offering patients personalized and dynamic treatment options. The integration of biotechnology into skincare and therapeutic products is enabling the development of formulations that do more than just treat symptoms—they actively promote skin regeneration and healing at the cellular level. The use of stem cells, growth factors, exosomes, and peptides is opening new avenues for repairing damaged skin and stimulating the body's natural healing processes. Stem cell-based formulations are being explored for their ability to regenerate skin cells and promote tissue repair. These formulations could have profound implications in the treatment of chronic wounds, burns, and even skin aging. Similarly, the use of exosomes—nano-sized vesicles derived from stem cells—has shown promise in promoting skin regeneration, reducing inflammation, and enhancing the skin's natural barrier function. In cosmetics, peptides are increasingly being used to stimulate collagen production and support the skin's elasticity, helping to reduce the appearance of fine lines and wrinkles. By delivering RNA molecules or gene-editing tools directly to the skin, it may be possible to correct mutations that cause disorders like epidermolysis bullosa or even reverse signs of aging toward cleaner, greener products that are both effective and environmentally responsible. The use of natural, biodegradable, and ethically sourced ingredients is on the rise, and many companies are focusing on reducing the environmental impact of their packaging. This includes adopting refillable containers, recyclable materials, and minimizing plastic use. In the realm of green chemistry, new methods of formulating products that reduce reliance on synthetic chemicals and solvents are being developed. This includes the use of plant-based oils, extracts, and essential fatty acids, which not only provide therapeutic benefits but also align with the increasing consumer demand for eco-friendly, cruelty-free products. Companies are also exploring more sustainable methods of producing active ingredients, such as biotechnological processes that use microorganisms or plant-based sources, reducing the environmental footprint of product manufacturing. Furthermore, transparency in ingredient sourcing and product testing is becoming increasingly important. Consumers are seeking brands that are transparent about their supply chains, ingredients, and sustainability practices, which is driving manufacturers to adopt cleaner, more ethical practices. This trend is influencing not only the cosmetic industry but also the pharmaceutical sector, where there is a growing demand for natural and sustainable alternatives to synthetic drugs. As these technologies continue to evolve, the ability to deliver more effective, personalized, and sustainable topical treatments will revolutionize skincare, dermatology, and wound care. The integration of smart delivery systems, bioactive ingredients, and real-time data will provide unprecedented levels of customization, offering consumers and patients a more dynamic, responsive, and targeted approach to skincare and therapeutic treatments. As these advancements unfold, they will not only improve the quality of life for individuals but also reshape the landscape of the global skincare and pharmaceutical industries.

REFERENCES

Anderson, L. T., & Brown, R. J. (2024). AI moderation frameworks in decentralized networks. In Patel, R. (Ed.), *AI and blockchain synergy in content control* (pp. 33–50). TechEdge Press., DOI: 10.4018/978-1-2345-6789-1.ch003

Athavale, V. A., Selvakumar, P., Poorani, S., Anand, T., & Rathore, D. S. (2025). Designing chatbots for educational leadership. In Musundire, A. (Ed.), *Chatbots in educational leadership and management* (pp. 181–204). IGI Global Scientific Publishing., DOI: 10.4018/979-8-3693-8734-4.ch008

Baker, M. A., & Sanchez, F. (2025). Deep learning ethics in recommendation engines. In Zhao, J. (Ed.), *Ethical perspectives on AI personalization* (pp. 19–42). DataVerse Publications., DOI: 10.4018/978-3-9876-5432-1.ch002

Chakrabarti, R., & Lin, K. (2023). Cross-cultural AI biases in content flagging. In Kumar, S. (Ed.), *Global AI moderation strategies* (pp. 71–96). Nova Academic., DOI: 10.4018/978-2-4567-1234-3.ch004

Chandel, P. S., & Ghosh, R. K. (2024). Reinventing online safety with ethical algorithms. In Desai, A. (Ed.), *AI interventions in digital harm reduction* (pp. 27–59). TechSphere., DOI: 10.4018/978-3-2025-4456-7.ch002

Das, M., & Tripathi, L. P. (2025). Ethical AI auditing practices for social networks. In Verma, N. (Ed.), *AI compliance and accountability online* (pp. 113–134). Insight Academic., DOI: 10.4018/978-9-8765-4321-0.ch006

Desai, T., & Anand, P. S. (2024). Sentiment analysis for hate speech detection. In Iyer, M. (Ed.), *AI tools for inclusive communication* (pp. 45–68). Scholarly Ink., DOI: 10.4018/978-1-1000-2938-4.ch005

Edwards, C. J., & Patel, H. (2023). Autonomous systems for misinformation tracking. In Green, M. (Ed.), *AI solutions in digital journalism* (pp. 101–122). FutureText., DOI: 10.4018/978-4-5678-9876-5.ch007

Fernandez, J., & Zhao, L. (2024). Reinforcement learning in ethical content curation. In Li, H. (Ed.), *AI agents in dynamic environments* (pp. 87–109). MetaScholars., DOI: 10.4018/978-1-1111-2222-3.ch004

Ghosh, A., & Pillai, M. N. (2025). AI-driven language filters for social platforms. In Mukherjee, D. (Ed.), *Multilingual AI safety mechanisms* (pp. 61–89). Informed AI Press., DOI: 10.4018/978-5-5555-6666-6.ch005

Gupta, R., & Bhatia, S. P. (2024). Digital well-being and ethical nudges. In Singh, N. (Ed.), *Behavioral AI for online harmony* (pp. 21–47). Cognitia Press., DOI: 10.4018/978-3-4444-7777-7.ch002

Hansen, V. T., & Ng, C. Y. (2025). Legal frameworks for AI governance in media. In Alami, M. (Ed.), *Policy and AI in the public sphere* (pp. 109–130). Juridica Publishing., DOI: 10.4018/978-6-7654-3210-9.ch006

Iqbal, R., & Nair, K. J. (2024). User-centric AI ethics in platform design. In Shah, B. (Ed.), *Ethics-first AI in digital experience* (pp. 55–84). PeopleFirst Books., DOI: 10.4018/978-0-1111-9999-9.ch004

Khan, S. T., & Rodrigues, V. (2023). Building trust in AI content filtering. In Venkatesan, S. (Ed.), *Trustworthy AI: Models and measures* (pp. 89–112). AI Insights., DOI: 10.4018/978-2-3344-5566-2.ch005

Lee, H. M., & Chen, Y. J. (2023). Inclusive dataset strategies for fair AI. In Wong, L. (Ed.), *AI training sets and ethical representation* (pp. 33–58). DataJustice Press., DOI: 10.4018/978-8-8888-2222-2.ch003

Malhotra, R., & Jain, I. (2024). Bias detection in social recommendation systems. In Sharma, M. (Ed.), *AI integrity in digital influence* (pp. 97–118). Equity Press., DOI: 10.4018/978-1-5555-8888-3.ch006

Mehta, A. K., Yashoda, L., Selvakumar, P., Mishra, B. R., Das, A., & C. T. C., M. (2025). Teaching methods: Techniques for disadvantaged learners. In S. Hai-Jew (Ed.), Mitigating learner disadvantages in teaching and learning (pp. 181–206). IGI Global Scientific Publishing. https://doi.org/DOI: 10.4018/979-8-3693-8623-1.ch007

Norris, K. D., & Ahmed, Z. (2024). Regulation of AI-powered political ads. In Choi, J. (Ed.), *Governance of AI in digital campaigns* (pp. 91–113). MediaEthics Press., DOI: 10.4018/978-3-764-3210-8.ch006

O'Connor, B., & Dubey, R. (2025). Deepfake detection and ethical implications. In Fraser, L. (Ed.), *Truth and trust in AI-generated media* (pp. 59–84). RealMedia Academic., DOI: 10.4018/978-9-3210-7654-3.ch004

Omar, F., & Wang, L. (2023). AI in flagging extremist content: Challenges and progress. In Becker, T. (Ed.), *Machine learning in content moderation* (pp. 103–125). SafeAI Press., DOI: 10.4018/978-3-2109-8754-1.ch007

Pradeep, E., Mukherjee, S. K., Selvakumar, P., Koppaka, A. K., Chandel, P. S., & Vats, C. (2025). Empowering social media users with ethical AI. In Chakraborty, S. (Ed.), *Ethical AI solutions for addressing social media influence and hate speech* (pp. 91–118). IGI Global Scientific Publishing., DOI: 10.4018/979-8-3693-9904-0.ch005

Pradeep, E., Mukherjee, S. K., Selvakumar, P., Koppaka, A. K., Chandel, P. S., & Vats, C. (2025). Empowering social media users with ethical AI. In Chakraborty, S. (Ed.), *Ethical AI solutions for addressing social media influence and hate speech* (pp. 91–118). IGI Global Scientific Publishing., DOI: 10.4018/979-8-3693-9904-0.ch005

Qureshi, L., & Dasgupta, T. (2024). AI fairness in targeting marginalized comunities. In Pillai, M. (Ed.), *Inclusive AI for social platforms* (pp. 29–55). Unity Press., DOI: 10.4018/978-6-1212-7777-1.ch003

Ranjitha, P. K., Selvakumar, P., Anute, N., Manjunath, T., Sureshkrishna, G., & Pougajendy, S. (2025). Transportation challenges in islands tourism. In Hassan, V. (Ed.), *Navigating mass tourism to island destinations: Preservation and cultural heritage challenges* (pp. 287–312). IGI Global Scientific Publishing., DOI: 10.4018/979-8-3693-9107-5.ch011

Sameer Babu, M., Karunakaran, N. B., Selvakumar, P., Sethumadhavan, R., & Chandel, P. S. (2025). The role of chatbots in educational leadership. In Musundire, A. (Ed.), *Chatbots in educational leadership and management* (pp. 321–346). IGI Global Scientific Publishing., DOI: 10.4018/979-8-3693-8734-4.ch013

Tanaka, Y., & Velasquez, C. (2024). Multi-agent AI and online safety. In Bennett, J. (Ed.), *Distributed AI in public discourse* (pp. 119–144). GridAI Publishers., DOI: 10.4018/978-9-9999-2222-3.ch007

Thomas, A. B., & Farooq, M. (2023). Ethical design patterns in content moderation. In Lee, R. (Ed.), *Architecting AI for human dignity* (pp. 51–76). DesignCode Press., DOI: 10.4018/978-3-2023-3030-1.ch003

Tiwari, R., & Ochieng, J. (2024). Youth safey and AI policy on social media. In Mendez, A. (Ed.), *AI regulation for vulnerable populations* (pp. 88–112). DigitalCare Publishing., DOI: 10.4018/978-0-9876-1000-5.ch005

Tripathi, L. P., & Deshmukh, A. (2025). Decoding algorithmic bias in AI filters. In Bhat, R. (Ed.), *AI ethics across cultures* (pp. 42–69). InsightBridge Press., DOI: 10.4018/978-3-3333-4444-6.ch004

Uddin, M. N., & Jensen, T. (2024). Preventing radicalization through AI moderation. In Das, K. (Ed.), *AI in extremism prevention* (pp. 121–144). PeaceTech Academic., DOI: 10.4018/978-1-5678-9999-0.ch006

Valdez, A., & Krishnan, M. S. (2023). AI ethics in meme and short-form content. In Ho, C. (Ed.), *Content formats and AI challenges* (pp. 36–63). PopTech Press., DOI: 10.4018/978-6-7777-8888-8.ch003

Vijayakumar, G., Muniyandi Rajkumar, Rajiv Chandar, N., Selvakumar, P., & Ramesh Duraisamy. (2024). Environmentally friendly TDS removal from wastewater by electrochemical ion exchange batch-type recirculation (EIR) technique. *Environmental Science. Water Research & Technology*, *10*, 826–835. DOI: 10.1039/D3EW00793F

Wagner, L., & Kumar, A. (2024). Bridging digital divides with ethical AI access. In Foster, D. (Ed.), *Equity in AI technologies* (pp. 51–77). FutureVision Press., DOI: 10.4018/978-5-1212-6543-2.ch004

Wang, Z., & Fernandes, J. (2023). Algorithmic explainability for content decisions. In Silva, M. (Ed.), *Understanding AI in social media governance* (pp. 67–93). Clarity Publishing., DOI: 10.4018/978-0-2310-3210-0.ch003

White, E. T., & Raman, R. (2024). Ethical dilemmas in AI nudging. In Noor, I. (Ed.), *Digital influence and ethical AI* (pp. 34–58). EthicAI Press., DOI: 10.4018/978

Chapter 8
Bioadhesive Films and Bandages

Yashvi Patel
https://orcid.org/0009-0004-9989-8005
Shobhaben Pratapbhai Patel School of Pharmacy and Technology Management, SVKM's NMIMS, India

Namita Juvale
https://orcid.org/0000-0001-7004-5675
Shobhaben Pratapbhai Patel School of Pharmacy and Technology Management, SVKM's NMIMS, India

ABSTRACT

Wounds can be of an acute type, such as minor cuts & abrasions, post-operative incisions, superficial burns, or chronic in nature, like diabetic ulcers, burns, or infected wounds. As not all synthetic polymers are bio-compatible and bio-degradable, herbal excipients and polymers-based bioadhesive films and bandages play a pivotal role in advanced wound management by focusing on prevention of complications, protecting against infections, and promoting healing. Bioadhesive films and bandages used for wound care are designed to adhere directly to skin or mucosal surfaces, providing both protective coverage and localized delivery of therapeutic agents. The goal of development of bioadhesive films based on biopolymers that are easily removable and non-toxic can be achieved by use of natural biopolymers. Various formulations like Pectin and Mucilage Patches, silk fibroin-chitosan film have been formulated and proven effective. Future efforts are required to address batch variability, stability, standardization and regulatory restrictions to accelerate clinical use for advanced wound care.

DOI: 10.4018/979-8-3373-3977-1.ch008

1. INTRODUCTION

The practice of wound dressing dates back to thousands of years when only natural materials were used. Ancient Mesopotamians cleaned wounds with water or milk and used honey and plant resins for dressing (Lopes et al., 2024). In 1600 BCE Egyptians commonly used linen or gauze strips soaked in oils or fats as per the texts (Dhivya et al., 2015). The germ theory was introduced in the 19th century and by the 20th century modern dressings such as occlusive films and hydrogels were engineered for wound treatment (Dhivya et al., 2015; Lopes et al., 2024). The historical progression from plant-derived dressings to synthetic gauze and foams laid the foundation for advanced bioadhesive films, many of which again employ natural polymers. The term "bioadhesion" was coined in 1970 to describe the adhesion of natural or synthetic polymers to biological tissues (Zhu et al., 2023). Bioadhesive films and bandages were engineered such that they can wet the wound surface and form interfacial bonds i.e. hydrogen bonding, van der Waals forces or chain interpenetration while retaining enough structural cohesion to resist deformation (Zhu et al., 2023). Plant-based polymers are generally biocompatible and biodegradable as they are derived from renewable sources. For example, cellulose derivatives are semi-synthetic polymers yet they retain favorable traits like non-toxicity and non-immunogenicity while being water-soluble (Tudoroiu et al., 2021). Recent reviews have emphasized that starch hydrogels are ideal matrices for wound therapeutics as they can absorb water and release drugs over time (Lee & Hwang, 2023). Similarly, natural mucoadhesive and non-toxic gums such as alginate form swellable matrices which absorb exudate released from wound. Pectin binds strongly with calcium, forming gel that provides good water absorption and mild adhesion to tissues (Patitucci et al., 2024). Modern research has developed plant-based bioadhesive dressings into "smart" technology. For example, pH-responsive films are being developed to monitor wound conditions. In recent advancement a cellulose-based nanocomposite embedded with pH-responsive indicators and nanoparticles allowed real-time colorimetric pH sensing while maintaining excellent conformability and moisture transport (Eskilson et al., 2023). A 3D-printed patch exhibited nearly 100% polyphenol release within 48 h and significantly enhanced fibroblast migration and collagen deposition during in vitro studies (Patitucci et al., 2024). Other emerging trends includes electrospun nanofibrous films that mimic the skin's extracellular matrix, and multilayer composites that combine barrier, adhesive and drug-delivery layers (Nada et al., 2020). In summary, the field is rapidly evolving toward multifunctional plant-based dressings that are not merely coverings, but active wound-healing systems.

2. BACKGROUND OF BIOADHESIVE FILMS AND BANDAGES

Bioadhesive films are thin polymeric membranes that adhere to epithelial membranes i.e. skin or mucosa for the purpose of wound dressing or drug delivery. Use of plant-based polymers (e.g. alginate, cellulose, pectin, guar gum, xanthan) in these films can help maintain moist environment for healing along with their biocompatible and biodegradable nature.(Fiorentini et al., 2021). Plant derived bioadhesives use special polysaccharide molecules containing high number of hydroxyl or carboxyl groups which can form films with good adhesion and controlled release properties (Isopencu et al., 2023; Priya et al., 2024). Consisting of one or more polymeric layers, the films are designed to respond to environmental stimuli. For therapeutic applications in wound management, classification of these films and bandages depends on the intended application site, their structural architecture, and their stimuli-responsiveness as shown in figure 1.

Figure 1. Classification of bioadhesive films and bandages

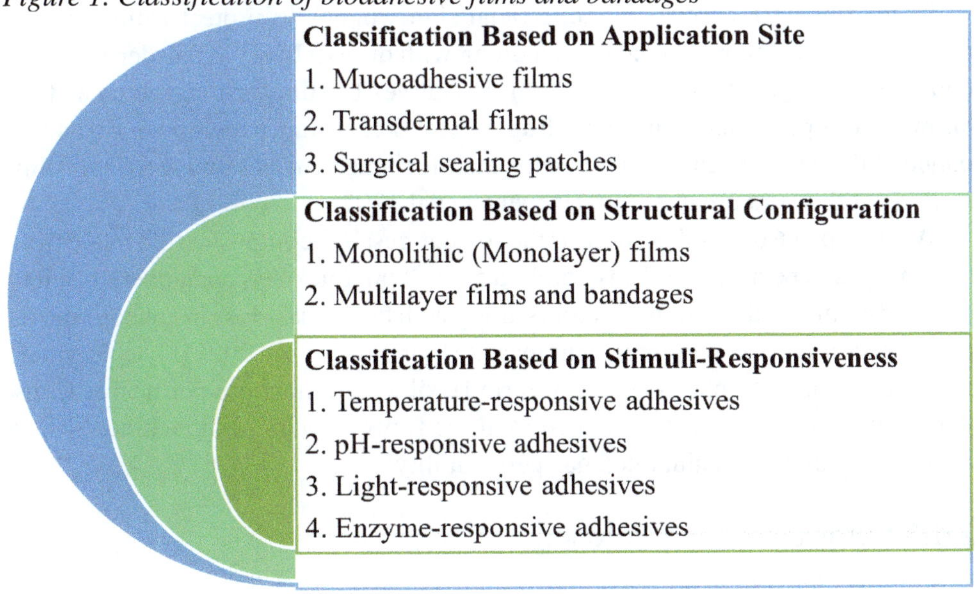

2.1 Classification by Application Site

2.1.1 Mucoadhesive Films

Thes films adhere to oral, sublingual, nasal or vaginal mucosa for topical wound healing or drug delivery. Plant mucilage are preferred for use as mucoadhesive agents due of presence hydrophilic polysaccharides having hydroxyl and carboxyl groups that form strong hydrogen bonds to bind with mucus membrane (Isopencu et al., 2023). For example, mucilage derived from *Mimosa pudica* or *Datura stramonium* seeds demonstrate the ability to extend residence time on the buccal mucosa and improve sustained drug release (Isopencu et al., 2023). When used for oral ulcers or vaginal wounds this can provide localized effect by moisture retention, strong adhesion, targeted and if required controlled drug delivery.

2.1.2 Transdermal Films

These films are applied for superficial skin wounds to protect from physical damage and provide microbial barrier along with drug delivery. Transdermal films commonly use herbal polymers, starch derivatives or film-forming gums as they allow water uptake and controlled drug release. For instance, cellulose fibers and nanocellulose have been widely used in patch-forming matrices owing to their film-forming ability and breathability (Isopencu et al., 2023).

Another plant-derived example is the solvent-cast bio-composite film made from zein and citrus pectin. The film exhibited 50-100 μm thickness and adhered well to skin and conformed to wound contours along with faster mass loss in aqueous media due to pectin released from the zein matrix (Fiorentini et al., 2021). The polymers in combination with plasticizers can form flexible and moisture-permeable films. A barrier against infection is created by these films through mild tackiness-based adhesion along with maintained gas permeability.

2.1.3 Surgical Sealing Patches

These are used to seal wounds and surgical incisions by adhering to tissue surfaces. Plant-based tissue adhesives are used in preparing films that help in closing wounds, prevent leaks or bleeding and promote healing by formation of strong bonds while maintained hemostasis. In situ crosslinking of polysaccharide hydrogels such as alginate or starch derivatives enables the formation of adherent seals directly on wounds. A tissue sealant film may contain calcium-crosslinked alginate or other natural polymers that can adhere strongly to wet tissue. Thus, plant-based polymers can be used to formulate films that provide adhesion and wound sealing without sutures (Ren et al., 2024).

2.2 Classification by Structural Configuration

2.2.1 Monolithic (Monolayer) Films

It is a single homogeneous layer of polymer or a polymer blend that is cast or extruded. They are formed by solvent casting or drying polymer solution. It can contain bioactive, plasticizer or nanoparticles throughout the film layer. In some cases, hydrophobic plasticizers may be added for extended release. For instance, a monolithic film composed of pectin and cellulose can be incorporated with an antiseptic agent to enable sustained release. These films typically exhibit consistent swelling behavior and uniform drug release kinetics (De Carvalho et al., 2023). Monolayer films composed of plant-derived polysaccharides are frequently employed for localized wound coverage in cases where a single functional layer is adequate.

2.2.2 Multilayer Films and Bandages

Multilayered films comprise of two or more polymer layers cast together for serving different functions. For example, a triple-layer film consisting of (i) an outer layer, acting as barrier made of carrageenan or alginate with antimicrobial nanoparticles for moisture control and avoiding infection, (ii) a middle layer for drug loading and mechanical strength prepared with polyvinyl alcohol (PVA)-chitosan combination, (iii) an inner layer that supports healing and regulates drug release (Alipour et al., 2025).

Multilayer bandages combine a supportive backing made of cotton fabric or an alginate sponge with one or more API layers. For example, alginate fibers can be freeze-dried into a porous dressing that not only absorbs wound exudate and swells but also serves as a scaffold for cell growth (Froelich et al., 2023). In Froelich et al. research, researchers created a "composite bandage" by freeze-drying a chitosan–alginate blend into a flexible, porous sheet, then infused it with zinc oxide nanoparticles to deliver antimicrobial protection (Froelich et al., 2023). By stacking different plant-derived polymers, these dressings harness each material's film-forming and gelling properties to work together: an alginate layer promotes hemostasis, while a cellulose nanofiber layer adds mechanical strength, and so on achieving multiple therapeutic functions within a single bandage (Froelich et al., 2023; Isopencu et al., 2023).

2.3 Classification by Stimuli-Responsiveness (Smart Adhesives)

Adhesive films can be formulated to respond to environmental triggers, known as "smart" behavior. In wound healing, four common stimuli are involved: temperature, pH, light, and enzymes (Ren et al., 2024). Stimuli-responsive adhesives adjust their adhesion or degradation properties in situ, which can enhance safety and healing.

2.3.1 Temperature-Responsive Adhesives

These smart adhesives are built from polymers that change their nature around body temperature. For instance, a material that's liquid at room temperature can firm up and grip tissue once it warms to 37 °C, then soften or release when cooled below or heated above that critical point. Researchers have even crafted hydrogels held together by reversible hydrogen or ionic bonds: they cling when warm but let go as they cool. While many of these thermo-responsive systems rely on synthetic blocks like (poly(N-isopropylacrylamide)), scientists are now grafting similar temperature-sensitive motifs onto plant-derived polymers, paving the way for wound glues that set on contact with warm skin and then release themselves when the temperature shifts (Liu et al., 2022). One research illustrates that we can impart temperature-switchability by using reversible crosslinks or blends like agarose which is thermo-responsive and could be blended with cellulose derivatives to produce a plant-only film that gels on heating. Regions of temperature difference can be narrow and sensitive to environmental salts, wound exudate or fever which can shift the transition temperature and change based on whether material is solid or fluid at skin temperature (Sekar et al., 2023).

2.3.2 pH-Responsive Adhesives

Wound environments often become more acidic especially if infection is present, pH-responsive films can be engineered to respond accordingly. By incorporating acid- or base-sensitive groups into biopolymer networks, these dressings can swell, dissolve, or change their crosslinking in response to local pH. For example, an alginate-chitosan film will expand and loosen more readily in acidic conditions, speeding up its release of embedded drug. Similarly, a pectin-based adhesive might stay intact at normal skin pH but break down and detach when the wound's acidity rises (Ren et al., 2024). A pH-responsive wound-healing film was developed using carboxyethyl chitosan and sodium alginate, incorporating a phenol red-based pH indicator. The embedded carboxyethylated phenol red-grafted chitosan imparts a distinct color change from orange to purple and when loaded with diclofenac sodium these films exhibited accelerated drug release at lower pH (Chalitangkoon et al., 2025). This approach allows dressings to cling securely to healthy skin yet loosen or degrade as per demand in an infected, acidic wound area. Certain properties such as ionic strength and acidic or basic functional groups alter swelling and can cause unpredictable release and adhesion in wounds (Ren et al., 2024).

2.3.3 Light-Responsive Adhesives

Photoresponsive adhesives take advantage of photo-sensitive compounds like coumarin, cinnamate, azobenzene or o-nitrobenzyl groups that can form or break bonds under specific wavelengths. On coming in contact with UV or visible light they either convert into a solid glue or cleave apart for removal. Imagine a surgeon spraying on a plant-based adhesive, locking it in place with a quick flash of light, and then later using a second light treatment to peel it away gently (Ren et al., 2024). A methylene blue loaded alginate film was developed for photodynamic wound treatment, upon illumination with red light generates reactive oxygen species with the controlled release of the photoactive agent into the wound cavity (Kuryanova et al., 2023; Solovieva et al., 2024). By combining natural polymer matrices with photochemistry, these photo-responsive systems offer precise spatial and temporal control over adhesion and peeling. Markedly, photosensitizers in presence of light can generate heat or reactive species that may damage healthy tissues so, repeated or high-doses raise safety concerns (Ren et al., 2024).

2.3.4 Enzyme-Responsive Adhesives

Enzyme-sensitive adhesives harness the very enzymes present in wounds i.e. proteases, esterases and trigger their own breakdown. These materials include biodegradable linkages such as peptide bonds, ester groups or glycosidic bonds that specific enzymes can cut. As healing progresses and enzyme levels shift, the adhesive steadily loosens or releases its contents. For instance, a polysaccharide film crosslinked with short peptides might stay firmly attached to healthy skin but selectively degrade in the presence of bacterial proteases at an infected site (Ren et al., 2024). A thin atelocollagen film cross-linked with metalloproteinase 8-cleavable peptide linker carries antimicrobial K4, releasing it slowly onto enzyme-rich wounds. The residual collagen scaffold remains bioadhesive and moist, supporting tissue regeneration while the liberated K4 provides targeted antimicrobial action (C.L. et al., 2023). This smart degradation means the dressing can fall away naturally, sparing patients the discomfort and trauma of manual removal. Microbial enzymes can cause premature loss of adhesion or unpredictable release profiles. Designing linkers that are specific, stable during storage and non-immunogenic is complex and increases cost as well as regulatory hurdles (Ren et al., 2024).

This classification assists in selection of appropriate bioadhesive dressing; such as for oral ulcers a mucoadhesive pectin film, a multilayer alginate-cellulose patch for dermal wounds or for on-demand adhesion use of a temperature-sensitive cellulose composite (Isopencu et al., 2023; Priya et al., 2024). Therefore, variety of plant-based biopolymers can provide supporting material for biocompatibility, biodegradability, and intrinsic bioadhesive properties of film and bandage used in dressing.

3. TYPES OF POLYMERS USED IN BIOADHESIVE FILMS AND BANDAGES

Herbal polymers are a rich, renewable resource combining biocompatibility, biodegradability and intrinsic bioactivity for bioadhesive films and bandages. Common plant-based polymers used in bioadhesive films include cellulose, alginate, pectin, guar and other gums, starch, konjac glucomannan, carrageenan, and xanthan gum. They can be prepared by crosslinking or chemical modifications to optimize viscosity, swelling behavior and mucoadhesion. They have hydrophilic bonds that not only deliver strong adhesion to wound surfaces but also assist in enhanced regeneration, they act as vehicle for drug delivery and in scaffold formation which is depicted in figure 2. Many herbal polymers possess inherent antioxidant or antimicrobial activities, further enhancing their therapeutic potential in wound-care. Some of them are discussed below and their source, properties and applications are summarized in table 1.

Figure 2. Schematic diagram of a bioadhesive polymer film on a wound bed

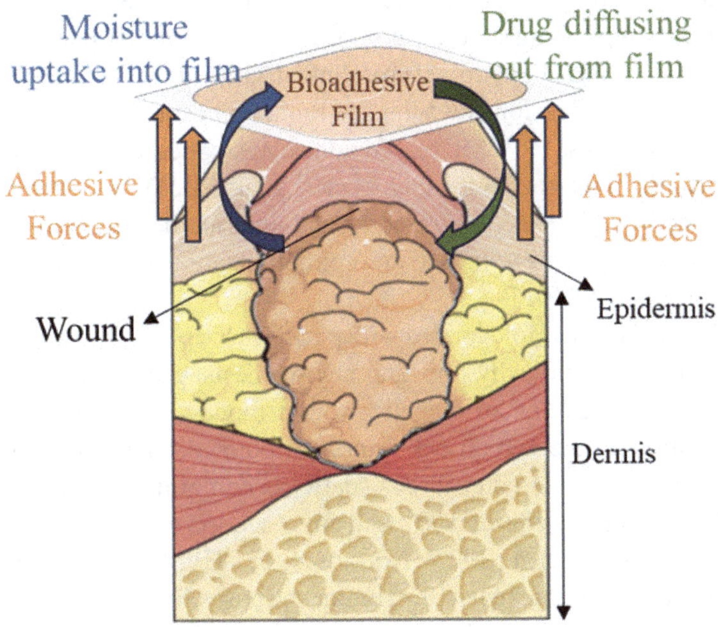

3.1 Cellulose

Cellulose is a natural polysaccharide (β-1,4-glucan) with free hydroxyl group and synthesized primarily by plant cell wall and bacteria (Ho et al., 2024). Native cellulose is insoluble but its semi-synthetic derivatives are widely used in wound dressings. Common derivatives include hydroxypropyl methylcellulose (HPMC), methylcellulose (MC), ethyl cellulose (EC), sodium carboxymethylcellulose (NaC-MC), hydroxyethyl cellulose (HEC) and esterified forms like cellulose acetate (CA). These derivatives are generally biocompatible and biodegradable and can be modified for enhanced solubility, gelation and mechanical properties (Tudoroiu et al., 2021).

Highly hydrophilic cellulose derivatives like NaCMC swell on absorbing large volume of fluid exudates from wound, hence it maintains a moist environment and prevents surrounding tissue dehydration (Tudoroiu et al., 2021). This property promotes healing by facilitating growth-factor activity and cell migration. Similarly, HPMC, MC and HEC help manage exudate by forming hydrophilic gels. Bioadhesivness of unmodified cellulose is poor but modified forms such as oxidized carboxymethyl-cellulose (CMC) on crosslinking with polyamines and catechols can provide strong bioadhesion (Tudoroiu et al., 2021). Oxidized carboxymethyl cellulose (OCMC) when blended with PVA and gelatin and electrospun into nanofibers they demonstrated

99.9% antibacterial efficacy and excellent cytocompatibility (91-92% viability) with full biodegradation over period of three weeks which is ideal for advanced antibacterial dressings (Jangra et al., 2025). A recent study prepared a dopamine containing oxidized NaCMC hydrogel crosslinked with polyallylamine, this complex showed vigorous wet adhesion and achieved rapid hemostasis in bleeding wounds. In rabbit ear model tests, the CMC-based adhesive stopped bleeding in short time period and promoted unscarred healing (Ameri et al., 2025). In a literature report, the NaCMC-pectin-cellulose composite film had superior mechanical properties and accelerated wound repairing with faster re-epithelialization and collagen deposition in vivo (Tudoroiu et al., 2021).

A 3D-printed CMC scaffold loaded with platelet-rich plasma provided sustained growth factor release, markedly boosting angiogenesis, granulation tissue formation, and re-epithelialization in diabetic wound models. Embedding zinc oxide nanoparticles into cellulose matrices improved both mechanical robustness and antibacterial activity, while nanofibrous scaffolds combining ulvan and cellulose supported fibroblast proliferation and rapid angiogenesis without eliciting foreign-body responses (Oliveira et al., 2023). Non-ionics like HPMC and MC are also used often as film-formers or thickeners for similar purposes. Insoluble EC is used as a backing layer in multilayer dressings (Tudoroiu et al., 2021).

3.2 Tannic Acid

Tannic acid is a plant-derived polyphenol in which hydroxyl groups of a D-glucose are esterified with multiple gallic acid dimers (Ali et al., 2024; Aliabadi et al., 2021). Tannic acid is a water-soluble and enable extensive hydrogen-bonding and metal-coordination crosslinking with biopolymers leading to tunable network formation and pH-responsive behavior (Jangra et al., 2025). It has strong antioxidant and astringent properties and it is a hemostatic and broad-spectrum antimicrobial agent with many phenolic hydroxyl groups that confer powerful bioactivities (Ali et al., 2024; Aliabadi et al., 2021). Historically, it was used to treat burn injuries as it reduced infection and mortality while in modern wound dressings it is used as both a bioactive agent and as a cross-linker.

The phenolics attack free radicals and chelate metal ions to protect tissues from oxidative stress and also disrupt microbial membranes. For example, a chitosan–carboxymethyl cellulose film incorporating just 1% tannic acid was able to neutralize approximately 95% of free radicals and inhibit around 81% of Staphylococcus aureus growth. The films exhibited remarkable in-vivo bioactivity in rabbit burn models, the tannic acid-enhanced films drove about 90% wound closure by day 7 (versus roughly 88% in the control group) and achieved full skin regeneration between days 10 and 12 (Ali et al., 2024). When combined with polymers such as chitosan, cellulose or gelatin, tannic acid forms extra crosslinks that boost a film's strength, porosity, and capacity to absorb water. These interactions also enhance adhesion: Tannic acid's catechol-like moieties and protein-binding ability enable the dressing to firmly adhere to tissue. For example, nanocellulose, chitosan and tannic acid composites self-assemble into lamellar, hydrogen-bonded networks that are both rigid and water-stable (Aliabadi et al., 2021).

A novel thin film combining chitosan, CMC and tannic acid with beeswax demonstrated excellent wound-healing performance. It was reported to have swelled 283%, released 89% of its drug payload in 24 hours (Ali et al., 2024). Tannic acid crosslinked films can provide hemostatic effects and potentially photothermal antimicrobial activity when combined with Fe^{3+} or other agents (Jangra et al., 2025). Crosslinking collagen or alginate matrices with tannic acid slows enzymatic degradation, prolonging residence time on the wound bed and supporting sustained therapeutic action (Oliveira et al., 2023). A researcher developed Tannic acid-collagen crosslinked films using a simple casting technique and reported enhanced mechanical strength and slowed degradation compared to uncrosslinked control group, hence underscoring tannic acid's value in collagen-based bandages (Natarajan et al., 2013).

3.3 Starch

Starch is a polysaccharide polymer of glucose (amylose and amylopectin) obtained from corn, potato, rice, etc. It is highly abundant and low-cost compared to other biopolymers. However, native starch films are brittle and highly water-soluble, which limits their direct use in moist wound care. Therefore, starch is usually plasticized or modified to improve film stability and mechanics. The optimized starch combined with PVA films, the combination can yield high uptake of exudate and inculcate adequate strength for dressing, making them viable for eco-friendly wound films (Delavari et al., 2022).

Starch is usually blended with synthetic polymers like PVA to improve its performance in wound dressings, other excipients like glycerol and citric acid are added as plasticizers and cross linker, respectively. The strategy to improve film flexibility, water resistance and adequate absorbance to manage exudate is by chemical modifications such as carboxymethylation that reduces starch's solubility. For instance, a starch–PVA film crosslinked with citric acid exhibited a high swelling index with about 344% increase in weight while maintaining respectable tensile strength (approximately 8.8 MPa). demonstrating that well-formulated starch films can function effectively as superabsorbent dressings (Delavari et al., 2022). Another example of type A gelatin (50 weight %) with high-amylose corn starch, plasticized with sorbitol resulted in improved flexibility due to sorbitol, rapid initial degradation assisted by gelatin and starch sustained structure (Kozłowska et al., 2023).

In one study, a blend of starch with PVA and plasticizer produced transparent and elastic film with appropriate wound dressing properties. In another study, antimicrobial nanoparticles like ZnO were introduced with starch to inculcate anti-microbial property. So, even though starch requires additional efforts to achieve desired properties it is valued for its low cost and biodegradability (Delavari et al., 2022). A corn starch film with micro-fibrillated cellulose and glycerol, infused with 5 weight % yerba mate extract was prepared and evaluated. The results showed anti-bacterial efficacy of >90 % growth reduction against *Staphylococcus aureus* and *Escherichia co*li along with >80 % radical scavenging shown in 2,2-diphenyl-1-picrylhydrazyl (DPPH) antioxidant assay (Aliabadi et al., 2020).

3.4 Pectin

Pectin is a naturally occurring plant polysaccharide, primarily made up of α-(1-4) linked D-galacturonic acid units, some of which are partially methyl-esterified (Nordin et al., 2022). It is a polyanionic compound commonly sourced from citrus peels or apple pomace. A highly hydrophilic polymer that readily forms gel-like structures in aqueous environments, especially under acidic conditions or in the presence of calcium ions (Said et al., 2023). Pectin's combined properties of high water uptake and anti-inflammatory action makes it valuable in moist wound dressings. In practice, pectin gels or drug films have been shown to accelerate healing especially in challenging diabetic burns by helping in absorption and removal of excess fluid and irritants, resulting in a soothing, protective barrier that reduces pain and supports healing (Nordin et al., 2022).

Likewise cellulose, pectin hydrogels can also encapsulate and gradually release therapeutic agents, because of their amorphous and hypoallergenic nature. Pectin possesses inherent anti-inflammatory and mild antimicrobial properties that are partly attributed to residual phenolic compounds making it apt for delivery and also a bioactivity for wound healing (Nordin et al., 2022). A study evaluated films prepared by pectin and chitosan blended at a 4:1 ratio and loaded with curcumin at 1.5 weight %. Results depicted that the films were superior compared to only pectin films and reduced dehydration of the wound bed. Moreover, thermal stability and mechanical strength both were added by chitosan and further improved by incorporated curcumin. In vivo studies revealed completely healed full-thickness rat wounds in 12 days, with well-organized collagen deposition and re-epithelialization (Muthulakshmi & Rajarajeswari, 2021).

Pectin films are generally prepared via solvent casting may it be with or without crosslinking agents. In one study, hydrogel films made with 2.5% and 5% pectin crosslinked with glutaraldehyde and plasticized with glycerol were evaluated on diabetic burn wounds in rats. The 5% pectin film achieved nearly 100% wound closure by day 20, performing on par with a standard herbal ointment. Notably, the films also demonstrated stronger in vitro antibacterial activity against Staphylococcus aureus than the ointment. These findings highlight pectin's promise as a multifunctional wound dressing material that is capable of managing moisture, delivering therapeutics, and actively promoting re-epithelialization (Nordin et al., 2022). Another example includes, composite films of chitosan and pectin extracted from passion-fruit peel, embedded with green-synthesized silver nanoparticles (AgNPs) at varying concentrations. The result is a slightly moist film that holds about 20 % water while swelling up to six times its weight to cushion and protect injured skin. It can kill over 90 % of common bacteria like *Staph aureus* and *Pseudomonas* and in animal tests it led to complete wound closure in 15 days (Nguyen et al., 2023).

3.5 Alginate

Alginate or alginic acid is a polysaccharide extracted from brown algae. It is a linear copolymer of β-D-mannuronic acid (M) and α-L-guluronic acid (G) residues, so these linear chains provide in-built biomimicry as it structurally resembles glycosaminoglycans, hence supporting cell adhesion and proliferation (Abourehab et al., 2022; Oliveira et al., 2023). Sodium alginate is widely used in wound dressings as it forms hydrogels on ionic crosslinking with multivalent cations like Ca^{2+}. Its remarkable biocompatibility, non-toxicity and natural adhesiveness to moist tissues make it a preferred choice for bioadhesives (Abourehab et al., 2022).

The standout feature of alginate dressings is their ability to gel on contact with wound fluid. As Ca-alginate fibers or films absorb exudate, Ca^{2+} ions diffuse out and swap places with Na^{+} in the wound bed, this triggers the polymer to swell into a soft compatible gel. This gel locks in fluid while maintaining a moist environment that promotes cell migration and autolytic debridement. It prevents leakage making alginate ideal for moderate-to-heavily exuding wounds. Additionally, a mild hemostatic boost from the released Ca^{2+} helps the blood to clot (Abourehab et al., 2022).

Alginate gels have porous hydrophilic network that makes it an excellent carrier for therapeutic agents, growth factors or even herbal extracts, providing for sustained and controlled release directly at the wound site. For instance, alginate–gelatin hydrogels and alginate–agar nanofiber mats have been explored for delivering drugs to chronic wounds. Because its structure closely resembles the extracellular matrix, alginate serves not only as a dressing but also as a biomimetic scaffold that actively supports tissue regeneration. Traditional alginate bandages are clinically used. Research demonstrates alginate hydrogel films fabricated by solvent casting or 3D-printing and crosslinked with $CaCl_2$ were flexible yet strong and can be loaded with antimicrobial agents (Abourehab et al., 2022).

In one study, a composite mucoadhesive film of Ca^{2+} crosslinked cellulose nanofibers with alginate effectively adhered to oral tissue and delivered pain-relieving and anti-inflammatory drugs to heal ulcers (Chang et al., 2024). A study reported that alginate and pectin were crosslinked with 0.5–1 % Ca^{2+} and mangosteen extract-niosomes loaded to form hydrogel film, it demonstrated swelling up to 1025 weight %, pH-sensitive release of 70-85 % over 7 days, strong bacterial inhibition, enhanced fibroblast migration, no cytotoxicity (Pooprommin et al., 2022). Alginate's Generally Recognized As Safe (GRAS) status and versatile chemistry (e.g. blending with gelatin, chitosan, nanocellulose) have led to numerous alginate-based film formulations (Abourehab et al., 2022; Pagano et al., 2021). Tromboguard a multi-layered dressing composed of a polyurethane foam, a semipermeable polyurethane film, and a hemostatic layer made from chitosan and alginate. It is designed for use in controlling bleeding in various types of wounds, including postoperative incisions, traumatic injuries, gunshot wounds, and skin graft donor sites (Ho et al., 2024).

Table 1. Summary of source, properties and applications of polymers

Polymer	Source	Main Properties	Applications in Bioadhesive Film Formulation
Cellulose (Ho et al., 2024; Jangra et al., 2025; Tudoroiu et al., 2021)	Native source: Plant cell walls and bacteria	Tailorable solubility, gelation, mechanical strength Highly hydrophilic, so better swelling capacity and exudate uptake Limited adhesion unless chemically modified	• Insoluble EC as moisture barrier or controlled-release membrane • Oxidized CMC–PVA-gelatin is antibacterial and biocompatibility • CMC with platelet-rich plasma for sustained growth-factor release • ZnO-cellulose for enhanced strength and antibacterial property.
Tannic acid (Ali et al., 2024; Aliabadi et al., 2021)	Plant derived polyphenol: D-glucose esterified with gallic acid units	Water-soluble, extensive H-bonding & metal-coordination crosslinker Strong antioxidant and astringent Hemostatic and broad-spectrum antimicrobial effect with enhanced adhesion	• Chitosan, cellulose, gelatin films with enhanced porosity, mechanical strength, water uptake • 1% tannic acid in CMC–chitosan films results in radical scavenging, S. aureus inhibition, faster wound closure • Complexation with Fe^{3+}gives collagen or alginate matrices • Chitosan-CMC-TA composite film for controlled swelling and drug release
Starch (Delavari et al., 2022)	Polysaccharide from corn, potato, rice (amylose, amylopectin)	Abundant, low-cost, biodegradable Brittle & highly water-soluble in native form Requires plasticizer (glycerol, sorbitol) and/or chemical modification	• For high exudate uptake and tensile strength starch and PVA plasticized with glycerol or sorbitol • Superabsorbent dressings obtained by citric acid-crosslinked starch-PVA with high swelling index • Transparent elastic films with starch-PVA blend • Antibacterial composite films with >90% bacterial reduction and >80% antioxidant activity

continued on following page

Table 1. Continued

Polymer	Source	Main Properties	Applications in Bioadhesive Film Formulation
Pectin (Muthulakshmi & Rajarajeswari, 2021; Nguyen et al., 2023; Nordin et al., 2022)	Plant polysaccharide from citrus peels or apple pomace	Polyanionic with high hydrophilicity Forms gels under acidic conditions or Ca^{2+} presence Anti-inflammatory and mild antimicrobial with good drug-encapsulation	• Improved mechanical strength, thermal stability, rapid re-epithelialization can be achieved in combination with chitosan and curcumin • Diabetic burn wounds had ~100% closure by day 20 can be achieved. • Can achieve 6 times swelling capacity, >90% bacterial kill, complete closure in 15 days
Alginate (Abourehab et al., 2022)	Brown-algae polysaccharide; sodium alginate commonly used	Ionic crosslinking suitable with Ca^{2+} to form hydrogels Biomimetic structure that supports cell adhesion and proliferation Instant gelation on exudate contact, high swelling and moisture retention	• Drug-delivery scaffolds like alginate-gelatin or alginate-agar can provide for sustained release • pH-sensitive release over 7 days • Suitable for oral and mucosal film formulations. • Mild hemostatic effect via Ca^{2+} release in hydrogel form.

4. IN-VITRO AND IN-VIVO CHARACTERIZATION METHODS

4.1 In-Vitro Characterization

A critical stage in development of biologically active films and bandages is in-vitro characterization, where they undergo a number of assays to evaluate its acceptability, robustness and quality for clinical application. It provides essential insights into the safety and therapeutic potential of these plant-based matrices. When performed in combination, these methods not only ensure that a given formulation possesses the requisite mechanical integrity and adhesive properties but also confirms that it can sustain controlled release of active compounds and support cellular processes to ensure wound healing. Thus, it establishes a robust foundation for subsequent in vivo evaluation and ultimately paves the way for eco-friendly wound dressings (Ahmad, 2022).

4.1.1 Physical and Morphological Tests

Initially for thickness, surface morphology, and porosity of films are assessed. Thickness of film ensures uniform drug distribution. It is measured at multiple points by using vernier caliper, digital micrometer, manual screw gauge or scanning electron microscopy (SEM) (Ahmad, 2022). Scanning electron microscopy and optical microscopy can be used for evaluating both thickness and surface morphology, which reveals surface characteristics such as wrinkles or roughness that is associated with increased surface area for adhesion (Pagano et al., 2021). For example, xanthan and alginate films were approximately 410-530 μm thick as per SEM (Pagano et al., 2021). Porosity may be quantified by SEM or atomic force microscopy (Ahmad, 2022; Kaczmarek-Szczepańska et al., 2025). A simpler method to determine porosity is to measure the quantity of solvent absorbed by the film after specified time interval (Gonçalves et al., 2020). Hence, suitable thickness and porosity of film dressing are important to allow cellular infiltration and proliferation, as well as for gas and fluid exchange (Gonçalves et al., 2020).

4.1.2 Swelling and Moisture Uptake

Gravimetric swelling tests are used to evaluate exudate absorbtion capacity of films. A simulated wound fluid or phosphate buffer used to immerse dried samples, weight gain is recorded over time and represented in percentage (Ahmad, 2022). For instance it was noted that films prepared using xanthan gum and alginate polymers absorbed up to 65-72% fluid rapidly till 48th hour (Pagano et al., 2021). To ensure the dressing is not excessively wet but has optimum moisture Water Vapor Transmission Rate can be measured (Ahmad, 2022). In one study, novel antimicrobial films were concluded to be semi-occlusive in nature on the basis of optimized Water Vapor Transmission Rate, moisture uptake and porosity (Gonçalves et al., 2020).

4.1.3 Mechanical Testing

Critical mechanical parameters include elastic modulus, tensile strength and elongation at break. Active Standard Test Method (ASTM) D882 is the standard testing method using Universal Testing Machine (UTM) after cutting of films in required dimensions (Ahmad, 2022; Gonçalves et al., 2020). For example, a xanthan–alginate film containing glycerol plasticizer had high elongation at break with elastic modulus of approximately 3 MPa (Pagano et al., 2021). In a study it was observed that glycerol addition improved flexibility on measuring the Young's modulus, tensile strength and elongation. Although mechanical strength of films can be sufficiently evaluated by tensile strength measurement but bandage materials require compression testing as well as dynamic rheology (Ahmad, 2022). Results are compared to healthy skin range e.g. 61-70% strain for skin (Pagano et al., 2021).

4.1.4 Chemical or Structural Analysis

Various analytical techniques like X-ray Diffraction (XRD), Fourier Transform Infrared Spectroscopy (FTIR), Differential Scanning Calorimetry (DSC) and Thermogravimetric Analysis (TGA) are used for chemical characterization of polymers. XRD is used for assessment of crystallinity, phase composition, structural characterization and assess strain and texture of thin film. FTIR can be used to identify functional groups, monitor changes due to processing and refractive index by detecting functional groups and crosslinking (Ali et al., 2024). Both DSC and TGA assess thermal transitions and residual moisture. The DSC quantifies heat flow within a sample to identify critical phase transitions such as the glass transition, melting point, and crystallization. On the other hand, TGA monitors the mass loss with increasing temperature as a result of decomposition and volatilization (Ahmad, 2022).

4.1.5 Adhesion Tests

For bioadhesive films and bandages prerequisite ex-vivo skin adhesion test is performed. animal skin from pig or rat is commonly used in a texture analyzer which pulls of the film while detachment force and time are recorded. One research reported that the detachment force of film containing higher concentration of alginate was around 0.20 N with adhesion time 14.7 seconds compared to xanthan-rich film having 0.07 N and 6.7 seconds detachment force and adhesion time, respectively. Hence, hydrophobicity of alginate is attributed to better adhesion to skin which can assist in optimum formulation modifications (Pagano et al., 2021).

4.1.6 Drug Content and Release

For drug-loaded dressings, content uniformity is often checked by dissolution of samples and High-Performance Liquid Chromatography or Ultraviolet assay. In vitro release is performed via dissolution or Franz diffusion. A model protocol involves immersion of the film in buffer and sampling over 24 hours. For example, ~58% of the drug was released by a pycnogenol–xanthan-alginate film in 1 hour and nearly 100% by 24 hour, fitting a Higuchi (diffusion) model (Pagano et al., 2021).

4.1.7 Cell Compatibility

Cytotoxicity is assessed using skin-relevant cell lines such as keratinocytes or fibroblasts. Standard assays include 3-(4,5-dimethyl-2-thiazolyl)-2,5-diphenyl-2H-tetrazolium bromide (MTT) and 3-bis-(2-methoxy-4-nitro-5-sulfophenyl)-2H-tetrazolium-5-carboxanilide (XTT) or AlamarBlue. The viability is measured against control group after dressings or their extracts are incubated with cells (Ahmad, 2022; Gonçalves et al., 2020). Non-toxic materials typically show ≥80% cell viability. In one study, the film had >70% viability in HaCaT keratinocytes exposed to dilutions of released pycnogenol at relevant doses. Blank films without drug prove to be non-cytotoxic (Pagano et al., 2021). Normal cell morphology is also confirmed by fluorescent staining or phase microscopy (Ahmad, 2022).

4.1.8 Cell Migration Assays

In vitro scratch or gap-closure assays are used to mimic wound closure. Confluent skin cell monolayers are scratched and then treated with film extracts or active drug. The imaging of closure of the artificial wound is performed over 6-24 hours. For instance, in a case complete scratch closure was achieved by a low-concentration film extract (0.015 mg/mL) in 24 hours, versus 93% closure achieved in untreated controls. Accelerated migration was indicated by differences at 6-12 hours (e.g. 62% vs 55% closure). Whether cell migration and proliferation were stimulated by the film's ingredients can be shown by these assays (Pagano et al., 2021).

4.1.9 Antimicrobial Testing

Antimicrobials are incorporated in many films used in dressing. Disk-diffusion and broth assays are standard in vitro tests (Ahmad, 2022). For disk diffusion, circular film samples are placed on bacteria-inoculated agar commonly *S. aureus* and *E. coli*. After incubation, zones of inhibition are measured (Ahmad, 2022; Gonçalves et al., 2020). In a chitosan, PVA and polylysine combination film study, zones of inhibition against *S. aureus* and *E. coli* were observed. In another study, *S. aureus*, *S. pyogenes* and *E. faecalis* were inhibited by pycnogenol-loaded films (Pagano et al., 2021). Potency can be quantified by MIC or CFU reduction assays, but disk diffusion is most common (Ahmad, 2022). Silver-based or natural antimicrobials like polylysine are often tested this way (Ahmad, 2022; Gonçalves et al., 2020).

4.2 In vivo (Animal) Wound Healing Evaluations

While in vitro tests ensure product stability and quality once those results are promising, tests are conducted on animal models to ascertain healing of wound. Commonly animal studies are conducted on rodents (mice, rats) or rabbits. It involves manually creating wounds under anesthesia and applying biopolymer film or bandage to monitor healing (Ahmad, 2022; Ali et al., 2024).

4.2.1 Wound Models

Typically, standardized model developed by excision of skin wounds (e.g., 1 × 1 cm, 2-4 mm deep) either via burn induced thermal-injury or bacteria-inoculated infection. For instance, a researcher created 1 × 1 cm excisional wounds and 1.5 × 1.5 cm burns on rabbits, then applied a cellulose–chitosan–tannic acid film daily under adhesive tape (Ali et al., 2024). Investigators usually initiate treatment immediately or within a few days post-burn and replace dressings on a daily basis.

4.2.2 Wound Closure Rate

During the healing period, teams photograph wounds at set intervals and quantify area using image-analysis software, calculating wound contraction relative to day 0 (Ahmad, 2022; Ali et al., 2024). In the rabbit study, the cellulose-based film accelerated closure across all experimental models (Ali et al., 2024). Likewise, in streptozotocin-induced diabetic rats, alginate–pectin films loaded with simvastatin achieved approximately 99 % closure by day 21, compared to markedly lower rates in untreated controls (Rezvanian et al., 2021).

4.2.3 Histological Analysis

At predetermined timepoints, researchers excise wounds for histological evaluation. They use hematoxylin and eosin staining to evaluate re-epithelialization, granulation tissue formation, and overall structural integrity (Ahmad, 2022). While Masson's trichrome or Sirius Red staining quantify collagen deposition via biochemical (Ahmad, 2022; Rezvanian et al., 2021). For example, the alginate-pectin film significantly enhanced collagen content and elevated Vascular Endothelial Growth Factor A (VEGF-A) expression, indicating higher angiogenesis and extracellular-matrix formation (Rezvanian et al., 2021).

4.2.4 Biochemical or Immunoassays

Assay of tissue or blood samples for biochemical markers like hydroxyproline content to assess collagen, measure of cytokines such as Interleukin-6 (IL-6) and Tumor Necrosis Factor alpha (TNF-α) via Enzyme-Linked Immunosorbent Assay (ELISA), and quantification of growth factors like VEGF (Ahmad, 2022; Rezvanian et al., 2021). Enzymatic myeloperoxidase assays reveal levels of inflammation. In the diabetic-rat model, treated wounds exhibited higher VEGF-A concentrations, underscoring accelerated biochemical progression of healing (Rezvanian et al., 2021).

5. CASE STUDIES OF BIOPOLYMER-BASED BIOADHESIVE FILMS FOR WOUND HEALING

Biodegradable and bioadhesive films are becoming a multifaceted sector in wound care. These films not only shield wounds from infection but with added natural polymers they provide healing compounds they actively support recovery by adapting to clinical needs. Here we describe three distinct case studies that illustrate this evolution and their key points are highlighted in table 2.

5.1 Multifunctional Starch Film with Anthocyanin-Rich Floral Extract and Zinc oxide (ZnO) Nanoparticles

The formulation had corn starch matrix along with glycerol as plasticizer and other active ingredient. The film strengthened by ZnO nanoparticles prepared by co-precipitation process which was followed by calcination. The anthocyanin rich active ingredient obtained from floral extract from *Torenia fournieri* (TFE) flowers was also incorporated (Koshy et al., 2023).

Preparation Method:

Firstly, starch was dissolved in water and glycerol, ZnO, TFE were added to yield ~0.5% extract by weight. The extract was separated by maceration of fresh flowers to obtain anthocyanin-rich solution (TFE). Final solution was dried and films prepared by solution-casting method at 50°C. The four variants prepared for evaluation were as follows: control starch-only (S), starch+ZnO (SZ), starch+extract (SE) and starch+extract+ZnO (SEZ) (Koshy et al., 2023).

Properties:

Scanning electron microscopy showed that ZnO nanoparticles had nanoflower-like morphology and were aggregated into clusters. On addition of ZnO, film thickness and tensile strength increased and water solubility reduced. This reinforces that ZnO strengthens the film matrix while maintaining flexibility and lesser water-permeability which enhances film barrier. Meanwhile, starch increased the surface wettability. The color imparted by anthocyanin extract caused the film to turn green in alkaline environment, making it acts as a visual pH-sensor. Starch, ZnO and anthocyanins each have known mild antimicrobial and antioxidant properties (Koshy et al., 2023).

Evaluation:

Thermogravimetric analysis inferred that in presence of ZnO second-stage decomposition temperature of the starch film shifts higher. The concentrations of cell migration had improved significantly with nearly complete scratch closure within 36 hours. These results confirmed that the film was non-toxic and the presence of bioactive components actively stimulated cell proliferation and migration. (Koshy et al., 2023)

Application:

The multifunctional starch-ZnO-anthocyanin film is positioned for both wound dressing and smart packaging roles. In wound care, its biocompatibility, moderate hydrophilicity, and pH-responsive antimicrobial and antioxidant nature suggested it could maintain a moist healing environment while identifying infection and promoting tissue repair. Its visible color change at high pH made it an eligible candidate for "smart" adhesive films (Koshy et al., 2023).

Similar to the above formulation, on addition of photosensitive compound like porphyrin tetraiodide (TMPyP), the physicochemical, mechanical and antimicrobial properties of starch-based film can be modified which enhances wound healing activity even without light. Although, addition of appropriate concentration of TMPyP is crucial as in case of 0.25% TMPyP remarkable decrease in elongation at break and tensile strength was noted (Lopes et al., 2023). Costa et al. prepared a blended film of starch with PVA and polyacrylic acid with incorporating pomegranate peel extract which proved effective anti-microbial activity at lower concentration of bioactive agent. The main challenge while formulating PVA and starch blend is controlling film hydrophilicity and dissolution. The extract incorporation enhances polymer interactions which in turn increases surface hydrophilicity, promoting aqueous contact and mass loss due to polymer dissociation on prolonged exposure (Costa et al., 2020). Likewise the extract was also used in a tapioca starch film which at optimum concentration displayed superior wound healing properties. The optimization of citric acid and β-cyclodextrin levels is necessary to attain acceptable physicochemical parameters (Savekar et al., 2024).

5.2 Chitosan–Tannic Acid–CMC Composite Film

The film is formulated from three biopolymers and additives; wherein key components were chitosan and CMC. Tannic acid served as a bioactive crosslinker, and beeswax was used in one variant. To improve film flexibility and emulsification, glycerol (0.2%) and Tween 80 (0.2%) were included as plasticizer and surfactant, respectively (Ali et al., 2024).

Preparation Method:

First, CMC was synthesized by alkali-chloroacetic acid treatment of cellulose with NaOH. For film formation, chitosan was dissolved in acetic acid solvent, with addition of CMC and tannic acid. The optimized composition (M4) contained 2% chitosan, 2% CMC, 1% tannic acid, plus 0.2% glycerol and 0.2% Tween 80. Films were casted using a solvent-evaporation approach (Ali et al., 2024).

Properties:

The optimal film (M4) was uniform in appearance, brownish in color due to tannic acid and easily peeled from the glass. The mechanical properties were recorded as tensile strength of 0.275 MPa, thickness of ~39.0 μm and enhanced flexibility due to the glycerol and Tween 80. Microscopy revealed excellent component compatibility. A low water contact angle of ~40.5° and high surface energy confirmed excellent wettability on both film sides. The film enables sustained release of incorporated agents, as demonstrated by the rapid yet constant elution of 89.4% of its tannic acid over 24 hours, indicating suitability for delivering bioactive compounds (Ali et al., 2024).

Evaluations:

Antioxidant activity revealed very strong free-radical scavenging attributed to the retained activity of incorporated tannic acid and chitosan. Antibacterial efficacy assessed via disk-diffusion testing showed strong inhibition against *Staphylococcus aureus* and moderate inhibition against *Escherichia coli*. Critically, in vivo evaluation showed almost 90% wound closure by day 7 as well as reaching ~98-99% re-epithelialization by day 10. Overall, the film significantly accelerates healing compared to expected rates for untreated dressings (Ali et al., 2024).

Application:

The high swelling and Water Vapor Transmission Rate regulate moisture balance at the wound site. Its strong antioxidant and antibacterial properties protect the wound from oxidative damage and infection. Most importantly, in vivo data confirm that the film actively enhances healing in burns and infected wounds, making it suitable as a topical wound dressing. The formulation could be adapted by adding specific drugs or growth factors for targeted therapy (Ali et al., 2024).

Additionally, Kim et al. developed nitric oxide releasing film with chitosan and S-nitrosoglutathione where nitric oxide release followed fickian diffusion and provided anti-bacterial effect against certain gram negative and positive bacteria. In this case, nitric oxide release from the films follows diffusion-controlled kinetics, so the drug released by passive diffusion may not be suitable when steady release is clinically required (Kim et al., 2015). A different study proved that chitosan film formulated by freeze-drying of hydroxypropylchitosan was effective in diabetic wound treatment. Importantly, the bFGF activity remained stable for 21 days when stored at 5 °C, but activity fell to about 86% at 25 °C, this stability under refrigeration is an important factor for formulation (Mizuno et al., 2003).

5.3 Biopolymer Film From Cola acuminata Gum (CAG)

The film material extracted from the pods of *Cola acuminata*. Fresh pods were cut and the endocarp pieces were soaked in distilled water for 24 hours. The viscous gum mucilage was filtered off then precipitated by adding acetone, then oven-dried at 60 °C, pulverized, and sieved to yield fine CAG powder (Ogeh, n.d.).

Preparation Method:

Films were prepared by aqueous casting of a CAG powder (10 g). For each film batch, 20 mL of this mucilage was poured into a petri dish and dried in an oven at 60°C for 12 hours. For study of plasticizer effects some mucilage batches included either propylene glycol (PPG) or glycerin at various concentrations. The formulations were labeled F1-F7. After drying, on examination the batches with 1-2% PPG were found to be smooth, flexible and form continuous transparent films with no cracks, hence they were selected for full evaluation. Batches with higher plasticizer remained tacky and rubbery even after drying that indicates over-plasticizing (Ogeh, n.d.).

Properties:

The films were light brown and odorless. The pH was slightly acidic due to uronic components of CAG. Both films absorb substantial moisture from humid air. At 75% relative humidity, F2 gains about 80.6% of its weight as water, and F3 about 85.2%. Tensile testing of F2 was higher compared to F3. The Young's modulus was lower for F2 and higher for F3 reflecting the softer more pliable nature of the more plasticized film (Ogeh, n.d.).

Evaluations:

The results of ex vivo test revealed films with 1-2% PPG required lower force to detach from gastric mucosa compared to intestinal mucosa. However, both films have significantly better adherence but the strength doubles at neutral pH because higher swelling at pH 7.4 lead to greater adhesion (Ogeh, n.d.).

Application:

The strong mucoadhesion at physiological pH implied it can adhere to mucosal tissues for extended periods making it useful for buccal, gastric or intestinal drug delivery systems. By selecting the pH environment, the release profile can be tuned via the pH-dependent swelling. Its pH-responsive swelling also suggests potential use as an enteric or colon-targeted carrier in the neutral or alkaline gut. On a moist skin or mucosal wound, the film would adhere, absorb exudate and gradually release any incorporated drug. Although, high moisture-sensitivity leads to softening, loss of mechanical integrity and necessitates refrigerated storage. The pH-dependent swelling of gum causes variability in drug release and adhesive performance. Over-hydration may promote polymer erosion at the interface, reducing mucoadhesive strength (Ogeh, n.d.).

Table 2. Summary of examples of biopolymer-based bioadhesive films for wound healing

Examples	*Starch + Anthocyanin Extract + ZnO (Koshy et al., 2023)*	*Chitosan–TA–CMC Composite (Ali et al., 2024)*	*Cola acuminata Gum Film (P.C. Ogeh, n.d.)*
Materials	Corn starch; glycerol (30%); ZnO (0.025 g); Torenia fournieri extract (0.5 %, 8.4 mL)	Chitosan (2 %); CMC (2 %); tannic acid (1 %); glycerol (0.2 %); Tween 80 (0.2 %)	CAG powder (10 %); propylene glycol (1-2 %); (glycerin studied)
Preparation	Dissolve starch + glycerol at 85 °C; add sonicated ZnO dispersion + floral extract; cast and dry at 50 °C	Dissolve chitosan in 1 % acetic acid + CMC, tannic acid; add glycerol, Tween; heat to 70 °C; cast on glass; dry 30 °C, 36 h	Soak pods, recover gum by acetone precipitation; make 10 % mucilage; add PPG; cast in 8.5 cm dish; dry 60 °C, 12 h
Key Properties	Thickness increases from 0.12 to 0.24 mm; Tensile strength is higher with ZnO; contact angle S~71°, SE~43°, SZ~76°, SEZ~64°; pH-sensitive color change (green at alkaline)	Thickness 39 ± 1 μm; Tensile strength 0.275 ± 0.003 MPa; swelling 283 ± 2 % (2 h); contact angle ~40.5°; Water Vapor Transmission Rate ~1,912 $g{\cdot}m^{-2}{\cdot}24\ h^{-1}$	F2: thickness ~0.15 mm, Tensile strength ~0.49 MN/m^2, elongation ~36.6 % F3: thickness ~0.17 mm, Tensile strength ~0.29 MN/m^2, elongation 63.6 %
Evaluations	In vitro scratch assay: 25-100 μg/mL, 100 μg nearly full closure at 36 hours; ammonia vapor produces green color	DPPH antioxidant ~95 % inhibition; antibacterial: *S. aureus* ~19.9 mm zone, *E. coli* ~14.5 mm; rabbit burn or infected wound ~90 % closure by day 7 and 100 % within 2 weeks.	Ex vivo mucoadhesion in sheep mucosa at pH 1.2 2.72-3.10 g/cm^2 and at pH 7.4, 5.46-6.38 g/cm^2; folding endurance: > 300 folds
Application	Biodegradable wound dressing, pH-identification	Advanced burn or wound dressing: moist-optimum barrier; sustained tannic acid release; antioxidant and antimicrobial therapy	Mucoadhesive delivery platform for buccal or gastrointestinal region; potential topical wound patch

6. ADVANTAGES AND CHALLENGES OF BIOADHESIVE FILMS AND BANDAGES

6.1 Advantages

(i) **Biocompatibility and Biodegradability**

Polymers like cellulose, alginate, starch and pectin are naturally biocompatible and biodegradable which makes them safe for skin contact and wound site (Tudoroiu et al., 2021; Valle et al., 2020). For instance, non-toxic, renewable and inexpensive polymers like cellulose and its derivatives or pectin (Tudoroiu et al., 2021). Another example includes, alginate and starch which are non-immunogenic and can readily break down in the body (Aderibigbe & Buyana, 2018). Even tannic acid is cheap, widely available, environmentally harmless and generally biocompatible (Chen et al., 2022). This proves that plant-based films and bandages cause negligible inflammation or allergy and eventually degrade harmlessly

(ii) **Moisture control and Promote Healing**

Most of these films can maintain moist microenvironment required to support healing process. Moist conditions aid reduced scarring with faster re-epithelialization. Alginate wound dressings absorb excess exudate by retaining moisture at the wound bed, while cellulose and starch are formulated by blending with hydrophilic agents to allow gas exchange and moisture control (Aderibigbe & Buyana, 2018; Tudoroiu et al., 2021). They block blood loss (hemostasis), deliver antibiotics or anti-inflammatories during inflammation, and support tissue regeneration and collagen remodeling during proliferation and remodeling (Lopes et al., 2024).

(iii) **Functional Bioactivity**

Many plant polymers bring extra therapeutic effects. Tannic acid, for example, has catechol and pyrogallol groups that confer strong adhesion and innate bioactivity (Chen et al., 2022). Tannic acid can be used to treat burns as it is a powerful antioxidant, antibacterial and hemostatic agent that can coagulate blood by binding proteins (Chen et al., 2022). Similarly, pectin has inherent anti-inflammatory activity (Yaşayan, 2020). Moreover, plant-based films can be easily loaded with natural extracts. For example, various studies have incorporated essential oils or phytochemicals into starch-, cellulose- or alginate-based films, yielding sustained antimicrobial and antioxidant action (Lopes et al., 2024). In short, plant-derived films can carry bioactive payloads (natural or synthetic) in addition to their own gentle healing effects.

(iv) **Strong Adhesion and Hemostatic Effect**

Some plant polymers have excellent adhesiveness. For example, a formulation combining alginate and chitosan resulted in films that were as smooth, flexible, robust, bioadhesive, and biocompatible (Abourehab et al., 2022). Tannic acid by forming stable complexes with proteins enhances adhesion even under wet conditions (Chen et al., 2022). In addition to its adhesive capabilities, alginate naturally exhibits hemostatic properties; upon contact with calcium ions in blood it rapidly gels and helps to cease bleeding. Both tannic acid-enriched hydrogels and alginate-based sheets have demonstrated rapid blood clotting and absorption proving their value in managing active wounds (Aderibigbe & Buyana, 2018; Chen et al., 2022).

(v) **Abundance and Low Cost**

Most of these polymers are extremely plentiful and inexpensive. Cellulose and its semi-synthetic derivatives are cheap to produce (Tudoroiu et al., 2021). Starch is abundantly available from corn, potato, rice and among the most affordable natural polymers for bioadhesion (Delavari et al., 2022). Alginate is derived from common seaweeds at industrial scale, and pectin is a byproduct of fruit processing. Tannic acid is extracted from oak, chestnut, sumac and other plants, making it readily available. This low cost encourages development of economically scalable dressings, important in global wound care (Aderibigbe & Buyana, 2018).

6.2 Challenges

(i) **Mechanical Weakness**

A common limitation is that plant-based films tend to be mechanically frail without additives. Native starch and alginate, for example, form brittle films with low tensile strength (Aderibigbe & Buyana, 2018; Delavari et al., 2022). Studies repeatedly note that alginate and starch have poor mechanical properties and unprocessed films can tear or deform easily under stress (Delavari et al., 2022; Lopes et al., 2024). In practice, researchers can blend them with synthetic polymers or plasticizers to achieve tolerable strength. Even cellulose esters like ethyl cellulose are stiff and brittle and might require plasticizers to become flexible (Tudoroiu et al., 2021). This need for additives complicates formulation and can raise manufacturing costs and regulatory complexity.

(ii) **Limited Fluid Absorption**

Although alginate excels at absorption, many of its plant-based films and bandages lack porosity for exudate absorbtion. One review warned that films have low porosity and cannot be used in high exudate wounds because they may not able to absorb high quantities of biological fluids (Lopes et al., 2024). In other words, a starch or pectin film dressing might maintain moisture but cannot soak up copious discharge. In case of heavy bleeding or large amount of extruding from wound alginate foam or hydrogel are often preferred over films over bandages.

(iii) **Susceptibility to Microbial Contamination and Stability**

The same hydrophilicity that helps wound healing also risks storage and contamination instability. Many plant gums and mucilage contain significant water content and are prone to spoilage (George & Suchithra, 2019). For example, traditional plant mucilages can ferment or lose viscosity over time. Likewise, hydrated starch or pectin films may have microbial growth if not properly sterilized or preserved (Lopes et al., 2024). Even after fabrication, they may require strict sterilization and anti-microbial additives to ensure safety. Moreover, natural polymers often vary with harvest conditions such as season, source plant, land type etc. so reproducibility can be an issue. Inter-batch variability can result in varying viscosity and tensile strength which complicated the manufacturing process and challenging to ensure quality control.

(iv) **Adhesion and Handling Difficulties**

While tannic acid can impart strong adhesion, many plant polymer films alone have only modest stickiness. Without crosslinkers like tannic acid or dopamine analogs, films may not adhere as strongly as synthetic medical adhesives (Chen et al., 2022). Also, some films like pure pectin or starch films they can be overly hydrophilic and may swell or dissolve if a wound is very wet, losing integrity (Sabando et al., 2020). Conversely, some cellulose derivatives resist water and might peel off. Balancing adhesion with ease of removal is tricky, if it is too sticky than removal hurts tissue, if too weak than the bandage might fall off. Achieving the right tackiness often requires chemical modification or blending, adding complexity.

(v) **Limited Shelf Life and Processing Constraints**

Natural films can be sensitive to environmental conditions. Starch- or pectin-based films may harden or crack upon drying, or conversely remain tacky in humid storage. They can be sensitive to temperature and humidity during processing (cast films can shrink unevenly) (George & Suchithra, 2019). There is a high probability of degradation of plant mucilage stored over longer period of time. Moreover, a minor shift in controls during sterilization methods like gamma irradiation or autoclaving can further damage natural polymers. Such handling and stability issues mean plant-based bandages may have shorter shelf lives or require cold storage compared to purely synthetic dressings.

To consolidate, plant-derived adhesive films are advantageous for their safety, property to promote wound healing, abundance and sustainability and ability to deliver bioactive agents (Aderibigbe & Buyana, 2018; Chen et al., 2022; Tudoroiu et al., 2021). However, challenges arise from their intrinsic material weaknesses like poor strength, limited exudate absorption and stability or sterilization issues (Aderibigbe & Buyana, 2018; A. I. Lopes et al., 2024).

7. FUTURE RESEARCH DIRECTIONS

Therefore, future research focusing on simpler and robust extraction process, advanced crosslinking or composite strategies to reinforce desired properties, development of antimicrobial preservation techniques and standardized quality controls to fully acquire the potential of plant-based bioadhesives in wound care. There should be standardize sustainable extraction with development of green processes. Researchers can aim to produce stable formulations that are easy to sterilize, have microbial smart-sensing and in vivo translational studies to support regulatory approval. Perform cost-effectiveness and life-cycle analyses to ensure manufacturing is economically viable and scalable.

8. CONCLUSION

Current chapter focuses on various classification, polymers, examples and performance of bioadhesive films and bandages formulated from plant-based polymers. Application of these polymers was illustrated using various examples and formulations such as monolayer or multilayer dressing, stimuli-responsive bandages or loading with herbal actives was discussed.

As synthetic films and bandages often lack biocompatibility and biodegradability they may release toxins upon degradation, causing inflammation or hypersensitivity at the wound site. Many of them require combination of excipients to achieve the right characteristics but risking wound dehiscence caused by brittleness or incompatibility to soft tissues.

Herbal polymers contain high amount of hydroxyl and carboxyl moieties that assist in strong adhesion with tissue by hydrogen bonding also ensuring safe and non-toxic degradation. Moreover, their hydrophilic nature confers optimum moisture retention at wound site. They are natural scaffold for administration of antibacterial or antimicrobial drugs that require localized sustained delivery at wound site. Although, herbal bioadhesives have certain challenges like processing variability due to inconsistent quality of raw materials. The increased hydrophilicity makes them susceptible to microbial contamination during storage hence maintain desired level of sterility and stability requires precise optimization.

REFERENCES

Abourehab, M. A. S., Rajendran, R. R., Singh, A., Pramanik, S., Shrivastav, P., Ansari, M. J., Manne, R., Amaral, L. S., & Deepak, A. (2022). Alginate as a Promising Biopolymer in Drug Delivery and Wound Healing: A Review of the State-of-the-Art. *International Journal of Molecular Sciences*, *23*(16), 9035. DOI: 10.3390/ijms23169035 PMID: 36012297

Aderibigbe, B., & Buyana, B. (2018). Alginate in Wound Dressings. *Pharmaceutics*, *10*(2), 42. DOI: 10.3390/pharmaceutics10020042 PMID: 29614804

Ahmad, N. (2022). In Vitro and In Vivo Characterization Methods for Evaluation of Modern Wound Dressings. *Pharmaceutics*, *15*(1), 42. DOI: 10.3390/pharmaceutics15010042 PMID: 36678671

Ali, M., Ullah, S., Ullah, S., Shakeel, M., Afsar, T., Husain, F. M., Amor, H., & Razak, S. (2024). Innovative biopolymers composite based thin film for wound healing applications. *Scientific Reports*, *14*(1), 27415. DOI: 10.1038/s41598-024-79121-8 PMID: 39521931

Aliabadi, M., Chee, B. S., Matos, M., Cortese, Y. J., Nugent, M. J. D., De Lima, T. A. M., Magalhães, W. L. E., & De Lima, G. G. (2020). Yerba Mate Extract in Microfibrillated Cellulose and Corn Starch Films as a Potential Wound Healing Bandage. *Polymers*, *12*(12), 2807. DOI: 10.3390/polym12122807 PMID: 33260883

Aliabadi, M., Chee, B. S., Matos, M., Cortese, Y. J., Nugent, M. J. D., De Lima, T. A. M., Magalhães, W. L. E., De Lima, G. G., & Firouzabadi, M. D. (2021). Microfibrillated cellulose films containing chitosan and tannic acid for wound healing applications. *Journal of Materials Science. Materials in Medicine*, *32*(6), 67. DOI: 10.1007/s10856-021-06536-4 PMID: 34117926

Alipour, A., Nejati, O., Yaşayan, G., Girgin, A., Zaman, B. T., Giray, B., Karal-Yılmaz, O., Bakırdere, S., & Bal-Öztürk, A. (2025). Multilayer Antibacterial Hydrogel Wound Dressings Incorporated With Green Synthesized Silver Nanoparticles. *Drug Development Research*, *86*(3), e70102. DOI: 10.1002/ddr.70102 PMID: 40341660

Ameri, Z., Shahabi, A., Farsinejad, A., Bardsiri, M. S., Javedani, H., Bagher, Z., Saraee, A., & Brouki Milan, P. (2025). A cellulose-based skin adhesive hydrogel incorporating N-acetyl-seryl-aspartyl-lysyl-proline peptide for enhanced wound healing and scar prevention in rabbit scar ear model in vivo. *International Journal of Biological Macromolecules*, *144981*. Advance online publication. DOI: 10.1016/j.ijbiomac.2025.144981 PMID: 40480579

Chalitangkoon, J., Ronte, A., Sintoppun, T., Manapradit, N., & Monvisade, P. (2025). Dual Cross-Linked Chitosan-Based Films with pH-Sensitive Coloration and Drug Release Kinetics for Smart Wound Dressings. *ACS Omega*, *10*(8), 7770–7782. DOI: 10.1021/acsomega.4c08089 PMID: 40060817

Chang, Y., Zhao, W., Li, W., Zhang, Q., & Wang, G. (2024). Bioadhesive and drug-loaded cellulose nanofiber/alginate film for healing oral mucosal wounds. *International Journal of Biological Macromolecules*, *276*, 133858. DOI: 10.1016/j.ijbiomac.2024.133858 PMID: 39009262

Chen, C., Yang, H., Yang, X., & Ma, Q. (2022). Tannic acid: A crosslinker leading to versatile functional polymeric networks: a review. *RSC Advances*, *12*(13), 7689–7711. DOI: 10.1039/D1RA07657D PMID: 35424749

C.L., V., Priya, P., Harikrishnan, K., & Kumar, G. S. V. (2023). Enhanced cutaneous wound healing through MMP-8-responsive release of antimicrobial peptide from a porous chitosan-based scaffold. *Journal of Drug Delivery Science and Technology*, *89*, 105069. DOI: 10.1016/j.jddst.2023.105069

Costa, N. N., De Faria Lopes, L., Ferreira, D. F., De Prado, E. M. L., Severi, J. A., Resende, J. A., De Paula Careta, F., Ferreira, M. C. P., Carreira, L. G., De Souza, S. O. L., Cotrim, M. A. P., Boeing, T., De Andrade, S. F., Oréfice, R. L., & Villanova, J. C. O. (2020). Polymeric films containing pomegranate peel extract based on PVA/starch/PAA blends for use as wound dressing: In vitro analysis and physicochemical evaluation. *Materials Science and Engineering C*, *109*, 110643. DOI: 10.1016/j.msec.2020.110643 PMID: 32229007

De Carvalho, A. C. W., Paiva, N. F., Demonari, I. K., Duarte, M. P. F., Do Couto, R. O., De Freitas, O., & Vicentini, F. T. M. D. C. (2023). The Potential of Films as Transmucosal Drug Delivery Systems. *Pharmaceutics*, *15*(11), 2583. DOI: 10.3390/pharmaceutics15112583 PMID: 38004562

Delavari, M. M., Ocampo, I., & Stiharu, I. (2022). Optimizing Biodegradable Starch-Based Composite Films Formulation for Wound-Dressing Applications. *Micromachines*, *13*(12), 2146. DOI: 10.3390/mi13122146 PMID: 36557445

Dhivya, S., Padma, V. V., & Santhini, E. (2015). Wound dressings – a review. *Biomedicine (Taipei)*, *5*(4), 22. DOI: 10.7603/s40681-015-0022-9 PMID: 26615539

Eskilson, O., Zattarin, E., Berglund, L., Oksman, K., Hanna, K., Rakar, J., Sivlér, P., Skog, M., Rinklake, I., Shamasha, R., Sotra, Z., Starkenberg, A., Odén, M., Wiman, E., Khalaf, H., Bengtsson, T., Junker, J. P. E., Selegård, R., Björk, E. M., & Aili, D. (2023). Nanocellulose composite wound dressings for real-time pH wound monitoring. *Materials Today. Bio*, *19*, 100574. DOI: 10.1016/j.mtbio.2023.100574 PMID: 36852226

Fiorentini, F., Suarato, G., Grisoli, P., Zych, A., Bertorelli, R., & Athanassiou, A. (2021). Plant-based biocomposite films as potential antibacterial patches for skin wound healing. *European Polymer Journal*, *150*, 110414. DOI: 10.1016/j.eurpolymj.2021.110414

Froelich, A., Jakubowska, E., Wojtyłko, M., Jadach, B., Gackowski, M., Gadziński, P., Napierała, O., Ravliv, Y., & Osmałek, T. (2023). Alginate-Based Materials Loaded with Nanoparticles in Wound Healing. *Pharmaceutics*, *15*(4), 1142. DOI: 10.3390/pharmaceutics15041142 PMID: 37111628

George, B., & Suchithra, T. V. (2019). Plant-derived bioadhesives for wound dressing and drug delivery system. *Fitoterapia*, *137*, 104241. DOI: 10.1016/j.fitote.2019.104241 PMID: 31201885

Gonçalves, M. M., Carneiro, J., Justus, B., Espinoza, J. T., Budel, J. M., Farago, P. V., & Paula, J. P. D. (2020). Preparation and characterization of a novel antimicrobial film dressing for wound healing application. *Brazilian Journal of Pharmaceutical Sciences*, *56*, e18784. DOI: 10.1590/s2175-97902020000118784

Ho, T. T., Tran, H. A., Doan, V. K., Maitz, J., Li, Z., Wise, S. G., Lim, K. S., & Rnjak-Kovacina, J. (2024). Natural Polymer-Based Materials for Wound Healing Applications. *Advanced NanoBiomed Research*, *4*(5), 2300131. DOI: 10.1002/anbr.202300131

Isopencu, G. O., Covaliu-Mierlă, C.-I., & Deleanu, I.-M. (2023). From Plants to Wound Dressing and Transdermal Delivery of Bioactive Compounds. *Plants*, *12*(14), 2661. DOI: 10.3390/plants12142661 PMID: 37514275

Jangra, N., Singla, A., Puri, V., Dheer, D., Chopra, H., Malik, T., & Sharma, A. (2025). Herbal bioactive-loaded biopolymeric formulations for wound healing applications. *RSC Advances*, *15*(16), 12402–12442. DOI: 10.1039/D4RA08604J PMID: 40248229

Kaczmarek-Szczepańska, B., Glajc, P., Chmielniak, D., Gwizdalska, K., Swiontek Brzezinska, M., Dembińska, K., Shinde, A. H., Gierszewska, M., Łukowicz, K., Basta-Kaim, A., D'Amora, U., & Zasada, L. (2025). Development and Characterization of Biocompatible Chitosan-Aloe Vera Films Functionalized with Gluconolactone and Sorbitol for Advanced Wound Healing Applications. *ACS Applied Materials & Interfaces*, *17*(10), 15196–15207. DOI: 10.1021/acsami.5c00715 PMID: 39999379

Kim, J. O., Noh, J.-K., Thapa, R. K., Hasan, N., Choi, M., Kim, J. H., Lee, J.-H., Ku, S. K., & Yoo, J.-W. (2015). Nitric oxide-releasing chitosan film for enhanced antibacterial and in vivo wound-healing efficacy. *International Journal of Biological Macromolecules*, *79*, 217–225. DOI: 10.1016/j.ijbiomac.2015.04.073 PMID: 25957720

Koshy, J. T., Vasudevan, D., Sangeetha, D., & Prabu, A. A. (2023). Biopolymer Based Multifunctional Films Loaded with Anthocyanin Rich Floral Extract and ZnO Nano Particles for Smart Packaging and Wound Healing Applications. *Polymers*, *15*(10), 2372. DOI: 10.3390/polym15102372 PMID: 37242946

Kozłowska, J., Skopińska-Wiśniewska, J., Kaczmarek-Szczepańska, B., Grabska-Zielińska, S., Makurat-Kasprolewicz, B., Michno, A., Ronowska, A., & Wekwejt, M. (2023). Gelatin and gelatin/starch-based films modified with sorbitol for wound healing. *Journal of the Mechanical Behavior of Biomedical Materials*, *148*, 106205. DOI: 10.1016/j.jmbbm.2023.106205 PMID: 37948920

Kuryanova, A. S., Kardumyan, V. V., Kaplin, V. S., Aksenova, N. A., Chernyak, A. V., Timofeeva, V. A., Glagolev, N. N., Timashev, P. S., & Solovieva, A. B. (2023). Effect of amphiphilic polymers and sodium alginate on the activity of methylene blue in photogeneration of singlet oxygen^1 O_2. *Laser Physics*, *33*(9), 095601. DOI: 10.1088/1555-6611/ace70e

Lee, C.-S., & Hwang, H. S. (2023). Starch-Based Hydrogels as a Drug Delivery System in Biomedical Applications. *Gels (Basel, Switzerland)*, *9*(12), 951. DOI: 10.3390/gels9120951 PMID: 38131937

Liu, W., Xie, R., Zhu, J., Wu, J., Hui, J., Zheng, X., Huo, F., & Fan, D. (2022). A temperature responsive adhesive hydrogel for fabrication of flexible electronic sensors. *NPJ Flexible Electronics*, *6*(1), 68. DOI: 10.1038/s41528-022-00193-5

Lopes, A. I., Pintado, M. M., & Tavaria, F. K. (2024). Plant-Based Films and Hydrogels for Wound Healing. *Microorganisms*, *12*(3), 438. DOI: 10.3390/microorganisms12030438 PMID: 38543489

Lopes, P., Joaquinito, A. S. M., Ribeiro, A., Moura, N. M. M., Gomes, A. T. P., Guerreiro, S. G., Faustino, M. A. F., Almeida, A., Ferreira, P., Coimbra, M. A., Neves, M. G. P. M. S., & Gonçalves, I. (2023). Starch-based films doped with porphyrinoid photosensitizers for active skin wound healing. *Carbohydrate Polymers*, *313*, 120894. DOI: 10.1016/j.carbpol.2023.120894 PMID: 37182978

Mizuno, K., Yamamura, K., Yano, K., Osada, T., Saeki, S., Takimoto, N., Sakurai, T., & Nimura, Y. (2003). Effect of chitosan film containing basic fibroblast growth factor on wound healing in genetically diabetic mice. *Journal of Biomedical Materials Research. Part A*, *64A*(1), 177–181. DOI: 10.1002/jbm.a.10396 PMID: 12483711

Muthulakshmi, V., & Rajarajeswari, G. R. (2021). *In vivo* wound healing efficiency of curcumin-incorporated pectin-chitosan biodegradable films. *New Journal of Chemistry*, *45*(38), 17918–17929. DOI: 10.1039/D1NJ03477D

Nada, A. A., Ali, E. A., Soliman, A. A. F., Shen, J., Abou-Zeid, N. Y., & Hudson, S. M. (2020). Multi-layer dressing made of laminated electrospun nanowebs and cellulose-based adhesive for comprehensive wound care. *International Journal of Biological Macromolecules*, *162*, 629–644. DOI: 10.1016/j.ijbiomac.2020.06.184 PMID: 32574744

Natarajan, V., Krithica, N., Madhan, B., & Sehgal, P. K. (2013). Preparation and properties of tannic acid cross-linked collagen scaffold and its application in wound healing. *Journal of Biomedical Materials Research. Part B, Applied Biomaterials*, *101B*(4), 560–567. DOI: 10.1002/jbm.b.32856 PMID: 23255343

Nguyen, T. T. T., Tran, N. T. K., Le, T. Q., Nguyen, T. T. A., Nguyen, L. T. M., & Tran, T. V. (2023). Passion fruit peel pectin/chitosan based antibacterial films incorporated with biosynthesized silver nanoparticles for wound healing application. *Alexandria Engineering Journal*, *69*, 419–430. DOI: 10.1016/j.aej.2023.01.066

Nordin, N. N., Aziz, N. K., Naharudin, I., & Anuar, N. K. (2022). Effects of Drug-Free Pectin Hydrogel Films on Thermal Burn Wounds in Streptozotocin-Induced Diabetic Rats. *Polymers*, *14*(14), 2873. DOI: 10.3390/polym14142873 PMID: 35890648

Ogeh, P.C., E. A. B. (n.d.). Evaluation of Physico-Mechanical and Mucoadhesive Properties of Biopolymer Films From Cola Acuminata Gum. *Nigerian Journal of Pharmaceutical Research*, *14*, 13.

Oliveira, C., Sousa, D., Teixeira, J. A., Ferreira-Santos, P., & Botelho, C. M. (2023). Polymeric biomaterials for wound healing. *Frontiers in Bioengineering and Biotechnology*, *11*, 1136077. DOI: 10.3389/fbioe.2023.1136077 PMID: 37576995

Pagano, C., Puglia, D., Luzi, F., Michele, A. D., Scuota, S., Primavilla, S., Ceccarini, M. R., Beccari, T., Iborra, C. A. V., Ramella, D., Ricci, M., & Perioli, L. (2021). Development and Characterization of Xanthan Gum and Alginate Based Bioadhesive Film for Pycnogenol Topical Use in Wound Treatment. *Pharmaceutics*, *13*(3), 324. DOI: 10.3390/pharmaceutics13030324 PMID: 33802607

Patitucci, F., Motta, M. F., Dattilo, M., Malivindi, R., Leonetti, A. E., Pezzi, G., Prete, S., Mileti, O., Gabriele, D., Parisi, O. I., & Puoci, F. (2024). 3D-Printed Alginate/Pectin-Based Patches Loaded with Olive Leaf Extracts for Wound Healing Applications: Development, Characterization and In Vitro Evaluation of Biological Properties. *Pharmaceutics*, *16*(1), 99. DOI: 10.3390/pharmaceutics16010099 PMID: 38258109

Pooprommin, P., Manaspon, C., Dwivedi, A., Mazumder, A., Sangkaew, S., Wanmasae, S., Tangpong, J., Ongtanasup, T., & Eawsakul, K. (2022). Alginate/pectin dressing with niosomal mangosteen extract for enhanced wound healing: Evaluating skin irritation by structure-activity relationship. *Heliyon*, *8*(12), e12032. DOI: 10.1016/j.heliyon.2022.e12032 PMID: 36506386

Priya, S., Choudhari, M., Tomar, Y., Desai, V. M., Innani, S., Dubey, S. K., & Singhvi, G. (2024). Exploring polysaccharide-based bio-adhesive topical film as a potential platform for wound dressing application: A review. *Carbohydrate Polymers*, *327*, 121655. DOI: 10.1016/j.carbpol.2023.121655 PMID: 38171676

Ren, H., Zhang, Z., Chen, X., & He, C. (2024). Stimuli-Responsive Hydrogel Adhesives for Wound Closure and Tissue Regeneration. *Macromolecular Bioscience*, *24*(3), 2300379. DOI: 10.1002/mabi.202300379 PMID: 37827713

Rezvanian, M., Ng, S.-F., Alavi, T., & Ahmad, W. (2021). In-vivo evaluation of Alginate-Pectin hydrogel film loaded with Simvastatin for diabetic wound healing in Streptozotocin-induced diabetic rats. *International Journal of Biological Macromolecules*, *171*, 308–319. DOI: 10.1016/j.ijbiomac.2020.12.221 PMID: 33421467

Sabando, C., Ide, W., Rodríguez-Díaz, M., Cabrera-Barjas, G., Castaño, J., Bouza, R., Müller, N., Gutiérrez, C., Barral, L., Rojas, J., Martínez, F., & Rodríguez-Llamazares, S. (2020). A Novel Hydrocolloid Film Based on Pectin, Starch and Gunnera tinctoria and Ugni molinae Plant Extracts for Wound Dressing Applications. *Current Topics in Medicinal Chemistry*, *20*(4), 280–292. DOI: 10.2174/15680266206662001241 00631 PMID: 31976835

Said, N. S., Olawuyi, I. F., & Lee, W. Y. (2023). Pectin Hydrogels: Gel-Forming Behaviors, Mechanisms, and Food Applications. *Gels (Basel, Switzerland)*, *9*(9), 732. DOI: 10.3390/gels9090732 PMID: 37754413

Savekar, P. L., Nadaf, S. J., Killedar, S. G., Kumbar, V. M., Hoskeri, J. H., Bhagwat, D. A., & Gurav, S. S. (2024). Citric acid cross-linked pomegranate peel extract-loaded pH-responsive β-cyclodextrin/carboxymethyl tapioca starch hydrogel film for diabetic wound healing. *International Journal of Biological Macromolecules*, *274*, 133366. DOI: 10.1016/j.ijbiomac.2024.133366 PMID: 38914385

Sekar, M. P., Budharaju, H., Sethuraman, S., & Sundaramurthi, D. (2023). Carboxymethyl cellulose-agarose-gelatin: A thermoresponsive triad bioink composition to fabricate volumetric soft tissue constructs. *SLAS Technology*, *28*(3), 183–198. DOI: 10.1016/j.slast.2023.04.005 PMID: 37149220

Solovieva, A., Kopylov, A., Cherkasova, A., Shershnev, I., Kaplin, V., Timofeeva, V., Akovantseva, A., Savko, M., Gulin, A., Zarkhina, T., Aksenova, N., & Timashev, P. (2024). Methylene Blue Solid Alginate Gels for Photodynamic Therapy: The Peculiarities of Production and Controlled Release of the Dye. *Polymers*, *16*(19), 2819. DOI: 10.3390/polym16192819 PMID: 39408531

Tudoroiu, E.-E., Dinu-Pîrvu, C.-E., Albu Kaya, M. G., Popa, L., Anu a, V., Prisada, R. M., & Ghica, M. V. (2021). An Overview of Cellulose Derivatives-Based Dressings for Wound-Healing Management. *Pharmaceuticals*, *14*(12), 1215. DOI: 10.3390/ph14121215 PMID: 34959615

Valle, K. Z. M., Saucedo Acuña, R. A., Ríos Arana, J. V., Lobo, N., Rodriguez, C., Cuevas-Gonzalez, J. C., & Tovar-Carrillo, K. L. (2020). Natural Film Based on Pectin and Allantoin for Wound Healing: Obtaining, Characterization, and Rat Model. *BioMed Research International*, *2020*(1), 6897497. DOI: 10.1155/2020/6897497 PMID: 33123582

Yaşayan, G. (2020). Chitosan films and chitosan/pectin polyelectrolyte complexes encapsulating silver sulfadiazine for wound healing. *İstanbul Journal of Pharmaceutics*, *50*(3). DOI: 10.26650/IstanbulJPharm.2020.0021

Zhu, J., Zhou, H., Gerhard, E. M., Zhang, S., Parra Rodríguez, F. I., Pan, T., Yang, H., Lin, Y., Yang, J., & Cheng, H. (2023). Smart bioadhesives for wound healing and closure. *Bioactive Materials*, *19*, 360–375. PMID: 35574051

KEY TERMS AND DEFINITIONS

Alginate: A polysaccharide derived from brown colored algae that forms ionically crosslinked hydrogels and gels on contact with wound exudate.

Bandage: A multilayer or structured dressing that provides mechanical support, absorption, and therapeutic delivery while adhering to tissue.

Bioadhesive Film: A thin polymer membrane designed to adhere to biological surfaces to protect wounds and/or deliver drugs.

Cellulose and Derivatives: Natural β-1,4 glucan used for film-forming or swelling with semi-synthetic derivatives like CMC, HPMC.

Pectin: A plant polysaccharide that forms gels and is used in moist wound dressings for its water uptake and mild bioactivity.

Swelling Index: The percentage increase in weight when a dry film absorbs simulated wound fluid; informs exudate handling.

Tannic Acid: A polyphenolic plant compound that acts both as an antioxidant agent and as a crosslinker to strengthen films.

Tensile Strength and Elongation at Break: Mechanical metrics measured by a universal testing machine (UTM) that indicate film robustness and flexibility under load.

Water Vapor Transmission Rate: A measure of the breathability of a dressing that affects moisture balance at the wound.

Chapter 9

Herbal Polymer-Infused Hydrogel Dressings for Enhanced Wound Healing

V. Aarthi
https://orcid.org/0009-0004-0177-7716
Vels Institute of Science, Technology, and Advanced Studies, India

R. Chandrasekaran
https://orcid.org/0000-0003-3975-3010
Vels Institute of Science, Technology, and Advanced Studies, India

Vivek Pazhamalai
Vels Institute of Science, Technology, and Advanced Studies, India

D. Yuvaraj
Vels Institute of Science, Technology, and Advanced Studies, India

S. Baskar
https://orcid.org/0009-0004-0859-1279
Vels Institute of Science, Technology, and Advanced Studies, India

S. Ivo Romauld
https://orcid.org/0000-0003-0610-0646
Vels Institute of Science, Technology, and Advanced Studies, India

ABSTRACT

This chapter explains the role and development of herbal-infused hydrogels in wound healing. This discussion starts with wounds; the wound healing mechanism and factors affecting wound healing and then focuses on the development of wound dressing from the ancient period. It also covers the evolution, and specialized characteristics. Hydrogels are classified based on composition, cross-linking, and functions. This chapter also explains the incorporation of herbal compounds into hydrogels. This chapter shows hydrogel development over the years in wound healing, even though it has challenges that will reduce by future innovation such as development of smart hydrogels in wound management.

DOI: 10.4018/979-8-3373-3977-1.ch009

INTRODUCTION TO WOUND HEALING

Innovative biomedical applications, particularly, in the field of wound care, have considered hydrogels as one of the key components owning to their modifiable-properties to maintain a moist environment as well as to facilitate cellular regeneration. The first use of hydrogels can be attributed to the 1960s when Wichterle and Lim fabricated crosslinked poly (2-hydroxyethyl methacrylate) hydrogels for contact lenses (Wichterle & Lim, 1960). Accordingly, hydrogels have been developed using a diverse set of materials ranging from synthetic polymers to natural biopolymers to hybrid systems each providing unique properties appropriate for specific clinical applications.

Moving away from dry traditional dressings to moist wound healing is a significant change in the science of wound repair. It is now well recognized that a moist wound environment not only protects a wound from drying out but can also promote the process of epithelialization, decrease scarring, and enhance the body's own autolytic debridement mechanism (Boateng et al., 2008). Hydrogels with high water content and a 3D porous network system are especially useful to achieve this perfect wound-healing microenvironment.

Furthermore, the progress towards more complex hydrogel chemistries has allowed for the creation of "smart" dressings that respond to stimuli, such as pH, temperature, or bacterial presence. These dynamic systems offer personalized medicine for challenging wounds, including diabetic ulcers, burns and surgical incisions. An emerging trend is the integration of herbal bioactive (e.g., curcumin, aloe vera, and neem) within hydrogel networks.

Smart hydrogels are development higher than traditional wound dressing they can specifically take care the wound healing.

Types of Wounds

Wounds fall into two types: acute and chronic. The type depends on how the wound happens how it recovers, and how much time healing takes. Acute wounds include things like surgical cuts, scratches, or injuries from accidents or medical treatments. These heal in a normal way without major issues (Rodrigues et al. 2019; Boateng & Catanzano 2015). Surgical wounds are classified under ICD-10 code T81, while trauma injuries are grouped in S01–S91 codes. Burns listed under T20–T32, are a more serious kind of acute wound. Their classification depends on depth. First-degree burns affect the outer skin layer second-degree burns go deeper, and third-degree burns damage every layer of the skin.

Hydrogel sheets, a type of special wound dressing, help by cooling the area and keeping it hydrated. Chronic wounds are unique since they fail to heal. They remain trapped in the inflammation stage of the healing process. Examples include pressure ulcers (ICD-10: L89). These often happen to older adults or People stuck in bed for a long time.

Diabetic foot ulcers (ICD-10: E11.621) – develop because of nerve damage and restricted blood flow.

Arterial ulcers (ICD-10: I70.233) – arise from limited blood supply linked to clogged arteries.

Venous leg ulcers (ICD-10: I83.0) – result from vein problems and fluid buildup in the legs.

Chronic wounds need special treatments like hydrogel dressings containing herbal extracts to lower microbes and support granulation tissue growth. Using the stage (I-IV) and type of exudate helps doctors pick the right hydrogel during treatment.

Phases of Wound Healing

Four stages of wound healing process that naturally occur in immune system as shown in Figure 1:

Figure 1. Four phases of wound healing

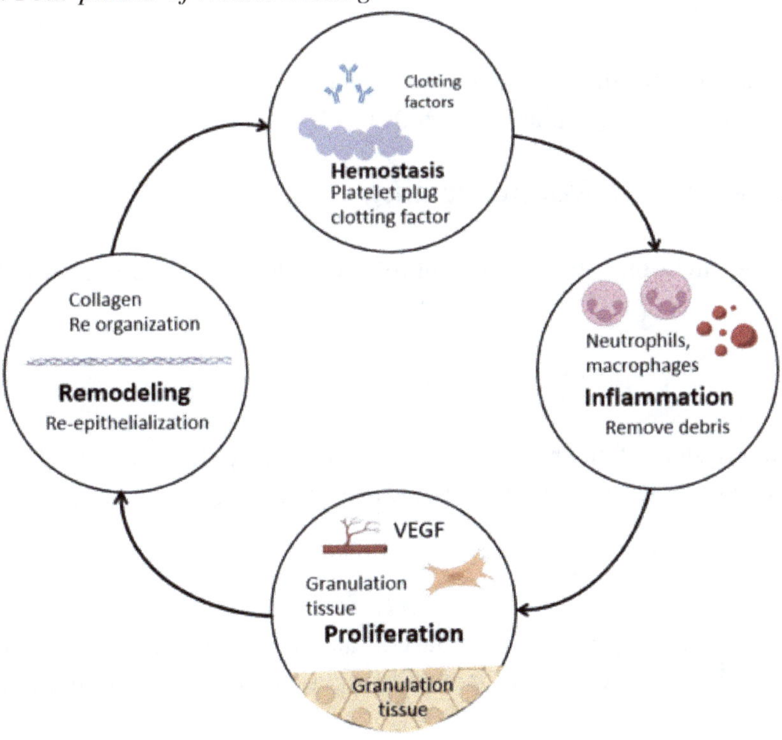

Wound healing happens in four steps: haemostasis, inflammation, proliferation, and remodelling. Each step depends on the role of immune cells, cytokines, and the activity of the extracellular matrix.

Haemostasis

Process of vasoconstriction (decrease in size of blood vessel), formation of clotting to stop the bleeding released by platelets and cytokines initiates the repairing process.

Inflammation

The body responses by involvement of macrophages and neutrophils to remove the debris and pathogens in wound area.

Proliferation

Formation of new tissues includes granulation tissue and capillaries in the wound by cells such as fibroblasts, keratinocytes and endothelial cells.

Remodelling

Remodeled extracellular matrix to improve tensile strength over time and collagen fibers are reorganized (Velnar et al., 2009).

Factors Affecting Wound Healing

Multiple environmental and patient related factors are affecting wound healing such as:

Age

Immune system of elder people is weak that delayed the wound healing process and also aged people have uneven immune response and decrease in cellular activity.

Infection

The wounds are affected by bacterial contamination that increases inflammation, and risk of chronic wound development by delaying tissue regeneration.

Comorbidities

Presence of one or more medical conditions in the same person such as diabetes, peripheral vascular disease, malnutrition, compromise in the oxygen supply, metabolic activity leads to impairing wound healing outcomes (Guo & Dipietro, 2010).

TRADITIONAL VS ADVANCED WOUND DRESSINGS

Overview of Conventional Dressings

Traditional wound dressing is the use of primarily designed material to protect a wound from some factors is also called as passive wound dressings like gauze, cotton pads and bandages. These are used for the protection from contamination and absorb exudate (Boateng et al., 2008). Gauze is the porous fabric of cotton or synthetic fibers that helps for sir circulation in the wound but it also affects the healing time by drying the wound quickly. For protection and secure of the gauze, the bandages are designed it offers the light compression to control bleeding (Gupta et al., 2010).

Even though these conventional dressings are low cost and easily accessible that doesn't have any features like antimicrobial properties, bioactivity, moisture holding capacity and don't provide an optimal healing environment which all of these are important to reduces infection and increases wound healing.

Limitations of Traditional Approaches

Even with historical importance of traditional methods affects in several limits like dehydration in the wounds due to poor water content maintenance leads to decreases rate of tissue generation which is called as epithelialization (Davis & Perez, 2009). Additionally, gauze dressings strongly attached to the wounds when its dries lead to trauma (pain, discomfort) to the patient during removal of dressings and also it has potential to reopening the wound (Dhivya et al., 2015).

Also, the traditional dressings don't provide antibacterial protection and develops risks of infection mainly in chronic wounds due to this the dressings have to change continuously that increases the contamination risks and costs in healthcare for long-term dressing procedure (Gupta et al., 2010).

Evolution of Advanced Dressings

These are the limits that led to the development of advanced wound dressings. These advanced materials are designed to improve healing, secure moist in the wound area, and act as a delivery system for the bioactive compounds such as antibiotics, herbal extract, and growth factor. It also protects the wounds from infection (Vowden & Vowden, 2017).

For advanced dressings specific materials like hydrogels, hydrocolloids, alginate and foam dressings are used to promote oxygen penetration, wetness in the wound site and also it manages the exudate from the wound. Compared to traditional dressings, advanced wound dressing materials are increasing the rate of tissue regeneration through innovative properties (Mogoşanu & Grumezescu, 2014).

Moreover, advanced wound dressing materials like hydrogels are incorporated with herbal extract such as neem, turmeric, aloe vera gel, honey to improve antioxidant and antibacterial activity for enhancing healing ability of dressings. The appearance of smart hydrogels in recent times developed especially as an environmental-stimuli such as pH, temperature and enzyme activity and advanced in drug release control adaptation of dynamic wounds (Li & Mooney, 2016).

INTRODUCTION TO HYDROGELS

Hydrogels are 3D and water loving polymer which is said to be hydrophilic compound, that polymer networks have capability to store huge amount of water inside its structure and also maintains the mechanical properties like biomedical application especially in wound healing. Hydrogels can be natural, synthetic, and semi-synthetic which have specific functionality like high water content, biocompatibility, soft and flexible in nature leads to response to environmental stimuli like ionic strength, temperature, and pH (Ahmed, 2015).

Out of many polymers, hydrogels especially used for wound healing due to their ability of moist wound maintenance, improve autolytic debridement, and accelerate cell motility (Kamoun et al., 2017). Hydrogels have most special features that specifically treat the wound and maintain the wound environment. Hydrogels can be customized depends on the injuries.

Definition and Characteristics

Hydrogels have hydrophilic character in nature and it has composition of polymer chains which can elaborate by storing water without mixing in it. Hydrogels have more than 90% of water content in their structure, which is helps to cell adherence, tissue regeneration, and nutrient transport (Ahmed, 2015).

Hydrogels is a material that have a porous nature, which helps in combination of delivering therapeutic agents, cell attachment and growth in the wound area. Hydrogels have many functional groups like hydroxyl (-OH), carboxyl (-COOH), and amide (-NH_2) helps in their swelling nature and its mechanical strength (Gholamali, 2019). Features like these improves hydrogels in the uses of wound dressings, contact lenses, and infusionable drug delivery in the immune systems.

Types of Hydrogels

Hydrogels can be classified into various types depends on the source and composition of hydrogels extracted or developed, divided as natural—which is derived from plants, animals or human's macromolecules like hyaluronic acid, alginate, chitosan and alginate. These polymers naturally have the ability of biodegradation, bioactivity and non-toxicity that helps cell adherence (attachment to the wall) and proliferation. For example, brown seaweed used in extraction of alginate which created ionic cross-linking in presence of calcium ions that develops the biocompatibility and soft matrix for suitable wound healing (Boateng et al., 2008).

Next type is synthetic hydrogels—that are engineered polymers from chemical compounds like polyacrylamide, and polyvinyl alcohol (PVA). These are modified specifically for the features of long-term usage, mechanical strength and degradation rate control. Synthetic hydrogels are more useful when the drug needs to integrate in particular desire, still they lack in bioactivity of natural hydrogels (Peppas et al., 2006).

The evolution of hydrogels leads to the innovation of semi-synthetic hydrogels—the combination of bioactivity feature of natural and strength & properties of synthetic hydrogels, both blends to form semi-synthetic polymer compounds (Li & Mooney, 2016). For example, PVA is a hydrogel that combines with aloe vera extract for antibacterial activities and quick tissue regeneration in chronic wounds (Hanif et al., 2021).

Hydrogels are highly varied in their composition and that may change the function and makes hydrogels more specific in wound healing. Natural hydrogels have high bio degradation and compatibility, on other hand synthetic hydrogels are great in strength and selectable properties (see table 1).

Classification of Hydrogels

Hydrogels are classified into different types based on their **structural** and **functional** activities.

Based on Composition

Hydrogels can be divided into three categories: natural, synthetic, and hybrid. Natural types like gelatin chitosan and alginate tend to be used because they are safe, work with living tissues, and break down. On the other hand, synthetic options such as polyethylene glycol (PEG), polyvinyl alcohol (PVA), and polyacrylamide (PAM) provide better control over their swelling breaking down, or resistance to stress.

Hybrid hydrogels mix natural and synthetic polymers to balance biological activity with mechanical strength. Recent examples use combinations like PVA with aloe vera, PEG with curcumin, and gelatin with turmeric. These blends include herbal compounds to offer antimicrobial and antioxidant benefits.

Based on Cross-Linking

Scientists group hydrogels by their structure in a few ways like, weak forces like hydrogen bonds or ionic ties allow physical cross-linking to create reversible structures. Strong covalent bonds drive chemical cross-linking giving hydrogels more durability and longer usage (Qiu & Park, 2012). Enzymatic cross-linking uses enzymes such as horseradish peroxidase or tyrosinase to help gels solidify.

These systems treat wounds effectively and are easy on the body since they avoid causing harm (Lei et al. 2023). Dual cross-linked hydrogels rely on both chemical and physical bonds. This combination allows the hydrogels to offer strength, flexibility, and a controlled way of breaking down. They perform well as dressings for joints or areas that experience frequent movement.

Based on Functionality

Hydrogels work in different ways such as, Passive ones that serve as moist covers for wounds, Active ones that deliver drugs to fight germs or promote healing, and Smart ones, which respond to changes such as pH levels, heat, or enzyme activity (Li & Mooney, 2016).

pH-sensitive hydrogels release medication in alkaline environments, like in infected wounds. Heat-sensitive hydrogels such as PNIPAM, shift their structure at body temperature letting them form gels on site. Enzyme-sensitive hydrogels break down when triggered by matrix metalloproteinases (MMPs) found in long-lasting wounds, which helps with controlled drug release and tissue repair.

The different hydrogels functions result the specific repair mechanism in the wound. The design of hydrogel properties depends on patients' conditions.

Table 1. Difference between natural and synthetic hydrogels in wound dressings

Features	Natural Hydrogels	Synthetic Hydrogels
Source	It is derived from biological materials like plants, animals or humans	It is developed using chemical compounds.
Biocompatibility	Fantastic in nature	Moderate, that is depends on the polymer.
Mechanical strength	Low in strength	It has high specific strength
Reproducibility	Varies depends on the batch production	It has high consistent synthesis using chemicals
Biodegradability	It has degradability naturally	It is non-degradable but it can degrade when modified
Cost	Usually high due to extraction process.	It cost is low and it can produce in high quantity.
Examples	Chitosan, Alginate and Gelatin	Polyacrylamide, PEG, PVA

Adapted from Boateng et al. (2008); Kamoun et al. (2017).

Clinical Notes. The study of Erdagi et al. (2020) innovates a Genipin-crosslinked gelatin-diosgenin-nanocellulose hydrogels, that shows great antibiotic release and mechanical activities in the wound area. These hydrogels are efficiently reducing the bacterial contamination, mainly in diabetic wounds explains its advanced care in wound healing.

ROLES OF HYDROGELS IN WOUND HEALING

Moist Wound Environment

Hydrogels are widely used due to their unique role of maintenance moist in wound environment that is increases healing rate and decreases scar evolution. Moisture is the one of the main environments needs to maintain in the wound site, that improves the epithelialization, and autolytic debridement process. This required also supports relocation of keratinocyte and increases in fibroblast, which is essential for regeneration of tissue (Jones et al., 2006). Hydrogels set this moist condition in the injured place that prevents wound desiccation and reduces pain when wound dressing changed.

Hydrogels act through several interdependent pathways which support all phases of the normal wound healing process, including four phases of wound healing. The most significant activity of hydrogel is moisture absorption as its application reduces exudate and desiccation and will support autolytic debridement, which is auto clean process due to action of body own enzymes to necrotic tissue (Okan et al., 2007). This absorbative capability also can reduce pain by protecting nerve endings.

Exudate Absorption

Hydrogels have exudate absorption feature that is main role to prevent infection from the fluid discharge in the wound. Moderate level of absorption done by hydrogels due to its porous matrix and it protects the new skin from maceration, reduces bacterial contamination, also maintain hydration in the wound (Gounden & Singh, 2024). Hydrogels also decrease the rate of changing the wound dressing and protects wound not damage furtherly. By this absorption, hydrogels prevent the wound from conversion from acute to chronic wound—which takes more time to heal.

Pain Reduction and Ease Removal

Hydrogels are not attached to the wounds deeply. So, the trauma reduces when the dressing removal and the chilling effect of hydrogels gives relief in inflamed chronic ulcers and burned wounds for the pediatrics—medicinal care for the infants and children, also for geriatrics—medicinal care of elder people (Thomas, 1990). Hydrogels are better than gauze or cotton pads, because unlike hydrogels they are stick to the wounds and make the pain even worse during wound dressing changes.

Barrier to Microbes

Hydrogels don't have an anti-microbial activity until they incorporate with some material which have anti-bacterial and anti-microbial properties. Even though hydrogels act like a semi-permeable barrier which protects the wounds from external contamination while serves gas exchange frequently. Recent studies and research from 2000's in hydrogels incorporate with silver nanoparticles or herbal extracts shows more effective in anti-microbial activity (Rujitanaroj et al., 2008). This feature of double action prevents colony formation of bacteria and disrupts the biofilm development in the wound bed surface.

Mechanistic Insights and Biofilm Disruption

From biochemical point of view, hydrogels adjust the wound pH to a degree, which may not be conducive for the growth of microorganisms. Indeed, many chronic wounds are characterised by an alkaline pH (>7.4) that promotes bacterial growth and hinders tissue healing. Acid hydrogel matrices contribute to correct these discrepancies, stimulating fibroblast migration and angiogenesis (Leveen et al., 1973).

In hydrogel systems based on plant hydrocolloids, further things have to be considered. Flavonoids and polyphenols, which are active plant compounds, have an antioxidant effect on the body. They clean up harmful oxygen molecules lowering stress on the wound as it heals. As an example, scientists have put curcumin in hydrogels. These gels block a signal called NF-κB, which cuts down on proteins that cause swelling, like IL-6 and TNF-α (Jirofti et al., 2021). Controlling how fast a drug comes out is also key.

Scientists can make hydrogels to release plant-based drugs. These gels might respond to outside changes like heat or inside factors like enzymes. Some plastics, like PNIPAM, can swell up or shrink based on body heat. This changes how the drug comes out. Breaking up biofilms has become a new focus in designing hydrogels. Harmful bacteria like *Pseudomonas aeruginosa* and *Staphylococcus aureus* form biofilms that fight off antibiotics and slow down healing.

Some hydrogels now include plant-based ingredients such as tea tree oil or clove extract. These have shown promise in breaking down the biofilm structure and helping antibiotics work better. To wrap up, the porous structure of hydrogels allows oxygen to flow through, cells to stick, and move around. These factors play a key role in helping skin grow back. Hydrogels also cut down on water loss through the skin. This keeps the wound area stable and helps the body heal itself.

SMART HYDROGELS AND THEIR BIOACTIVE FUNCTIONS

Smart hydrogels is advanced development of hydrogels which is basically response to environment of wounds like temperature, pH, or enzyme activities and most smart hydrogels have bioactive in function that means the wound dressing can carry drugs, antibiotics, herbal extract and some factors which helps to improve the wound healing. This section is about the different types of smart hydrogels as shown in Figure 2.

Drug-Loaded Hydrogels

Hydrogels act as a drug carrier to the wounds, drugs like antibiotics, pain relief medicines—known as analgesics and even be a growth factor for wound healing. These smart hydrogels are specifically designed for direct delivery of drug to the wound site and it serves as an advantage in sustainable drug release control, maintain the therapeutic levels of drug at the wound. By using this hydrogel, the continuous use of drugs can be reduced.

Ampicillin, azithromycin and gentamicin are drugs used to control infections, speed up the wound repair by the growth factors like EGF, VEGF and analgesics like paracetamol or acetaminophen are given to reduce pain in wound area (Lin et al., 2024). Also, hydrogels are loaded with natural and herbal based medicines such as curcumin, neem, aloe vera to improve patient comfort zone, drug stability, bioactivity, and reduces pain along with decrease in side effects.

Stimuli-Responsive Hydrogels

These hydrogels are designed especially for response to the changes in the wound environment. These smart hydrogels are change the drug release and its structure involuntarily corresponding to the conditions like temperature, pH, and enzymes metabolism. For instance, when temperature changed in the wounds, hydrogel dressings can sense it in real-time and release needed antibiotic that loaded in it (Zhang et al., 2025).

Recently, the smart hydrogels are tested in burn wounds and diabetic ulcers for enzyme-responsive. because in such burn wounds, the activity of enzymes changed, and these hydrogels are helps to control the situation in injured area. By this method, the overuse of drug in wound is avoided and maintain healing process, these smart hydrogels act like intelligent system for drug release at right place in needed time without disturbing patient's comfort.

Figure 2. Controlled release from herbal-infused hydrogels

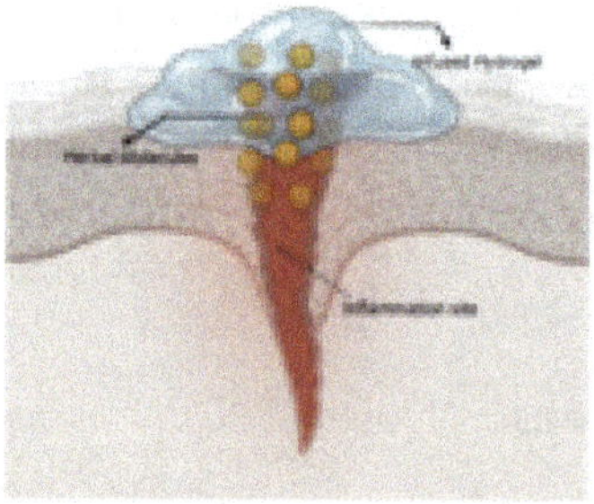

A hydrogel matrix tailored to wounds reacts to triggers like pH levels or enzymes and controls how medication is dispensed. Herbal agents like curcumin focus on the injured area to promote healing while minimizing impact on the rest of the body.

Self-Healing and Shape-Memory Hydrogels

These smart hydrogels can heal itself, when its broken or torn apart that is most helpful in chronic wounds due to its long-term usage and these polymers called as self-healing hydrogels (Zhang et al., 2024).

They have the capacity to maintain their structure by rejoining polymer chains naturally after a mechanical breakage.

Other hand, shape-memory hydrogels which can change it structure based on temperature, pH, or even in light (Xuan et al., 2023). This type hydrogels are still in studies and research but definitely these polymers are amazing use to fill an uneven wound, some unreachable areas and also provide customized dressing to wound site. In results of research, the shape-memory hydrogels give promising variations in regenerative medicine and some personal wound dressing care.

Both self-healing and shape-memory hydrogels are significantly useful in various medicine fields and so much convenient to the patient's pain and healing at the wound site. Recently the incorporation of herbal and other compounds like drugs, with smart hydrogels becomes more powerful.

Some Examples and Uses of Smart Hydrogels are Shown Below

- pH-responsive hydrogels are maintaining pH when it becomes alkaline, by antibiotics releasing
- Temperature responsive hydrogels controls heat in the immune system by using drug
- Enzyme-responsive hydrogels are releasing growth factors to control and heal the chronic wounds
- Self-healing hydrogels can rejoin itself after the breakage in the structure.
- Shape-memory hydrogels can change its structure in uneven wound and return to its normal shape

Adapted from Lin et al. (2024); Zhang et al. (2024); Xuan et al. (2023); Zhang et al. (2025).

SOURCES AND FABRICATION TECHNIQUES

Natural Polymers in Hydrogels

Natural polymers are used in wound dressings because of its biodegradability and compatibility in nature. For example, alginate developed from brown seaweed for hydrogel production by using calcium ions and alginate is more effective in exudate absorption (Lee & Mooney, 2012).

Chitosan is another example of natural polymer which is produced from crustacean shells, reveals antibacterial and hemostatic properties that is making chitosan useful in wound healing progress (Dutta et al., 2004). The other example which is normally used by people that is gelatin, created from hydrolysis of collagen, mostly used for supporting in cell attachment, and proliferation to promote wound healing (Van Den Bulcke et al., 2000).

Hyaluronic acid that is a polymer widely known for its hydration properties and a particle of an extracellular matrix, which is helps in angiogenesis process, improves cell migration and important for tissue regeneration (Collins & Birkinshaw, 2013).

Even though, natural hydrogels lack in mechanical strength—to improve its stability, properties and functionalities these hydrogels combine with synthetic hydrogels or modified using chemicals for enhancement (Peppas et al., 2000).

Synthetic Polymers in Hydrogels

Synthetic hydrogels are chemically synthesis with specific modification like polyvinyl alcohol (PVA), which is used to form hydrogels by physical cross-linking methods such as frost-thaw weathering— that means expansion by using water filling in the gap then freeze it to get great elasticity and also water retention (Peppas et al., 2000). Polylactic-co-glycolic acid (PLGA) which has biodegradability in nature and it is mainly used for drug release control in drug-loaded hydrogels, particularly used in chronic wounds (Jain, 2000).

Polyethylene glycol (PEG) that is a polymer, and it is highly hydrophilic, also biocompatible. It is used to improve bioavailability, solubility and more used in modification of natural polymers (Zhu, 2010). Synthetic polymers also have a negative because its lacks in biological activity, even though synthetic hydrogels provide consistency and with tunable functions. So, these polymers also incorporated with natural polymers or some bioactive compounds to enhance in wound healing process (Hoffman, 2002).

Fabrication Techniques

Varieties of fabrication methods are used in innovative production of hydrogels in specific properties or even in the way of hydrogel wound dressing usage:

Freeze-Drying

This method is used to develop porous hydrogel dressing to improve mechanical structure and its stability.

3D-Printing

This technique helps to create customized wound matrices for adaptation to uneven wounds and allows to combination of cells or drugs (Murphy & Atala, 2014).

In-situ Gelation

This process produces hydrogels that significantly used for irregular and deep wounds by directly forming hydrogels at wound area in response to the physical conditions like temperature, pH (Ruel-Gariepy & Leroux, 2004).

Electrospinning

This procedure helps to make nanofiber mats with high surface area, to enhance drug release control and drug-loading into the polymer for better wound healing (Bhardwaj & Kundu, 2010).

These are the techniques widely used for hydrogels influence in activity and properties of polymers.

ANTIBACTERIAL AND ANTIOXIDANT PROPERTIES IN WOUND HEALING

The combination of antioxidant and antibacterial with hydrogels, to improve wound healing by prevents microbial infections, reducing biofilm formation and stress. Traditional wounds are don't have sustainable antimicrobial activity, but modern smart hydrogels specifically designed to protect the wound site by direct delivery of antimicrobial agents, this provides stable control in infection and avoid side effects.

Antibacterial and Antioxidant Agents

There are many compounds provides antimicrobial activity and recent development in nanotechnology gives a way in wound healing like silver nanoparticles which is widely used antimicrobial agent for healing applications. These nanoparticles easily incorporate with hydrogel scaffolds improves antibacterial property without toxicity production. The AgNPs mechanism is disturbs microbial membrane, produce ROS (reactive oxygen species) and disrupts DNA replication in the cells (Rigo et al., 2013). Silver nanoparticles are mostly loaded into polymer due to its activity against both gram-negative and gram-positive bacteria such as *pseudomonas aeruginosa, staphylococcus aureus.*

The continuous production of Ag+ ions from hydrogel scaffolds provides long-term protection and reduces inflammation, cytotoxicity and improves re-epithelialization. For examples, chitosan hydrogels loaded with silver nanoparticles increasing rate of healing in wounds (Paladini & Pollini, 2019). As well, the porous material of hydrogels distributes the nanoparticles evenly in the wound and improves the contact with surface microorganism.

Another example is zinc oxide (ZnO) nanoparticles, which has many types of antibacterial property. Also, zinc oxide supports angiogenesis process, fibroblast proliferation and increases the ROS generation and disruption of bacterial cell membrane makes it useful of tissue regeneration. Zinc oxides are cost-effective and has low toxicity, which is suitable for long-term wound management (Raghupathi et al., 2011).

Next one is honey, which is widely used in food products as a sweetener and it has antibacterial with antioxidant property. Honey can develop an unpleasant surrounding for bacterial growth because it has acidic pH, high osmolarity, and hydrogen peroxide. When honey combined with hydrogels, which is improved antimicrobial activity as well water retention and manuka honey is well-known documented for chronic wound treatment (Molan, 2001).

Recently, hydrogels are incorporate with herbal extracts such as neem, aloe vera, green tea and curcumin, due to their duality of both antimicrobial and antioxidant activities. For example, aloe vera infused hydrogels are supports re-epithelialization and wound closure (Maan et al., 2018). Also, curcumin loaded hydrogels are improves collagen production, maintains anti-inflammatory activity and neem extract, which is other side provides antimicrobial agent along with reduces the odor from the wound site.

Role of Antibacterial and Antioxidant Properties

Antibacterial is a process of protecting wounds from inflammation and antioxidant is the way of removing free radicals, to prevent cell damages.

This antioxidant is important in ischemic and diabetic wounds, where oxidative level is high, those cell damage by free radicals reduces the rate of healing, causing by the destruction of proteins, lipids and nuclei acid. Some herbal extracts have phenolic, flavonoids, terpenoids compounds have antioxidant property. For instance, resveratrol, grape seed extract and green tea catechins are mostly infused in hydrogels because they show high antioxidant property (Salehi et al., 2018).

These compounds reduce scars by control collagen deposition, activity of fibroblast, and improves vascularization in addition of tissue regeneration.

Duality of antibacterial and antioxidant activity is more effective in inflammation, infection and it increases the rate of wound healing in chronic injuries, that duality effects come from the combination of both agents like zinc-resveratrol, silver-curcumin.

Biofilm Prevention

Biofilm is a bacterial consortium that fixed to the polymer and attached to the wound, it has antibiotic resistance function. Biofilms are protecting bacteria in the wound and makes bacteria strong against action of drugs, immune responses, and delayed the healing process. Incorporation of hydrogels with zinc, silver, as well herbal extracts affects the bacterial attachment, quorum sensing and breakdown the formation of biofilm.

For example, silver nanoparticles are disturbing the gene expression in *pseudomonas aeruginosa* by inhibiting biofilm-association (Percival & McCarty, 2015). Hydrogels are keeping the wound in moist environment and prevents biofilm formation by protecting wounds from crusting and scabbing. Recent studies of hydrogels showing some of them have DNase and proteases which breakdown the biofilm scaffolds.

CASE STUDIES AND CLINICAL TRIALS OF HYDROGELS

Hydrogel wound dressings are clinically tested, showed promising results in both acute and chronic wounds. Recent cases and clinical trials proved the real-life evolution of traditional dry wound dressings to advanced customized wound dressings, also hydrogel dressings become commercially successful and many case studies in the documents of patient's recovery shows the unimaginable features of hydrogels.

Commercial Hydrogel Dressings

A shapeless hydrogel dressings are commercialized successfully in a different form. For example, Intrasite® Gel fabricated by Smith & Nephew, it contains carboxymethylcellulose, propyl glycol that helps in autolytic wound care, provides moisture and removes necrotic tissue without affecting healthy tissue in the wound.

By use of hydrogels, reports increased in rate of healing along with decrease in pain and increasing in cosmetic results in clinical evaluations (Jones, A., & Vaughan, D. (2005).

On the other hand, hydrogel sheets are providing extra structural integrity, used in chronic superficial wounds and its easier for application. For instance, Vigilon® and DermaFilm® are useful in moist maintenance in wound area till proper healing.

Another example, NuGel® is produced by Johnson & Johnson, which is widely used for pressure ulcers and burns treatment. It is a hydrogel have cross-linking polymer structure improves bacterial barrier, water retention and healing activity (Aswathy et al., 2020).

Case Studies of Wound Healing

Various case studies proves that hydrogel based advanced wound dressings is way better than traditional dressings. There are two different types of hydrogels case studies mentioned below for example:

Silver Nanoparticle Infused Hydrogels. In severe burns patients are treated with silver nanoparticle infused hydrogels because, AgNPs hydrogels are heal the wounds faster and reduces pain compared to silver sulfadiazine cream. This study explains that hydrogels can develop re-epithelialization and bacterial colonies reduction (Nguyen et al., 2019).

Aloe Vera-Gelatin Hydrogels. In clinical case of skin scrapping, hydrogels completely heal the skin within 10 days. This case shows the biocompatibility and tissue regeneration activities, also patients gave feedback about hydrogels which reduces the itching, scarring, and the rate increases in crust detachment (Saenchoopa et al., 2025). These case studies highlight the development of hydrogels healing process in chronic wounds like donor sites, infected surgical cuts, and venous leg ulcers.

Curcumin-Chitosan Hydrogels. Researchers tested a curcumin-loaded chitosan hydrogel to heal diabetic foot ulcers infected with *Staphylococcus aureus*. In 28 days, the hydrogel group showed more closed wounds and formed more granulation tissue than the group treated with saline. They also felt less pain, noticed less odor, and experienced less fluid discharge. When researchers studied the tissue, they found increased blood vessel growth and more collagen buildup. This highlighted the antioxidant and germ-fighting effects of curcumin combined with the biopolymer traits of chitosan (Li et al. 2019).

Clinical Trials and Practice Performance

The efficacy of hydrogels is tested in large number of people and runs a number of randomized controlled trials (RCTs). Two examples are followed below:

Hydrocolloids vs Hydrogels Dressings

For pressure ulcers, multiple studies are done to compare hydrogel dressings with other kind of dressings by Cochrane review. This review explains hydrogels are more effective than others in pressure ulcers, but there is no solid proof to confirm if hydrogels are more effective than all other various types of dressings (Dumville et al., 2015).

Honey-Infused Hydrogels

This study proves the honey-infused hydrogels are more efficient in wound healing. Because these hydrogels have antimicrobial activity and also maintain moisture in the wound site (El-Kased et al., 2017). In high level meta-analyses of wound dressing trials, hydrogels topped in one due to reduction dressings change frequency and patients' satisfaction. As for now, many hospitals use hydrogel-based procedures in part of wound debridement by improvement in clinical results.

Graphene Oxide–Gelatin Smart Hydrogel

Researchers carried out a double-blind randomized trial to test a graphene oxide–gelatin hydrogel on burns classified as second-degree. This smart hydrogel responded to heat by releasing silver ions when the local temperature rose above 38°C, mimicking the body's inflammation. The study shows that it sped up re-epithelialization by 30%. Pain levels dropped, and infections came back compared to using standard silver sulfadiazine cream. Its electric conductivity and ability to adapt drug release proved useful to treat burns caused by heat (Chen et al., 2024).

Emerging Clinical Use

Along with the products and trials we talked about earlier, a few important clinical uses of hydrogel-based dressings have shown how well they work. A recent study with 80 people who had diabetic foot ulcers tested a hydrogel containing Centella asiatica extract. It healed wounds 40% faster than salt water over six weeks (Chen,

2022). People in the study said they had less fluid coming out less pain, and better tissue growth.

This shows that herbal hydrogels can help with long-lasting wounds where swelling won't go away and normal antibiotics don't work well. Another study looked at an aloe vera-gelatin hydrogel to treat skin damage from radiation in breast cancer patients. The hydrogel reduced skin peeling and redness. Patients said they felt much more comfortable during their radiation treatment (Farrugia et al. 2019). One less-talked-about but important use of hydrogel sheets is in healing donor sites after skin grafts.

Researchers compared paraffin gauze to hydrogel dressings and found that sites treated with hydrogel healed in half the time and showed less hyperpigmentation (Kujur & D'Souza, 2019). These examples back the idea that active hydrogel matrices not only cover wounds but also help deliver phytopharmaceuticals boosting recovery in various wound types. More studies with bigger groups and multiple centers are needed to confirm this and push hydrogel into standard treatments.

LIMITS AND CHALLENGES OF HYDROGELS

Hydrogels wound dressing have various advantages as well specific properties. Mainly, hydrogel infused with drugs and herbal extract dressings have smart functions in wound healing. But still in real-life, these smart hydrogels have many challenges in industrial scale-up, clinical applications and some regulatory schemes.

The Relation of Economic Issues to Cost Effectiveness

The use of hydrogel dressings is still limited in low-middle-income countries due to the high cost compared to traditional gauze and foam dressings. There are multiple factors contributing to the overall cost of hydrogels that include:

Sterilization, infusion of nanoparticles, incorporation of natural extracts, and synthesis of crosslinking networks (Al-Gharibi et al., 2018). Despite the reduction in healing time and hospital stays with the use of hydrogels, the initial cost is still an obstacle for public healthcare systems to overcome.

In an attempt to improve cost, biopolymers derived from biomass waste like Cellulose and Pectin Gels, along with low-cost biosynthesis from plant waste material is being researched (Hamed et al., 2025). Although, these methods are in early stages of development and lack standard operating procedures, inhibiting their efficacy.

Limited Shelf-Life and Stability Concerns

Any gels containing live bioactive such as probiotics, enzymes and herbal oils tend to degrade quickly in uncontrolled environments; so, do hydrogels containing natural polymers. Unpreserved gels have a shelf-life of only two weeks.

In addition, microbial contamination and hydrolytic instability are primary concerns which make cold-chain logistics a necessity (Luong et al., 2014). Preservation techniques such as UV sterilization or lyophilization change one form of preservation for another by compromising physical integrity and active compound bioavailability.

Allergenicity and Patient Differences

Some components of hydrogels, especially acrylates and glutaraldehyde (preservatives), synthetic monomers, and herbal infusions, have been reported to induce allergic type reactions or delayed type hypersensitivity among sensitive patients (Küçük et al., 2025).

While herbal extracts type irritable are biocompatible, if not properly standardized for purity and dosage, contact dermatitis can ensue.

Because of these reasons, thorough background checks and preclinical testing for immunogenicity is required for safe clinical use. In addition, formal-checked medical herb blends lack dose consistency from batch to batch which is difficult due to the unpredictable composition of plant compounds.

Biodegradability vs Mechanical Strength

The trade-off between mechanical stability and biodegradability poses one of the greatest difficulties. Natural hydrogels such as gelatin, chitosan, or alginate readily undergo in vivo biodegradation, but do not possess the requisite tensile strength and elasticity for irregular or deep wounds.

On the other hand, some synthetic hydrogels like PEGDA and polyacrylamide possess mechanical strength but do not metabolize; instead, they burden the tissues and necessitate surgery for extraction (Dodda et al., 2023). The focus is on hybrid systems which incorporate natural biopolymers with tunable synthetic crosslinkers, providing better equilibria of the aforementioned properties. However, the degradation rates in biological environment are still not easily predictable and may change due to the wound's pH, moisture level, or enzymatic activities.

Scientists have developed biodegradable synthetic monomers such as polylactic acid and polycaprolactone to create a mix of strength and resorption. They are also studying bio-inks with bonds that break down based on how a wound is healing.

Regulatory Barriers and Clinical Translation

The majority of herbal-infused or bioactive hydrogels falls under the combination products category of the FDA, requiring separate assessments as a medical device and as a drug (Pawar et al., 2025).

This bifurcation leads to longer approval pathways and increased time to market. In addition, there are no universal protocols for wound care that advise the use of a specific type of hydrogel. XL Clinical guidelines vary from hospital to hospital and from one country to another, leading to diluted usage regardless of efficacy.

There are few training courses available for clinicians and nursing staff on proper application of hydrogel dressings.

FUTURE TRENDS AND KEY RESEARCH AREAS

The rapid evolution of hydrogel wound dressings is mostly derived from the integration of biotechnology, additive manufacturing, and digital health monitoring. Emerging trends are focusing on overcoming existing limitations by adding real-time biosensing, targeted drug release, and personalized scaffolds for wound care.

Customized Hydrogel Dressings Through 3D Printing

Additive manufacturing or 3D printing has transformed the design and production of hydrogel dressings by allowing customization to the wound's geometry, depth, and individual biology. Bioinks containing gelatin methacrylate, alginate, or fibrinogen can be mixed with cells, drugs, or herbal extracts, and such bioinks are printable and can generate layered structures fitting anatomical sites (Chia & Wu, 2015). The complex healing needs of chronic wounds can be simulated by 3D hydrogels incorporating several zones with different release profiles. Also, it is possible to bio print vascular channels or oxygen reservoirs. Some examples are specified (see Table 2).

Table 2. Examples of 3D-printed hydrogels

Type of Hydrogel	Additional Function	Application
Alginate–Gel MA	VEGF & fibroblasts	Diabetic ulcers
PVA–Curcumin	Herbal Extract	Burn Injuries
Gelatin–PEGDA	Antibiotics	Infected Wounds

Adapted from Kumi et al. (2024); Li et al. (2021); Thapa et al. (2021).

Integration with Wearable Sensor Technologies

The future of wound care lies in intelligent dressings with embedded biosensors that continuously track parameters like: pH and temperature - to identify infection, Oxygenation levels – to evaluate ischemia, and Exudate composition – to analyse inflammation.

Intelligent hydrogels can wirelessly send feedback to clinicians or on-the-go apps, which allow remote wound monitoring, particularly useful for diabetic patients, bedridden patients, or geriatric populations (Tang et al., 2021). Using Bluetooth Low Energy (BLE) modules or Near-Field Communication (NFC) allows immediate data sharing without needing large external gadgets.

These advances help patients follow treatments better and cut down on hospital trips leading to a move toward personalized wound care at home.

Regenerative Medicine and Tissue Engineering

Hydrogels act as a biological scaffold for cell migration, attachment, and differentiation. Infused with mesenchymal stem cells (MSCs), exosomes, or platelet-rich plasma, such scaffolds can stimulate angiogenesis, collagen remodelling, and tissue regeneration (Khayambashi et al., 2021).

Advanced research addresses CRISPR-edited MSCs to create hydrogels that deliver gene-controlled healing cues. Another trend is 3D bio printed skin patches with incorporated hydrogel layers for stratified skin healing and limited scarring.

AI-Driven Hydrogel Design

Artificial intelligence and machine learning codes are being employed to develop hydrogel formulations that can forecast: Swelling ratio, Drug diffusion profile, Degradation time, and Mechanical strength.

This computational simulation largely decreases laboratory experimentation and opens the door for customized hydrogel formulation kits (Memon et al., 2025). In the future, pharmacies will provide AI-designed hydrogel matrices based on a patient's wound information and treatment objectives.

Emerging Innovations in Smart Hydrogel Systems

One less-talked-about but important use of hydrogel sheets is in healing donor sites after skin grafts. Researchers compared paraffin gauze to hydrogel dressings and found that sites treated with hydrogel healed in half the time and showed less hyperpigmentation (Kujur & D'Souza, 2019). These examples back the idea that active hydrogel matrices not only cover wounds but also help deliver phytopharmaceuticals boosting recovery in various wound types. More studies with bigger groups and multiple centers are needed to confirm this and push hydrogel into standard treatments.

A new trend is self-healing hydrogels. These can fix themselves through dynamic bonds like Schiff base connections or hydrogen bonds and can repair damage (Devi et al., 2021). This is good for wounds in flexible areas like joints over time. Another cool thing is using blockchain in hydrogel supply chain to verify the authenticity and traceability of herbal bioactive. Problem of variability and contamination in plant extracts has always been an issue in making herbal hydrogels. Blockchain can document where materials are sourced, batch test results and handling details so clinicians can follow regulations and get trust from clinicians.

The living wound dressings is widely on-going research which is bacterial wound dressing infused with hydrogels like lactobacillus strains produce growth factors when inflammation occurs (Yu et al., 2022). Researchers are also looking into voice assisted AI systems to monitor wounds. These systems work with hydrogel sensors. They can be helpful to elderly or blind patients by giving spoken updates using data from smart dressings. Experts predict a move towards smarter, more versatile and patient specific wound care solutions. Although researchers are still testing these in labs and on prototypes initial clinical trials suggest they will work in real life.

Researchers are looking into combining adaptive hydrogels with wearable energy sources or systems that can recharge themselves to keep sensors running without breaks. These are opening up possibilities for future "autonomous healing platforms". These systems bring together monitoring, decision making and treatment into one functional unit.

GLOBAL MARKET AND SOCIETAL IMPACT OF HERBAL HYDROGELS

Herbal hydrogel wound dressings are becoming more popular worldwide because they are safe for the body, have fewer side effects, and are eco-friendly. Allied Market Research reports that the global hydrogel wound dressing market could hit USD 1.5 billion by 2030. This growth comes from an increase in chronic wounds older populations, and interest in using advanced natural materials.

Role in Rural and Low-Resource Settings

Herbal hydrogels provide a cheap method to heal wounds in areas with low income. People in regions like South Asia, Africa, and Latin America often depend on plants such as neem, turmeric, and aloe vera to treat skin problems. Combining these natural options with hydrogel materials creates an affordable treatment that is simple to use and trusted by the community.

Research shows aloe–chitosan and curcumin–gelatin hydrogels can be made from leftover crops on farms (Arshad et al. 2023). This reduces the need to bring in medical supplies from other countries. These hydrogels are easy to store and break down. This makes them helpful to take to mobile clinics or for health professionals working in local areas.

Public Health and SDG Impact

Herbal hydrogels align with SDG-3, which aims to boost health and well-being. They provide effective ways to treat long-term wounds easing pain for patients and raising their quality of life. Using hydrogels instead of antibiotics also helps fight the rising issue of antimicrobial resistance, a major global health concern today.

Local Manufacturing and Job Creation

Producing herbal hydrogels creates jobs in villages and connects biotechnology with old systems of medicine. Strict rules and proper quality checks can help these small community-based units thrive while supporting the growth of Ayurveda or Unani medicine with proof-based methods.

In short herbal hydrogel wound dressings are more than a new invention. They blend advanced biotech with ancient knowledge to move society forward. This mix supports new ideas and makes healthcare easier to reach for all.

CONCLUSION

Wound dressings based on hydrogel have revolutionized the approach to wound treatment by integrating the effects of moisture retention, antimicrobial coverage, and regenerative capacity into a unifying therapeutic modality. This chapter summarized the characterization, formulation, mechanisms, and clinical effects of conventional and intelligent hydrogels.

Herbal-infused and bioactive hydrogels are the new generation of natural therapeutics that harness centuries of traditional medicine with a science-optimized mode. Clinical trials and commercial success have substantiated their efficacy in angiogenesis, infection reduction, and epithelialization enhancement. There still exist hurdles in the form of expense, short shelf-life, risk of allergic reaction, and regulative issues. These need to be overcome by means of biotechnological advancement, training in clinics, and policy initiatives for widespread use.

Futures directions are thrilling. From 3D-printed personalized hydrogels to smart dressings embedded with biosensors, wound care is turning highly personalized, data-driven, and regenerative. With the convergence of machine learning, synthetic biology, and material science, we may see fully autonomous hydrogel systems with real-time sensing, adaptation of drug release, and scaffold-driven regeneration soon. Thus, hydrogel dressings for wounds—especially those which are mixed with herbal medicine—have the potential to sharply reduce health costs, improve outcomes of recovery, and provide equal care to communities.

Hydrogels have revolutionized wound care from the state of being just passive cover-ups to active healing tools. They maintain wound hydration, they transport drugs, and they assist in the functions of cells. These properties make them a valuable ingredient in wound treatments for long-term and short-term wounds. The inclusion of plant extracts made them safer to use. It also augmented their germ-killing power as well as their role in eliminating swelling without triggering drug resistance.

This chapter has reviewed the production of hydrogels how they work, and how they are taken to actual applications in the form of clinical conditions. It also mentioned challenges like cost and regulation while giving a glimpse of new developments like AI for customized solutions, blockchain to verify products, and scaffolds that respond to body response. Hydrogel dressings can decrease hospitalization, conserve unnecessary antibiotic use, and increase patient compliance with therapy if used with remote monitoring devices. For the treatment of wounds in resource-poor settings, herbal hydrogels offer a low-cost fit, and a welcoming choice. But to move forward in developing hydrogel dressings several challenges require attention.

Reducing manufacturing costs, establishing clinical guidelines, and training healthcare personnel will be key. Teamwork between biotechnologists herbal medicine experts, and doctors will help move these solutions from research labs to patient care. With the development of fourth-generation hydrogels, which sense, react, repair, and report, these materials are set to not just help with wound care but also cause a major shift in how healing is approached.

REFERENCES

Ahmed, E. M. (2015). Hydrogel: Preparation, characterization, and applications: A review. *Journal of Advanced Research*, *6*(2), 105–121. DOI: 10.1016/j.jare.2013.07.006 PMID: 25750745

Al-Gharibi, K. A., Sharstha, S., & Al-Faras, M. A. (2018). Cost-Effectiveness of Wound Care: A concept analysis. *Sultan Qaboos University Medical Journal*, *18*(4), e433–e439. DOI: 10.18295/squmj.2018.18.04.002 PMID: 30988960

Arshad, R., Razlansari, M., Hosseinikhah, S. M., Pandey, A. T., Ajalli, N., Manicum, A. L. E., & Tabish, T. A. (2023). Antimicrobial and anti-biofilm activities of bio-inspired nanomaterials for wound healing applications. *Drug Discovery Today*, *28*(9), 103673. DOI: 10.1016/j.drudis.2023.103673 PMID: 37331691

Aswathy, S. H., Narendrakumar, U., & Manjubala, I. (2020). Commercial hydrogels for biomedical applications. *Heliyon*, *6*(4). Advance online publication. DOI: 10.1016/j.heliyon.2020.e03719 PMID: 32280802

Bhardwaj, N., & Kundu, S. C. (2010). Electrospinning: A fascinating fiber fabrication technique. *Biotechnology Advances*, *28*(3), 325–347. DOI: 10.1016/j.biotechadv.2010.01.004 PMID: 20100560

Boateng, J., & Catanzano, O. (2015). Advanced Therapeutic Dressings for Effective Wound Healing—A Review. *Journal of Pharmaceutical Sciences*, *104*(11), 3653–3680. DOI: 10.1002/jps.24610 PMID: 26308473

Boateng, J. S., Matthews, K. H., Stevens, H. N., & Eccleston, G. M. (2008). Wound healing dressings and drug delivery systems: A review. *Journal of Pharmaceutical Sciences*, *97*(8), 2892–2923. DOI: 10.1002/jps.21210 PMID: 17963217

Chen, S. (2022). *Dermal delivery of Centella asiatica using hyaluronic acid niosomal system for wound healing* (Doctoral dissertation, University of Auckland).

Chen, Y., Chang, L., Zhang, Z., Zhou, M., Gao, Y., Wang, Y., & Qin, J. (2024). Biodegradable pectin-based thermo-responsive composite GO/hydrogel with mussel inspired tissue adhesion for NIR enhanced burn wound healing. *Chemical Engineering Journal*, *480*, 148067. DOI: 10.1016/j.cej.2023.148067

Chia, H. N., & Wu, B. M. (2015). Recent advances in 3D printing of biomaterials. *Journal of Biological Engineering*, *9*, 4. DOI: 10.1186/s13036-015-0001-4 PMID: 25866560

Collins, M. N., & Birkinshaw, C. (2013). Hyaluronic acid-based scaffolds for tissue engineering—A review. *Carbohydrate Polymers*, *92*(2), 1262–1279. DOI: 10.1016/j.carbpol.2012.10.028 PMID: 23399155

Davis, S. C., & Perez, R. (2009). Cosmeceuticals and natural products: Wound healing. *Clinics in Dermatology*, *27*(5), 502–506. DOI: 10.1016/j.clindermatol.2009.05.015 PMID: 19695483

Devi, V. K. A., Shyam, R., Palaniappan, A., Jaiswal, A. K., Oh, T. H., & Nathanael, A. J. (2021). Self-Healing Hydrogels: Preparation, Mechanism and Advancement in Biomedical Applications. *Polymers*, *13*(21), 3782. DOI: 10.3390/polym13213782 PMID: 34771338

Dhivya, S., Padma, V. V., & Santhini, E. (2015). Wound dressings - a review. *Biomedicine (Taipei)*, *5*(4), 22. DOI: 10.7603/s40681-015-0022-9 PMID: 26615539

Dodda, J. M., Deshmukh, K., & Bezuidenhout, D. (Eds.). (2023). *Multicomponent hydrogels: smart materials for biomedical applications* (Vol. 15). Royal Society of Chemistry., DOI: 10.1039/9781837670055

Dumville, J. C., Keogh, S. J., Liu, Z., Stubbs, N., Walker, R. M., & Fortnam, M. (2015). Alginate dressings for treating pressure ulcers. *Cochrane Database of Systematic Reviews*, *2015*(5), CD011277. Advance online publication. DOI: 10.1002/14651858.CD011277.pub2 PMID: 25994366

Dutta, P. K., Dutta, J., & Tripathi, V. S. (2004). Chitin and chitosan: Chemistry, properties and applications. *Journal of Scientific and Industrial Research*, *63*, 20–31.

El-Kased, R. F., Amer, R. I., Attia, D., & Elmazar, M. M. (2017). Honey-based hydrogel: In vitro and comparative In vivo evaluation for burn wound healing. *Scientific Reports*, *7*(1), 9692. DOI: 10.1038/s41598-017-08771-8 PMID: 28851905

Farrugia, C. E., Burke, E. S., Haley, M. E., Bedi, K. T., & Gandhi, M. A. (2019). The use of aloe vera in cancer radiation: An updated comprehensive review. *Complementary Therapies in Clinical Practice*, *35*, 126–130. DOI: 10.1016/j.ctcp.2019.01.013 PMID: 31003648

Gholamali, I. (2019). Stimuli-responsive polysaccharide hydrogels for biomedical applications: A review. *Regenerative Engineering and Translational Medicine*, *7*, 91–114. DOI: 10.1007/s40883-019-00134-1

Gounden, V., & Singh, M. (2024). Hydrogels and Wound Healing: Current and Future Prospects. *Gels (Basel, Switzerland)*, *10*(1), 43. DOI: 10.3390/gels10010043 PMID: 38247766

Guo, S., & Dipietro, L. A. (2010). Factors affecting wound healing. *Journal of Dental Research, 89*(3), 219–229. DOI: 10.1177/0022034509359125 PMID: 20139336

. Gupta, B., Agarwal, R., & Alam, M. S. (2010). Textile-based smart wound dressings.

Hamed, R., Magamseh, K. H., Al-Shalabi, E., Hammad, A., Abu-Sini, M., Abulebdah, D. H., Tarawneh, O., & Sunoqrot, S. (2025). Green Hydrogels Prepared from Pectin Extracted from Orange Peels as a Potential Carrier for Dermal Delivery Systems. *ACS Omega, 10*(17), 17182–17200. DOI: 10.1021/acsomega.4c08449 PMID: 40352493

Hanif, W., Hardiansyah, A., Randy, A., & Asri, L. A. T. W. (2021). Physically cross-linked PVA/graphene-based materials/aloe vera hydrogel with antibacterial activity. *RSC Advances, 11*(46), 29029–29041. DOI: 10.1039/d1ra04992e PMID: 35478571

Hoffman, A. S. (2002). Hydrogels for biomedical applications. *Advanced Drug Delivery Reviews, 54*(1), 3–12. DOI: 10.1016/s0169-409x(01)00239-3 PMID: 11755703

Ilkar Erdagi, S., Asabuwa Ngwabebhoh, F., & Yildiz, U. (2020). Genipin crosslinked gelatin-diosgenin-nanocellulose hydrogels for potential wound dressing and healing applications. *International Journal of Biological Macromolecules, 149*, 651–663. DOI: 10.1016/j.ijbiomac.2020.01.279 PMID: 32006574

Jain, R. A. (2000). The manufacturing techniques of various drug loaded biodegradable poly(lactide-co-glycolide) (PLGA) devices. *Biomaterials, 21*(23), 2475–2490. DOI: 10.1016/S0142-9612(00)00115-0 PMID: 11055295

Jirofti, N., Golandi, M., Movaffagh, J., Ahmadi, F. S., & Kalalinia, F. (2021). Improvement of the Wound-Healing Process by Curcumin-Loaded Chitosan/Collagen Blend Electrospun Nanofibers: In Vitro and In Vivo Studies. *ACS Biomaterials Science & Engineering, 7*(8), 3886–3897. DOI: 10.1021/acsbiomaterials.1c00131 PMID: 34256564

Jones, A., & Vaughan, D. (2005). Hydrogel dressings in the management of a variety of wound types: A review. *Journal of Orthopaedic Nursing, 9*, S1–S11. DOI: 10.1016/S1361-3111(05)80001-9

Jones, V., Grey, J. E., & Harding, K. G. (2006). Wound dressings. *BMJ (Clinical Research Ed.), 332*(7544), 777–780. DOI: 10.1136/bmj.332.7544.777 PMID: 16575081

Kamoun, E. A., Kenawy, E. S., & Chen, X. (2017). A review on polymeric hydrogel membranes for wound dressing applications: PVA-based hydrogel dressings. *Journal of Advanced Research, 8*(3), 217–233. DOI: 10.1016/j.jare.2017.01.005 PMID: 28239493

Khayambashi, P., Iyer, J., Pillai, S., Upadhyay, A., Zhang, Y., & Tran, S. D. (2021). Hydrogel Encapsulation of Mesenchymal Stem Cells and Their Derived Exosomes for Tissue Engineering. *International Journal of Molecular Sciences*, *22*(2), 684. DOI: 10.3390/ijms22020684 PMID: 33445616

Küçük, K., Van Gysel, J., Del Marmol, V., & White, J. M. L. (2025). Allergic Contact Dermatitis Induced by Modern Wound Dressings: A Comprehensive Analysis of Risks and Allergenic Components. *International Wound Journal*, *22*(3), e70153. DOI: 10.1111/iwj.70153 PMID: 40069101

Kujur, A. R., & D'Souza, N. T. (2019). Comparison of Three Methods of Dressings for Split Thickness Skin Graft Donor Site-Non-Woven Dressing Impregnated with Amorphous Hydrogel, Amorphous Hydrogel with Colloidal Silver and Conventional Paraffin Gauze Dressing. *International Journal of Contemporary Medical Research*, *6*(12), 17–22.

Kumi, M., Chen, T., Zhang, Z., Wang, A., Li, G., Hou, Z., & Li, P. (2024). Integration of Hydrogels and 3D Bioprinting Technologies for Chronic Wound Healing Management. *ACS Biomaterials Science & Engineering*, *10*(10), 5995–6016. PMID: 39228365

Lee, K. Y., & Mooney, D. J. (2012). Alginate: Properties and biomedical applications. *Progress in Polymer Science*, *37*(1), 106–126. DOI: 10.1016/j.progpolymsci.2011.06.003 PMID: 22125349

Lei, X. X., Zou, C. Y., Hu, J. J., Jiang, Y. L., Zhang, X. Z., Zhao, L. M., & Xie, H. Q. (2023). Click-crosslinked in-situ hydrogel improves the therapeutic effect in wound infections through antibacterial, antioxidant and anti-inflammatory activities. *Chemical Engineering Journal*, *461*, 142092. DOI: 10.1016/j.cej.2023.142092

Leveen, H. H., Falk, G., Borek, B., Diaz, C., Lynfield, Y., Wynkoop, B. J., Mabunda, G. A., Rubricius, J. L., & Christoudias, G. C. (1973). Chemical acidification of wounds. An adjuvant to healing and the unfavorable action of alkalinity and ammonia. *Annals of Surgery*, *178*(6), 745–753. DOI: 10.1097/00000658-197312000-00011 PMID: 4759406

Li, F., Shi, Y., Liang, J., & Zhao, L. (2019). Curcumin-loaded chitosan nanoparticles promote diabetic wound healing via attenuating inflammation in a diabetic rat model. *Journal of Biomaterials Applications*, *34*(4), 476–486. DOI: 10.1177/0885328219860929 PMID: 31280635

Li, J., & Mooney, D. (2016). Designing hydrogels for controlled drug delivery. *Nature Reviews. Materials*, *1*, 16071. DOI: 10.1038/natrevmats.2016.71 PMID: 29657852

Li, R., Song, Y., Fouladian, P., Arafat, M., Chung, R., Kohlhagen, J., & Garg, S. (2021). Three-dimensional printing of curcumin-loaded biodegradable and flexible scaffold for intracranial therapy of glioblastoma multiforme. *Pharmaceutics*, *13*(4), 471. PMID: 33807243

Lin, X., Zhang, X., Wang, Y., Chen, W., Zhu, Z., & Wang, S. (2024). Hydrogels and hydrogel-based drug delivery systems for promoting refractory wound healing: Applications and prospects. *International Journal of Biological Macromolecules*, *285*, 138098. DOI: 10.1016/j.ijbiomac.2024.138098 PMID: 39608543

Luong, P. T., Browning, M. B., Bixler, R. S., & Cosgriff-Hernandez, E. (2014). Drying and storage effects on poly (ethylene glycol) hydrogel mechanical properties and bioactivity. *Journal of Biomedical Materials Research. Part A*, *102*(9), 3066–3076. DOI: 10.1002/jbm.a.34977 PMID: 24123725

Maan, A. A., Nazir, A., Khan, M. K. I., Ahmad, T., Zia, R., Murid, M., & Abrar, M. (2018). The therapeutic properties and applications of Aloe vera: A review. *Journal of Herbal Medicine*, *12*, 1–10. DOI: 10.1016/j.hermed.2018.01.002

Memon, A. Q., Shah, A., Rana, N. A., & Bangash, S. A. (2025). AI for Wound Healing and Management. *Prospects*, *29*(6), 378–385.

Mogoşanu, G. D., & Grumezescu, A. M. (2014). Natural and synthetic polymers for wounds and burns dressing. *International Journal of Pharmaceutics*, *463*(2), 127–136. DOI: 10.1016/j.ijpharm.2013.12.015 PMID: 24368109

Molan, P. C. (2001). Potential of honey in the treatment of wounds and burns. *American Journal of Clinical Dermatology*, *2*(1), 13–19. DOI: 10.2165/00128071-200102010-00003 PMID: 11702616

Murphy, S. V., & Atala, A. (2014). 3D bioprinting of tissues and organs. *Nature Biotechnology*, *32*(8), 773–785. DOI: 10.1038/nbt.2958 PMID: 25093879

Nguyen, T. D., Nguyen, T. T., Ly, K. L., Tran, A. H., Nguyen, T. T. N., Vo, M. T., & Nguyen, T. H. (2019). In vivo study of the antibacterial chitosan/polyvinyl alcohol loaded with silver nanoparticle hydrogel for wound healing applications. *International Journal of Polymer Science*, *2019*(1), 7382717. DOI: 10.1155/2019/7382717

Okan, D., Woo, K., Ayello, E. A., & Sibbald, G. (2007). The role of moisture balance in wound healing. *Advances in Skin & Wound Care*, *20*(1), 39–55. DOI: 10.1097/00129334-200701000-00013 PMID: 17195786

Paladini, F., & Pollini, M. (2019). Antimicrobial Silver Nanoparticles for Wound Healing Application: Progress and Future Trends. *Materials (Basel, Switzerland)*, *12*(16), 2540. DOI: 10.3390/ma12162540 PMID: 31404974

Pawar, S. R., Patel, P., & Jain, K. (2025). Herbal Formulations: Development, Challenges, Testing, Stability, and Regulatory Guidelines. In *Advances in Pharmaceutical Product Development* (pp. 379-397). Singapore: Springer Nature Singapore. https://doi.org/DOI: 10.1007/978-981-97-9230-6_15

Peppas, N. A., Bures, P., Leobandung, W. S., & Ichikawa, H. (2000). Hydrogels in pharmaceutical formulations. *European Journal of Pharmaceutics and Biopharmaceutics*, *50*(1), 27–46. DOI: 10.1016/S0939-6411(00)00090-4 PMID: 10840191

Peppas, N. A., Hilt, J. Z., Khademhosseini, A., & Langer, R. (2006). Hydrogels in biology and medicine: From molecular principles to bionanotechnology. *Advanced Materials*, *18*(11), 1345–1360. DOI: 10.1002/adma.200501612

Percival, S. L., & McCarty, S. M. (2015). Silver and Alginates: Role in Wound Healing and Biofilm Control. *Advances in Wound Care*, *4*(7), 407–414. DOI: 10.1089/wound.2014.0541 PMID: 26155383

Qiu, Y., & Park, K. (2012). Environment-sensitive hydrogels for drug delivery. *Advanced Drug Delivery Reviews*, *64*, 49–60. DOI: 10.1016/j.addr.2012.09.024 PMID: 11744175

Raghupathi, K. R., Koodali, R. T., & Manna, A. C. (2011). Size-dependent bacterial growth inhibition and mechanism of antibacterial activity of zinc oxide nanoparticles. *Langmuir*, *27*(7), 4020–4028. DOI: 10.1021/la104825u PMID: 21401066

Rigo, C., Ferroni, L., Tocco, I., Roman, M., Munivrana, I., Gardin, C., Cairns, W. R., Vindigni, V., Azzena, B., Barbante, C., & Zavan, B. (2013). Active silver nanoparticles for wound healing. *International Journal of Molecular Sciences*, *14*(3), 4817–4840. DOI: 10.3390/ijms14034817 PMID: 23455461

Rodrigues, M., Kosaric, N., Bonham, C. A., & Gurtner, G. C. (2019). Wound Healing: A Cellular Perspective. *Physiological Reviews*, *99*(1), 665–706. DOI: 10.1152/physrev.00067.2017 PMID: 30475656

Ruel-Gariepy, E., & Leroux, J. C. (2004). In situ-forming hydrogels—Review of temperature-sensitive systems. *European Journal of Pharmaceutics and Biopharmaceutics*, *58*(2), 409–426. DOI: 10.1016/j.ejpb.2004.03.019 PMID: 15296964

Rujitanaroj, P. O., Pimpha, N., & Supaphol, P. (2008). Wound-dressing materials with antibacterial activity from electrospun gelatin fiber mats containing silver nanoparticles. *Polymer*, *49*(21), 4723–4732. DOI: 10.1016/j.polymer.2008.08.021

Saenchoopa, A., Plaeyao, K., Talodthaisong, C., Thet Tun, W. S., Nasomjai, P., Lapmanee, S., Somsakeesit, L. O., Hutchison, J. A., & Kulchat, S. (2025). Development of Antibacterial Hydrogels Based on Biopolymer Aloe Vera/Gelatin/Sodium Alginate Composited With SM-AgNPs Loaded Curcumin-Nanoliposomes. *Macromolecular Bioscience*, *25*(4), e2400504. DOI: 10.1002/mabi.202400504 PMID: 39748596

Salehi, B., Mishra, A. P., Nigam, M., Sener, B., Kilic, M., Sharifi-Rad, M., Fokou, P. V. T., Martins, N., & Sharifi-Rad, J. (2018). Resveratrol: A Double-Edged Sword in Health Benefits. *Biomedicines*, *6*(3), 91. DOI: 10.3390/biomedicines6030091 PMID: 30205595

Tang, N., Zheng, Y., Jiang, X., Zhou, C., Jin, H., Jin, K., Wu, W., & Haick, H. (2021). Wearable Sensors and Systems for Wound Healing-Related pH and Temperature Detection. *Micromachines*, *12*(4), 430. DOI: 10.3390/mi12040430 PMID: 33919752

. Thapa, R. K., Winther-Larsen, H. C., Ovchinnikov, K., Carlsen, H., Diep, D. B., & Tønnesen, H. H. (2021). Hybrid hydrogels for bacteriocin delivery to infected wounds. *European journal of pharmaceutical sciences: official journal of the European Federation for Pharmaceutical Sciences, 166*, 105990. https://doi.org/DOI: 10.1016/j.ejps.2021.105990

Thomas, S. (1990). *Wound management and dressings*. Pharmaceutical Press.

Van Den Bulcke, A. I., Bogdanov, B., De Rooze, N., Schacht, E. H., Cornelissen, M., & Berghmans, H. (2000). Structural and rheological properties of methacrylamide modified gelatin hydrogels. *Biomacromolecules*, *1*(1), 31–38. DOI: 10.1021/bm990017d PMID: 11709840

Velnar, T., Bailey, T., & Smrkolj, V. (2009). The wound healing process: An overview of the cellular and molecular mechanisms. *The Journal of International Medical Research*, *37*(5), 1528–1542. DOI: 10.1177/147323000903700531 PMID: 19930861

Vowden, P., & Vowden, K. (2017). Wound dressings: Principles and practice. *Surgery (Oxford)*, *35*(9), 489–494. DOI: 10.1016/j.mpsur.2017.06.005

Wichterle, O., & Lim, D. (1960). Hydrophilic gels for biological use. *Nature*, *185*(4706), 117–118. DOI: 10.1038/185117a0

Xuan, H., Du, Q., Li, R., Shen, X., Zhou, J., Li, B., & Yuan, H. (2023). Shape-memory-reduced graphene/chitosan cryogels for non-compressible wounds. *International Journal of Molecular Sciences*, *24*(2), 1389. DOI: 10.3390/ijms24021389 PMID: 36674906

Yu, S., Sun, H., Li, Y., Wei, S., Xu, J., & Liu, J. (2022). Hydrogels as promising platforms for engineered living bacteria-mediated therapeutic systems. *Materials Today. Bio*, *16*, 100435. PMID: 36164505

Zhang, W., Hu, J., Wu, H., Lin, X., & Cai, L. (2025). Stimuli-responsive hydrogel dressing for wound healing. *APL Materials*, *13*(1), 010601. DOI: 10.1063/5.0245545

Zhang, X., Liang, Y., Huang, S., & Guo, B. (2024). Chitosan-based self-healing hydrogel dressing for wound healing. *Advances in Colloid and Interface Science*, *332*, 103267. DOI: 10.1016/j.cis.2024.103267 PMID: 39121832

Zhu, J. (2010). Bioactive modification of poly (ethylene glycol) hydrogels for tissue engineering. *Biomaterials*, *31*(17), 4639–4656. DOI: 10.1016/j.biomaterials.2010.02.044 PMID: 20303169

Chapter 10
Nanotechnology in Herbal-Based Wound Care

Tarun Kumar Patel
https://orcid.org/0009-0003-3002-8100
Department of Biotechnology, Sant Guru Ghasidas Government P.G. College, Kurud, India

ABSTRACT

This chapter explores the transformative potential of integrating nanotechnology with herbal medicine to advance wound care, addressing challenges like chronic wounds and antimicrobial resistance. It examines how nanoscale systems enhance the delivery, stability, and bioavailability of herbal constituents overcoming limitations like poor solubility and low bioavailability. The discussion covers mechanisms of action, including targeted drug delivery and controlled release, and their applications. Safety concerns, including nanomaterial toxicity and variability in herbal extracts, are analyzed alongside clinical evidence gaps. Future directions, such as green nanotechnology and personalized nanotherapies, are highlighted for their eco-friendly and precision medicine potential. By bridging traditional herbal wisdom with modern nanotechnology, the chapter aims to inspire researchers and clinicians to develop sustainable, effective wound healing therapies, improving patient outcomes while aligning with global healthcare trends.

INTRODUCTION

Wound healing is a complex physiological process involving hemostasis, inflammation, proliferation, and remodeling, yet it often fails in chronic conditions

DOI: 10.4018/979-8-3373-3977-1.ch010

like diabetic ulcers and burns. For centuries, herbal remedies have been integral to wound care across diverse cultures, from ancient Egyptian papyrus records describing plant-based poultices to traditional Chinese and Ayurvedic practices using herbs for tissue repair. This historical reliance on natural sources highlights humanity's early recognition of plants' healing potential, setting the foundation for modern explorations in eco-friendly therapies.

Herbal remedies, in the context of wound care, can be defined as plant-derived substances or extracts used to promote healing, typically administered topically or systemically to leverage their natural bioactive properties. These remedies encompass a wide array of structural features, chemical compositions, and classification methods that underpin their therapeutic effects. Structurally, herbal constituents often feature complex macromolecular architectures, such as polymeric chains in polysaccharides or aromatic rings in flavonoids, which influence their interaction with biological tissues—for instance, the gel-like matrix of Aloe vera polysaccharides enables moisture retention at wound sites. Chemically, they are composed of diverse secondary metabolites, including alkaloids, terpenoids, and phenolic compounds, which confer antimicrobial, anti-inflammatory, and antioxidant activities. Classification of herbal remedies is typically based on phytochemical profiles or functional roles: polysaccharides (e.g., from Aloe vera) are grouped for their hydrating and regenerative properties; flavonoids (e.g., curcumin from turmeric) for anti-inflammatory effects via inhibition of pathways like NF-κB; and essential oils (e.g., from tea tree) for antimicrobial action through membrane disruption. These classifications aid in standardizing applications, though variability in plant sources can affect consistency.

Despite these beneficial characteristics, the therapeutic potential of herbal remedies is limited by inherent challenges, such as poor solubility, low bioavailability, and inconsistent delivery to wound sites. For instance, curcumin's anti-inflammatory properties are hindered by its hydrophobicity, reducing its effectiveness in raw forms. Globally, chronic wounds exacerbate these issues, affecting millions with rising prevalence due to aging populations and increasing diabetes rates. These wounds incur significant healthcare costs, estimated in billions annually, due to prolonged treatment and complications. Antibiotic resistance further complicates management, as infections hinder healing and increase morbidity. Conventional therapies, often reliant on synthetic drugs, face sustainability challenges, prompting the need for innovative, eco-friendly solutions that enhance healing, combat resistance, and reduce environmental impact.

Nanotechnology revolutionizes wound care by overcoming these limitations through precise, targeted, and controlled delivery systems that amplify herbal efficacy. Nanomaterials exist in various forms (Figure 1), including nanoparticles, nanofibers, nanoporous structures, nano-emulsions, and nanostructured bulk materials, each with unique properties and applications. These nanomaterials enhance the properties of herbal constituents, enabling deeper tissue penetration and sustained release. This synergy combines the natural healing properties of herbs with nanoscale precision, offering sustainable and biocompatible solutions. For example, curcumin-loaded nanoparticles demonstrate superior anti-inflammatory effects compared to free curcumin. The chapter explores this interdisciplinary approach, examining mechanisms, applications, and challenges like safety and scalability. By bridging traditional herbal wisdom with modern science, it aims to inspire researchers and clinicians to develop personalized, effective wound care therapies that address chronic wounds and antimicrobial resistance sustainably.

FUNDAMENTALS OF NANOTECHNOLOGY IN WOUND HEALING

Nanoparticles, nanofibers, nanoemulsions, and nanocomposites are nanoscale systems with distinct structures and properties, each uniquely suited for applications like wound healing. **Nanoparticles** are solid particles with dimensions between 1 and 100 nanometer (nm), characterized by tunable size, and surface chemistry, enabling efficient drug delivery and antimicrobial activity (Baig et al., 2021). **Nanofibers** are elongated structures with nanoscale diameters, resembling the extracellular matrix, offering high porosity and flexibility for tissue scaffolds (Mekuye & Abera, 2023). **Nanoemulsions** are colloidal dispersions of liquid droplets (typically 20–200 nm) stabilized by surfactants, recognized for stability and bioavailability, ideal for delivering hydrophobic drugs (Barhoum et al., 2022). **Nanocomposites** are hybrid materials combining nanomaterials (e.g., nanoparticles, nanofibers) within a matrix, providing enhanced mechanical strength and bioactivity (Paras et al., 2022). A summary of different nanomaterial along with their property, mechanism, applications, advantages and limitations is given in Table 1.

Table 1. Comparison of nanomaterial in wound healing

Nanomaterial type	Structure	Properties	Mechanism in Wound Healing	Applications	Advantages and Challenges
Nanoparticles	Solid particles, spherical or varied shapes	High surface-to-volume ratio, tunable size and surface chemistry, customizable for drug encapsulation	endocytosis, antimicrobial action (ROS generation), stimuli-responsive release	Infection control in chronic wounds; anti-inflammatory effects (Pormohammad et al., 2021; Krausz et al., 2015)	**Advantages**: Precise targeting, high drug loading capacity, versatility in functionalization. **Challenges**: Potential cytotoxicity, bioaccumulation risks
Nanofibers	Fibrous, elongated structures, web-like matrices	High porosity, mimics ECM, flexible and biodegradable	adhesion and proliferation, sustained drug release, supports tissue regeneration during proliferation phase	Aloe vera-loaded poly(ethylene oxide)/polyurethane nanofibers for diabetic wound healing; electrospun scaffolds with growth factors for angiogenesis (Ghosh et al., 2024; Kushwaha et al., 2022)	**Advantages**: ECM-like structure promotes cell growth, high drug elution capacity. **Challenges**: High production costs via electrospinning, limited scalability (Arida et al., 2021)
Nanoemulsions	Colloidal dispersions, liquid droplets stabilized by surfactants	High stability, low viscosity, enhanced solubility for hydrophobic drugs, deep tissue penetration	Uniform drug distribution, enhanced bioavailability, controlled release	burn wound infections; diabetic ulcers (Kumari & Nanda, 2023; Chhabra et al., 2023)	**Advantages**: Biocompatible, minimizes irritation, effective for hydrophobic bioactives. **Challenges**: Surfactant optimization needed, high production costs (Chhabra et al., 2023)
Nanocomposites	Hybrid materials combining nanomaterials	Enhanced mechanical strength, multifunctionality,	Dual action: antimicrobial effects & regenerative support from matrix	chronic wounds; burn wound regeneration (Iqbal et al., 2024; Dam et al., 2023)	**Advantages**: Synergistic properties, customizable for multiple therapeutic roles. **Challenges**: Complex synthesis, potential biocompatibility issues (Paras et al., 2022)

Nanoparticles are discrete, solid entities, unlike nanoemulsions, which are liquid droplets, making nanoparticles better for targeted drug release while nanoemulsions excel in deep tissue penetration due to their fluidity (Barhoum et al., 2022). Nanofibers, with their fibrous, web-like structure, differ from nanoparticles' spherical or varied shapes, offering structural support for cell growth, whereas nanoparticles focus on cellular interactions (Mekuye & Abera, 2023). Nanocomposites integrate multiple nanomaterials, unlike the singular nature of nanoparticles or nanofibers, combining properties like strength and bioactivity for multifunctional applications (Paras et al., 2022). Nanoemulsions, being liquid-based, contrast with the solid nature of nanofibers and nanocomposites, providing superior solubility but less structural integrity. These distinctions solid vs. liquid, singular vs. composite, and structural vs. carrier roles define their specialized uses, with nanoparticles and nanoemulsions focusing on delivery, nanofibers on scaffolding, and nanocomposites on hybrid functionality, all leveraging nanoscale properties for enhanced therapeutic outcomes.

MECHANISMS OF ACTION

Nanotechnology enhances wound healing by leveraging the unique properties of nanoscale systems nanoparticles, nanofibers, nanoemulsions, and nanocomposites to optimize drug delivery, controlled release, and cellular uptake, aligning with the four phases of wound healing: hemostasis, inflammation, proliferation, and remodeling. **Drug delivery** is improved due to the high surface-to-volume ratio of nanoparticles, which allows precise targeting of therapeutic agents to the wound sites. For instance, silver nanoparticles encapsulated in hydrogels deliver antimicrobial agents directly to infected tissues, minimizing systemic toxicity (Dam et al., 2023). During hemostasis, nanoparticles like chitosan-based systems promote clot formation by enhancing platelet adhesion (Wang et al., 2021). **Controlled release** is achieved through stimuli-responsive nanomaterials, such as pH-sensitive nanoemulsions or temperature-responsive nanofibers, which release drugs like growth factors or antibiotics in a sustained manner. In chronic or infected wounds with an acidic pH (4-6) due to bacterial metabolism, inflammation, or hypoxia, pH-sensitive nanoemulsions achieve controlled release by responding to this microenvironment. The acidic pH triggers protonation of ionizable groups in pH-responsive polymers or surfactants, inducing a conformational change that destabilizes the nanoemulsion's structure. This causes the nanoscale droplets to swell, rupture, or dissolve, releasing encapsulated therapeutic agents like curcumin or antibiotics. The controlled, sustained release ensures optimal drug concentrations, enhancing antimicrobial and anti-inflammatory effects while minimizing systemic exposure, precisely targeting the wound site's pathological conditions. This is critical during the inflammation phase, where prolonged release of anti-inflammatory agents reduces excessive immune responses (Sangnim et al., 2024). Nanofibers, mimicking the extracellular matrix, provide a scaffold for controlled drug elution, ensuring therapeutic levels throughout proliferation (Kushwaha et al., 2022). **Cellular uptake** is enhanced by nanoparticles' small size and tunable surface chemistry, facilitating endocytosis by fibroblasts and keratinocytes, key cells in the proliferation and remodeling phases. For example, gold nanoparticles conjugated with growth factors stimulate collagen synthesis and angiogenesis, accelerating tissue regeneration (Nandhini et al., 2024). Nanocomposites, combining nanoparticles with hydrogels, enhance mechanical stability and bioactivity, supporting remodeling by promoting organized collagen deposition (Blanco-Fernandez et al., 2021). These mechanisms collectively address wound healing challenges by delivering therapeutics efficiently, maintaining optimal drug concentrations, and promoting cellular activities essential for each healing phase, though limitations like potential cytotoxicity require careful design (Hamed et al., 2023).

RELEVANCE TO WOUND MANAGEMENT

Nanoscale systems are highly relevant to wound management, addressing critical challenges such as infection, delayed healing, and chronic inflammation through targeted and multifunctional approaches. **Infection control** is a primary benefit, with nanoparticle-mediated antimicrobial action being a cornerstone. Silver nanoparticles, for instance, disrupt bacterial cell membranes and inhibit biofilm formation, effectively combating multidrug-resistant pathogens like *Staphylococcus aureus* in infected wounds (Pormohammad et al., 2021). This is vital for chronic wounds, where persistent infections delay healing. **Delayed healing**, common in diabetic or burn wounds, is mitigated by nanomaterials like nanofibers and nanocomposites, which provide structural support and deliver bioactive molecules. Electrospun nanofiber scaffolds loaded with growth factors, such as epidermal growth factor, enhance fibroblast proliferation and angiogenesis, accelerating the proliferation phase (Kushwaha et al., 2022). Nanoemulsions improve the delivery of hydrophobic drugs, such as curcumin, to deep wound tissues, reducing inflammation and promoting tissue repair (Sangnim et al., 2024). **Chronic inflammation** is addressed by nanoparticles that modulate immune responses; for example, cerium oxide nanoparticles scavenge reactive oxygen species, reducing oxidative stress and facilitating progression from inflammation to proliferation (Wang et al., 2021). Nanocomposites, integrating antimicrobial nanoparticles with biocompatible hydrogels, offer dual functionality preventing infection while supporting tissue regeneration (Dam et al., 2023). These systems also tackle wound-specific challenges like poor vascularization, with gold nanoparticles promoting angiogenesis in ischemic wounds (Nandhini et al., 2024). However, challenges like scalability and long-term biocompatibility remain, necessitating rigorous clinical validation (Hamed et al., 2023). By addressing infection, enhancing tissue regeneration, and modulating inflammation, nanoscale systems revolutionize wound management, offering tailored solutions for acute and chronic wounds.

HERBAL POLYMERS IN NANOTECHNOLOGY

Key Herbal Polymers and Extracts

Herbal polymer refers to a biopolymer obtained from plant sources (herbal origin) that exhibits polymeric properties such as high molecular weight, structural complexity, and ability to form gels, films, or matrices. These are naturally occurring macromolecules derived from herbs, shrubs, or trees and are composed of repeating units of carbohydrates, proteins or other biopolymers. Herbal polymers and extracts, such as chitosan, alginate, turmeric, and ginseng, are widely utilized in wound healing due to their bioactive properties, including antimicrobial, anti-inflammatory, and regenerative effects. **Chitosan**, a deacetylated derivative of chitin, exhibits potent antimicrobial activity by disrupting bacterial cell membranes and promotes tissue regeneration by stimulating fibroblast proliferation (Rajinikanth et al., 2024; Feng et al., 2021). Its hemostatic properties enhance clot formation, making it ideal for acute wounds (Singh et al., 2017). **Alginate**, a polysaccharide from brown algae, forms hydrogels that maintain a moist wound environment, supporting granulation and epithelialization (Aderibigbe & Buyana, 2018; Zarei & Hassanzadeh-Tabrizi, 2023). Its anti-inflammatory effects reduce excessive immune responses, while its biocompatibility aids regenerative processes (Ishfaq et al., 2023). **Turmeric**, rich in curcumin, offers robust anti-inflammatory and antioxidant properties by inhibiting pro-inflammatory cytokines and scavenging reactive oxygen species (ROS), accelerating wound closure (Kumari et al., 2022; Tejada et al., 2016). Its antimicrobial action targets pathogens like *Staphylococcus aureus* (Akbik et al., 2014). **Ginseng**, containing saponins and protopanaxadiol, promotes angiogenesis and collagen synthesis via VEGF-ERK pathways, enhancing proliferation and remodeling phases (Park & Park, 2019; Wang et al., 2023). These materials' bioactive properties antimicrobial for infection control, anti-inflammatory for reducing chronic inflammation, and regenerative for tissue repair make them cornerstone constituents in wound healing, with their efficacy further amplified when integrated with nanotechnology (Iqbal et al., 2024; Hwang et al., 2023). Details of some herbal constituents and their nanotechnological enhancements are given in Table 2.

Table 2. Herbal constituents and their nanotechnological enhancements

Herbal Constituent	Bioactive Properties	Challenges in Raw Form	Nanotechnology Solution	Outcome
Chitosan	Antimicrobial, hemostatic, promotes fibroblast proliferation	Poor solubility, aggregation in physiological environments	Encapsulation in nanoparticles, surface modification with hydrophilic groups	Enhanced fibroblast uptake, increase in bioavailability, improved infection control (Loo et al., 2022)
Alginate	Anti-inflammatory, maintains moist environment, supports granulation	Limited drug release, high molecular weight reduces uptake	Nanoparticle-loaded hydrogels, co-delivery with bioactives	Faster granulation and epithelialization in diabetic wounds (Ishfaq et al., 2023)
Curcumin (Turmeric)	Anti-inflammatory, antimicrobial, antioxidant via NF-κB inhibition	Poor solubility, instability under light/heat	PLGA nanoparticles, nanoemulsions	Faster wound closure in burns, reduced bacterial load (Kumari & Nanda, 2023)
Ginseng (Saponins)	Angiogenic, regenerative, promotes collagen synthesis via VEGF-ERK	Oxidative degradation, low bioavailability	Nanoemulsions, liposomal encapsulation	Improved VEGF expression, accelerated healing in rat models (Park et al., 2023)
Neem (Azadirachtin)	Antimicrobial, anti-inflammatory, inhibits biofilm formation	Low water solubility, rapid degradation	Silver nanoparticles, hydrogel-coated nanoemulsions	Reduction in bacterial load, suppressed TNF-α in chronic wounds (Raju et al., 2024; Nguyen et al., 2022)
Aloe Vera (Acemannan)	Anti-inflammatory, regenerative, stimulates fibroblast activity	Poor stability, limited penetration through skin barriers	Electrospun nanofiber scaffolds, hydrogel encapsulation	Enhanced angiogenesis, reduced IL-6, faster diabetic wound closure (Ghosh et al., 2024; Wang et al., 2023)
Tea Tree Oil (Terpinen-4-ol)	Antimicrobial against MDR pathogens, anti-inflammatory	Volatility, skin irritation at high doses	Nanoemulsions, liposomal carriers	Reduced infection rates in diabetic ulcers, sustained release over 72 hours (Chhabra et al., 2023)
Astragalus Polysaccharides	Immunomodulatory, promotes vascularization, antioxidant	High molecular weight, poor cellular uptake	Nanoparticle-loaded hydrogels, co-delivery with growth factors	Improved granulation, enhanced VEGF expression in ischemic wounds (Yang et al., 2024)

Challenges with Raw Herbal Materials

Raw herbal materials, despite their therapeutic potential, face significant challenges that limit their efficacy in traditional wound healing formulations. **Poor solubility** is a major issue, particularly for hydrophobic compounds like curcumin, which has low water solubility, hindering its absorption and bioavailability at wound sites (Kumari et al., 2022; Akbik et al., 2014). This restricts its ability to penetrate skin layers effectively. **Instability** further complicates their use; curcumin degrades under light, heat, or alkaline conditions, losing its anti-inflammatory and antioxidant properties (Tejada et al., 2016). Similarly, ginseng's bioactive saponins are susceptible to oxidative degradation, reducing their regenerative effects (Park & Park, 2019). **Low bioavailability** is another critical barrier, as herbal extracts like alginate and chitosan often exhibit limited cellular uptake due to their high molecular weight or poor interaction with biological membranes (Zarei & Hassanzadeh-Tabrizi, 2023; Liu et al., 2018). For instance, alginate's gelation properties can impede drug release in non-nanoscale forms, while chitosan's cationic nature may cause aggregation in physiological environments (Feng et al., 2021). These challenges result in suboptimal therapeutic outcomes, such as delayed wound closure or inadequate infection control, particularly in chronic wounds where sustained drug delivery is essential (Ishfaq et al., 2023). Additionally, variability in herbal extract composition due to source differences further complicates standardization, reducing reproducibility in clinical applications (Iqbal et al., 2024). These limitations underscore the need for advanced delivery systems to enhance the therapeutic potential of herbal constituents.

Nanotechnology Solutions

Nanotechnology addresses the limitations of raw herbal materials by enhancing their solubility, stability, and bioavailability through encapsulation, surface modification, and synergistic effects, significantly improving their efficacy in wound healing. **Encapsulation** in nanoscale systems like nanoparticles, nanoemulsions, and hydrogels protects herbal constituents from degradation and improves delivery. For example, **curcumin nanoparticles**, encapsulated in polymeric matrices like PLGA or chitosan, exhibit enhanced stability against light and pH changes, with studies showing a 10-fold increase in bioavailability compared to free curcumin (Dai et al., 2017; Kumari et al., 2022). These nanoparticles facilitate controlled release, ensuring sustained anti-inflammatory and antimicrobial effects during the inflammation and proliferation phases (Akbik et al., 2014). Similarly, **alginate-based nanoparticles** loaded with *Betula utilis* extract demonstrate improved solubility and sustained release, accelerating wound closure in diabetic models compared to raw extracts (Ishfaq et al., 2023; Froelich et al., 2023). **Surface modification** enhances cellular uptake and targeting; chitosan nanoparticles modified with hydrophilic groups improve their interaction with fibroblasts, boosting collagen synthesis (Loo et al., 2022; Pramanik et al., 2024). **Ginseng-loaded nanoemulsions**, with droplet sizes of 50–100 nm, enhance protopanaxadiol's bioavailability, promoting angiogenesis via VEGF pathways, with in vivo studies showing faster wound healing in rats (Park et al., 2023; Hwang et al., 2023). **Synergistic effects** are achieved by combining herbal extracts with nanomaterials; for instance, alginate hydrogels incorporating iron oxide nanoparticles and turmeric extracts exhibit enhanced antimicrobial activity and ROS scavenging, reducing infection rates in burn wounds (Nqoro et al., 2024). Nanotechnology also enables co-delivery of multiple bioactives, as seen in chitosan-alginate nanocomposites loaded with ginseng and curcumin, which synergistically reduce inflammation and promote remodeling (Iqbal et al., 2024). These advancements overcome the instability and poor solubility of raw herbal materials, ensuring consistent therapeutic outcomes. However, challenges like scalability and potential nanotoxicity require further optimization (Shah et al., 2025). By bridging herbal medicine with nanotechnology, these solutions revolutionize wound healing, offering precise, efficient, and multifunctional therapies.

APPLICATIONS IN WOUND CARE

Herbal-Loaded Nanoparticles

Herbal-loaded nanoparticles, such as silver nanoparticles with neem extract and curcumin-loaded systems, have emerged as powerful tools in wound care, leveraging their antimicrobial and anti-inflammatory properties to enhance healing. **Silver nanoparticles with neem extract** combine the inherent antibacterial activity of silver with neem's bioactive compounds, like azadirachtin, to combat wound infections. Studies demonstrate that neem-induced silver nanoparticles disrupt bacterial cell membranes and inhibit biofilm formation, effectively targeting pathogens like *Staphylococcus aureus* and *Pseudomonas aeruginosa* (Raju et al., 2024; Nguyen et al., 2022). In vitro studies show these nanoparticles reduce oral biofilm viability, attributed to silver's release of reactive oxygen species (ROS) and neem's disruption of bacterial adhesion (Raju et al., 2024). Their anti-inflammatory effects, mediated by neem's suppression of pro-inflammatory cytokines like TNF-α, further reduce chronic inflammation, promoting progression from the inflammatory to the proliferative phase of wound healing (Nguyen et al., 2022). **Curcumin-loaded nanoparticles**, encapsulated in polymeric matrices like PLGA or liposomes, enhance curcumin's poor solubility and stability, delivering potent antimicrobial and anti-inflammatory effects. Curcumin nanoparticles inhibit bacterial growth by damaging cell walls and reduce inflammation by downregulating NF-κB pathways, as evidenced by significant reduction in inflammatory markers in infected wounds (Krausz et al., 2015; Trigo-Gutierrez et al., 2021). *In vivo* studies show curcumin-loaded nanoparticles accelerate wound closure in murine models, attributed to enhanced fibroblast proliferation and collagen deposition (Krausz et al., 2015). Additionally, curcumin combined with copper nanoparticles exhibits synergistic effects, reducing bacterial load and inflammation in infected wounds, due to copper's catalytic enhancement of curcumin's ROS scavenging (Rajkumari et al., 2023). These systems also promote angiogenesis, critical for the proliferative phase, by upregulating VEGF expression (Serini et al., 2025). However, challenges like potential cytotoxicity of silver and scalability of nanoformulations require further optimization. These herbal-loaded nanoparticles offer a multifaceted approach, addressing infection and inflammation while supporting tissue regeneration, making them a cornerstone of advanced wound care.

Nanofiber Scaffolds and Hydrogels

A nanofiber scaffold is a three-dimensional, porous structure composed of fibers with diameters in the nanoscale range (typically 50–500 nm), often produced through techniques like electrospinning. These scaffolds mimic the extracellular matrix (ECM), providing a biocompatible framework that supports cell adhesion, proliferation, and migration. Their high surface area and porosity facilitate nutrient diffusion, drug delivery, and tissue regeneration, making them ideal for applications like wound healing and tissue engineering (Arida et al., 2021; Ghosh et al., 2024).

A hydrogel is a cross-linked network of hydrophilic polymers capable of absorbing large amounts of water while maintaining structural integrity. Hydrogels create a moist environment, ideal for wound healing, by managing exudate and promoting autolytic debridement. Their tunable mechanical and swelling properties allow incorporation of bioactive compounds, supporting tissue repair and drug delivery in applications like chronic wound management (Chelu et al., 2024; Zhang et al., 2024).

Nanofiber scaffolds and hydrogels, particularly those incorporating bioactive compounds like aloe vera, have revolutionized wound care by promoting tissue regeneration and maintaining moist wound environments, especially for chronic wounds such as diabetic ulcers and burns. **Nanofiber scaffolds**, produced via electrospinning, are fibrous matrices with nanoscale diameters (50–500 nm) that mimic the ECM, providing a biocompatible scaffold for cell adhesion, proliferation, and migration (Arida et al., 2021; Ghosh et al., 2024). Their high porosity and surface area facilitate nutrient diffusion and drug delivery, critical for the proliferative phase of wound healing. For instance, aloe vera extract-loaded poly(ethylene oxide)/polyurethane nanofibers, combined with cerium oxide nanoparticles, enhance diabetic wound healing by promoting angiogenesis and collagen deposition, reducing wound closure time in rat models (Ghosh et al., 2024). Aloe vera's polysaccharides, such as acemannan, exhibit anti-inflammatory and regenerative properties, downregulating pro-inflammatory cytokines like IL-6 and stimulating fibroblast activity (Chelu et al., 2023). These scaffolds also provide mechanical support, preventing wound contraction, and their biodegradability ensures gradual integration with regenerating tissue, making them ideal for chronic wounds where ECM degradation is a barrier (Arida et al., 2021).

Hydrogels, composed of cross-linked polymer networks with high water content, maintain a moist wound environment, essential for preventing desiccation and promoting autolytic debridement in chronic wounds (Chelu et al., 2024; Zhang et al., 2024). Aloe vera-based hydrogels, often combined with herbal extracts like Astragalus polysaccharides, absorb exudate, reduce bacterial load, and accelerate epithelialization (Yang et al., 2024). Their swelling capacity ensures effective exudate management, while their softness minimizes trauma during dressing changes (Lin et al., 2025). In chronic wound models, aloe vera hydrogels loaded with bioactive compounds reduce inflammation and enhance granulation tissue formation, attributed to aloe's antioxidant effects and stimulation of VEGF expression (Chelu et al., 2023; Zhu et al., 2024). Smart-response hydrogels, incorporating pH- or temperature-sensitive polymers, release antimicrobials like berberine in response to infection cues, reducing bacterial counts in infected wounds (Fan et al., 2024). These hydrogels also support the remodeling phase by providing a hydrated matrix for organized collagen alignment (Zhang et al., 2024).

In chronic wound applications, both systems address specific challenges. Nanofiber scaffolds excel in providing structural support and sustained drug release, crucial for diabetic wounds with impaired angiogenesis. For example, electrospun scaffolds loaded with traditional Chinese herbs like Rehmannia root enhance vascularization in ischemic wounds (Yang et al., 2024). Hydrogels, meanwhile, are superior for exudate-heavy wounds, such as venous ulcers, where their high absorbency and cooling effect reduce pain and inflammation (Lin et al., 2025). Combined approaches, like hydrogel-coated nanofiber scaffolds, integrate the strengths of both, offering mechanical stability and moisture retention, with studies showing faster healing in burn wounds (Yan et al., 2024). However, challenges like high production costs for nanofibers and potential cytotoxicity of synthetic polymers require further optimization (Zhu et al., 2024). By leveraging aloe vera's regenerative and anti-inflammatory properties within nanofiber scaffolds and hydrogels, these systems provide tailored solutions for chronic wound management, significantly improving healing outcomes.

Nanoemulsions and Topical Formulations

Nanoemulsions, colloidal dispersions of nanoscale droplets (20-200 nm) stabilized by surfactants, have emerged as promising topical formulations for burns and chronic wounds due to their enhanced penetration, stability, and ability to deliver bioactive compounds. In burn wound infections, **curcumin nanoemulsions** demonstrate significant antimicrobial and anti-inflammatory effects, reducing bacterial load in *Staphylococcus aureus*-infected burns in mice (Kumari & Nanda, 2023). Curcumin's poor solubility is overcome by nanoemulsion encapsulation, which enhances its bioavailability by 10-fold, allowing deep penetration into wound tissues to combat infection and reduce inflammation via NF-κB pathway inhibition (Kumari & Nanda, 2023). The small droplet size ensures uniform distribution across irregular burn surfaces, promoting faster re-epithelialization by compared to conventional curcumin gels (Chhabra et al., 2023). For chronic wounds, such as diabetic ulcers, nanoemulsions incorporating **tea tree oil** offer potent antimicrobial activity against multidrug-resistant pathogens like *Pseudomonas aeruginosa*. A case study showed tea tree oil nanoemulsions reducing wound infection rates in diabetic rat models, attributed to enhanced stability and sustained release over 72 hours (Chhabra et al., 2023). The high stability of nanoemulsions, resistant to phase separation under physiological conditions, ensures consistent therapeutic delivery, unlike traditional emulsions (Kumari & Nanda, 2023). Their low viscosity and high surface area facilitate deeper skin penetration, delivering bioactives to the dermal layer, which is critical for chronic wounds with impaired vascularity. Additionally, nanoemulsions' biocompatibility minimizes irritation, a key advantage for sensitive burn wounds. However, challenges like high production costs and the need for optimized surfactant ratios persist (Chhabra et al., 2023). These formulations excel in providing a moist healing environment, reducing scarring, and accelerating proliferation, making them a transformative approach for managing complex wounds.

ASSOCIATED CHALLENGES

Potential Toxicity of Nanomaterials

The application of nanomaterials in wound healing, while promising, raises significant safety concerns due to their potential toxicity, including cytotoxicity, bioaccumulation, and oxidative stress, necessitating comprehensive toxicological studies. **Cytotoxicity** is a primary concern, as nanomaterials like silver nanoparticles can induce cell death by disrupting cellular membranes and inhibiting mitochondrial function. Studies show silver nanoparticles (AgNPs) cause dose-dependent cytotoxicity in human fibroblasts, reducing cell viability at concentrations above 50 μg/mL, which may impair wound healing by damaging regenerative cells (Bahadar et al., 2016; Thu et al., 2023). **Bioaccumulation** poses another risk, as nanomaterials' small size enables penetration through biological barriers, leading to accumulation in organs like the liver and kidneys. For instance, AgNPs have been detected in rat livers after topical application, raising concerns about long-term systemic effects (Xuan et al., 2023). This bioaccumulation is particularly alarming in chronic wound treatments requiring repeated applications, potentially exacerbating tissue damage

(Kumah et al., 2023). **Oxidative stress**, triggered by nanomaterials' high surface reactivity, generates reactive oxygen species (ROS), causing lipid peroxidation and DNA damage. AgNPs, widely used for their antimicrobial properties, induce ROS-mediated oxidative stress in keratinocytes, increasing inflammation and delaying healing in high doses (Thu et al., 2023). Other nanomaterials, like titanium dioxide nanoparticles, amplify oxidative stress, with in vitro studies showing a significant increase in ROS levels in human cell lines (Bahadar et al., 2016). These risks are compounded by factors like nanoparticle size, shape, and surface chemistry, which influence toxicity; smaller AgNPs (<20 nm) exhibit higher toxicity due to greater cellular uptake (Xuan et al., 2023). The lack of standardized toxicological models further complicates risk assessment, as current in vitro and in vivo models often fail to replicate human exposure scenarios (Kumah et al., 2023). Comprehensive toxicological studies, including long-term exposure assessments and human-relevant models, are critical to establish safe dosage thresholds and mitigate risks. These studies must address nanomaterial-specific properties and their interactions with biological systems to ensure safe application in wound care, balancing efficacy with minimal toxicity.

Good Manufacturing Practices for Herbal Medicines

Good Manufacturing Practices (GMP) for herbal medicines ensure consistent quality, safety, and efficacy of plant-based products used in applications like wound healing. These practices address the inherent variability in herbal extracts, which arises from differences in plant genotypes, environmental conditions, and processing methods. A well-structured GMP framework is critical to overcoming challenges such as inconsistent phytochemical profiles and ensuring regulatory compliance. This section outlines conventional GMP approaches, highlights recent innovations, and discusses ongoing challenges, emphasizing their relevance to nanotechnology-enhanced herbal products for wound care.

Conventional GMP Approaches

Traditional GMP for herbal medicines focuses on standardizing raw materials, processing, and final products to ensure reproducibility and safety. Key practices include sourcing plants from controlled environments, using validated analytical methods like High-Performance Liquid Chromatography (HPLC) to quantify active compounds, and adhering to pharmacopoeial standards. For instance, HPLC is widely used to measure markers like rosmarinic acid in *Thymus carnosus* extracts, ensuring consistent antioxidant activity critical for wound repair (Martins-Gomes et al., 2024). Batch-to-batch consistency is achieved through standardized cultivation and harvesting protocols, such as specifying soil conditions and harvest times to minimize variability in phenolic content of *Adenophora triphylla* (Ajayi et al., 2023). Quality control also involves microbial testing and heavy metal screening to ensure safety, particularly for topical wound healing products like curcumin or aloe vera formulations (Dhami & Mishra, 2015). However, these methods often fail to account for synergistic effects among multiple phytochemicals, and the reliance on single-marker compounds limits comprehensive standardization. Additionally, conventional GMP struggles with scalability and cost, as manual processes and basic analytical tools cannot fully address the complexity of herbal extracts.

Recent Innovations in GMP

Recent advancements in GMP for herbal medicines leverage cutting-edge technologies to enhance standardization, traceability, and quality control, particularly for nanotechnology-based herbal products. **Metabolomics** has emerged as a powerful tool, enabling comprehensive profiling of phytochemicals to capture synergistic interactions. For example, liquid chromatography-mass spectrometry (LC-MS)-based metabolomics identified over 50 bioactive compounds in *Panax ginseng*, ensuring consistent angiogenic effects in wound healing formulations (Wang et al., 2023). This approach surpasses traditional HPLC by providing a holistic chemical fingerprint, improving reproducibility. **Genetic profiling** of plant genotypes, such as *Adenophora triphylla*, allows manufacturers to select strains with optimal phenolic content, reducing variability and enhancing therapeutic efficacy (Ajayi et al., 2023). **Blockchain-based traceability** systems track herbal materials from cultivation to final product, ensuring transparency and compliance with GMP standards. A 2023 study demonstrated blockchain's ability to reduce batch variability in an eight-herb formulation by providing verifiable data on sourcing and processing (Wang et al., 2023). For nanotechnology applications, GMP innovations include **in-line monitoring** during nanoparticle synthesis, such as real-time spectroscopy to ensure uniform particle size in curcumin-loaded nanoparticles, critical for consistent drug release in wound care (Awlqadr et al., 2025). Additionally, **green synthesis protocols**, using plant extracts like *Azadirachta indica* for nanoparticle production, align GMP with sustainable practices, minimizing environmental impact while maintaining product quality (Verma et al., 2019). These innovations enhance precision and scalability, addressing limitations of conventional methods.

Regulatory Frameworks for Herbal Nanomedicines in Wound Healing

The integration of nanotechnology with herbal medicines for wound healing introduces unique regulatory challenges due to the complex nature of nanomaterials and the variability of herbal extracts. Regulatory frameworks, such as those established by the World Health Organization (WHO) and country-specific agencies, aim to ensure the safety, efficacy, and quality of these products. This section provides a critical analysis and comparison of regulatory approaches in the United States, European Union, India, and China, focusing on their application to herbal nanomedicines for wound healing. It highlights gaps, emerging trends, and potential future challenges, supported by recent literature, to strengthen the understanding of regulatory landscapes and their implications.

Comparative Analysis of Regulatory Approaches

United States (FDA): The U.S. Food and Drug Administration (FDA) regulates herbal nanomedicines as combination products, requiring compliance with both drug and medical device regulations. The FDA's Center for Drug Evaluation and Research (CDER) evaluates herbal components under the Dietary Supplement Health and Education Act (DSHEA) for non-drug claims, while nanomaterials are assessed for safety under nanotechnology-specific guidance (FDA, 2014). For wound healing products like curcumin-loaded nanoparticles, the FDA mandates rigorous preclinical and clinical data to demonstrate safety, particularly addressing nanomaterial toxicity risks like bioaccumulation (Kumah et al., 2023). However, the lack of specific guidelines for herbal nanomedicines creates ambiguity, as herbal extracts are not evaluated as stringently as synthetic drugs, leading to delays in approval for products like aloe vera-based nanoemulsions (Jalili et al., 2023).

European Union (EMA). The European Medicines Agency (EMA) regulates herbal nanomedicines under the Directive 2004/24/EC for traditional herbal medicinal products, combined with nanomaterial-specific guidelines from the European Commission. The EMA emphasizes Good Manufacturing Practices (GMP) compliance and requires detailed toxicological profiles for nanomaterials, such as silver nanoparticles used in wound dressings, to address risks like cytotoxicity (Thu et al., 2023). Unlike the FDA, the EMA allows simplified registration for herbal products with a history of safe use, facilitating market entry for products like Panax ginseng-loaded nanofibers. However, the EMA's stringent nanomaterial testing requirements can conflict with the variability of herbal extracts, complicating standardization (Parveen et al., 2015).

India (AYUSH). India's Ministry of AYUSH regulates herbal medicines under the Drugs and Cosmetics Act, 1940, with specific guidelines for Ayurvedic formulations like turmeric-based nanoemulsions. The Central Drugs Standard Control Organization (CDSCO) oversees nanotechnology products, but lacks dedicated regulations for herbal nanomedicines, resulting in reliance on general drug standards (Teja et al., 2022). This approach supports rapid development of herbal wound care products, leveraging India's traditional knowledge, but the absence of nanomaterial-specific guidelines risks inconsistent safety assessments, particularly for chronic wound applications (Awlqadr et al., 2025).

China (NMPA). China's National Medical Products Administration (NMPA) regulates herbal medicines under the Chinese Pharmacopoeia, which includes standards for traditional Chinese medicine (TCM) like Astragalus polysaccharides in wound dressings. Nanotechnology products face additional scrutiny under the NMPA's 2021 nanotechnology guidelines, requiring extensive safety and efficacy data. China's regulatory framework is stringent, with a focus on clinical evidence, but its integration of TCM facilitates approval of herbal nanomedicines compared to Western systems (Zhang et al., 2021). However, variability in herbal sourcing can lead to batch inconsistencies, challenging GMP compliance (Wang et al., 2023).

Gaps in Regulatory Frameworks

A major gap across all regions is the lack of harmonized guidelines specifically for herbal nanomedicines. The FDA and EMA provide nanomaterial-specific guidance, but these do not address the unique challenges of herbal variability, such as fluctuating phytochemical profiles in Adenophora triphylla (Ajayi et al., 2023). India and China, while supportive of traditional medicine, lag in nanotechnology-specific regulations, risking inadequate safety assessments for products like neem-based nanoparticles (Verma et al., 2019). The WHO's guidelines on herbal medicines emphasize quality control but lack enforceable standards for nanomaterials, leading to inconsistent global practices (WHO, 2013). Additionally, the scarcity of clinical trial data for herbal nanomedicines, particularly in humans, hinders regulatory approval, as most studies rely on in vitro or animal models (Namuga et al., 2023). These gaps result in delayed market access and potential safety risks for wound healing applications.

Emerging Trends

Recent trends indicate progress toward harmonization and innovation. The International Council for Harmonisation (ICH) is developing guidelines to standardize nanomaterial testing, potentially bridging gaps between the FDA and EMA (Jalili et al., 2023). Green nanotechnology is gaining traction, with regulatory bodies like the

EMA incorporating sustainability criteria into GMP assessments, supporting eco-friendly wound care products like Azadirachta indica-derived nanoparticles (Kumar et al., 2024). Digital tools, such as blockchain for supply chain traceability, are being integrated into regulatory frameworks in China and India to ensure consistent herbal sourcing (Wang et al., 2023). Additionally, the rise of personalized nanotherapies for wound healing is prompting regulators to explore adaptive licensing models, allowing faster approval based on patient-specific data (López-Estévez et al., 2024).

Future Challenges

Future challenges include scalability of regulatory processes, as small-scale producers of herbal nanomedicines struggle with costly compliance requirements, particularly in India and developing regions (Teja et al., 2022). Ensuring long-term safety of nanomaterials, such as silver nanoparticles' potential cytotoxicity, requires standardized toxicological models that current frameworks lack (Kumah et al., 2023). Global harmonization remains elusive due to differing priorities - Western agencies prioritize safety, while India and China emphasize traditional knowledge - complicating multinational approvals (Zhang et al., 2021). The integration of digital health technologies, like smart dressings, introduces new regulatory complexities, as agencies must address data privacy and real-time monitoring compliance (Derakhshandeh et al., 2018). Addressing these challenges requires collaborative efforts to develop universal standards, invest in scalable testing methods, and align regulations with innovations in green and personalized nanotherapies.

Regulatory frameworks for herbal nanomedicines in wound healing vary significantly across the USA, EU, India, and China, with each region balancing safety, efficacy, and traditional knowledge differently. Gaps in harmonization, clinical evidence, and nanomaterial-specific guidelines pose barriers, while trends like green nanotechnology and digital integration offer solutions. Future challenges include scalability, safety validation, and global standardization. By addressing these issues, regulators can support the safe and effective use of herbal nanomedicines, advancing wound care innovation.

The implementation of GMP ensures quality and safety in herbal medicines, but it is closely tied to ethical considerations in sourcing and production. Regulatory frameworks, such as WHO guidelines and country-specific standards, provide a foundation for GMP compliance, yet ethical issues like fair trade, indigenous rights, and environmental sustainability are equally critical. These concerns influence the responsible development of herbal nanomedicines, ensuring equitable and eco-friendly practices in wound care applications.

Ethical Considerations

Ethical considerations in herbal medicine and nanotechnology for wound healing encompass fair trade, indigenous rights, and environmental sustainability, ensuring responsible sourcing and production. These issues are critical as herbal medicines rely on plant materials often harvested from indigenous lands, and nanotechnology introduces additional concerns about environmental impact. The following table (Table 3) summarizes key ethical considerations, their implications, and proposed solutions to distill the core messages and avoid reiteration.

Table 3. The key ethical considerations, their implications, and proposed solutions

Ethical Issue	Implications for Wound Healing	Proposed Solutions	References
Fair Trade	Inequitable compensation for farmers in developing regions can lead to unsustainable harvesting, reducing availability of herbs like Aloe vera for wound dressings.	Implement fair trade certification; ensure equitable profit sharing with local communities.	Wang et al., 2023; Dhami & Mishra, 2015
Indigenous Rights	Unauthorized harvesting from indigenous lands risks cultural exploitation and loss of traditional knowledge for herbs like Panax ginseng.	Engage indigenous communities in sourcing decisions; obtain prior informed consent; integrate traditional knowledge into R&D.	Wang et al., 2023; Parveen et al., 2015
Environmental Sustainability	Overharvesting and chemical-based nanoparticle synthesis deplete resources and increase carbon footprint, impacting eco-friendly wound care solutions.	Adopt green nanotechnology (e.g., phyto-synthesis using Azadirachta indica); promote sustainable cultivation practices.	Verma et al., 2019; Kumar et al., 2024
Regulatory Compliance	Lack of ethical oversight in GMP can lead to unsafe or inconsistent herbal nanomedicines, risking patient safety in wound care applications.	Align with WHO guidelines and country-specific regulations (e.g., FDA, EMA); develop ethical auditing frameworks.	Jalili et al., 2023; Parveen et al., 2015

This structured approach ensures ethical sourcing and production of herbal nanomedicines, aligning with global sustainability goals and supporting equitable access to advanced wound care therapies. By addressing these ethical challenges, the integration of herbal medicine with nanotechnology can achieve both therapeutic efficacy and social responsibility.

Clinical Evidence Gaps

The integration of nanotechnology with herbal medicines for applications like wound healing is promising, but significant clinical evidence gaps, primarily due to the scarcity of human trials compared to in vitro and animal studies, hinder its widespread adoption. Most research, such as studies on curcumin-loaded nanoparticles or aloe vera nanoemulsions, relies heavily on in vitro models or animal models like rats and mice, which demonstrate enhanced antimicrobial and regenerative effects but lacks direct applicability to humans (Bonifácio et al., 2014; Namuga et al., 2023). For instance, while herbal nanoliposomes show improvement in wound closure in diabetic rat models, human trials are sparse, with only limited studies in a recent systematic review involving human subjects (Namuga et al., 2023). This gap raises concerns about translational validity, as human physiological responses, including immune reactions and skin barrier functions, differ significantly from animal models (Teja et al., 2022).

FUTURE DIRECTIONS AND INNOVATIONS

Personalized Nanotherapies

Personalized nanotherapy refers to the use of nanotechnology-based therapeutic systems tailored to an individual patient's specific physiological, genetic, or molecular profile to optimize treatment efficacy and minimize adverse effects. By leveraging nanomaterials such as nanoparticles, nanoliposomes, or nanofibers, these therapies deliver drugs, growth factors, or bioactive molecules with precision, targeting specific cells, tissues, or disease characteristics. In wound healing, personalized nanotherapies are designed based on wound type (e.g., diabetic vs. burn), patient-specific biomarkers (e.g., glucose levels, microbial profiles), or genetic predispositions, enabling customized drug release, enhanced cellular uptake, and real-time monitoring through theranostic capabilities. This approach integrates advanced diagnostics, like single-cell sequencing, to align nanomaterial properties with individual needs, advancing precision medicine (Fornaguera & García-Celma, 2017; López-Estévez et al., 2024). Personalized nanotherapies represent a transformative frontier in wound care, offering tailored treatments for specific wound types and patient profiles, such as diabetic versus burn wounds, by leveraging precision medicine principles. **Diabetic wounds**, characterized by impaired angiogenesis and chronic inflammation, benefit from nanotherapies tailored to individual metabolic profiles. For instance, nanoparticles loaded with growth factors like VEGF, designed with patient-specific surface modifications, enhance vascularization in diabetic mouse models, addressing delayed healing (Fornaguera & García-Celma, 2017; López-Estévez et al., 2024). These systems use biomarkers, such as glucose levels, to adjust drug release, ensuring optimal therapeutic efficacy for patients with varying glycemic control (Kaushik et al., 2017). In contrast, **burn wounds**, prone to infection and excessive scarring, require nanotherapies focused on antimicrobial action and tissue remodeling. Silver nanoparticle-loaded hydrogels, customized to patient microbial profiles, reduce bacterial load in burn wounds, with theranostic capabilities allowing real-time monitoring of infection via pH-sensitive fluorescence (Mura & Couvreur, 2012). Personalized nanotherapies also account for genetic and proteomic differences; for example, liposomes engineered to target specific integrin expressions on fibroblasts improve collagen deposition in patients with hypertrophic scarring tendencies (Pala et al., 2019). **Precision medicine** integration involves advanced diagnostics, such as single-cell RNA sequencing, to identify patient-specific wound healing deficits, enabling nanoparticle designs with tailored payloads, like anti-inflammatory miRNAs for diabetic patients or ROS-scavenging enzymes for burn victims (López-Estévez et al., 2024). These therapies overcome biological barriers, such as the skin's stratum corneum, via size-optimized nanoparticles (<50 nm) for enhanced intracellular delivery (Fornaguera & García-Celma, 2017). However, challenges like high costs and regulatory hurdles for patient-specific formulations persist, requiring scalable production and standardized biomarkers (Kaushik et al., 2017). By aligning nanomaterial properties with individual wound characteristics and patient needs, personalized nanotherapies promise to revolutionize wound care, improving outcomes through targeted, efficient, and adaptive treatments.

Green Nanotechnology

Green nanotechnology, leveraging plant-derived nanomaterials and sustainable production methods, is poised to revolutionize wound care by aligning with eco-friendly healthcare trends. **Plant-derived nanomaterials**, synthesized using extracts from plants like *Azadirachta indica* (neem) or *Aloe vera*, offer biocompatible and non-toxic alternatives to conventional nanomaterials. These extracts, rich in polyphenols and flavonoids, act as reducing and stabilizing agents, producing nanoparticles with antimicrobial and anti-inflammatory properties ideal for wound healing. For instance, neem extract-mediated silver nanoparticles exhibit a significant reduction in bacterial load in infected wounds, attributed to their ROS-generating capacity (Verma et al., 2019; Alqarni et al., 2022). Similarly, *Curcuma longa*-derived nanoparticles enhance collagen deposition in diabetic wound models, promoting tissue regeneration without synthetic chemicals (Kanwar et al., 2019). **Sustainable production methods**, such as phyto-synthesis, utilize renewable plant resources, minimizing energy consumption and hazardous waste compared to traditional chemical synthesis, which often involves toxic solvents like sodium borohydride (Dutta & Mech Das, 2021). Phytosynthesis refers to the eco-friendly, biological synthesis of nanomaterials, particularly nanoparticles, using plant extracts as reducing and stabilizing agents. This green nanotechnology approach leverages phytochemicals, such as polyphenols, flavonoids, and alkaloids, present in plant materials (e.g., leaves, roots, or fruits) to reduce metal ions (e.g., silver or gold) into nanoscale particles, eliminating the need for toxic chemical reagents or high-energy processes. The plant extracts also act as capping agents, enhancing nanoparticle stability and biocompatibility. Phytosynthesis is sustainable, cost-effective, and aligns with environmental goals by utilizing renewable plant resources, reducing hazardous waste, and minimizing energy consumption compared to conventional chemical synthesis methods (Verma et al., 2019; Dutta & Mech Das, 2021). These methods reduce the carbon footprint and align with Sustainable Development Goals (SDGs), particularly SDG 12 (Responsible Consumption and Production) (Kumar et al., 2024). Green nanotechnology also employs biodegradable carriers, like chitosan-based nanogels, which degrade naturally, reducing environmental persistence (Nasrollahzadeh et al., 2019). In wound care, these systems support eco-friendly healthcare by offering scalable, cost-effective solutions; for example, plant-based nanoemulsions are economical to produce than synthetic counterparts (Alqarni et al., 2022). Innovations like microwave-assisted phyto-synthesis further enhance efficiency, reducing synthesis time while maintaining nanoparticle stability (Kanwar et al., 2019). However, challenges such as variability in plant extract composition and regulatory gaps for green nanomaterials persist, requiring standardized protocols (Verma et al., 2019). By integrating renewable resources and sustainable practices, green nanotechnology not only enhances wound healing outcomes but also supports a circular bioeconomy, aligning with global demands for environmentally conscious healthcare solutions.

Smart Dressings and Integration

Smart dressings integrated with pH-responsive herbal nanosystems and digital health technologies are revolutionizing wound care by enabling dynamic, real-time monitoring and tailored therapeutic delivery. **pH-responsive herbal nanosystems** leverage the acidic microenvironment of infected or chronic wounds (pH 4–6) to trigger controlled drug release, enhancing efficacy while minimizing systemic toxicity. For instance, curcumin-loaded pH-sensitive nanoparticles, encapsulated in PEGylated silica matrices, release their payload in acidic conditions, reducing bacterial load in infected wounds compared to non-responsive systems (Mohan et al., 2024; Li et al., 2022). These systems, often incorporating plant-derived extracts like aloe vera or turmeric, improve stability and bioavailability, with studies showing faster wound closure in diabetic models due to enhanced anti-inflammatory and regenerative effects (Awlqadr et al., 2025; Teja et al., 2022). The dynamic boronic acid/ester transformations in these nanosystems allow precise release modulation, ensuring optimal dosing during the inflammation and proliferation phases (Chen et al., 2023). **Smart dressings**, embedded with sensors and nanomaterials, monitor wound parameters like pH, temperature, and exudate levels, transmitting data to digital health platforms for real-time analysis. For example, magnetic nanoparticle-based dressings with pH-responsive polymers, integrated with IoT sensors, detect infection cues and release antimicrobials like neem extract, reducing infection rates in burn wounds (Mai et al., 2018; Pang et al., 2023). These dressings align with green nanotechnology by using biodegradable, plant-based nanomaterials, reducing environmental impact compared to synthetic alternatives (Garima et al., 2025). **Integration with digital health technologies**, such as mobile apps and cloud-based dashboards, enables clinicians to adjust treatments remotely, improving patient outcomes. The future of wound healing technologies is poised for transformative advancements, driven by smart bandages and integrated nanosystems as outlined in Derakhshandeh et al. (2018). These intelligent dressings, embedded with sensors and pH-responsive nanomaterials, enable real-time monitoring of wound parameters like pH, temperature, and infection status, facilitating dynamic therapeutic responses. For instance, smart bandages incorporating herbal nanoparticles, such as curcumin or aloe vera, can release antimicrobials on-demand in acidic wound environments, reducing bacterial load and accelerating healing in chronic wounds. Integration with digital health platforms, including IoT sensors and mobile apps, allows clinicians to tailor treatments remotely, potentially reducing hospital readmissions. Additionally, green nanotechnology using plant-derived nanomaterials aligns with sustainable healthcare, minimizing environmental impact. However, challenges like high production costs and regulatory hurdles for personalized formulations persist. Advances in scalable phyto-synthesis and standardized biomarkers could overcome these barriers, making smart bandages a cornerstone of precision wound care. By merging nanotechnology, digital health, and eco-friendly practices, they promise enhanced outcomes for complex wounds, revolutionizing patient care with adaptive, efficient solutions (Derakhshandeh et al., 2018).

CONCLUSION

The integration of nanotechnology with herbal medicine marks a transformative era in wound care, addressing critical challenges in chronic wound management while aligning with sustainable and personalized healthcare trends. Nanoscale systems, including nanoparticles, nanofibers, nanoemulsions, and nanocomposites, enhance the delivery, stability, and bioavailability of herbal constituents like chitosan, alginate, turmeric, and ginseng, overcoming limitations such as poor solubility and low bioavailability inherent in raw herbal materials. These systems facilitate precise drug delivery, controlled release, and enhanced cellular uptake, aligning with the hemostasis, inflammation, proliferation, and remodeling phases of wound healing. For instance, curcumin-loaded nanoparticles and aloe vera-based nanofiber scaffolds demonstrate superior antimicrobial, anti-inflammatory, and regenerative effects, significantly reducing bacterial load and accelerating wound closure in diabetic and burn wounds. Nanoemulsions, with their deep tissue penetration, and smart dressings, integrated with pH-responsive nanosystems and digital health technologies, further revolutionize treatment by enabling real-time monitoring and adaptive therapy, reducing hospital readmissions.

Safety and efficacy concerns, however, remain critical. The potential toxicity of nanomaterials, such as cytotoxicity and bioaccumulation from silver nanoparticles, necessitates rigorous toxicological studies to establish safe dosages. Variability in herbal extracts due to environmental and genetic factors poses standardization challenges, risking inconsistent therapeutic outcomes. Clinical evidence gaps, with limited human trials compared to in vitro and animal studies, underscore the need for standardized testing and robust clinical data to validate translational efficacy. Green nanotechnology, utilizing phyto-synthesis and plant-derived nanomaterials, offers a sustainable solution, minimizing environmental impact and aligning with Sustainable Development Goals. Personalized nanotherapies, tailored to patient-specific profiles and wound types, promise precision medicine advancements, though scalability and regulatory hurdles require attention.

Future innovations, including smart dressings and green nanotechnology, will drive the field forward by combining eco-friendly practices with digital health integration. These advancements hold immense potential to transform wound care into a precise, efficient, and sustainable discipline, addressing global health challenges like antibiotic resistance and chronic wound prevalence. By bridging traditional herbal wisdom with cutting-edge nanotechnology, this interdisciplinary approach paves the way for next-generation wound healing therapies, inspiring researchers and clinicians to develop solutions that are both effective and environmentally conscious, ultimately improving patient outcomes worldwide.

REFERENCES

Aderibigbe, B. A., & Buyana, B. (2018). Alginate in Wound Dressings. *Pharmaceutics, 10*(2), 42. DOI: 10.3390/pharmaceutics10020042 PMID: 29614804

Ajayi, O. E., Yoon, S. Y., Moon, S., Kim, K. H., Kim, J. H., Chung, J.-W., Jang, K.-I., & Hyun, T. K. (2023). Variability in Phytochemical Contents and Biological Activities among *Adenophora triphylla* Genotypes. *Applied Sciences (Basel, Switzerland), 13*(20), 11184. DOI: 10.3390/app132011184

Akbik, D., Ghadiri, M., Chrzanowski, W., & Rohanizadeh, R. (2014). Curcumin as a wound healing agent. *Life Sciences, 116*(1), 1–7. DOI: 10.1016/j.lfs.2014.08.016 PMID: 25200875

Alqarni, L. S., Alghamdi, M. D., Alshahrani, A. A., & Nassar, A. M. (2022). Green nanotechnology: Recent research on bioresource-based nanoparticle synthesis and applications. *Journal of Chemistry, 4030999.* Advance online publication. DOI: 10.1155/2022/4030999

Arida, I. A., Ali, I. H., Nasr, M., & El-Sherbiny, I. M. (2021). Electrospun polymer-based nanofiber scaffolds for skin regeneration. *Journal of Drug Delivery Science and Technology, 64*, 102623. DOI: 10.1016/j.jddst.2021.102623

Awlqadr, F. H., Majeed, K. R., Altemimi, A. B., Hassan, A. M., Qadir, S. A., Saeed, M. N., Faraj, A. M., Salih, T. H., Abd Al-Manhel, A. J., Najm, M. A. A., Tsakali, E., Van Impe, J. F. M., Abd El-Maksoud, A. A., & Abedelmaksoud, T. G. (2025). Nanotechnology-based herbal medicine: Preparation, synthesis, and applications in food and medicine. *Journal of Agriculture and Food Research, 19*, 101661. DOI: 10.1016/j.jafr.2025.101661

Baig, N., Kammakakam, I., & Falath, W. (2021). Nanomaterials: A review of synthesis methods, properties, recent progress, and challenges. *Materials Advances, 2*(6), 1821–1871. DOI: 10.1039/d0ma00807a

Barhoum, A., García-Betancourt, M. L., Jeevanandam, J., Hussien, E. A., Mekkawy, S. A., Mostafa, M., Omran, M. M. S., Abdalla, M., & Bechelany, M. (2022). Review on Natural, Incidental, Bioinspired, and Engineered Nanomaterials: History, Definitions, Classifications, Synthesis, Properties, Market, Toxicities, Risks, and Regulations. *Nanomaterials (Basel, Switzerland), 12*(2), 177. DOI: 10.3390/nano12020177 PMID: 35055196

Blanco-Fernandez, B., Castaño, O., Mateos-Timoneda, M. Á., Engel, E., & Pérez-Amodio, S. (2021). Nanotechnology Approaches in Chronic Wound Healing. *Advances in Wound Care*, *10*(5), 234–256. DOI: 10.1089/wound.2019.1094 PMID: 32320364

Bonifácio, B. V., Silva, P. B., Ramos, M. A., Negri, K. M., Bauab, T. M., & Chorilli, M. (2014). Nanotechnology-based drug delivery systems and herbal medicines: A review. *International Journal of Nanomedicine*, *9*, 1–15. DOI: 10.2147/IJN.S52634 PMID: 24363556

Chelu, M., Calderon Moreno, J. M., Musuc, A. M., & Popa, M. (2024). Natural Regenerative Hydrogels for Wound Healing. *Gels (Basel, Switzerland)*, *10*(9), 547. DOI: 10.3390/gels10090547 PMID: 39330149

Chelu, M., Musuc, A. M., Popa, M., & Calderon Moreno, J. (2023). *Aloe vera*-Based Hydrogels for Wound Healing: Properties and Therapeutic Effects. *Gels (Basel, Switzerland)*, *9*(7), 539. DOI: 10.3390/gels9070539 PMID: 37504418

Chen, W., Xie, W., Zhao, G., & Shuai, Q. (2023). Efficient pH-Responsive Nano-Drug Delivery System Based on Dynamic Boronic Acid/Ester Transformation. *Molecules (Basel, Switzerland)*, *28*(11), 4461. DOI: 10.3390/molecules28114461 PMID: 37298937

Chhabra, J., Chopra, H., Pahwa, R., Raina, N., Wadhwa, K., Saini, S., Negi, P., Gupta, M., Singh, I., Dureja, H., & Emran, T. B. (2023). Potential of nanoemulsions for accelerated wound healing: Innovative strategies. *International Journal of Surgery*, *109*(8), 2365–2377. DOI: 10.1097/JS9.0000000000000460 PMID: 37158143

Dai, X., Liu, J., Zheng, H., Chen, Y., Wang, X., Chen, D., & Zhang, H. (2017). Nano-formulated curcumin accelerates acute wound healing through Dkk-1-mediated fibroblast mobilization and MCP-1-mediated anti-inflammation. *NPG Asia Materials*, *9*, e368. DOI: 10.1038/am.2017.31

Dam, P., Celik, M., Ustun, M., Saha, S., Saha, C., Kacar, E. A., Kugu, S., Karagulle, E. N., Tasoglu, S., Buyukserin, F., Mondal, R., Roy, P., Macedo, M. L. R., Franco, O. L., Cardoso, M. H., Altuntas, S., & Mandal, A. K. (2023). Wound healing strategies based on nanoparticles incorporated in hydrogel wound patches. *RSC Advances*, *13*(31), 21345–21364. DOI: 10.1039/d3ra03477a PMID: 37465579

Derakhshandeh, H., Kashaf, S. S., Aghabaglou, F., Ghanavati, I. O., & Tamayol, A. (2018). Smart Bandages: The Future of Wound Care. *Trends in Biotechnology*, *36*(12), 1259–1274. DOI: 10.1016/j.tibtech.2018.07.007 PMID: 30197225

Dhami, N., & Mishra, A. D. (2015). Phytochemical variation: How to resolve the quality controversies of herbal medicinal products? *Journal of Herbal Medicine*, *5*(2), 118–127. DOI: 10.1016/j.hermed.2015.04.002

Dutta, D., & Mech Das, B. (2021). Scope of green nanotechnology towards amalgamation of green chemistry for cleaner environment: A review on synthesis and applications of green nanoparticles. *Environmental Nanotechnology, Monitoring & Management*, *15*, 100418. DOI: 10.1016/j.enmm.2020.100418

Fan, Y., Wang, H., Wang, C., Xing, Y., Liu, S., Feng, L., Zhang, X., & Chen, J. (2024). Advances in Smart-Response Hydrogels for Skin Wound Repair. *Polymers*, *16*(19), 2818. DOI: 10.3390/polym16192818 PMID: 39408528

Feng, P., Luo, Y., Ke, C., Qiu, H., Wang, W., Zhu, Y., Hou, R., Xu, L., & Wu, S. (2021). Chitosan-based functional materials for skin wound repair: Mechanisms and applications. *Frontiers in Bioengineering and Biotechnology*, *9*, 650598. DOI: 10.3389/fbioe.2021.650598 PMID: 33681176

Fornaguera, C., & García-Celma, M. J. (2017). Personalized Nanomedicine: A Revolution at the Nanoscale. *Journal of Personalized Medicine*, *7*(4), 12. DOI: 10.3390/jpm7040012 PMID: 29023366

Froelich, A., Jakubowska, E., Wojtyłko, M., Jadach, B., Gackowski, M., Gadziński, P., Napierała, O., Ravliv, Y., & Osmałek, T. (2023). Alginate-Based Materials Loaded with Nanoparticles in Wound Healing. *Pharmaceutics*, *15*(4), 1142. DOI: 10.3390/pharmaceutics15041142 PMID: 37111628

Garima, Sharma, D., & Mittal, N. (2025). Greener nanomaterials for soft tissue regeneration: Diagnostic and therapeutic advances. *Journal of Drug Delivery Science and Technology*, *106*, 106747. DOI: 10.1016/j.jddst.2025.106747

Ghosh, A., Saha, K., Bhattacharya, T., Sarkar, S., Sengupta, D., Maiti, A., Ghoshal, D., Dey, S., & Chattopadhyay, D. (2024). Electrospun cerium oxide nanoparticle/aloe vera extract-loaded nanofibrous poly(ethylene oxide)/polyurethane mats as diabetic wound dressings. *ACS Applied Bio Materials*, *7*(8), 5268–5278. DOI: 10.1021/acsabm.4c00475 PMID: 39093691

Hamed, S. H., Azooz, E. A., & Al-Mulla, E. A. J. (2023). Nanoparticles-assisted wound healing: A review. *Nano Biomedicine and Engineering*, *15*(4), 425–435. DOI: 10.26599/NBE.2023.9290039

Hwang, J., Kang, Y., Park, H.-J., Kim, S., Lee, S.-H., Kim, H., Nam, S.-J., & Lim, K.-M. (2023). Skin wound healing effects of (+)-syringaresinol from ginseng berry. *Journal of Ginseng Research, 47*(5), 654–661. DOI: 10.1016/j.jgr.2023.04.003 PMID: 37720576

Iqbal, Y., Amin, F., Fatima, M., Khalid, M., Kanwal, N., Abdel Hafez, A. A., Farooq, A. S., Issa, S. A. M., Zakaly, H. M. H., & Alam, M. (2024). Chitosan-based functional materials combined with plant extract: A promising strategy in the stimulation of wound healing process. *Journal of Drug Delivery Science and Technology, 101*(Part B), 106314. https://doi.org/DOI: 10.1016/j.jddst.2024.106314

Ishfaq, B., Khan, I. U., Khalid, S. H., & Asghar, S. (2023). Design and evaluation of sodium alginate-based hydrogel dressings containing *Betula utilis* extract for cutaneous wound healing. *Frontiers in Bioengineering and Biotechnology, 11*, 1042077. DOI: 10.3389/fbioe.2023.1042077 PMID: 36777244

Jalili, A., Bagherifar, R., Nokhodchi, A., Conway, B., & Javadzadeh, Y. (2023). Current Advances in Nanotechnology-Mediated Delivery of Herbal and Plant-Derived Medicines. *Advanced Pharmaceutical Bulletin, 13*(4), 712–722. DOI: 10.34172/apb.2023.087 PMID: 38022806

Kanwar, R., Rathee, J., Salunke, D. B., & Mehta, S. K. (2019). Green nanotechnology-driven drug delivery assemblies. *ACS Omega, 4*(5), 8804–8815. DOI: 10.1021/acsomega.9b00304 PMID: 31459969

Kaushik, A., Jayant, R. D., & Nair, M. (Eds.). (2017). *Advances in personalized nanotherapeutics* (1st ed.). Springer Cham., DOI: 10.1007/978-3-319-63633-7

Krausz, A. E., Adler, B. L., Cabral, V., Navati, M., Doerner, J., Charafeddine, R. A., Chandra, D., Liang, H., Gunther, L., Clendaniel, A., Harper, S., Friedman, J. M., Nosanchuk, J. D., & Friedman, A. J. (2015). Curcumin-encapsulated nanoparticles as innovative antimicrobial and wound healing agent. *Nanomedicine; Nanotechnology, Biology, and Medicine, 11*(1), 195–206. DOI: 10.1016/j.nano.2014.09.004 PMID: 25240595

Kumar, A., Tyagi, P. K., & Tyagi, S. (2024). Integrating green nanotechnology with sustainable development goals: A pathway to sustainable innovation. *Discover Sustainability, 5*, 364. DOI: 10.1007/s43621-024-00610-x

Kumari, A., Raina, N., Wahi, A., Goh, K. W., Sharma, P., Nagpal, R., Jain, A., Ming, L. C., & Gupta, M. (2022). Wound-Healing Effects of Curcumin and Its Nanoformulations: A Comprehensive Review. *Pharmaceutics, 14*(11), 2288. DOI: 10.3390/pharmaceutics14112288 PMID: 36365107

Kumari, M., & Nanda, D. K. (2023). Potential of curcumin nanoemulsion as antimicrobial and wound healing agent in burn wound infection. *Burns, 49*(5), 1003–1016. DOI: 10.1016/j.burns.2022.10.008 PMID: 36402615

Kushwaha, A., Goswami, L., & Kim, B. S. (2022). Nanomaterial-Based Therapy for Wound Healing. *Nanomaterials (Basel, Switzerland), 12*(4), 618. DOI: 10.3390/nano12040618 PMID: 35214947

Li, D., Tang, G., Yao, H., Zhu, Y., Shi, C., Fu, Q., Yang, F., & Wang, X. (2022). Formulation of pH-responsive PEGylated nanoparticles with high drug loading capacity and programmable drug release for enhanced antibacterial activity. *Bioactive Materials, 16*, 47–56. DOI: 10.1016/j.bioactmat.2022.02.018 PMID: 35386319

Lin, X., Zhang, X., Wang, Y., Chen, W., Zhu, Z., & Wang, S. (2025). Hydrogels and hydrogel-based drug delivery systems for promoting refractory wound healing: Applications and prospects. *International Journal of Biological Macromolecules, 285*, 138098. DOI: 10.1016/j.ijbiomac.2024.138098 PMID: 39608543

Liu, H., Wang, C., Li, C., Qin, Y., Wang, Z., Yang, F., Li, Z., & Wang, J. (2018). A functional chitosan-based hydrogel as a wound dressing and drug delivery system in the treatment of wound healing. *RSC Advances, 8*(14), 7533–7549. DOI: 10.1039/c7ra13510f PMID: 35539132

Loo, H. L., Goh, B. H., Lee, L.-H., & Chuah, L. H. (2022). Application of chitosan-based nanoparticles in skin wound healing. *Asian Journal of Pharmaceutical Sciences, 17*(3), 299–332. DOI: 10.1016/j.ajps.2022.04.001 PMID: 35782330

López-Estévez, A. M., Lapuhs, P., Pineiro-Alonso, L., & Alonso, M. J. (2024). Personalized cancer nanomedicine: Overcoming biological barriers for intracellular delivery of biopharmaceuticals. *Advanced Materials, 36*(n/a), 2309355. https://doi.org/DOI: 10.1002/adma.202309355

Mai, B. T., Fernandes, S., Balakrishnan, P. B., & Pellegrino, T. (2018). Nanosystems based on magnetic nanoparticles and thermo- or pH-responsive polymers: An update and future perspectives. *Accounts of Chemical Research, 51*(5), 999–1013. DOI: 10.1021/acs.accounts.7b00549 PMID: 29733199

Martins-Gomes, C., Nunes, F. M., & Silva, A. M. (2024). Linking Variability in Phytochemical Composition with Safety Profile of *Thymus carnosus* Boiss. Extracts: Effect of Major Compounds and Evaluation of Markers of Oxidative Stress and Cell Death. *International Journal of Molecular Sciences, 25*(10), 5343. DOI: 10.3390/ijms25105343 PMID: 38791385

Mekuye, B., & Abera, B. (2023). Nanomaterials: An overview of synthesis, classification, characterization, and applications. *Nano Select*, *4*(8), 486–501. DOI: 10.1002/nano.202300038

Mekuye, B., & Abera, B. (2023). Nanomaterials: An overview of synthesis, classification, characterization, and applications. Nano Select, 4(8), 486–501. Portico. https://doi.org/DOI: 10.1002/nano.202300038

Mohan, A., Santhamoorthy, M., & Lee, Y.-C. (2024). Recent advances in the pH-responsive organic–inorganic mesoporous hybrid silica for targeted drug delivery. *European Polymer Journal*, *206*, 112783. DOI: 10.1016/j.eurpolymj.2024.112783

Mura, S., & Couvreur, P. (2012). Nanotheranostics for personalized medicine. *Advanced Drug Delivery Reviews*, *64*(13), 1394–1416. DOI: 10.1016/j.addr.2012.06.006 PMID: 22728642

Namuga, C., Ocan, M., Kinengyere, A. A., Richard, S., Namisango, E., Muwonge, H., Kirabira, J. B., Lawrence, M., & Obuku, E. A. (2023). Efficacy of nano encapsulated herbal extracts in the treatment of induced wounds in animal models: A systematic review protocol. *Systematic Reviews*, *12*(1), 215. DOI: 10.1186/s13643-023-02370-7 PMID: 37968731

Nandhini, J., Karthikeyan, E., & Rajeshkumar, S. (2024). Nanomaterials for wound healing: Current status and futuristic frontier. *Biomedical Technology*, *6*, 26–45. DOI: 10.1016/j.bmt.2023.10.001

Nasrollahzadeh, M., Sajjadi, M., Sajadi, S. M., & Issaabadi, Z. (2019). Green nanotechnology. In Nasrollahzadeh, M., Sajadi, S. M., Sajjadi, M., Issaabadi, Z., & Atarod, M. (Eds.), *Interface science and technology* (Vol. 28, pp. 145–198). Elsevier., DOI: 10.1016/B978-0-12-813586-0.00005-5

Nguyen, T. L. C., Narayanan, M., Chinnathambi, A., Govindasamy, C., Subramani, B., Brindhadevi, K., Pimpimon, T., & Pikulkaew, S. (2022). Fabrication, characterization, anti-inflammatory, and anti-diabetic activity of silver nanoparticles synthesized from *Azadirachta indica* kernel aqueous extract. *Environmental Research*, *208*, 112684. DOI: 10.1016/j.envres.2022.112684 PMID: 34995544

Nqoro, X., Adeyemi, S. A., & Ubanako, P.. (2024). Wound healing potential of sodium alginate-based topical gels loaded with a combination of essential oils, iron oxide nanoparticles and tranexamic acid. *Polymer Bulletin*, *81*, 3459–3478. DOI: 10.1007/s00289-023-04879-2

Pala, R., Mohieldin, A. M., Shamloo, K., Sherpa, R. T., Kathem, S. H., Zhou, J., Luan, Z., Zheng, J. G., Ahsan, A., & Nauli, S. M. (2019). Personalized Nanotherapy by Specifically Targeting Cell Organelles To Improve Vascular Hypertension. *Nano Letters, 19*(2), 904–914. DOI: 10.1021/acs.nanolett.8b04138 PMID: 30582331

Pang, Q., Jiang, Z., Wu, K., Hou, R., & Zhu, Y. (2023). Nanomaterials-based wound dressing for advanced management of infected wound. *Antibiotics (Basel, Switzerland), 12*(2), 351. DOI: 10.3390/antibiotics12020351 PMID: 36830262

Paras, Yadav, K., Kumar, P., Teja, D. R., Chakraborty, S., Chakraborty, M., Mohapatra, S. S., Sahoo, A., Chou, M. M. C., Liang, C. T., & Hang, D. R. (2022). A Review on Low-Dimensional Nanomaterials: Nanofabrication, Characterization and Applications. *Nanomaterials (Basel, Switzerland), 13*(1), 160. DOI: 10.3390/nano13010160 PMID: 36616070

Park, D. H., Park, J. Y., Shin, M.-S., & Hwang, G. S. (2023). Wound Healing Effect of 20(*S*)-Protopanaxadiol of Ginseng Involves VEGF-ERK Pathways in HUVECs and Diabetic Mice. *Processes (Basel, Switzerland), 11*(3), 692. DOI: 10.3390/pr11030692

Park, K. S., & Park, D. H. (2019). The effect of Korean Red Ginseng on full-thickness skin wound healing in rats. *Journal of Ginseng Research, 43*(2), 226–235. DOI: 10.1016/j.jgr.2017.12.006 PMID: 30976160

Parveen, A., Parveen, B., Parveen, R., & Ahmad, S. (2015). Challenges and guidelines for clinical trial of herbal drugs. *Journal of Pharmacy & Bioallied Sciences, 7*(4), 329–333. DOI: 10.4103/0975-7406.168035 PMID: 26681895

Pormohammad, A., Monych, N. K., Ghosh, S., Turner, D. L., & Turner, R. J. (2021). Nanomaterials in Wound Healing and Infection Control. *Antibiotics (Basel, Switzerland), 10*(5), 473. DOI: 10.3390/antibiotics10050473 PMID: 33919072

Pramanik, S., Aggarwal, A., Kadi, A., Alhomrani, M., Alamri, A. S., Alsanie, W. F., Koul, K., Deepak, A., & Bellucci, S. (2024). Chitosan alchemy: Transforming tissue engineering and wound healing. *RSC Advances, 14*(27), 19219–19256. DOI: 10.1039/d4ra01594k PMID: 38887635

Rajkumari, N. P., Roy, P., Siddika, S., Adhikary, K., & Goswami, P. (2023). Enhancing anti-inflammatory and antibacterial activity of curcumin by nano composing with curcumin reduced copper nano for the treatment of bacterial infection. *Materials Science and Engineering B, 292*, 116416. DOI: 10.1016/j.mseb.2023.116416

Raju, R., & Prasad, A. S., & S, R. K. (2024). Anti-inflammatory and Antioxidant Activity of Neem and Kirata-Induced Silver Nanoparticles Against Oral Biofilm: An In Vitro Study. *Cureus, 16*(8), e67708. DOI: 10.7759/cureus.67708 PMID: 39318902

Rajinikanth B, S., Rajkumar, D. S. R., K, K., & Vijayaragavan, V. (2024). Chitosan-Based Biomaterial in Wound Healing: A Review *Cureus*, *16*(2), e55193. DOI: 10.7759/cureus.55193

Sangnim, T., Puri, V., Dheer, D., Venkatesh, D. N., Huanbutta, K., & Sharma, A. (2024). Nanomaterials in the Wound Healing Process: New Insights and Advancements. *Pharmaceutics*, *16*(3), 300. DOI: 10.3390/pharmaceutics16030300 PMID: 38543194

Serini, S., Trombino, S., Cassano, R., Marino, M., & Calviello, G. (2025). Anti-inflammatory effects of curcumin-based nanoparticles containing α-linolenic acid in a model of psoriasis in vitro. *Nutrients*, *17*(4), 692. DOI: 10.3390/nu17040692 PMID: 40005020

Shah, J., Patel, D., Rananavare, D., Hudson, D., Tran, M., Schloss, R., Langrana, N., Berthiaume, F., & Kumar, S. (2025). Recent advancements in chitosan-based biomaterials for wound healing. *Journal of Functional Biomaterials*, *16*(2), 45. DOI: 10.3390/jfb16020045 PMID: 39997579

Singh, R., Shitiz, K., & Singh, A. (2017). Chitin and chitosan: biopolymers for wound management. International Wound Journal, 14(6), 1276–1289. Portico. https://doi .org/DOI: 10.1111/iwj.12797

Teja, P. K., Mithiya, J., Kate, A. S., Bairwa, K., & Chauthe, S. K. (2022). Herbal nanomedicines: Recent advancements, challenges, opportunities and regulatory overview. *Phytomedicine*, *96*, 153890. DOI: 10.1016/j.phymed.2021.153890 PMID: 35026510

Teja, P. K., Mithiya, J., Kate, A. S., Bairwa, K., & Chauthe, S. K. (2022). Herbal nanomedicines: Recent advancements, challenges, opportunities and regulatory overview. *Phytomedicine*, *96*, 153890. DOI: 10.1016/j.phymed.2021.153890 PMID: 35026510

Tejada, S., Manayi, A., Daglia, M., Nabavi, S. F., Sureda, A., Hajheydari, Z., Gortzi, O., Pazoki-Toroudi, H., & Nabavi, S. M. (2016). Wound Healing Effects of Curcumin: A Short Review. *Current Pharmaceutical Biotechnology*, *17*(11), 1002–1007. DOI: 10.2174/1389201017666160721123109 PMID: 27640646

Trigo-Gutierrez, J. K., Vega-Chacón, Y., Soares, A. B., & Mima, E. G. O. (2021). Antimicrobial Activity of Curcumin in Nanoformulations: A Comprehensive Review. *International Journal of Molecular Sciences*, *22*(13), 7130. DOI: 10.3390/ijms22137130 PMID: 34281181

Verma, A., Gautam, S. P., Bansal, K. K., Prabhakar, N., & Rosenholm, J. M. (2019). Green Nanotechnology: Advancement in Phytoformulation Research. *Medicines (Basel, Switzerland)*, *6*(1), 39. DOI: 10.3390/medicines6010039 PMID: 30875823

Wang, F., Liu, J., An, Q., Wang, Y., Yang, Y., Huo, T., Yang, S., Ju, R., & Quan, Q. (2023). Aloe Extracts Inhibit Skin Inflammatory Responses by Regulating NF-κB, ERK, and JNK Signaling Pathways in an LPS-Induced RAW264.7 Macrophages Model. *Clinical, cosmetic and investigational*

Wang, H., Chen, Y., Wang, L., Liu, Q., Yang, S., & Wang, C. (2023). Advancing herbal medicine: Enhancing product quality and safety through robust quality control practices. *Frontiers in Pharmacology*, *14*, 1265178. DOI: 10.3389/fphar.2023.1265178 PMID: 37818188

Wang, M., Huang, X., Zheng, H., Tang, Y., Zeng, K., Shao, L., & Li, L. (2021). Nanomaterials applied in wound healing: Mechanisms, limitations and perspectives. *Journal of Controlled Release*, *337*, 236–247. DOI: 10.1016/j.jconrel.2021.07.017 PMID: 34273419

Wang, Z., Xie, X., Wang, M., Ding, M., Gu, S., Xing, X., & Sun, X. (2023). Analysis of common and characteristic actions of *Panax ginseng* and *Panax notoginseng* in wound healing based on network pharmacology and meta-analysis. *Journal of Ginseng Research*, *47*(4), 493–505. DOI: 10.1016/j.jgr.2023.02.005 PMID: 37397412

Yan, M., Hu, S.-Y., Wang, Z.-G., Hong, R., Peng, X., Kuzmanović, M., Yang, M., Dai, R., Wang, Y., Gou, J., Li, K., Xu, J.-Z., & Li, Z.-M. (2024). Antibacterial, fatigue-resistant, and self-healing dressing from natural-based composite hydrogels for infected wound healing. *Biomacromolecules*, *25*(4), 2438–2448. DOI: 10.1021/acs.biomac.3c01385 PMID: 38502912

Yang, D., Chen, H., Wei, H., Liu, A., Wei, D.-X., & Chen, J. (2024). Hydrogel wound dressings containing bioactive compounds originated from traditional Chinese herbs: A review. *Smart Materials in Medicine*, *5*(1), 153–165. DOI: 10.1016/j.smaim.2023.10.004

Zarei, N., & Hassanzadeh-Tabrizi, S. A. (2023). Alginate/hyaluronic acid-based systems as a new generation of wound dressings: A review. *International Journal of Biological Macromolecules*, *253*(Part 6), 127249. DOI: 10.1016/j.ijbiomac.2023.127249 PMID: 37802435

Zhang, J., Hu, K., Di, L., Wang, P., Liu, Z., Zhang, J., Yue, P., Song, W., Zhang, J., Chen, T., Wang, Z., Zhang, Y., Wang, X., Zhan, C., Cheng, Y.-C., Li, X., Li, Q., Fan, J.-Y., Shen, Y., & Qiao, H. (2021). Traditional herbal medicine and nanomedicine: Converging disciplines to improve therapeutic efficacy and human health. *Advanced Drug Delivery Reviews*, *178*, 113964. DOI: 10.1016/j.addr.2021.113964 PMID: 34499982

Zhang, W., Liu, L., Cheng, H., Zhu, J., Li, X., Ye, S., & Li, X. (2024). Hydrogel-based dressings designed to facilitate wound healing. *Materials Advances*, *5*(4), 1364–1394. DOI: 10.1039/d3ma00682d

Zhu, H., Ao, H. T., Fu, Y., Zou, C., Chen, Z., Jin, Z., Zhou, H., Sun, B., & Guo, S. (2024). Optimizing alginate dressings with allantoin and chemical modifiers to promote wound healing. *International Journal of Biological Macromolecules*, *275*(Part 1), 133524. DOI: 10.1016/j.ijbiomac.2024.133524 PMID: 38945316

Zhu, J., Cheng, H., Zhang, Z., Chen, K., Zhang, Q., Zhang, C., Gao, W., & Zheng, Y. (2024). Antibacterial Hydrogels for Wound Dressing Applications: Current Status, Progress, Challenges, and Trends. *Gels (Basel, Switzerland)*, *10*(8), 495. DOI: 10.3390/gels10080495 PMID: 39195024

Chapter 11
Nanotechnology in Herbal-Based Wound Care

P. Selvakumar
https://orcid.org/0000-0002-3650-4548
Department of Science and Humanities, Nehru Institute of Technology, Coimbatore, India

Maurya Manjunath
https://orcid.org/0000-0001-9563-9269
JSS Academy of Higher Education and Research, Mysuru, India

T.C. Manjunath
https://orcid.org/0000-0003-2545-9160
Rajarajeswari College of Engineering, India

Chitra Rengarajan
https://orcid.org/0009-0005-2425-910X
Tamilnadu Agricultural University, Coimbatore, India

Prita Pillai
https://orcid.org/0009-0003-5517-7698
Sree Vidhyadhi Raja NSS College, Vazhoor, India

ABSTRACT

Wound care stands as a fundamental pillar in the healthcare system, playing a critical role in patient recovery, the prevention of complications, and the enhancement of overall quality of life. Whether resulting from surgical procedures, traumatic injuries, burns, pressure ulcers, or chronic conditions like diabetes, wounds represent

DOI: 10.4018/979-8-3373-3977-1.ch011

a significant medical concern that requires meticulous attention, timely intervention, and specialized careThe impact of inadequate wound management extends beyond individual suffering; it places a substantia. l burden on healthcare systems worldwide in terms of prolonged hospital stays, increased readmission rates, and rising treatment costs. Consequently, effective wound care is not merely a supportive measure but a central component of comprehensive healthcare delivery.At its core, wound care aims to promote healing, reduce the risk of infection, alleviate pain, and restore functionality. It encompasses a wide range of practices, from basic first aid and dressing changes to advanced therapies such.

THE IMPORTANCE OF WOUND CARE IN HEALTHCARE

Wound care stands as a fundamental pillar in the healthcare system, playing a critical role in patient recovery, the prevention of complications, and the enhancement of overall quality of life. Whether resulting from surgical procedures, traumatic injuries, burns, pressure ulcers, or chronic conditions like diabetes, wounds represent a significant medical concern that requires meticulous attention, timely intervention, and specialized care. The impact of inadequate wound management extends beyond individual suffering; it places a substantia. l burden on healthcare systems worldwide in terms of prolonged hospital stays, increased readmission rates, and rising treatment costs. Consequently, effective wound care is not merely a supportive measure but a central component of comprehensive healthcare delivery. At its core, wound care aims to promote healing, reduce the risk of infection, alleviate pain, and restore functionality. It encompasses a wide range of practices, from basic first aid and dressing changes to advanced therapies such. Wound care stands as a fundamental pillar in the healthcare system, playing a critical role in patient recovery, the prevention of complications, and the enhancement of overall quality of life. Whether resulting from surgical procedures, traumatic injuries, burns, pressure ulcers, or chronic conditions like diabetes, wounds represent a significant medical concern that requires meticulous attention, timely intervention, and specialized care. The impact of inadequate wound management extends beyond individual suffering, (Augustine et al., 2021). It places a substantial burden on healthcare systems worldwide in terms of prolonged hospital stays, increased readmission rates, and rising treatment costs. Consequently, effective wound care is not merely a supportive measure but a central component of comprehensive healthcare delivery. At its core, wound care aims to promote healing, reduce the risk of infection, alleviate pain, and restore functionality. It encompasses a minimizes complications such as infection, necrosis, and sepsis, which are not only detrimental to the patient's health but can also be life-threatening (Babenko et al., 2012).

Conversely, poor wound management can lead to delayed healing, chronic wound formation, or even amputation in extreme cases, especially among vulnerable populations like the elderly or those with comorbid conditions. From a clinical perspective, proper wound care contributes to improved patient outcomes in several key ways. Firstly, it accelerates rates and extended hospitalizations. Thirdly, efficient wound care protocols support early mobility and rehabilitation, particularly after surgeries or injuries, enabling patients to regain independence and resume daily activities sooner. All of these factors collectively enhance the patient's physical well-being and reduce the psychological stress that often accompanies chronic or severe wounds. The psychological and emotional dimensions of wound care are often overlooked but are equally important. Living with a wound, particularly a chronic or disfiguring one, can lead to anxiety, depression, social isolation, and diminished self-esteem. Patients may experience embarrassment due to visible wounds or the odor associated with infected wounds, leading to social withdrawal. Effective wound care alleviates these concerns by promoting faster healing and providing reassurance through continuous monitoring and support. (Augustine et al., 2020). Moreover, the establishment of a trusting relationship between healthcare providers and patients during wound treatment can significantly improve adherence to care plans and foster a more positive healthcare experience., specialized dressings, and sometimes surgical interventions. In the United States alone, chronic wound care costs an estimated \$28 to \$31 billion annually. By investing in early intervention, patient education, and advanced wound care techniques, healthcare systems can significantly reduce these costs and allocate resources more efficiently.

Preventive strategies, such as pressure injury prevention programs in hospitals or routine foot care for diabetic patients, have demonstrated substantial cost savings and improved clinical outcomes. In addition, wound care plays a pivotal role in specific clinical populations and settings. For example, of pressure injuries among immobile or bedridden patients. In community and home-based care settings, proper wound care training for caregivers and patients themselves can help reduce the need for hospital readmissions and allow for more effective management of wounds in non-clinical environments. This highlights the need for interdisciplinary collaboration, ongoing education, and the integration of wound care into all levels of healthcare services, (Bai et al., 2020). The advancement of wound care science has brought forth a range of innovative products and technologies that have revolutionized traditional practices. Modern wound dressings, such as hydrocolloids, alginates, and foam dressings, are designed to promote optimal healing environments. Antimicrobial dressings infused with silver or iodine help manage infection risk, while smart wound dressings equipped with sensors can monitor wound conditions in real time.

Additionally, bioengineered skin substitutes and tissue regeneration technologies offer hope for patients with complex or non-healing wounds. These innovations not only enhance the effectiveness of wound care but also reflect the growing recognition of wound care as a specialized field requiring dedicated research and clinical expertise. Training and education of healthcare professionals in wound care are crucial to ensure evidence-based practices are consistently applied. This includes understanding wound etiology, proper assessment techniques, infection control, dressing selection, and patient-centered care planning. Incorporating wound care into medical and nursing curricula, offering continuing education programs, and promoting certification in wound management can elevate the standard of care and empower professionals to deliver high-quality, individualized treatment. Moreover, patient education is a vital component of successful wound care. Empowering patients with the knowledge and skills to care for their wounds at home, recognize signs of complications, and maintain overall health can significantly improve outcomes and reduce recurrence rates. In conclusion, that profoundly influences patient outcomes, quality of life, and healthcare resource utilization. By prioritizing effective wound management strategies. Recognizing its importance and integrating it seamlessly into all levels of healthcare is essential to achieving better health outcomes for individuals and communities alike.

THE POTENTIAL OF NANOTECHNOLOGY IN WOUND CARE

While wound care is a fundamental aspect of healthcare, the traditional methods that have been employed for decades are increasingly being scrutinized for their limitations, particularly in the face of complex, chronic, or non-healing wounds. Traditional wound care typically involves basic interventions such as cleaning the wound with saline or antiseptics, applying gauze or cotton dressings, and relying on natural healing processes over time. Although these methods may be sufficient for minor, acute wounds, they often fall short when addressing the multifaceted needs of more severe or persistent wound types. As the understanding of wound pathophysiology has evolved, so too has the recognition that conventional approaches may not only be limited in efficacy but also pose potential risks to patient outcomes. One of the primary limitations of traditional wound care is its lack of adaptability to different wound types and healing stages, (Cheng et al., 2019). Wounds vary significantly in terms of etiology, depth, tissue involvement, infection status, and healing potential. Yet, traditional care methods often apply a "one-size-fits-all" approach that fails to account for these variables. For instance, the routine use of dry gauze dressings, though inexpensive and widely available, can adhere to the wound bed and cause trauma upon removal, disrupting newly formed tissue and delaying the healing process. This mechanical trauma may also increase the risk of secondary infections, pain, and bleeding—particularly detrimental for patients with fragile or compromised skin integrity. Another significant drawback of traditional wound care is its limited capacity to manage moisture balance—an essential component of optimal wound healing. (Chigurupati et al., 2013). The principle of moist wound healing, first introduced in the 1960s, underscores the importance of maintaining a balanced environment that is neither too dry nor overly saturated. Traditional dressings like dry gauze or cotton often absorb too much exudate, leaving the wound bed desiccated and inhibiting cellular activity crucial for regeneration.

Conversely, they may become overly saturated in heavily exuding wounds, leading to maceration of the surrounding skin and promoting bacterial growth. Without the capability to regulate moisture effectively, these basic dressings create suboptimal healing conditions that prolong recovery and increase the likelihood of complications. Infection control is another area where traditional wound care methods reveal their shortcomings. Although basic antiseptics and topical antibiotics are sometimes used, their overuse can contribute to antimicrobial resistance and cytotoxicity, damaging healthy tissue in the process. such as diabetic foot ulcers or pressure injuries, where infection control is not only about treating visible symptoms but also about disrupting these entrenched bacterial communities. Pain management is another aspect often neglected in traditional wound care. The removal of dry dressings, application of irritating antiseptics, or frequent dressing changes can cause significant discomfort for patients. Pain not only reduces patient compliance with treatment plans but also has physiological impacts that may impair the healing process by triggering stress responses that hinder tissue repair. Modern wound care practices emphasize atraumatic dressing materials, soothing agents, and pain assessment protocols—features largely absent in traditional approaches. Without adequately addressing pain, traditional wound care may contribute to a diminished patient experience and reduced engagement in their own recovery. Moreover, traditional wound care often lacks a holistic, patient-centered approach that considers comorbidities, nutritional status, mobility, and psychosocial factors—all of which play critical roles in wound healing. For example, patients with diabetes, vascular disease, or immune suppression may require tailored interventions that go beyond standard cleaning and dressing techniques. (Clark et al., 2011). In such cases, failure to incorporate systemic considerations into the wound management plan can lead to poor outcomes and recurrent wounds. Traditional methods, with their limited scope, rarely integrate multidisciplinary care, patient education, or preventive strategies—all of which are essential for effective long-term wound management. Documentation and monitoring are also areas where traditional wound care falls behind. Accurate and consistent wound assessment is crucial for evaluating healing progress and adjusting treatment plans accordingly. However, traditional care often relies on subjective observation and limited metrics, which may result in inconsistent documentation and misinterpretation of wound status. In contrast, modern wound care incorporates objective measurement tools, imaging technologies, and digital documentation systems that enhance accuracy and enable data-driven decision-making. Without such capabilities, traditional wound care risks under- or over-treating wounds, leading to either unnecessary interventions or dangerous neglect. Another challenge lies in the sustainability and efficiency of traditional wound care, especially in resource-limited or high-demand healthcare settings. Frequent dressing changes, longer healing times, and recurrent wound complications increase the workload for healthcare providers and contribute to higher overall treatment costs. In hospitals, this can translate into prolonged hospital stays and higher readmission rates. In home care or outpatient settings, it burdens caregivers and patients, both financially and logistically.

Advanced wound care solutions, while often more expensive initially, have demonstrated greater cost-effectiveness in the long run due to faster healing rates and reduced complications—advantages not typically offered by traditional methods. Cultural and institutional inertia also play a role in the continued reliance on outdated wound care practices. Many healthcare professionals continue to use traditional methods simply because of habit, lack of training in advanced techniques, or institutional protocols that have not kept pace with current evidence-based guidelines. (Damle et al., 2019). This adherence to outdated practices can hinder the adoption of more effective, patient-centered interventions. Moreover, patients themselves may be unaware of better alternatives and may not advocate for or access advanced care unless informed and supported by their healthcare providers. These demographic and epidemiological trends necessitate a shift away from conventional, reactive wound care toward proactive, personalized, and technologically supported strategies. Continuing to rely solely on traditional methods in this context risks exacerbating health disparities, increasing healthcare costs, and compromising patient outcomes on a systemic level.In summary, while traditional wound care methods have served as the foundation for treating wounds for centuries, they are increasingly inadequate for meeting the demands of modern healthcare. Their limited efficacy, potential for adverse effects, and lack of customization render them unsuitable for many contemporary wound care challenges. From poor moisture and infection control to insufficient pain management and lack of holistic patient care, these methods fall short of the comprehensive, science-driven approach required to address today's complex wound care needs. As healthcare continues to advance, it is imperative that wound care practices evolve as well—embracing innovation, interdisciplinary collaboration, and evidence-based strategies that offer better outcomes for patients and more sustainable solutions for healthcare systems.

NANOPARTICLES IN HERBAL-BASED WOUND CARE

By harnessing the unique properties of nanoparticles and nanostructures, this technology introduces innovative solutions that go far beyond conventional wound management, offering precision, efficiency, and bioactivity that traditional materials cannot match. antimicrobial activity without promoting resistance. Infection is a major barrier to wound healing and a common cause of prolonged treatment, hospitalization, and even mortality. Nanomaterials such as silver nanoparticles, zinc oxide nanoparticles, target a single site and are susceptible to resistance development, nanoparticles can attack pathogens through multiple pathways, reducing the likelihood of resistance. Furthermore, these nanoparticles can be integrated directly into wound dressings, gels, or sprays, enabling continuous antimicrobial activity at the wound site and minimizing the need for systemic antibiotics, (Darby et al., 2014). Beyond infection control, nanotechnology offers promising solutions for enhancing the wound healing process itself. cell proliferation, and tissue regeneration. Such precision delivery not only improves the bioavailability and stability of these therapeutic agents but also reduces side effects by minimizing systemic exposure. The potential of nanotechnology in promoting tissue regeneration is further amplified by which combine nanoparticles with polymeric materials, offer superior mechanical strength, moisture retention, and responsiveness to environmental stimuli, further optimizing the wound microenvironment for healing.

Another or signaling the need for clinical intervention. Some prototypes even integrate wireless communication capabilities, allowing healthcare providers to remotely monitor wound conditions in real time. This level of monitoring and responsiveness represents a paradigm shift in wound care, enabling earlier detection of complications and more personalized, proactive treatment strategies. The biocompatibility and safety of nanomaterials are crucial considerations in wound care applications. While certain nanoparticles, such as silver or gold, have been extensively studied and shown to have favorable safety profiles when used appropriately, others may pose risks of cytotoxicity, oxidative stress, or long-term accumulation in tissues. (Ellis et al., 2018). Therefore, r by producing more environmentally friendly and biologically benign nanoparticles. The application of nanotechnology in wound care also aligns with the goals of personalized medicine. By designing nanocarriers that respond to specific wound characteristics—such as the presence of certain enzymes, ectly to the wound site, counteracting the local effects of hyperglycemia and oxidative stress.of healthcare costs due to their prolonged healing times, frequent clinic visits, and the high risk of complications. By accelerating healing and reducing infection rates, nanotechnology can decrease the need for long-term care and hospital readmissions. Although the initial costs of nanotechnology-based products may be higher than traditional alternatives, the long-term cost-effectiveness is expected to be favorable due to improved outcomes and reduced treatment duration. Despite its promise, the widespread adoption of nanotechnology in wound care faces several challenges. Manufacturing scalability, regulatory approval, and integration into existing clinical workflows are significant hurdles. safety without stifling innovation. Education and training of healthcare professionals are also necessary to familiarize them with the use and benefits of nanotechnology-based wound care products, promoting acceptance and optimal usage in clinical settings. The integration of artificial intelligence and machine learning with nanotechnology is also being investigated to optimize treatment protocols based on data from smart dressings and patient records. These advancements signal a shift toward a more intelligent, responsive, and efficient wound care paradigm.

HERBAL EXTRACTS AND NANOTECHNOLOGY IN WOUND HEALING

The poor water solubility, low bioavailability, rapid degradation, and inconsistent efficacy. The advent of nanotechnology has provided an effective solution to these limitations by enabling the encapsulation, stabilization, and targeted delivery of herbal bioactives through nanoparticles. This convergence—commonly referred to as are research and clinical application. Herbal-based nanoparticles are typically created by incorporating plant-derived bioactive compounds into nanocarriers barriers such as the skin and wound bed. For instance, curcumin, a well-known compound derived from turmeric (Curcuma longa), exhibits powerful antioxidant, anti-inflammatory, and antimicrobial properties, making, (Eriksson et al., 2018). It highly suitable for wound healing. However, its poor water solubility and rapid metabolism limit its effectiveness in conventional formulations. By incorporating curcumin into nanoparticles—such as polymeric nanocarriers or nanoemulsions—its stability is improved, and it can be released in a controlled manner directly at the site of the wound, significantly enhancing its therapeutic effects. For example, silver nanoparticles synthesized using neem extract or green tea polyphenols demonstrate superior bactericidal activity compared to either the plant extract or the silver nanoparticles alone, due to a synergistic effect. This dual action, combining the antimicrobial properties of both the metallic core and the phytochemicals, is particularly valuable in managing infected wounds and preventing biofilm formation—one of the major challenges in chronic wound care.which are critical aspects of wound healing. Many plant-derived bioactives, such as quercetin (from onions, apples), resveratrol (from grapes), and asiaticoside (from Centella asiatica), exhibit anti-inflammatory and collagen-stimulating properties. When encapsulated in nanoparticles, these compounds can be delivered precisely to the inflamed tissue, downregulating pro-inflammatory cytokines and promoting the proliferation of fibroblasts and keratinocytes—cells essential for tissue remodeling and repair. Nanocarriers protect these sensitive compounds from degradation and ensure their sustained release over time, thereby maintaining therapeutic concentrations in the wound environment for longer durations compared to conventional herbal ointments or extracts.r films, which can be directly applied to the wound. Such dressings not only deliver herbal bioactives locally but also provide physical protection, maintain moisture balance, and facilitate gas exchange—ideal conditions for wound healing. These approaches are especially promising in diabetic foot ulcers, where traditional therapies often fail to deliver satisfactory (Fisichella et al., 2014). results. surface contribute additional therapeutic effects. For example, gold or silver nanoparticles synthesized using clove, ginger, or tulsi (holy basil) extracts have demonstrated remarkable wound healing properties with minimal toxicity. The sustainability and scalability of green synthesis methods make them highly attractive for both laboratory research and industrial-scale production. Education and awareness are also key factors in the adoption of these novel therapies. Healthcare professionals must be trained in the mechanisms, benefits, and limitations of herbal nanotechnology in wound care to make informed decisions and ensure appropriate usage. Likewise, public perception and acceptance play a role, as patients may be more receptive to natural, plant-based therapies when they are confident in their efficacy and safety.

NANOFIBERS AND NANOCOMPOSITES IN WOUND CARE

The integration of herbal extracts with nanotechnology in wound healing represents a promising frontier in modern medicine, combining the therapeutic richness of traditional botanical remedies with the precision and efficiency of nanoscience. Herbal extracts have long been valued for their potent biological properties—including anti-inflammatory, antimicrobial, antioxidant, and tissue-regenerative effects—making them ideal candidates for managing and accelerating wound repair. However, conventional delivery methods for herbal compounds often suffer from limitations such as poor bioavailability, rapid degradation, and low penetration into deeper tissue layers. Nanotechnology offers a transformative solution by enhancing the delivery, stability, and effectiveness of these plant-based agents, thereby unlocking their full therapeutic potential in wound care. Herbal extracts are derived from various parts of medicinal plants—leaves, roots, stems, seeds, or flowers—they can reduce inflammation by modulating cytokine activity, promote collagen synthesis, enhance angiogenesis, combat microbial infections, and neutralize free radicals.(Futosi et al., 2013) For instance, curcumin from turmeric (Curcuma longa), asiaticoside from Centella asiatica, aloin from Aloe vera, and quercetin from various fruits and vegetables are widely studied for their pro-healing properties. Yet, these phytochemicals often exhibit poor water solubility, chemical instability, and rapid systemic elimination, limiting their clinical efficacy when used in traditional formulations such as creams, ointments, or extracts. Nanotechnology addresses these challenges by allowing herbal compounds to be encapsulated. This targeted delivery not only increases the local concentration of the therapeutic agent where it is most needed but also reduces the risk of systemic side effects. For instance, curcumin-loaded nanoparticles have shown significantly higher wound healing efficacy than free curcumin due to better absorption and prolonged retention at the site of injury. with nanocarriers that can independently enhance wound penetration or offer intrinsic antimicrobial action—such as silver nanoparticles—the resulting formulations are significantly more effective than their individual components. For example, silver nanoparticles synthesized using neem (Azadirachta indica) or green tea (Camellia sinensis) extracts not only exhibit strong antimicrobial activity but also benefit from the wound-healing properties of the phytochemicals present in the extract, offering dual-functionality in infection control and tissue repair. alternative. Antioxidant-rich herbal nanoparticles can scavenge reactive oxygen species (ROS), modulate the inflammatory response, and stimulate tissue regeneration at the molecular level. For instance, nanoparticles herbal-nano systems further exemplify the practical application of this technology. These dressings, which include hydrogels, electrospun nanofibers, films, and sponges, serve both as a physical barrier and a drug delivery system.

Herbal nanoparticles embedded within these materials provide localized, sustained release of bioactives while maintaining a moist, oxygen-rich environment conducive to healing. For example, a hydrogel wound dressing loaded with green tea extract nanoparticles has demonstrated superior healing outcomes in animal studies, including reduced inflammation, enhanced granulation tissue formation, and accelerated re-epithelialization. Electrospun nanofiber mats containing curcumin or Centella asiatica extracts have also shown promise in enhancing fibroblast proliferation and collagen deposition Systems optimize therapeutic action while minimizing drug wastage and potential toxicity. eliminating the need for harmful chemicals. These biosynthesized nanoparticles are not only environmentally friendly but also inherently more biocompatible, (Gabbiani, 2003). For instance, gold or silver nanoparticles synthesized using clove, tulsi (Ocimum sanctum), or ginger (Zingiber officinale) have demonstrated low toxicity profiles and potent healing effects in preclinical models. to validate preclinical findings and establish efficacy in diverse patient populations. Regulatory frameworks must also evolve to accommodate the unique nature of these hybrid therapies, which combine elements of natural medicine and nanotechnology. To overcome these challenges, interdisciplinary collaboration is crucial. Botanists, pharmacologists, nanotechnologists, and clinicians must work together to develop standardized extraction protocols, optimize nanoformulation parameters, and design comprehensive safety and efficacy studies. In parallel, increased awareness and education among healthcare providers regarding the benefits and use of herbal-nano wound care products will help integrate them into mainstream clinical practice. In addition to clinical potential, the use of herbal extracts and nanotechnology also holds socioeconomic and environmental appeal, especially in low-resource settings. Many medicinal plants used in nanoformulations are locally available and cost-effective. When combined with scalable green synthesis methods, herbal-based nanotherapies can provide affordable and sustainable wound care solutions in communities with limited access to modern pharmaceuticals.

NANOTECHNOLOGY-ENHANCED HERBAL WOUND DRESSINGS

As chronic wounds and complex skin injuries continue to challenge traditional treatments, nanofibers and nanocomposites emerge as transformative solutions that can enhance healing outcomes, reduce complications, and improve the quality of patient care gaseous exchange while preventing microbial infiltration, and their ECM-like architecture provides a favorable scaffold for cellular activities critical to wound repair. or platelet-derived growth factor (PDGF) have demonstrated accelerated wound closure and enhanced tissue integrity in preclinical models. In parallel, nanocomposites—materials composed of a matrix embedded with nanoscale fillers—offer a different but complementary set of advantages. In wound care, nanocomposites are typically formed by incorporating nanoparticles (e.g., silver, zinc oxide, gold, silica, graphene oxide) into a biocompatible polymeric matrix.(Hirst et al., 2009) These composite materials are designed to combine the physical benefits of the polymer base (such as flexibility, strength, and moisture retention) with the functional properties of the nanoparticles, including antimicrobial activity, oxidative stress reduction, or stimuli responsiveness. Nanocomposites can be processed into various forms, including films, hydrogels, sponges, or foams, depending on the wound type and clinical requirements. One of the most critical contributions of nanocomposites to wound healing is their antimicrobial activity. Infection is a major obstacle to wound resolution and can prolong inflammation, impair tissue repair, and increase the risk of systemic complications. Nanoparticles such as silver and, the sustained release of antimicrobial agents from nanocomposites minimizes the frequency of dressing changes and reduces the risk of cytotoxicity associated with burst-release formulations. Both nanofibers and nanocomposites contribute to moisture management, a critical factor in optimizing the wound healing environment. Maintaining an appropriate moisture level promotes cellular activity, enhances autolytic debridement, and prevents desiccation of newly formed tissue. Nanofiber excess fluid or releasing moisture as needed. This self-regulating capacity makes them especially useful in chronic wounds with fluctuating exudate levels. Another notable benefit of nanofibers and nanocomposites is their potential for multifunctionality. These materials can be designed to serve not only as protective barriers but also as drug delivery systems, diagnostic tools, and stimuli-responsive platforms. (Hosseini et al., 2020). For instance, smart nanofibers or nanocomposites may incorporate pH- or temperature-sensitive polymers that release therapeutic agents in response to infection or inflammation. Some nanocomposite dressings are being developed to include colorimetric sensors that change color when infection is detected, providing real-time visual cues for clinicians and reducing the need for invasive inspections or laboratory tests. Furthermore, structural support and mechanical strength provided by nanofibers and nanocomposites play a vital role in wound management, especially in areas subjected to tension or shear forces (e.g., joints, pressure points). These materials can reinforce the wound site, prevent re-injury, and provide a stable platform for new tissue formation. By modulating the elasticity, degradation rate, and tensile strength of the dressing material, researchers can tailor its performance to match different wound types and healing stages, (Ilina and Friedl, 2009). In addition to their functional advantages, the biocompatibility and biodegradability of nanofibers and nanocomposites make them attractive for clinical use. Many formulations are based on natural polymers or FDA-approved synthetic materials that degrade into non-toxic byproducts, eliminating the need for dressing removal and minimizing patient discomfort. This property is especially beneficial for burn victims or patients with highly sensitive skin, where repeated dressing changes can be traumatic and

NANOPARTICLE-BASED DELIVERY SYSTEMS FOR HERBAL WOUND CARE

Herbal medicine has long been revered for its anti-inflammatory, antimicrobial, antioxidant, and tissue-regenerative properties. Plants such as *Curcuma longa* (turmeric), *Centella asiatica*, *Aloe vera*, *Azadirachta indica* (neem), *Ocimum sanctum* (holy basil), and *Camellia sinensis* (green tea) are rich in bioactive compounds like flavonoids, polyphenols, tannins, terpenoids, and alkaloids. These compounds have shown great promise in promoting wound repair by modulating inflammation, stimulating collagen production, enhancing angiogenesis, and combating oxidative stress. (Ji et al., 2012). However, challenges like poor water solubility, rapid degradation, and low permeability across the skin barrier have historically limited the clinical use of herbal remedies in modern wound care. A prime example of this technology is curcumin-loaded nanofiber wound dressings. Curcumin, the principal curcuminoid in turmeric, has powerful antioxidant and anti-inflammatory effects but suffers from poor aqueous solubility and rapid systemic elimination. When curcumin is encapsulated into electrospun nanofibers composed of biocompatible polymers like polycaprolactone (PCL) or polyvinyl alcohol (PVA), it forms a wound dressing capable of gradually releasing curcumin into the wound environment. Studies have shown that such curcumin-loaded nanofiber mats accelerate wound contraction, promote fibroblast proliferation, and enhance collagen deposition in animal models of full-thickness wounds. The nanofibers mimic the extracellular matrix, further facilitating cell migration and tissue regeneration. Another widely studied system is the Aloe vera–based hydrogel embedded with nanoparticles. Aloe vera contains aloin and other polysaccharides that support hydration, reduce inflammation, and promote epithelial cell growth, (Yang et al., 2022). Aloe vera extract into a nanocomposite hydrogel matrix (for example, one that contains zinc oxide or silver nanoparticles) results in a multifunctional wound dressing that offers moisture retention, antimicrobial activity, and sustained herbal drug release.

Zinc oxide nanoparticles, in particular, enhance epithelialization and collagen synthesis, while Aloe vera maintains a soothing, protective barrier that encourages regeneration, (Xue et al., 2024). Together, these elements form a synergistic environment conducive to healing chronic wounds, including diabetic foot ulcerscombat a broad range of pathogens, including antibiotic-resistant bacteria, while neem and tea tree contribute additional antifungal and anti-inflammatory properties. When embedded into a polymeric film or nanofiber scaffold, these biosynthesized nanoparticles provide continuous antimicrobial action while maintaining biocompatibility. This makes them particularly useful in managing infected (Johnson and Wilgus, 2014) or high-risk wounds where bacterial colonization is a major concern. asiatica contains asiaticoside and madecassoside—triterpenoids that have been shown to stimulate collagen synthesis and angiogenesis. Nanogels loaded with Centella asiatica extracts offer excellent skin adhesion, moisture retention, and controlled drug release, making them ideal for topical application on chronic or slow-healing wounds. These nanogels can be designed to respond to pH or temperature changes, releasing the herbal active only when inflammation or infection is present, thus maximizing therapeutic impact and minimizing wastage. When infection occurs and the wound becomes more alkaline, the dressing responds by releasing antimicrobial and antioxidant compounds directly at the site. Some smart dressings also include visual indicators—such as a color change—that alert healthcare providers to changes in wound status without the need to remove the dressing, thus preventing unnecessary disruption of the healing tissue. electrospun nanofiber mats loaded with herbal extracts has also expandedin various preclinical models. Their ease of customization makes them adaptable to different wound types—from superficial abrasions to deep, chronic ulcers.

NANOTECHNOLOGY AND HERBAL-BASED WOUND CARE FOR CHRONIC WOUNDS

The development of nanoparticle-based delivery systems for herbal wound care represents a significant innovation at the intersection of traditional medicine and nanotechnology. Herbal remedies, long known for their wound healing capabilities, are often rich in natural compounds such as flavonoids, tannins, terpenoids, alkaloids, and polyphenols—many of which have proven anti-inflammatory, antioxidant, antimicrobial, and tissue-regenerative properties. Despite these therapeutic advantages, the clinical application of herbal extracts remains limited due to several pharmacokinetic challenges, including poor solubility, low skin penetration, instability under physiological conditions, and rapid systemic clearance. Nanoparticle-based systems offer solutions to these limitations by providing enhanced delivery, protection, and controlled release of herbal actives, thus significantly improving both their efficacy and safety in wound healing applications.(Kaarniranta et al., 2019) The fundamental advantage of these nanosystems lies in their ability to protect fragile phytochemicals from premature degradation, improve their solubility and permeability across skin barriers, and enable their sustained or stimuli-responsive release directly at the wound site dramatically. (Yildizbakan et al., 2023). For instance, curcumin-loaded PLGA nanoparticles have demonstrated better wound closure rates, increased collagen synthesis, and improved angiogenesis in animal wound models compared to free curcumin. Chitosan-based nanoparticles, in particular, are highly favored for wound applications due to their inherent antimicrobial activity, hemostatic properties, and ability to promote fibroblast proliferation and keratinocyte migration., or essential oils and releasing them slowly over extended periods. Their occlusive properties help retain skin moisture and improve skin permeability, which is essential for dry or necrotic wound beds. Moreover, lipid nanoparticles can easily be incorporated into gels, creams, or spray formulations for ease of topical application. studied as carriers for herbal wound healing agents. They mimic biological membranes, making them particularly effective for skin delivery. Herbal compounds like Centella asiatica, tea tree oil, or neem extract, when encapsulated in liposomes, show enhanced skin retention and reduced irritation. Liposomal systems can also be modified with surface ligands to target specific cell types in the wound bed, such as macrophages or fibroblasts, for improved therapeutic outcomes.

These nanoparticles exhibit combined effects—leveraging the antimicrobial properties of the metal and the biological activities of the herbal compounds. For example, green-synthesized silver nanoparticles using neem or clove extracts have shown superior antimicrobial efficacy and biocompatibility compared to chemically synthesized ones, (Kamalipooya et al., 2024) These systems are particularly effective against multidrug-resistant bacteria, which are a major concern in chronic and infected wounds. Nanogels are three-dimensional, water-swollen, crosslinked polymeric networks that can encapsulate both hydrophilic and hydrophobic compounds. Their high-water content makes them ideal for hydrating wound environments, while their nanoscale size allows for enhanced skin penetration. Herbal nanogels containing extracts of licorice (*Glycyrrhiza glabra*), tulsi (*Ocimum sanctum*), or moringa (*Moringa oleifera*) have been reported to reduce inflammation and oxidative stress in wound sites, supporting faster and cleaner healing. Dendrimers, due to their highly branched structure and surface functionality, offer precise control over drug loading and release, though their use in herbal wound care is still emerging release drugs slowly over hours or days, depending on the material composition and wound environment.(Li et al., 2023) This reduces the need for repeated dressing changes, minimizes patient discomfort, and maintains effective therapeutic levels in the wound bed for longer periods. systemic exposure and toxicity. systems offer improved safety profiles over synthetic drugs due to the biocompatibility of both the herbal active and the carrier material. For example, herbal-metallic nanoparticles often show reduced cytotoxicity because the phytochemicals on their surfaces modulate the interaction with human cells. However, comprehensive toxicological evaluations are necessary, stringent safety standards for human use. injectable solutions, depending on the wound type and treatment goals. For instance, electrospun nanofiber mats containing herbal-loaded nanoparticles provide structural support and a bioactive surface for cell migration. Sprayable nanoparticle suspensions can offer convenient application over large wound areas, particularly in burns or surgical wounds. Injectable nanogels are being explored for deep tissue injuries where surface application may be insufficient. Standardization of herbal extracts, scalable manufacturing of nanoparticles, regulatory approval pathways, and long-term safety assessments remain significant hurdles. Nevertheless, numerous preclinical studies and a growing number of early-phase clinical trials show strong evidence of the potential benefits of nano-herbal wound care systems.

NANOTECHNOLOGY IN HERBAL-BASED WOUND CARE:

Traditional wound care strategies frequently fail to address the complex pathophysiology of chronic wounds, resulting in recurrent infections, patient discomfort, increased hospitalization, and even amputations. In this context, the integration of nanotechnology and herbal-based medicine has emerged as a promising and innovative approach, offering new possibilities to accelerate wound healing and significantly improve patient outcomes.*Azadirachta indica* (neem), and *Camellia sinensis* (green tea)—have shown considerable promise in promoting the wound healing cascade. They aid in reducing inflammation, inhibiting microbial growth, stimulating fibroblast proliferation, enhancing angiogenesis, and promoting collagen synthesis, (Zeng et al., 2022). However, despite their efficacy, the clinical application of herbal therapies is often limited due to poor solubility, instability under physiological conditions, and rapid metabolism or clearance from the wound environment. Nanotechnology offers a highly effective solution to these limitations. By encapsulating or incorporating herbal extracts into nanoscale delivery systems—including nanoparticles, nanofibers, liposomes, nanogels, and nanocomposites—it becomes possible to protect bioactive compounds from degradation, enhance their solubility, control their release over time, and target them directly to the wound site.(Li et al., 2018) These advanced delivery mechanisms improve the bioavailability of herbal compounds and enable a more consistent, effective therapeutic response in chronic wound environments. and pro-angiogenic—is particularly beneficial in chronic wounds that are marked by tissue hypoxia and insufficient blood supply. membranes, inhibit quorum sensing, and prevent biofilm maturation—critical actions in managing infected chronic wounds like *Centella asiatica*, *Aloe vera*, or *Moringa oleifera*, these nanofibers deliver both structural support and continuous therapeutic exposure. For instance, (Ma et al., 2019) *Centella asiatica*-loaded nanofibers have shown enhanced fibroblast activity and faster epithelial regeneration in preclinical studies.

The ability to tailor fiber diameter, porosity, and drug loading makes nanofibers ideal for adapting to different wound conditions and healing stages effects, along with controlled release properties.(Zhao et al., 2023) These gels can be directly applied to wound beds, filling irregular wound cavities and forming a moist, bioactive interface that supports healing and reduces pain. release of active ingredients, providing a more predictable and sustained therapeutic profile. Another study demonstrated the efficacy of an *Aloe vera*-silver nanoparticle composite dressing in managing pressure ulcers, with patients reporting reduced pain and faster healing times. However, the widespread adoption of these therapies still faces challenges. (Madgule et al., 2023). These include the standardization of herbal extracts (which can vary by region, season, and preparation method), the complexity of nanoparticle synthesis and scale-up, regulatory hurdles, and the need for robust clinical trials to confirm safety and efficacy. Ensuring product consistency, reproducibility, and cost-effectiveness is critical for successful commercialization and integration into mainstream wound care protocols. Future directions in this field include the development of personalized and precision medicine approaches, where nano-herbal therapies are tailored based on patient-specific wound characteristics, microbiome profiles, and genetic markers. Advances in wearable sensors and smart bandage technologies may also be integrated with nano-herbal dressings to provide real-time monitoring of wound healing, drug release, and infection

HERBAL-BASED WOUND CARE PRODUCTS WITH NANOTECHNOLOGY

The integration of nanotechnology with herbal medicine has led to transformative advancements in wound care, particularly for chronic and hard-to-heal wounds. As the limitations of conventional treatments have become more evident—especially in managing infections, inflammation, and impaired healing—researchers and clinicians have turned to nanotechnology-enhanced herbal formulations for more effective, safer, and holistic solutions. These novel systems have not only demonstrated remarkable preclinical efficacy but have also progressed into clinical trials and real-world applications, (Purohit et al., 2020) where they have shown tangible improvements in healing outcomes, patient satisfaction, and healthcare cost reduction. The following case studies and success stories underscore the significant impact of this innovative therapeutic approach. A Phase II randomized clinical trial conducted in India evaluated the effect of this nanoformulation on patients with diabetic foot ulcers (DFUs). The study enrolled 60 patients with non-infected grade II ulcers. Half received standard care, while the other half received topical application of the curcumin nanoparticle gel once daily for four weeks. The nano-herbal therapy group exhibited significantly faster wound contraction, enhanced epithelialization, and reduced pain scores compared to the control group. Histological analysis revealed increased collagen deposition and neovascularization, confirming the regenerative effects of the treatment. Notably, no adverse effects were reported, highlighting the safety of the formulation. This case stands as a landmark example of how nanotechnology can overcome herbal medicine's delivery limitations and achieve clinical relevance. The resulting nanoformulation was incorporated into a hydrogel and used to treat infected chronic wounds in patients with post-surgical complications.

In a small observational study involving 12 patients, daily application of the neem-AgNP hydrogel resulted in significant bacterial load reduction within one week, including eradication of *Staphylococcus aureus* and *Escherichia coli*. Complete wound closure was achieved in an average of 18 days, compared to the typical 30–40 days with conventional treatment. Patients reported reduced odor, inflammation, and discomfort. This success story not only highlights the synergistic effects of combining herbal extracts with nanometals but also showcases the scalability and sustainability of green nanotechnology. *Aloe vera* is a well-established herbal remedy used for treating burns due to its cooling, hydrating, and regenerative properties. These results suggest that herbal nanofiber systems may be superior alternatives to synthetic topical antimicrobials in burn care*Centella asiatica* is rich in triterpenoids likeasiaticoside and madecassoside, compounds that stimulate fibroblast proliferation, collagen synthesis, reduction in wound area, compared to 40% in the control group receiving standard hydrocolloid dressings. Furthermore, the smart nanogel responded to the slightly alkaline pH of chronic wounds by enhancing release of the active compound precisely when needed. Patients tolerated the treatment well, with no allergic reactions or adverse skin responses reported, (Raja and Fathima, 2018) This case demonstrates how smart nanotechnology can improve herbal drug delivery in complex wound environments.

NANOTECHNOLOGY AND HERBAL-BASED WOUND CARE IN VETERINARY MEDICINE

The intersection of herbal medicine and nanotechnology in wound care represents an innovative approach aimed at overcoming the limitations of conventional wound healing treatments. the wound site, improving healing outcomes. While the benefits of these nano-enhanced herbal formulations are substantial, there are also certain limitations that must be carefully considered when developing these products. One of the primary challenges in using herbal extracts for wound healing is their poor solubility and bioavailability, especially for hydrophobic compounds such as curcumin, resveratrol, and many essential oils. Nanotechnology addresses this issue by encapsulating these herbal compounds into nanoparticles or nanostructured carriers that increase their solubility in aqueous environments, thus enhancing their absorption through the skin barrier and increasing their therapeutic concentration at the wound site. For instance, liposomes or dendrimer-based systems containing, (Ramakrishnan et al., 2022) herbal compounds like Centella asiatica or Aloe vera can be engineered to enhance drug retention and release in the affected tissue, promoting faster recovery. leading to suboptimal concentrations at the wound site or the need for frequent reapplication. Nanoparticles, nanofibers, and nanogels can be designed to release herbal actives over an extended period, providing consistent therapeutic effects with fewer applications. For example, hyaluronic acid-based nanogels containing herbal extracts like Calendula officinalis or Arnica montana provide sustained anti-inflammatory and antimicrobial activity, reducing the need for frequent dressing changes and ensuring that the wound remains continuously protected and treated Tea Tree Oil (*Melaleuca alternifolia*), have demonstrated superior antibacterial activity(Sugumaran et al., 2024), particularly against antibiotic-resistant bacteria such as *Staphylococcus aureus* and *Pseudomonas aeruginosa*. absorbed into the bloodstream. Moreover, biodegradable and biocompatible materials like chitosan or polymeric nanoparticles derived from natural sources ensure that the formulations are non-toxic, even with prolonged use. This is particularly important in managing sensitive populations such as the elderly, immunocompromised individuals, and children, for whom systemic toxicity or skin irritation can be a major concern use of nanoformulated gels, sprays, and dressings reduces the need for frequent applications and dressing changes, which can be painful and distressing for patients. Furthermore, (Sreenivasulu et al., 2022) the moisture-retentive properties of many nanoformulations help maintain an optimal wound environment, preventing desiccation and promoting faster healing.

THE CHALLENGES OF DEVELOPING NANOTECHNOLOGY-BASED HERBAL WOUND CARE PRODUCTS

Another promising application of nanotechnology is in the development of nanoemulsions or nanogels containing herbal extracts. These can be used in topical formulations that provide enhanced penetration into the skin and wound tissue. For instance, nanoemulsions containing antimicrobial herbal compounds like Tea Tree Oil (*Melaleuca alternifolia*) or Turmeric (*Curcuma longa*) have shown efficacy in reducing infection and inflammation in animal wounds. Nanofibers, particularly those made from biodegradable materials such as chitosan or collagen, are also gaining attention as wound dressings. These nanofibers can mimic the extracellular matrix, providing a scaffold for tissue regeneration while simultaneously releasing healing agents like Aloe Vera or Centella Asiatica (gotu kola)In veterinary applications, the combination of herbal medicine and nanotechnology offers numerous advantages, such as reduced application frequency, enhanced healing speeds, and better management of chronic and infected wounds. For example, in the case of equine wounds, which are often difficult to treat due to the horse's movement, the use of herbal-based nanocomposite dressings allows for targeted delivery of active agents that can reduce inflammation, prevent infection, and promote healing, all while minimizing the need for frequent changes of dressings. Nanoparticles containing neem oil (known for its antifungal and antibacterial properties) and honey (with natural antimicrobial and healing properties) can be used in a topical gel or ointment to treat skin abrasions, lacerations, or infected wounds in animals. Applications in Veterinary Medicine:hoof abscesses, and pressure sores. Traditional treatments for these types of wounds may be slow to promote healing, with horses requiring prolonged treatment regimens.

Nanoformulations of herbal extracts such as Aloe Vera or Calendula, when used in conjunction with nanoparticle-based dressings, have shown enhanced healing properties. The nanotechnology allows these herbal agents to be released steadily over time, reducing the frequency of dressing changes and improving healing outcomes. A study conducted in equine veterinary care demonstrated that nanoparticle-incorporated Aloe Vera gel applied to chronic ulcers in horses promoted faster healing compared to traditional Aloe Vera-based creams. (Thakur et al., 2019). The nanoencapsulation of Aloe Vera ensured deeper penetration into the wound bed and provided a controlled release of active compounds, enhancing cellular regeneration and accelerating tissue repair. of Turmeric have shown promise in managing post-surgical wounds in dogs, significantly reducing inflammation and infection rates. Curcumin, the active compound in Turmeric, is known for its powerful anti-inflammatory properties. However, it is poorly absorbed through the skin. When encapsulated in polymeric nanoparticles, it is able to penetrate deeper into the wound bed and maintain therapeutic levels of the drug for a longer period, reducing the frequency of applications and improving patient comfort.-honey dressings were used in treating burn injuries in dogs. (Tracy et al., 2016). The nano-honey promoted antimicrobial activity while also accelerating the regeneration of epithelial tissue, reducing scar formation, and improving the overall healing process. Furthermore, the nanofiber scaffolds, designed to hold the herbal ingredients in place, allowed for more effective dressing and less discomfort during recovery.

THE OPPORTUNITIES OF NANOTECHNOLOGY IN HERBAL-BASED WOUND CARE

However, the development of nanotechnology-based herbal wound care products faces several significant challenges, including regulatory hurdles, manufacturing difficulties, scalability issues, toxicological concerns, and the variability of herbal extracts. These challenges must be addressed before these products can be successfully commercialized and widely adopted in clinical practice. This section delves into these critical obstacles, exploring the regulatory, scientific, and practical barriers that need to be overcome in the creation of effective and safe nano-enhanced herbal wound care formulations. are still in the early stages and often lack the specificity required for safe and efficient market introduction. nanomaterials in medicines and devices, these regulations often do not account for the unique characteristics and behaviors of nano-herbal formulations. For example, nanomaterials in the accepted framework to evaluate the synergy between nanotechnology and herbal ingredients, which complicates the regulatory approval process.erm safety evaluations are necessary to address these concerns, which can be time-consuming and costly. difficult. Moreover, the standardization of herbal extracts for use in combination with nanomaterials is essential to guarantee that each batch of the product delivers the same therapeutic effect, which adds another layer of complexity.-scale manufacturing without compromising the quality, consistency, and cost-effectiveness of the products is one of the most significant challenges in this fieldignificantly. (Velnar and Bailey, 2009). This could make nano-herbal wound care products prohibitively expensive, especially when compared to traditional wound care treatments is particularly critical when the active herbal ingredients are incorporated into the formulation, as variability in the concentration of the herbal extract can lead to inconsistent therapeutic outcomes. This issue is exacerbated by the inherent variability in herbal extracts, which adds another layer of complexity to the manufacturing process, (Veith et al., 2019) Furthermore, the need for good manufacturing practices (GMP), stringent quality control protocols, and clinical trials to demonstrate the efficacy and safety of the final product adds to the financial burden. The overall cost of developing, manufacturing, and bringing a nano-herbal wound care product to market can be substantial, which may limit its accessibility, particularly in resource-constrained settings. Ensuring the biocompatibility of nanoformulations is crucial, especially when the product is used in sensitive populations such as infants, the elderly, or patients with compromised immune systems.

RECOMMENDATIONS FOR FUTURE RESEARCH AND DEVELOPMENT

As we conclude our exploration of nanotechnology in herbal-based wound care, it is clear that this innovative intersection of nanoscience and traditional herbal medicine holds tremendous promise for transforming the landscape of wound management. The combination of nanomaterials with bioactive herbal compounds offers an exciting array of opportunities to overcome the limitations of conventional wound care treatments and provide more effective, efficient, and personalized solutions for patients across diverse medical settings.(Vijayakumar et al., 2024) The convergence of these two powerful fields is not only revolutionizing how we approach wound healing but also creating a paradigm shift in the way we view drug delivery, patient outcomes, and overall healthcare improvement. absorption of herbal active ingredients. This ability to enhance the bioavailability of key herbal bioactives is particularly important for chronic wounds, where inflammation and infection often delay healing processes. Moreover, nano-engineered scaffolds made from biocompatible materials such as collagen or chitosan, when combined with herbal extracts that stimulate collagen synthesis (like Centella Asiatica) or promote angiogenesis (like green tea), can support the regeneration of tissue and the formation of new blood vessels. Nanofibrous scaffolds, in particular, create a 3D(Wang et al., 2015). Nanotechnology allows these compounds to be delivered effectively to the wound site, ensuring their continuous therapeutic action over extended periods. The controlled release of herbal agents also enables better management of chronic wounds by reducing the frequency of application and improving patient adherence to treatment regimens. personalized wound care, addressing a wide range of wound types, including those associated with chronic conditions, diabetes, vascular insufficiencies, and trauma. fungi, and viruses, and their combination with herbal antimicrobial agents can provide an enhanced, broad-spectrum solution to infection, (Walkey et al., 2015). With nanoparticles, however, it is possible to design formulations that are capable of delivering herbal compounds directly to specific areas of the wound or even targeting particular cellular receptors involved in the healing process. By functionalizing nanoparticles with ligands or antibodies, nanotechnology can facilitate precise targeting of damaged tissue, ensuring that bioactive herbal molecules are delivered where they are needed most, thus improving the efficiency of the healing process and minimizing the risks of systemic side effects.

CONCLUSION

This ability to tailor treatments to the specific needs of an individual patient opens the door to more personalized, effective care, especially for complex or chronic wounds that are difficult to manage with standard treatments. By nano-encapsulating or nano-formulating these compounds, their therapeutic efficacy is enhanced, and their ability to work together in combination therapies can be better exploited. The use of nanoparticles to combine multiple herbal extracts in a single formulation creates a synergistic effect, where the combined therapeutic properties of the ingredients enhance the wound-healing process. For example, the combination of nano-silver, with its potent antimicrobial effects, and herbal bioactives like aloe vera or turmeric, which provide anti-inflammatory and collagen-boosting properties, creates a dual-action product that addresses both the infection and healing aspects of wound care simultaneously. This synergistic antimicrobial effect is invaluable in reducing the incidence of wound infection, which remains one of the most common complications in wound care, particularly for patients with immunocompromised conditions. These bioactive nanomaterials could be especially valuable for treating complex, non-healing wounds that result from vascular issues, diabetes, or pressure ulcers, applications of topical treatments, which can be inconvenient, painful, and disruptive to the patient's daily life. With nanotechnology, smart dressings and nanoformulations can release active ingredients over a longer duration, reducing the need for frequent changes. Nanoparticle-based dressings can offer both moisture retention and antimicrobial protection, while also maintaining biocompatibility with the skin, which can significantly enhance comfort for patients with chronic wounds or sensitive skin wound's status, adjusting the release of herbal compounds based on environmental changes (e.g., changes in pH, temperature, or infection markers). This level of precision ensures that the wound receives the appropriate treatment without unnecessary intervention, leading to a more comfortable and efficient healing experience for the patient. This is particularly valuable in elderly patients or those with limited mobility, where ease of application and fewer dressing changes can significantly improve quality of life. In addition to reducing treatment costs, nanotechnology-enhanced herbal wound care products could also improve accessibility. As manufacturing costs decrease, these advanced wound care solutions could become more widely available to healthcare providers and patients, especially in resource-limited settings. This accessibility is critical, as chronic wounds often affect the most vulnerable populations, including the elderly, those with diabetes, and individuals living in developing regions with limited access to modern healthcare infrastructure. In conclusion, the future of nanotechnology in herbal-based wound care holds transformative potential for improving the efficacy, safety, and accessibility of wound healing treatments.

REFERENCES

Augustine, R., Hasan, A., Patan, N. K., Dalvi, Y. B., Varghese, R., & Antony, A.. (2020). Cerium oxide nanoparticle incorporated electrospun poly(3-hydroxybutyrate-Co-3-Hydroxyvalerate) membranes for diabetic wound healing applications. *ACS Biomaterials Science & Engineering*, *6*, 58–70. DOI: 10.1021/acsbiomaterials.8b01352 PMID: 33463234

Augustine, R., Zahid, A. A., Hasan, A., Dalvi, Y. B., & Jacob, J. (2021). Cerium oxide nanoparticle-loaded gelatin methacryloyl hydrogel wound-healing patch with free radical scavenging activity. *ACS Biomaterials Science & Engineering*, *7*, 279–290. DOI: 10.1021/acsbiomaterials.0c01138 PMID: 33320529

Babenko, L. P., Zholobak, N. M., Shcherbakov, A. B., Voychuk, S. I., Lazarenko, L. M., & Spivak, M. Y. (2012). Antibacterial activity of cerium colloids against opportunistic microorganisms in vitro. *Mikrobiolohichnyi Zhurnal (Kiev, Ukraine)*, *74*, 54–62. PMID: 22830198

Bai, Q., Han, K., Dong, K., Zheng, C., Zhang, Y., & Long, Q.. (2020). Potential applications of nanomaterials and technology for diabetic wound healing. *International Journal of Nanomedicine*, *15*, 9717–9743. DOI: 10.2147/ijn.s276001 PMID: 33299313

Cheng, Y., Chang, Y., Feng, Y., Jian, H., Wu, X., & Zheng, R.. (2019). Hierarchical acceleration of wound healing through intelligent nanosystem to promote multiple stages. *ACS Applied Materials & Interfaces*, *11*(37), 33725–33733. DOI: 10.1021/acsami.9b13267 PMID: 31449386

Chigurupati, S., Mughal, M. R., Okun, E., Das, S., Kumar, A., & McCaffery, M.. (2013). Effects of cerium oxide nanoparticles on the growth of keratinocytes, fibroblasts and vascular endothelial cells in cutaneous wound healing. *Biomaterials*, *34*(9), 2194–2201. DOI: 10.1016/j.biomaterials.2012.11.061 PMID: 23266256

Clark, A., Zhu, A., Sun, K., & Petty, H. R. (2011). Cerium oxide and platinum nanoparticles protect cells from oxidant-mediated apoptosis. *Journal of Nanoparticle Research*, *13*, 5547. DOI: 10.1007/s11051-011-0544-3 PMID: 22039334

Damle, M. A., Jakhade, A. P., & Chikate, R. C. (2019). Modulating pro- and antioxidant activities of nanoengineered cerium dioxide nanoparticles against Escherichia coli. *ACS Omega*, *4*, 3761–3771. DOI: 10.1021/acsomega.8b03109

Darby, I. A., Laverdet, B., Bonté, F., & Desmoulière, A. (2014). Fibroblasts and myofibroblasts in wound healing. *Clinical, Cosmetic and Investigational Dermatology*, *7*, 301–311. DOI: 10.2147/CCID.S50046 PMID: 25395868

Ellis, S., Lin, E. J., & Tartar, D. (2018). Immunology of wound healing. *Current Dermatology Reports*, *7*, 350–358. DOI: 10.1007/s13671-018-0234-9 PMID: 30524911

Eriksson, P., Tal, A. A., Skallberg, A., Brommesson, C., Hu, Z., & Boyd, R. D.. (2018). Cerium oxide nanoparticles with antioxidant capabilities and gadolinium integration for MRI contrast enhancement. *Scientific Reports*, *8*, 6999. DOI: 10.1038/s41598-018-25390-z PMID: 29725117

Fisichella, M., Berenguer, F., Steinmetz, G., Auffan, M., Rose, J., & Prat, O. (2014). Toxicity evaluation of manufactured CeO2 nanoparticles before and after alteration: Combined physicochemical and whole-genome expression analysis in Caco-2 cells. *BMC Genomics*, *15*(1), 700. DOI: 10.1186/1471-2164-15-700 PMID: 25145350

Futosi, K., Fodor, S., & Mócsai, A. (2013). Neutrophil cell surface receptors and their intracellular signal transduction pathways. *International Immunopharmacology*, *17*, 638–650. DOI: 10.1016/j.intimp.2013.06.034 PMID: 23994464

Gabbiani, G. (2003). The myofibroblast in wound healing and fibrocontractive diseases. *The Journal of Pathology*, *200*, 500–503. DOI: 10.1002/path.1427 PMID: 12845617

Hirst, S. M., Karakoti, A. S., Tyler, R. D., Sriranganathan, N., Seal, S., & Reilly, C. M. (2009). Anti-inflammatory properties of cerium oxide nanoparticles. *Small*, *5*(24), 2848–2856. DOI: 10.1002/smll.200901048 PMID: 19802857

Hosseini, M., Amjadi, I., Mohajeri, M., & Mozafari, M. (2020). Sol-gel synthesis, physico-chemical and biological characterization of cerium oxide/polyallylamine nanoparticles. *Polymers*, *12*(7), 1444. DOI: 10.3390/polym12071444 PMID: 32605197

Ilina, O., & Friedl, P. (2009). Mechanisms of collective cell migration at a glance. *Journal of Cell Science*, *122*, 3203–3208. DOI: 10.1242/jcs.036525 PMID: 19726629

Ji, Z., Wang, X., Zhang, H., Lin, S., Meng, H., & Sun, B.. (2012). Designed synthesis of CeO2 nanorods and nanowires for studying toxicological effects of high aspect ratio nanomaterials. *ACS Nano*, *6*(6), 5366–5380. DOI: 10.1021/nn3012114 PMID: 22564147

Johnson, K. E., & Wilgus, T. A. (2014). Vascular endothelial growth factor and angiogenesis in the regulation of cutaneous wound repair. *Advances in Wound Care (New Rochelle, N.Y.)*, *3*, 647–661. DOI: 10.1089/wound.2013.0517 PMID: 25302139

Kaarniranta, K., Pawlowska, E., Szczepanska, J., Jablkowska, A., & Blasiak, J. (2019). Role of mitochondrial DNA damage in ROS-mediated pathogenesis of age-related macular degeneration (AMD). *International Journal of Molecular Sciences*, *20*, 2374. DOI: 10.3390/ijms20102374 PMID: 31091656

Kamalipooya, S., Fahimirad, S., Abtahi, H., Golmohammadi, M., Satari, M., & Dadashpour, M.. (2024). Diabetic wound healing function of PCL/cellulose acetate nanofiber engineered with chitosan/cerium oxide nanoparticles. *International Journal of Pharmaceutics*, *653*, 123880. DOI: 10.1016/j.ijpharm.2024.123880 PMID: 38350498

Li, J., Wang, X., Yao, Z., Yuan, F., Liu, H., & Sun, Z.. (2023). NLRP3-Dependent crosstalk between pyroptotic macrophage and senescent cell orchestrates trauma-induced heterotopic ossification during aberrant wound healing. *Advanced Science (Weinheim, Baden-Wurttemberg, Germany)*, *10*(19), e2207383. DOI: 10.1002/advs.202207383 PMID: 37204068

Li, J. H., Wen, J., Li, B., Li, W., Qiao, W., & Shen, J.. (2018). Valence state manipulation of cerium oxide nanoparticles on a titanium surface for modulating cell fate and bone formation. *Advanced Science (Weinheim, Baden-Wurttemberg, Germany)*, *5*(2), 1700678. DOI: 10.1002/advs.201700678 PMID: 29610729

Ma, X., Cheng, Y., Jian, H., Feng, Y., Chang, Y., & Zheng, R.. (2019). Hollow, rough, and nitric oxide-releasing cerium oxide nanoparticles for promoting multiple stages of wound healing. *Advanced Healthcare Materials*, *8*(16), e1900256. DOI: 10.1002/adhm.201900256 PMID: 31290270

Madgule, M., Vinayaka, N., Sonkhaskar, Y. M., Patel, D. R., Karthikeyan, R., & Selvakumar, P. (2023). Mechanical properties and microstructure of activated TIG welded similar joints of Inconel alloys by desirability approaches. *Materials Today: Proceedings*, *77*, 528–533.

Purohit, S. D., Singh, H., Bhaskar, R., Yadav, I., Chou, C.-F., & Gupta, M. K.. (2020). Gelatin—alginate—cerium oxide nanocomposite scaffold for bone regeneration. *Materials Science and Engineering C*, *116*, 111111. DOI: 10.1016/j.msec.2020.111111 PMID: 32806319

Raja, I. S., & Fathima, N. N. (2018). Gelatin-cerium oxide nanocomposite for enhanced excisional wound healing. *ACS Applied Bio Materials*, *1*(2), 487–495. DOI: 10.1021/acsabm.8b00208 PMID: 35016389

Ramakrishnan, T., Mohan Gift, M. D., Chitradevi, S., Jegan, R., & Subha Hency Jose, P. Nagaraja, Rajneesh Sharma H.N., Selvakumar P., Sintayehu Mekuria Hailegiorgis, (2022). "Study of Numerous Resins Used in Polymer Matrix Composite Materials", Advances in Materials Science and Engineering, vol. 2022, Article ID 1088926, 8 pages, 2022. https://doi.org/DOI: 10.1155/2022/1088926

Sreenivasulu, A., & Manimozhi, T. Satheesh kumar P., Selvakumar P. and Singh P.,(2022). "The Model of Smart Sensing Device For Sensitive Nanoclusters Modification in Sensing Properties," 2022 2nd International Conference on Advance Computing and Innovative Technologies in Engineering (ICACITE), Greater Noida, India, 2022, pp. 1043-1047, doi: DOI: 10.1109/ICACITE53722.2022.9823846

Sugumaran, K. M. D., Pandiyarajan V., Y. B S, Selvakumar P. and M. S, (2024). "Analysis of Electromyography Signals for Control of Mechanical Prosthesis using Machine Learning Techniques," 2024 2nd International Conference on Intelligent Data Communication Technologies and Internet of Things (IDCIoT), Bengaluru, India, 2024, pp. 1059-1067, doi: DOI: 10.1109/IDCIoT59759.2024.10467707

Thakur, N., Manna, P., & Das, J. (2019). Synthesis and biomedical applications of nanoceria, a redox active nanoparticle. *Journal of Nanobiotechnology*, *17*(1), 84. DOI: 10.1186/s12951-019-0516-9 PMID: 31291944

Tracy, L. E., Minasian, R. A., & Caterson, E. J. (2016). Extracellular matrix and dermal fibroblast function in the healing wound. *Advances in Wound Care (New Rochelle, N.Y.)*, *5*, 119–136. DOI: 10.1089/wound.2014.0561 PMID: 26989578

Veith, A. P., Henderson, K., Spencer, A., Sligar, A. D., & Baker, A. B. (2019). Therapeutic strategies for enhancing angiogenesis in wound healing. *Advanced Drug Delivery Reviews*, *146*, 97–125. DOI: 10.1016/j.addr.2018.09.010 PMID: 30267742

Velnar, T., & Bailey, T. (2009). The wound healing process: An overview of the cellular and molecular mechanisms. *The Journal of International Medical Research*, *37*, 1528–1542. DOI: 10.1177/147323000903700531 PMID: 19930861

Vijayakumar, G., Rajkumar, M., Chandar, N. R., Selvakumar, P., & Duraisamy, R. (2024). Environmentally friendly TDS removal from waste water by electrochemical ion exchange batch-type recirculation (EIR) technique. *Environmental Science. Water Research & Technology*, *10*(4), 826–835.

Walkey, C., Das, S., Seal, S., Erlichman, J., Heckman, K., & Ghibelli, L.. (2015). Catalytic properties and biomedical applications of cerium oxide nanoparticles. *Environmental Science. Nano*, *2*(1), 33–53. DOI: 10.1039/c4en00138a PMID: 26207185

Wang, L., Ai, W., Zhai, Y., Li, H., Zhou, K., & Chen, H. (2015). Effects of nano-CeO with different nanocrystal morphologies on cytotoxicity in HepG2 cells. *International Journal of Environmental Research and Public Health, 12*(9), 10806–10819. DOI: 10.3390/ijerph120910806 PMID: 26404340

Xue, Y., Yang, F., Wu, L., Xia, D., & Liu, Y. (2024). CeO2 nanoparticles to promote wound healing: A systematic review. *Advanced Healthcare Materials, 13*(6), e2302858. DOI: 10.1002/adhm.202302858 PMID: 37947125

Yang, B. Y., Zhou, Z. Y., Liu, S. Y., Shi, M. J., Liu, X. J., & Cheng, T. M.. (2022). Porous Se@SiO2 nanoparticles enhance wound healing by ROS-PI3K/akt pathway in dermal fibroblasts and reduce scar formation. *Frontiers in Bioengineering and Biotechnology, 10*, 852482. DOI: 10.3389/fbioe.2022.852482 PMID: 35387298

Yildizbakan, L., Iqbal, N., Ganguly, P., Kumi-Barimah, E., Do, T., & Jones, E.. (2023). Fabrication and characterisation of the cytotoxic and antibacterial properties of chitosan-cerium oxide porous scaffolds. *Antibiotics (Basel, Switzerland), 12*(6), 1004. DOI: 10.3390/antibiotics12061004 PMID: 37370323

Zeng, Q., Qi, X., Shi, G., Zhang, M., & Haick, H. (2022). Wound dressing: From nanomaterials to diagnostic dressings and healing evaluations. *ACS Nano, 16*(2), 1708–1733. DOI: 10.1021/acsnano.1c0841 PMID: 35050565

Zhao, R., Zhao, C., Wan, Y., Majid, M., Abbas, S. Q., & Wang, Y. (2023). In vitro and in vivo evaluation of alginate hydrogel-based wound dressing loaded with green chemistry cerium oxide nanoparticles. *Frontiers in Chemistry, 11*, 1298808. DOI: 10.3389/fchem.2023.1298808 PMID: 38075491

Chapter 12
Case Studies of Successful Herbal-Based Wound Formulation:
Wound Healing

Ekata Prajapati
https://orcid.org/0009-0002-1920-2035
Oriental University, Russia

ABSTRACT

The process of wound healing involves a number of biochemical processes. Utilizing herbal remedies for wound healing serves to preserve the knowledge of traditional medicine, given its immune-regulating and anti-inflammatory properties, while also aligning with advancements in contemporary biopharmaceutical technology, including the development of innovative biomaterials like hydrogels. Initially, this article presents the innate structural features of healthy skin and the physiological traits associated with chronic wounds in individuals suffering from diabetes and burns. The article goes on to explore the most recent progress in both clinical and experimental research regarding the effects of active constituents in herbal medicine on wound tissue regeneration. It also summarizes current studies investigating the mechanisms of different herbal medicines in healing diabetic and burn wounds. Disruptions in skin integrity contribute to its disorientation, while tissue annihilations lead to the formation of acute or chronic wounds.

DOI: 10.4018/979-8-3373-3977-1.ch012

INTRODUCTION

Acute wound healing occurs through the seamless advancement through four overlapping phases: haemostasis, inflammation, proliferation, and remodeling; every phase is marked by the arrival at the wound site of particular types of cells, which all interact and communicate through chemical signals to enhance repair, (Albahri et al., 2023). Unlike acute healing, chronic wounds necessitate a lengthy healing period, do not heal at all, or happen to recur often. These injuries usually arise when the typical wound healing process is disrupted, such as due to infection, metabolic issues, or an underlying condition. Pressure ulcers, venous leg ulcers, and diabetic ulcers are the most common examples, all marked by a relative inability to generate new tissue, (Mukherjee et al., 2003; Budovsky, Yarmolinsky, & Ben-Shabat, 2015). Impaired healing incurs significant societal costs and reduces the quality of life for millions globally. Consequently, there has been a recent focus on exploring alternative therapeutic strategies that are both cost-effective and accessible. Traditional medicine, practiced for hundreds of years in Africa and Asia, is undergoing scientific examination to assess its potential for treating wounds and related ailments, (Krishnan, 2006; Gendrisch et al., 2021). Most of these studies have utilized in vitro models involving fibroblasts, keratinocytes, and endothelial cells to represent the different phases. 5 A recent review of such studies acknowledged that, although the in vitro approach has its advantages, the pharmacological validation of herbal medicines ultimately relies on demonstrable effects in animals and humans, (Lone et al., 2012). The only traditional herbal remedy for wound healing that has undergone a range of studies involving cell cultures, animals, and humans is aloe vera. The herb is a cactus-like species that thrives in hot and dry environments, (Olisova et al., 2018). The gel extracted from the mucilaginous tissue at the center of the aloe vera leaf has been used for therapeutic purposes for hundreds of years and is the primary component in commercial products, (Huemer et al., 2020). Describing the scientific methodologies applied to Aloe vera as a way of exemplifying the study of herbal medicines for wound healing was considered worthwhile. Herbal treatments and the plant materials used to create them account for a considerable share of the worldwide medicinal market. Medicinal plants and pharmaceuticals have had a major part in the treatment of illnesses across human history. A vast body of literature exists regarding their healing properties; however, there are no established protocols for quality control of plant materials concerning their identification (phytochemical, pharmacological, and therapeutic activity). To guarantee their reliability and therapeutic efficacy, medicinal plants must be standardized. To assess their therapeutic efficacy and pharmacological action for authenticity verification, herbal products are examined for their identity (characterization), quality, and the quality of the extracts they contain. Herbal medicines can treat and cure ailments such as ulcers, wound healing issues, skin infections, inflammation, scabies, leprosy, and venereal diseases. Herbal remedies used in wound treatment or care involve disinfection, debridement, and creating a moist environment that promotes the development of suitable natural healing conditions. A considerable number of plants are used in folklore cultures to treat cuts, wounds, and burns.

A wound occurs when living tissue's cellular, anatomical, and functional integrity is compromised by physical, chemical, electrical, or microbial threats. Wound healing is a multifaceted process that involves either the regeneration or reconstruction of damaged tissue. Burns and wounds can result in a loss of many productive hours and be one of the main causes of physical incapacity. In essence, wounds occur when the anatomical structure and functional continuity of cells and tissues at the sites of injury are disrupted. They may be brought on by physical, chemical, microbiological, or immunological insults to the tissue. Over 80 percent of the 14 million persons who are thought to get burns and wounds each year reside in low- and middle-income nations . However, since wounds are common and can happen to anyone at any moment, and because individuals do not always seek medical attention for minor burns and wounds, this may go unreported. Age, dessication, necrosis, pressure at the wound site, body type (e.g., obesity), chronic diseases (e.g., diabetes mellitus, cancer, peripheral vascular disease, etc.), immunosuppression, nutritional status, vascular insufficiency, and infection with microbes like bacteria can all slow down or impair the aforementioned capabilities. Thus, intervention in the form of treatment is required. Antimicrobial medicines, such as Neomycin Sulphate (NS) cream and Silver Sulfadiazine (SSD) cream, are extensively used to treat burns and wounds in Uganda, (Lone et al., 2012). Although it hasn't been documented as standard procedure, our clinical practice observations indicate that utilizing metronidazole powder or intravenous solutions to treat burns and wounds is standard procedure at Mulago Hospital. A vital component of healthcare is traditional medicine. According to the WHO Traditional Medicine Strategy 2002–2005, one study states One major factor contributing to TCAM's broad adoption is the high per capita distribution of TCAM practitioners in developing nations. The WHO study uses Uganda, Tanzania, and Zambia as examples, where the population to healer ratio is between 1200 and 1400, and the allopathic practitioner to population ratio is 1:20,000, (Olisova et al., 2018). A recent source reports that these percentages remain unchanged, (Huemer et al., 2020). Furthermore, it is believed that 60% of Uganda's healthcare system uses traditional medicine, (Huemer et al., 2020). Traditional medicine is practiced all across the world and is becoming increasingly significant economically. Wounds heal more quickly when treated with herbal remedies because they increase collagen concentration and fibro-genetics, (Krishnan, 2006). We developed a polyherbal topical preparation with extracts from Aloe barbadensis and Bidens pilosa and evaluated its wound-healing capacity on experimentally induced cutaneous wounds in rat models due to the increasing popularity of natural and herbal medications, their easy accessibility of raw materials, their affordability, and the rarity of reported adverse reactions. Aloe barbadensis (Liliaceae), commonly referred to as aloe vera, possesses analgesic, antibacterial, and anti-inflammatory qualities that make it a valuable tool for wound care. It is indigenous to the Canary Islands, southern Europe's Mediterranean region, and North Africa, (Saraswathy et al., n.d.). This resilient perennial semi-tropical plant can also flourish in regions that are prone to drought, (Gopinath et al., 2004). One of the biggest issues facing the globe today is wound care, and infections linked to wounds have a big effect on the global healthcare economy. Acute or chronic wounds, diabetes, trauma, burns, minor cuts, bruises, rashes, etc., can all be considered. Using appropriate dressing materials to cover the wound and hasten the healing process is one of the main therapeutic options available for these disorders. Archaeological ideas suggest that medicinal herbs and oils have been used to cure wounds from prehistoric times. Researchers worldwide are currently concentrating their efforts on creating innovative dressing materials that can offer the best possible care, facilitate nutrition exchange, and absorb wound exudate. They offer the perfect environment for the healing process since they include a variety of bioactive substances that can influence the different stages of the wound healing process. The several methods used to prepare dressing materials containing phytoconstituents or extracts obtained from plants are covered in the current review. The healing process and wound-healing compounds made from medicinal herbs and oils are also discussed in this review. Researchers in this field can use the review as a database to help them choose the best dressing material for the efficient administration of herbal medications in wound care.

Diabetics are more susceptible to infections and other consequences because their wounds may take longer to heal. Diabetic foot ulcers, a serious side effect of diabetes mellitus, are the most prevalent sores in diabetic individuals. The annual cost of treating these wounds, including pain and infection control, is $18.7 billion in the US alone. Amputation may be necessary for infected lesions if they are not appropriately treated. The necessity to create methods to hasten the healing of diabetic foot ulcers is highlighted by the high expense of wound treatment and the severe outcomes if left untreated. Extracted from the rubber tree, Hevea brasiliensis, natural rubber latex (NRL) has been used extensively as a vehicle for a number of pharmacologically active substances. Moreover, it has been demonstrated to promote angiogenesis and aid cells adhere. Because it supplies the nutrients, proteins, cells, and environment needed for regeneration, exudate production is crucial to wound healing. Despite its advantages, excessive exudate must be managed to prevent lesion formation, maceration of the wound margins, and protracted healing brought on by dermatitis. We sought to control humidity by absorbing excess exudate and enhancing water vapor transport in order to address the issue of excessive exudate release brought on by the application of NRL membranes. We created a permeable, alginate-loaded NRL dressing that is highly absorbent. NRL membranes swelled up to 80 times when alginate was added, absorbing 4.80 g of water for every gram of dry membrane. Furthermore, the material conveyed 480% more water vapor than pure NRL membranes, significantly improving water vapor transmission. Keratinocytes multiply ten times more quickly than they should in psoriasis, a condition that causes persistent inflammation and immune cell infiltration in the skin. Because aloe vera (A. vera) creams include a number of antioxidant species, they have been used topically to treat psoriasis; however, they have a number of drawbacks. By encouraging cell division, neoangiogenesis, and the production of extracellular matrix, natural rubber latex (NRL) has been utilized as an occlusive dressing to aid in wound healing. In order to load A. vera into NRL, we created a new A. vera-releasing NRL dressing in this work using a solvent casting technique. There were no covalent interactions between A. vera and NRL in the dressing, according to FTIR and rheological analyses. After four days, we noticed that 58.8% of the loaded A. vera that was inside the dressing and on the surface had been discharged. Hemocompatibility and biocompatibility were confirmed in vitro using sheep blood and human skin fibroblasts, respectively. The overall phenolic concentration was 2.31 times higher than NRL alone, and we found that almost 70% of A. vera's free antioxidant qualities were retained. In conclusion, we developed a novel occlusive dressing that may be indicated for the easy and affordable control and/or treatment of psoriasis symptoms by combining the antipsoriatic qualities of A. vera with the healing activity of NRL. Creating a glycerol antimicrobial peptide natural latex film (NRL-GI-AMP film) to treat skin wound infections was the goal of this project. This study examines how the physical and chemical characteristics of natural latex (NRL) are affected by the addition of glycerol (GI) and an antimicrobial peptide (AMP). It also examines the cytocompatibility, bacteriostatic activity, and infected wound healing promotion of the NRL-GI-AMP film. The findings demonstrated that while the addition of G(LLKK)3L AMP did not alter the structure or characteristics of the NRL film, the addition of GI increased the number of pores in the internal structure of the film. in contrast to the NRL movie.

BACKGROUND

The usual methods for curing wounds in humans or animals, as is well-known in the prior art, involve certain clearly specified steps. The methods involved are curettage (elimination of infected/dead tissue), disinfection (using disinfectants with hydrogen peroxide or iodine) and antibiotic treatment (local or systemic, in the form of cream, spray or powder). Finally, to prevent skin hardening and crust formation, gauzes soaked in fatty humectants made from Vaseline, silicone oils, or glycerol are used. The wound is usually dressed with sterile gauze not only to protect it from exposure to infectious agents. In nations with aging demographics, such as the United States, patients with leg ulcers present significant challenges. Leg ulcers cause an estimated loss of 2 million workdays in the US. In addition to the loss of man-days, the expense involved in treating these non-healing wounds can have a tremendous impact. It is estimated that the prevalence of pressure ulcers (also known as pressure sores or bed sores) in the lower body among the elderly ranges from 3% to 11%. Pressure ulcers are linked to considerable morbidity and mortality. Patients with pressure ulcers have a death rate that is four times higher than that of those without. Moreover, the hospital mortality rate for septic elderly patients with pressure ulcers exceeds 50%. Treatment costs can be high due to the inclusion of intensive nursing care and adjunctive therapies. In diabetics, wounds are nearly impossible to manage and are typically viewed as incurable. Diabetes is, in fact, a significant underlying factor in leg ulcers. Diverse therapy. There are various methods for treating leg ulcers, such as multi-layer compression bandage systems, topical recombinant human platelet-derived growth factor, and human skin equivalents for skin grafting. These options may assist in the healing of wounds. Nonetheless, these treatments come with a high price tag and could be beyond one's financial means a lot of patients. It happens quite often that, due to wounds not being treated, the infected limbs have to be amputated. It is more difficult to manage wounds in animals. In contrast to humans, chances when wounds are exposed to environmental infestations, the risk for animals is significantly greater. Attacks by flies, particularly myiasigenic ones (sarcophagidae, cally phoridae) and others (muscidae), are of special concern as they can worsen wounds and cause complications. A common practice to prevent fly infestations in wounded animals is to pour creolina (a mixture of phenols and tar) on the wound. Whether in humans or animals, the healing and management of wounds presents significant challenges. Current therapies based on modern science have limitations regarding care and remedy for specific injuries. In animals, wounds and lesions present practical difficulties, particularly in the tropical heat and humidity when flies are especially active. Such circumstances impact wound care in people as well, particularly in developing nations where hygiene standards are frequently insufficient. The danger of complications arising from parasites, bacteria, and so on is a grim reality, particularly for weak and malnourished individuals, especially children. The present invention offers a new herbal composition that includes neem bark aqueous extracts combined with various herbs in a blend of natural oils. The formulation intended for external or topical use only, displays extraordinary antibiotic effects and wound-healing capabilities. Its effectiveness in treating and curing wounds is notable, especially considering that these are deemed incurable with current methods. The herbal formulation's effectiveness and strong antimicrobial action stem from the synergistic effects of its components, primarily plant extracts. The prior art describes several herbal formulations for wound healing and injuries. US patent application no. 2006/0134229 describes a herbal formulation comprising the organic extract from the Geum Japoni cum Thunb variant plant. The invention is specifically aimed at curing skeletal muscle injuries and facilitating soft tissue healing, rather than addressing wounds. The herbal composition disclosed in PCT application no. WO2005/115090A2 exhibits powerful antimicrobial effects and promotes wound healing. The composition features extracts of solely Ficus species and Azadirachta indica, formulated using a combination of aqueous and organic solvents with pharmaceutically acceptable carriers, excipients, and adjuvants. The bark of the respective plants is emphasized for use. No other components are added to the herbal formulation in the invention described.

INFECTION OF THE WOUND AND PAIN

Infection of the Wound

The presence of microorganisms, such as bacteria and fungus, can cause infection in the wounded areas and impair the host's natural immune system. Common bacterial causes of delayed wound healing include Streptococcus pyogenes, Staphylococcus aureus, Pseudomonas aeruginosa, and certain species of Clostridium. Hypoxia, ischemia, and immunological deficits (e.g., virus and chemotherapy) are other factors that contribute to wound infection. Neglected wound care can also eventually result in septicemia and bacteraemia-related deaths, (Apel et al., 2021). Microorganisms will grow on the surface of a wound in healthy people, but this does not cause the host immune system to react or cause any outward signs, (Chaudhary, Goyal, & Poonia, 2010). Unfortunately, a number of local and systemic reactions are set off when the wound colonizes the host's living tissues. Purulent drainage and clinical cellulitis may follow, which can further result in soft tissue damage. According to some reports, the increased microbial load on the wound site causes bacterial biofilms to form, which delays wound healing.

Wounds Pain

For damaged people to recuperate, pain management is essential. Because anxiety causes stress hormones to build up, excessive pain can impede the healing process, resulting in lengthy hospital stays and physical and mental strain, (Garcia-Orue et al., 2017). Because the pain process mostly depends on each patient's perspective, not what professionals think it should be, it is important to note that each patient's manifestation of pain must be addressed individually. Nociceptive pain and neuropathic pain are the two categories of wound pain. A normal physiological reaction to tissue injury is nociceptive discomfort. This kind of discomfort usually goes away after a certain amount of time, but the inflammatory reaction may persist if the healing process slows down. in this situation. In order to reduce local inflammation and modulate pain at the spinal cord level, non-steroidal anti-inflammatory drugs (NSAIDs) and mild opioids can be used in hospitals to treat primary hyperalgesia, which is heightened sensitivity to the wound and surrounding area brought on by prolonged inflammation or repeated stimuli. Wound dressings have two fundamental purposes. To stop infection, the first step is to cover the wound. By lowering the bacterial burden and, consequently, the inflammatory response to the neurological system, the second goal is to lessen wound pain. On the other hand, it may take a few days for oral treatment to significantly reduce pain.

Hemostasis, inflammation, proliferation, and remodeling are some of the phases that make up the intricate process of wound healing. The integrity and function of the skin depend on this dynamic and strictly controlled process. Chronic wounds are a major health burden that can result from disruptions in this process.

IMPORTANT PHASES OF WOUND HEALING

1. **Hemostasis:** The first step is creating a blood clot and narrowing blood arteries to stop bleeding. To stop additional blood loss, platelets and fibrin temporarily patch the hole.
2. **Inflammation:** Signals released by injured cells draw immune cells, such as macrophages, to the area of the wound. By removing germs and debris, this procedure starts the subsequent phase.
3. **Proliferation:** Rebuilding the injured tissue is the goal of this step. Epithelial cells from the surrounding skin move to cover the wound, while fibroblasts create collagen to fill it.
4. **Remodeling**: The goal of the last stage is to refine the tissue and reinforce the wound. The wound becomes more robust as a result of the structured collagen fibers.

Sampling and Preparing Tissue

- **Wound biopsy:**

A tiny sample of tissue is extracted from the wound site.

- **Fixation:**

To preserve tissue structure, the sample is kept in a fixative solution, such as formalin.

- **Processing:**

To get the tissue ready for sectioning, it goes through a number of processes, including drying, cleaning, and embedding.

- **Partitioning:**

A microtome is used to cut the tissue into thin slices, typically 5–10 micrometers.

Mounting and Staining: To improve the visibility of cellular features, the sections are placed on microscope slides and stained with particular dyes, such as hematoxylin and eosin.

- **Mounting and Staining:**

To improve the visibility of cellular features, the sections are placed on microscope slides and stained with particular dyes, such as hematoxylin and eosin.

Microscopic Analysis

- **Qualitative Assessment:** Using a microscope, the histopathologist visually inspects the tissue sections to look for indications of collagen deposition, inflammation, angiogenesis, fibroplasia, and epithelialization.
- **Quantitative Assessment:** In certain situations, measures can be taken, such as the area of epithelialization, the quantity of collagen, or the number of inflammatory cells.
- **Scoring Systems**: The many facets of wound healing can be graded using scoring systems, which range from qualitative to semi-quantitative.

Interpreting the Findings

- **Stages of Healing Wounds:** The predominant stage of wound healing inflammation, proliferation, or remodeling is determined in part by the histological evaluation.
- **Inflammation:** Inflammatory cells (neutrophils, lymphocytes, and macrophages) are among the indicators of inflammation that are assessed.

- **Angiogenesis:** The growth of new blood vessels is evaluated since it is essential for supplying the wound with oxygen and nutrients.
- **Fibroplasia:** The development of scar tissue is indicated by the evaluation of collagen and fibroblast production. In order to restore the skin barrier, epithelialization the process of new skin formation is evaluated.
- **Collagen Deposition:** Since collagen is the main structural protein of scar tissue, its type and quantity are evaluated.

Clinical Significance

- **Tracking Healing Progress:** Over time, wound healing can be tracked by histopathological evaluation.
- **Recognizing Complications:** It can assist in recognizing issues like infection, severe scarring, or delayed healing.
- **Assessing Treatment Effectiveness:** It can assist in assessing the efficacy of various wound care procedures, including topical drugs and surgery.
- **Comprehending Wound Healing Mechanisms:** It can shed light on the molecular and cellular processes that underlie wound healing.

WOUND CLASSIFICATION

Generally, wounds are classified based on the underlying cause that led to their development.

Acute Wounds

Acute wounds involve tissue damage that typically progresses through a structured and timely reparative phase, leading to a sustainable restoration of anatomical and functional integrity. Acute wounds are usually the result of cuts or surgical incisions

Closed Wounds

In closed wounds, blood leaves the circulatory system but remains within the body. It manifests as bruises.

Open Wounds

An open wound allows blood to escape the body, making bleeding evident. The exposed wound could be further subdivided into categories based on the source of the injury.

Incised Wounds

This type of wound does not involve tissue loss and results in only slight damage to the tissue. It is mainly caused by sharp items such as a scalpel or knife. Tear or laceration injuries These are non-surgical injuries that occur alongside other forms of trauma, leading to tissue loss and harm.

Puncture Wounds

These occur when an object, such as a needle or nail, penetrates the skin. Because dirt can get deep into the wound, these wounds often have a high risk of infection. Abrasive or superficial injuries Sliding a slip onto a coarse surface causes abrasion. Throughout this period, abrasion removes material from the skin's surface layer (the epidermis), thereby exposing nerve endings and causing a painful injury.

Penetration Wounds

These injuries are primarily inflicted by an object, such as a knife, that punctures the skin and then withdraws.

Tear or Laceration Injuries

These are non-surgical injuries that occur alongside other forms of trauma, leading to tissue loss and harm.

Puncture Wounds

These occur when an object, such as a needle or nail, penetrates the skin. Because dirt can get deep into the wound, these wounds often have a high risk of infection.

Abrasive or Superficial Injuries

Sliding a slip onto a coarse surface causes abrasion. Throughout this period, abrasion removes material from the skin's surface layer (the epidermis), thereby exposing nerve endings and causing a painful injury.

Penetration Wounds

These injuries are primarily inflicted by an object, such as a knife, that punctures the skin and then withdraws.

Gunshot Wounds

These injuries are usually caused by a bullet or another comparable projectile that penetrates through or into the body.

Chronic Wounds

Are those that have failed to progress through the normal stages of healing, resulting in a condition of pathological inflammation. They require an extended duration for healing.

Figure 1. Wound healing classification (Jain et al., n.d.)

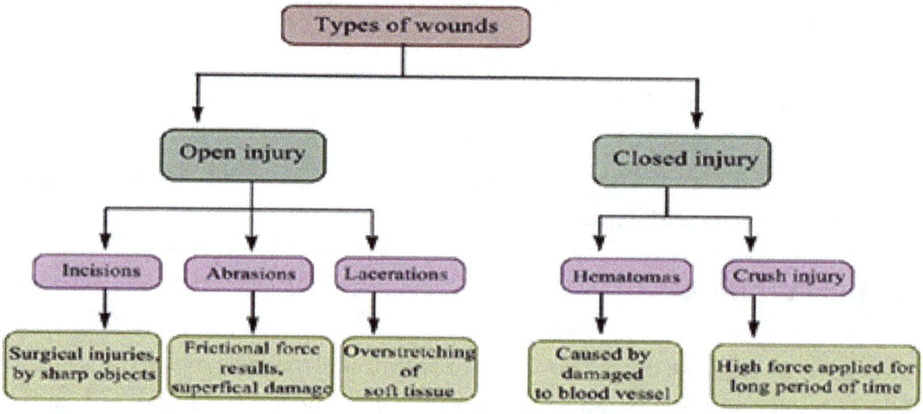

HERBAL FORMULATION FOR WOUND HEALING FIELD OF INVENTION

The present invention pertains to herbal formulations with therapeutic properties. In particular, it pertains to a herbal preparation with strong antimicrobial, antifungal, and wound-healing abilities that is very effective in treating external wounds of all kinds in humans, particularly non-healing diabetic wounds and those known as bedsores. Herbal formulation is also very effective for treating animal wounds. The use of natural plant-derived substances to speed up and improve wound healing is known as herbal formulations for wound healing, and it frequently addresses problems including infection, inflammation, and scar formation. By adding them to lotions, gels, or other topical preparations, this field makes use of the therapeutic qualities of different herbs and plants.

Homeostasis, inflammation, proliferation, and tissue remodeling are the four interconnected and overlapping phases that make up the complicated and dynamic physiological process of wound healing. Following an acute injury, the wound healing process is started by a highly coordinated series of events that coordinate the wound healing process' passage through the overlapping but separate phases of healing indicated above . During the several stages of wound healing, a number of tightly controlled processes take place, including phagocytosis, chemotaxis, collagen remodeling with neo collagen production, collagen breakdown, and the cellular release of different growth factors (GFs) and cytokines. Since adults' healing processes are slower than those of children and frequently lead to scarring (fibrosis healing) rather than regeneration, creative approaches to scarless, high-quality wound healing are also required. In the case of chronic or non-healing wounds, the healing process usually halts and is unable to precisely repair skin tissue because of the huge lesion size or depth, which results in keloid formation with undesired scars . Hemostasis is the first stage of wound healing that occurs right after an injury. During this phase, the body tries to halt the bleeding by constricting the blood vessels and forming a scab through platelet aggregation. When the platelets reach the area, they encourage blood coagulation without interfering with regular blood flow.

ESSENTIAL FEATURES OF THE COMPONENT

Herbal Ingredients

Aloe vera, calendula, centella asiatica, curcuma longa, and other plants and herbs with proven wound-healing qualities are used in the field.

Formulations

To facilitate topical application and skin absorption, herbal formulations are frequently created as creams, gels, or ointments.

Mechanism of Action

These formulations' herbal ingredients function in a number of ways, such as antibacterial activity to stop infections, anti-inflammatory qualities to lessen pain and swelling, and antioxidant actions to shield the area from harm.

Benefits

Faster wound closure, less scarring, and a more comfortable healing process are just a few advantages that herbal wound healing formulas can provide.

Traditional and Modern Approaches

To maximize wound healing results, the area integrates contemporary research and formulation techniques with traditional knowledge of herbal treatments.

EXAMPLES OF FORMULATIONS FOR HERBAL WOUND HEALING

Creams

An extract of Argyreia nervosa may be included in a cream formulation along with additional substances such as cetostearyl alcohol, cetomacrogol, and other emollients.

Hydrogels

Hydrogel formulations can promote wound healing and aid in efficient wound care, especially when they contain extracts from plants like Terminalia arjuna.

Ointments

Topical application of ointments containing herbs such as aloe vera or calendula can aid in inflammation reduction and healing.

PLANT PARTS UTILIZED FOR HEALING PURPOSES HEALING ATTRIBUTES CAN BE OBTAINED FROM THE SUBSEQUENT

Bark

The protective covering of a tree trunk, consisting of layers of living cells situated above the wood. The bark often contains higher concentrations of active ingredients. Bark with medicinal properties includes quinine bark, oak bark, pepper bark, and willow bark.

Bulb

A bulb is characterized as a fleshy entity made up of multiple layers of leaf bases, referred to as bulb scales. Onion species and garlic bulbs are widely used for medicinal purposes.

Essential Oil

These oils are characterized by their volatility and are typically obtained from plants via steam distillation. Camphor and peppermint oil are among the examples.

Fatty Oil

This term refers to non-volatile vegetable oils that are extracted from the seeds or fruits of plants and do not dissolve in water. Castor oil, olive oil, and safflower oil are examples of fatty oils utilized in medicine. Some fatty oils possess direct medicinal properties, while others serve as carriers in liquid formulations and ointments.

Flowers

In traditional medicine, the flowers of plants have always been valued. Instances comprise clove and chamomile flowers. Parts of flowers are also utilized, including saffron stamens, maize stigmas, or pollen.

Fruit

Fruits have served as a cornerstone of medicinal applications. Whole dried fruits or fruit pieces can be utilized. Numerous members of the carrot family possess fruits utilized in medicine, such as fennel. Some relevant part of the herb used in the formulation is provided below in Table 1.

Table 1. Plant parts utilized for healing purposes healing attributes

S.No.	Scientific Name	Part used in the formulation
1	*Catharanthus roseus*	Periwinkle
2	quinine	Bark
3	Aloe Vera	Leaves
4	Cardamom	Flowers
5	Zingiber officinale	Roots
6	Curcuma longa	Rhizomes
7	Matricaria chamomilla	Flowers

Those with expertise in the field will recognize that the approximate weight percentages mentioned above generally rely on the anticipated potencies of the individual components.

where the relative weight percentages will differ, at times significantly, from the individual amounts mentioned above. The skilled person, in light of this disclosure, will understand that the aims of the present invention necessitate that each of the components be included in relative approximate weight percentages as specified above.

FACTORS INFLUENCING THE HEALING OF WOUNDS

The process of oxygenation cell metabolism, especially the synthesis of ATP for energy, depends on oxygen, which is also required for practically every aspect of wound healing. It prevents infections, promotes angiogenesis, boosts keratinocyte differentiation, migration, and re-epithelialization, enhances fibroblast proliferation and collagen synthesis, and makes wound contraction easier. Due to consumption by metabolically active cells, the early wound's microenvironment is severely hypoxic and oxygen-depleted. Reduced vascular flow is a result of several systemic conditions, such as diabetes and aging, which pave the way for insufficient tissue oxygenation. In the concept of recovery, this superposition of insufficient perfusion results in a hypoxic wound. Chronic wounds are particularly hypoxic; transcutaneous measurements of tissue oxygen concentrations showed that they ranged from 5 to 20 mm Hg, compared to control tissue concentrations of 30 to 50 mm Hg.

Infections

Usually isolated on the skin's surface, microorganisms penetrate the underlying tissues till the skin is injured. The condition of infection and the status of the microorganisms' replication are determined by whether the wound is classified as having inflammation, colonization, local invasion/critical colonization, and/or spreading invasive infection. Whereas colonization is defined as the presence of replicating microorganisms on a wound without causing tissue damage, contamination is defined as the presence of non-replicating germs on a wound. Local infection/critical colonization, which includes microbial growth and the onset of local tissue reactions, is an intermediate stage. However, because germ clearance is insufficient, inflammation may persist even if cleaning is unsuccessful. The Prolonged increases in pro-inflammatory cytokines like TNF-alpha and interleukin-1 (IL-1) will prolong the inflammatory process and aid in the growth of germs and endotoxins. If this continues, the wound may become chronic and not heal. Furthermore, an increased concentration of matrix metalloproteases (MMPs), a protease family that can break down the ECM, is a result of this protracted inflammation. Together with the increasing protease content, there is a decrease in the naturally occurring protease inhibitors. The quick degradation of growth factors that takes place in chronic wounds could be brought on by this shift in protease equilibrium.

Age

The number of elderly persons (those over 60) is increasing faster than that of any other age group (a notable High age and the World Health Organization are risk factors for delayed wound healing. Age-related alterations and delays in wound healing have been investigated in a number of human and animal investigations at the cellular and molecular level.

It is generally acknowledged that aging causes stable older adults to experience a brief halt in wound healing, but not a true impairment in terms of healing consistency.

Anxiety

Stress significantly affects social behavior and personal well-being. Stress is linked to a number of conditions such diabetes, cancer, heart disease, and impaired wound healing. According to numerous studies, stress-induced disruption of neuroendocrine immune homeostasis is essential for overall health.

Category of Body

Wound healing can also be influenced by body form. An obese patient, for example, may suffer a compromise. In wound healing as a result of inadequate blood flow to adipose tissue.

Additionally, some obese people suffer from protein deficiency, which makes recovery much more difficult. On the other hand, when a patient is underweight, the lack of oxygen and nutrition storage may impede the healing of wounds.

Chronic Illnesses

Chronic illnesses that might hinder the healing of wounds include peripheral arterial disease, coronary heart disease, diabetes mellitus, stroke, and vascular disease. Patients with chronic illnesses should be continuously evaluated throughout their treatment in order to have the best strategy.

Vascular Inadequacy

The lower extremities may be affected by a variety of wounds or ulcers, including venous, diabetic, arterial, and pressure ulcers. One of the most frequent causes of these ulcers is a reduced blood flow. To guarantee that the right topical and supportive medicines are used, the clinician must determine the type of ulcer.

Nutrition

For over a century, it has been known that food plays a major role in wound healing.

The most obvious is that wound healing can be significantly impacted by malnutrition or certain nutritional deficiencies after trauma and surgery. Patients with nutritional deficiencies and persistent or non-healing wounds also require special nutrients. The healing process will be impacted by the metabolism of energy, carbs, proteins, lipids, vitamins, and minerals.

PATHOPHYSIOLOGY AND MECHANISM OF WOUND HEALING

The intricate process of wound healing can be divided into three categories: remodeling, allergic reaction, and proliferation. in three stages that are concurrent. A proliferative wound repair response, which is further defined by vascular reactions including blood coagulation and hemostasis, is triggered by the inflammatory process. Leukocyte invasion accompanied by the release of cytokines and antibiotics is one example of cellular activity. Granulation tissue grows to fill the wound space after the epithelium forms to cover the wound surface during the proliferative process. Fibroblast proliferation, collagen deposition along with other extracellular matrix, and the formation of new blood vessels are all components of granulation tissue creation.

Following the establishment of the new tissue, the remodeling process starts to restore the tissue's structural integrity and functional competency. within the injury. However, the three phases of wound healing are not straightforward, sequential processes; rather, they change throughout time. Burns, other serious injuries, and surgical wounds are examples of acute wounds, which are related to injuries that heal rapidly. A clean, uninfected incisional surgical wound that is roughly represented by operating sutures is an example of a normal acute wound. Although tissue synthesis with a structure and function comparable to that of retained skin is the intended outcome of organized healing, regeneration is uncommon (with notable exceptions, such as early fetal healing). As a result, the outcome of healing is not equal but is physically and functionally appropriate.

MEDICINAL PLANT USAGE FOR WOUND HEALING

In the past Egyptians, native populations in Africa, Asia, the Americas, and the Romans have all used medicinal herbs as a first-line treatment for surgical wounds, ulcers, burns, and inflammation. They include a variety of naturally occurring bio-active substances that promote tissue regeneration at the wound site and hasten the healing process. The following is a list of some medicinal plant examples and how they might help heal wounds.

(Centella Asiatica) Centella

Known by another name, Asian pennywort, it was used to promote wound healing. To aid in the recovery of the Extracts from Centella asiatica aerial sections are described, along with information on the distance, depth, and extent of chronic ulcers. It has been demonstrated that Asiaticoside, which is extracted from Centella Asiatica, stimulates collagen deposition and epithelialization in punch-type wounds. Isolated triterpenes from Centella astica enhance glycosaminoglycan production and collagen remodeling. Furthermore, it has been demonstrated that oral administration of Centella asiatica's madecassoside stimulates angiogenesis and collagen synthesis at the wound site.

(Wedelia Trilobata) Bay

Bay was formerly indigenous to the tropical Americas; However, it is currently one of the most invasive plants in the world and is found throughout in the tropics. Rheumatism, chronic wounds, and aching arthritic joints have all been treated with alcohol extracts made from the leaves of Wedelia trilobata. Wedelia trilobata leaves contain luteolin, a flavonoid that has been demonstrated to have anti-cancer, antioxidant, immunomodulatory, and neuroprotective properties. Wedelia trilobata leaves are used by traditional healers to cure skin wounds. One of the hallmarks of psoriasis and skin infections is the inhibition of NF-κB-regulated proinflammatory cytokine production by luteolin.

(Arctium Lappa) Burdock

This perennial weed is commonly grown and is commonly called burdock. The use of Arctium lappa in the treatment of skin conditions such acne, rashes, and boils as well as sore throats across North America, Europe, and Asia. Arctium lappa was found to have hepatoprotective, antiviral, anti-inflammatory, anti-diabetic, antibacterial, and antioxidant properties in a clinical experiment. Root extract from Arctium lappa has been demonstrated to significantly improve dermal ECM metabolism, influence glycosaminoglycan turnover, and reduce evident in vivo wrinkles in human skin. Additionally, it has been documented that Arctium lappa regulates gene expression and cell adhesion in canine dermal fibroblasts, impacting the Wnt/β-catenin signaling pathway, which is a crucial regulator of wound healing.

(Panax Ginseng) Ginseng

One of the most widely used medicinal plants in China, Japan, Korea, and Eastern Siberia is ginseng (Panax ginseng). Additionally, it is believed that memory improves physical agility, immunity, and fatigue levels. Panax ginseng is therefore used to treat chronic fatigue, anxiety, and depression. Panax ginseng has been demonstrated to have anti-inflammatory, anti-cancer, antibacterial, anti-allergic, anti-aging, and immunomodulatory properties in addition to causing vasodilatation and blood lipid regulation.

(Aloe Barbadensis Miller) Aloe Vera

Aloe vera, or aloe, Numerous naturally occurring bioactive substances, including complex and basic ones like glycosides, are found in aloe vera. polysaccharides, water-soluble polysaccharides, pyrocatechol, anthraquinones, acemannan, phytol, and oleic acid.

Compared to alcohol and aqueous extracts, aloe vera leaf acetone extracts exhibit stronger antibacterial activity. Gram-positive bacteria are generally more likely to infect aloe vera than gram-negative ones. Compounds having demonstrated antibacterial action include anthraquinone derivatives, acemannan, and saponins. Acemannan, a sizable Aloe vera mucopolysaccharide (mesoglycan), stimulates the production of proinflammatory mRNAs (such as IL-1af, IL-1β, IL-6, TNF-af, PGE2, and nitrous oxide) and effectively boosts the function of macrophages and T cells.

(Curcuma Longa) Turmeric

For many years, curcumin has been utilized as a food flavor and medicine since it is an active ingredient in the root of Curcuma longa and a ginger tribe member. Practitioners of traditional Ayurvedic medicine utilize curcumin to treat skin injuries, diabetes, liver problems, respiratory illnesses, and asthma. In traditional Chinese medicine, curcumin is a common treatment for stomachaches. Curcumin is one of the most extensively researched nutraceuticals and has been utilized for decades by various ethnic groups. It has been demonstrated that a highly pleiotropic molecule interacts with important biological pathways at the transcription, translation, and post-translation stages.

(Chamomilla Recutita) Chamomile

Chamomile (Chamomilla recutita) from Germany Researchers investigated the impact of electrospun polycaprolactone/polystyrene nanofibrous membranes.(PCL/PS) as active wound dressings that contain chamomile.Qualities of therapy The presence of C. Recutita (L.) Rauschert, a member of the Asteraceae family, is due to certain flavonoids and phenolics, including luteolin, patuletin, quercetin, apigenin, and their glucosides. The rarest flavonoid found in chamomile plants, apigenin, has a profound impact on the healing process of wounds. Nanofibers' effectiveness against bacteria, S. aureuas, and C. albicans (fungi) was proven by in vitro antibacterial and antifungal studies. Their inhibitory zones measured about 7.6 mm in diameter.

(Azadirachta Indica) Neem

It was widely recognized for its anti-ulcer, antifungal, antibacterial, antiviral, anticancer, and antioxidant properties in wound dressings. The content of nitric oxide was discovered to be 10 μg/mL in collagen-integrated wells containing 1000 μg/mL of neem extract. The biocomposite film exhibits strong nitric oxide scavenging and anti-inflammatory properties. The scientists used the neem-incorporated collagen film RAW 264.7 cell lines to conduct additional studies, including the biocompatibility and antioxidant activity tests. The MTT experiment revealed that the integrated collagen films of the neem extract (400 μg/mL) exhibited a cell viability of above 80% and an 80% increase in DPPH scavenging activity. Four distinct plant extracts were tested for electrospinning capability. Some ideal plant based constituents and their properties are given below

Table 2. Ideal candidate plants based constituents for treating wounds

S.No.	Types of dressings	Properties
1	**Curcumin**	From turmeric, it has anti-inflammatory and antimicrobial properties
2	**Honey**	Lavender, chamomile, tea tree, and thyme oils have antimicrobial and anti-inflammatory properties.
3	**Aloe Vera**	Honey has antibacterial and wound-healing properties.
4	**Centella Asiatica**	Known for its soothing and wound-healing properties
5	**Essential Oils**	Centella Asiatica is a medicinal plant used to promote epithelialization and collagen deposition.

SPECIES OF PLANTS AND THEIR POSSIBLE MEDICAL USES

Achille amillefolium L

Many species of yarrow (Achillea millefolium L.) have long been utilized in ethnopharmacology. a while. For the treatment of wounds, bleeding, stomachaches, gastrointestinal diseases, colds, flu, and stomach problems, A. millefolium is one of the most commonly used natural plant species, (Burusapat et al., 2018). It is said that during the Trojan War, the Greek warrior Achilles used this plant to track his blood flow and heal his wounds. Thus, the species name "millefolium" refers to the finely split, feather-like leaves, while the genus name might have been derived from his name. Many cultures have used various Achillea species as traditional herbal remedies since prehistoric times. The yarrow plant, Achillea millefolium L., is one of the most important and widely used medicinal plants in the world. It grows naturally in North America, Asia, Europe, and North Africa, (Hekmatpou et al., 2019). Native to the Northern Hemisphere, the flowering plant has been used in traditional medicine as an astringent, antibacterial, anti-inflammatory, and antispasmodic agent to hasten the healing process of cuts, wounds, burns, and ulcers. Figure 2 lists the main antioxidant phytochemical components of Achillea. A. millefolium's flavonoid content has been connected to its anti-inflammatory and antioxidant properties, (Gupta, Patchva, & Aggarwal, 2013). The significant antioxidant, tyrosinase-inhibiting, and Achillea extracts' antibacterial properties make them attractive options for usage as active components in medications and cosmetics that shield the skin from the harm caused by external stressors, (Vollono et al., 2019). After two months of in vivo administration of A. millefolium extracts, the expression patterns of cytokeratin 10, transglutaminase-1, and filaggrin have improved in cultured skin biopsies, and the thickness of the epidermis has also increased in comparison to placebo.

Figure 2. Bioactive phytochemical components of Achillea millefolium L (Chaudhary, Goyal, & Poonia, 2010)

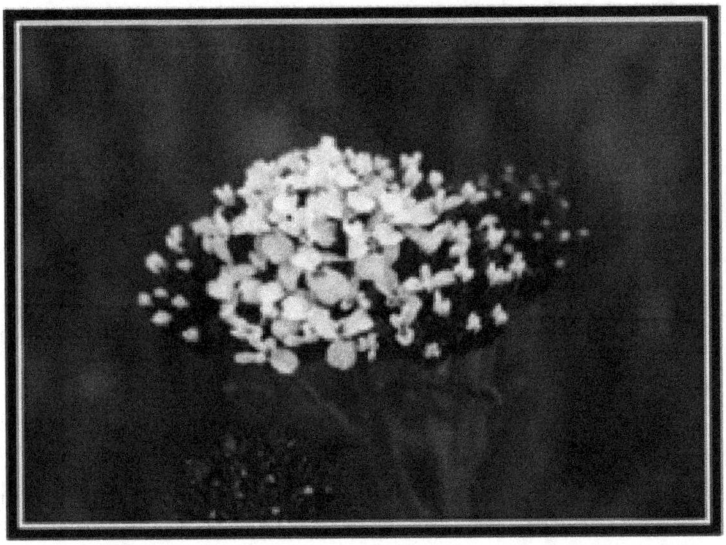

Aloe barbadensis

Aloe barbadensis, another name for aloe vera, belongs to the Lilaceae family. The Arabic word "alloeh," which meaning "bitter," is where the term "aloe" originates. Aloevera is currently utilized more often in the creation of novel food items because of its therapeutic and practical properties, (Cruceriu, Balacescu, & Rakosy, 2018). Aloe vera was known as the "plant of immortality" by the ancient Egyptians, and for over 2,000 years, Arab, Chinese, Egyptian, Greek, Indian, Japanese, and Korean societies have utilized it as a traditional medicine to treat conditions like diabetes, hyperlipidemia, skin problems, constipation, and internal and external ulcers. The cultivation of aloe vera has expanded due to the plant's numerous purported health advantages. It is utilized in the production of cosmetics, laxative drugs, and functional foods such lotions, foundations, face and hand creams, cleansers, lipsticks, and Shampoos and hair tonics, shaving supplies, bath items, and cosmetic and scent preparations. The bioactive effects of aloe vera on clinical trials conducted over specified time periods are displayed in Figure 3.

Figure 3. Bioactive of A. arborescens and A. barbadensis (Leitgeb et al., 2021)

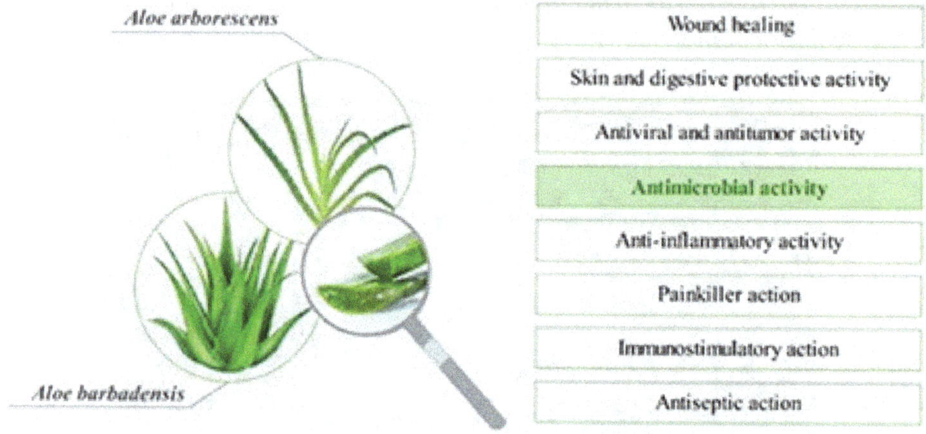

Both aloes are most frequently used as anti-inflammatory and antibacterial agents, to cure wounds and burns, and to treat skin, stomach, and digestive issues, (Xiong et al., 2019; Sharma, Jeyabalan, & Singh, 2013). As a result, the food industry capitalized on the usage of aloes in traditional medicine by incorporating aloe extracts into foods and dietary supplements as functional foods, (Ayoobi et al., 2017; Chaudhary, Goyal, & Poonia, 2010). The gel made from aloe has grown in popularity recently. It is typically utilized as a nutraceutical in the food sector, as well as in the pharmaceutical and cosmetics industries.

Turmeric

The brilliant yellow chemical compound curcumin is derived from the Zingiberaceae family's Curcuma longa L. (turmeric) plants. About 200 years in the past, Harvard College Curcumin was initially discovered in the rhizomes of Curcuma longa (turmeric) by lab scientists Vogel and Pelletier, (Asif et al., 2007). Turmeric has been used in traditional herbal therapy to treat weight loss, gastrointestinal and skin inflammation, and digestive issues, (Mulyaningsih et al., 2010). Turmeric contains curcumin, demethoxycurcumin, and bisdemethoxycurcumin, which are bioactive curcuminoids that have been proven to have anti-inflammatory, anti-cancer, and anti-aging properties. A prior study demonstrated that mice's wounds quickly healed with well-formed granulation tissue, primarily made up of deposited collagen and a regenerated epithelium, after receiving topical Curcumin treatment. Additionally, curcumin therapy greatly decreased tumor necrosis factor alpha and matrix metallopeptidase-9 and accelerated wound healing in mice by regulating the levels of several cytokines, (Mumtaz et al., 2022). Figure 4 shows a number of possible impacts of curcumin essential oils.

Figure 4. Some active components of curcumin essential oils and their potential effects (Hamid & Soliman, 2015)

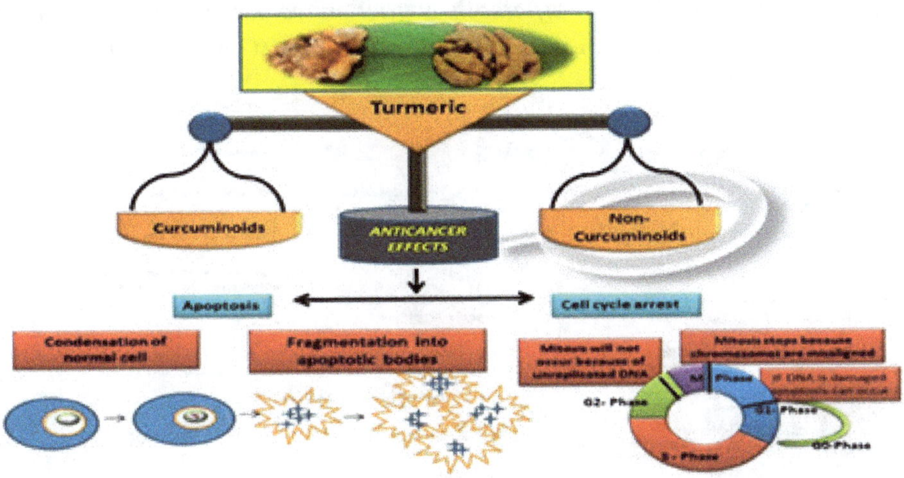

The Calendula Plant

Ethnopharmacology has a long history of using Calendula officinalis (pot marigold) flower extracts. Conventional treatments for minor skin irritation and encouraging the Aqueous and lipophilic Calendula alcoholic extracts are used to treat small wounds, (Brandão et al., 2016). The most important pharmacological effects associated with C. officinalis extracts are their anti-inflammatory, anti-edematous, antioxidant, antibacterial, antifungal, and immunostimulant qualities. The majority of C. officinalis's chemical makeup is composed of terpenoids, flavonoids, phenolic acids, carotenoids, coumarins, quinones, volatile oils, amino acids, and lipids, (Brandão et al., 2016). Antimicrobial, antiviral, anti-immunomodulatory, antioxidant, and effective treatment for breast cancer are among the additional pharmacological characteristics of C. officinalis. It also has strong anti-gastric ulcer, anti-acne, wound-healing, hepatoprotective, and renoprotective effects. Rat excision wounds were treated topically and orally with calendula officinalis to investigate its effects. The findings demonstrated that the extract-treated group had a 90.0% wound closure rate on the eighth day following the formation of the wound (compared to the control group's 51.1% wound closure), and the extract-treated group had noticeably larger levels of hydroxyproline and hexosamine than the untreated group (Figure 5), (Cicua & Racovita, 2023). Furthermore, because calendula ointment greatly speeds up the healing of cesarean wounds, it can be used to hasten the recovery from cesarean sections.

Figure 5. Effects of Calendula officinalis extract on wound closure, regeneration, hydroxyl proline, and hexosamine content in rat modles (Gunasekaran, Nayagam, & Natarajan, 2020)

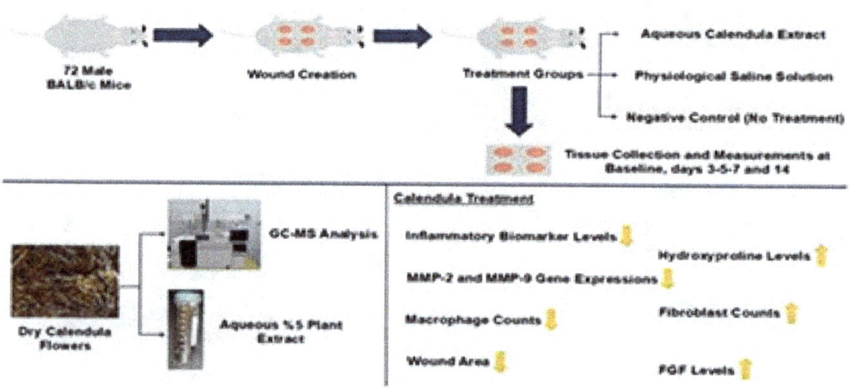

HISTOPATHOLOGICAL ASSESSMENT

Significant variations in the tissue responses across the different treatment groups were found by a histological examination of the representative skin biopsies. A thorough grasp of the tissue healing and response mechanisms was made possible by the scoring of the histopathological characteristics, such as inflammation, hyperkeratosis, and epidermal hyperplasia. The biopsies of the control group showed a high level of inflammatory infiltration, as evidenced by the presence of poly morphonuclear leukocytes, plasma cells, and lymphocytes. Additionally, some epidermal hyperplasia was noted. In comparison to the vehicle group, the vehicle-treated group displayed intense inflammatory infiltration together with noticeable hyperkeratosis. While the resin 5% group was linked to severe inflammatory reactions, the 10% resin treatment produced only mild inflammatory components and no discernible hyperkeratosis in the epidermis. providing more proof about the spectrum of therapeutic doses. There were sporadic clusters of a few inflammatory cells in the healing area, but the inflammatory infiltration was less severe in the 0.5% and 1% sapwood extract groups (Scores of 10 and 9, respectively). In comparison to the 0.5% sapwood treatment, the 1% sapwood therapy had a marginally improved healing profile with reduced inflammation. At 0.5% and 1% concentrations (Scores: 9 and 8, respectively), the heartwood extract groups showed signs of inflammation across the entire dermal thickness. But there was no sign of parakeratosis, unlike the sapwood extract and 5% resin groups, (Ali-Obaidi et al., 2017).

Case 1

A male patient, age 27, came in with several plantar warts on his feet and toes. The left thumb developed a lesion two months later. It was assumed that the lesion was a wart that had spread from the feet. The lesion was not healed with topical antiviral cream debridement with 5% Cimetidine, 5% 5-Fluoracil, and 10% Salicylic acid. The fingers got more lesions. The patient was referred to a dermatologist who unsuccessfully administered injections of Candida. The HIV test came back negative. The patient was sent back to get topical antiviral cream and debridement treatment. But now, the cause of the injuries is being questioned. The lesions only developed on the left hand's fingers, and they affected all four fingers but the middle one. The contact transmission logics did not seem to be followed by the lesions. PCR was used to culture the wound (HealthTrackRx, Denton, TX). Cutibacterium acnes and Peptostreptococcus anaerobius were found in high concentrations. The patient admitted to having a nail-biting habit. Following two weeks of topical antibiotic ointment and seven days of azithromycin, all of the finger lesions disappeared, (Dubey & Dixit, 2023).

Case 2

A 47-year-old woman came in with an incidental complaint of athlete's foot and an ingrown toenail. The lesions were found in the left fourth interspace, according to the patient, and they had been resistant to over-the-counter antifungals for a few weeks. There were vesicles and open skin in the erythematous webspace. Since she had received a double transplant because of a rare desmin-related myopathy, suspicion was quickly aroused. PCR was used to culture the wound (HealthTrackRx, Denton, TX). Trichophyton mentagraphophytes, Staphylococcus species, Enterococcus faecalis, E. faecium, Klebsiella pneumoniae, K. Oxytoca, P. anaerobius, and C. acnes were found in high concentrations. The patient acknowledged experiencing problems with her stomach pouch. The patient called her transplant team right away. Levofloxacin was administered for seven days to close open wounds. The patient kept using topical antifungal medication for tinea pedis. The patient returned six weeks later with cellulitis and an abscess in the same spot. PCR was used to culture the wound. The findings revealed no enterobacteria but a moderate level of Trichophyton and a high amount of C. acnes.

Microscopically analyzing tissue samples to analyze the various stages of the healing process, such as inflammation, angiogenesis, fibroplasia, and epithelialization, is known as histopathological assessment of wound healing, (Nagoba & Dayane, 2019).

DETAILED WOUND HEALING PROGRESS

Week 1

- **Debridement:** Non-viable slough was successfully removed by the first round of enzymatic and sharp debridement

Look of the Wound

- Slough decreased by around 30% Adequate vascular supply is indicated by minimal bleeding during debridement.
- The exudate is moderate and serous (clean, showing no symptoms of infection).
- Pain: 4/10 (better with leg elevation).
- surrounding skin: slight erythema, no spreading cellulitis.
- Interventions: Hydrocolloid dressings, compression therapy, and improved blood sugar control (Hormozi & Baharyand, 2024).

Week 2

50% of the wound bed was covered by healthy red granulation tissue; exudate had decreased to mild serous

- Wound Size: Reduced by approximately 25% to 3.5 cm × 2.5 cm

Surrounding Skin: Reduced erythema, improved texture and color

- Pain: 2–3/10, mostly felt when changing clothes.
- Patient Compliance: Good adherence to insulin dosage, clothing changes, and quitting smoking, (Leitgeb et al., 2021).

Week 3

- Wound Edges: There is observable migration of the epithelium from the wound margins.
- Gradulation: The wound bed is now about 80% covered.
- Exudate: Very little
- The wound measures 2.5 cm by 2 cm, which is about 50% smaller than the baseline.
- Clothes: To control moisture and promote healing, a foam dressing was used instead.
- Compression: Persisted successfully using a multilayer system; Glycemic Control: HbA1c is declining, and glucose levels are improving, (Saberianpour et al., 2018).

Week 4

- Wound Status: >90% granulation, epithelial cells covering 40% of surface
- Wound Size: 2 cm x 1.5 cm
- Pain: 1–2/10, mild discomfort only during prolonged standing
- Skin Integrity: Periwound skin intact, minimal maceration
- Mobility: Patient encouraged to walk short distances with support, (Wahedi et al., 2017).

Week 5

- Epithelialization: Continually growing, spanning the wound area; Size of wound: 1.2 cm by 1 cm
- Nutrition: Dietitian involved to increase protein intake (wound healing support)
- Compression therapy continued with increased patient tolerance
- Dressing: changed to silicone-based low-adherence dressing to protect new skin, (Brandão et al., 2016).

Week 6

- About 80–90% of the wounds are closed.
- About 90% of the epithelium is covered; only a little granulating region is left.
- No exudate
- Patient Report: Pain-free, increased mobility, and motivated to stop smoking altogether Skin Condition: Healthy pink skin surrounding wound, no indications of infection or recurrence
- Plan: Continue weekly dressing for a further two weeks; assess if compression garments are necessary for maintenance. Summary of healing metrics mentioned in Table 3, (Hamid & Soliman, 2015).

This evaluation aids in identifying possible side effects and evaluating how well a medication is working. Here's a more thorough explanation:

Table 3. Summary of healing metrics

Week	Wound Size (cm)	Granulation	Epithelialization	Exudate	Pain (0–10)
1	4 x 3	~10%	None	Moderate	4
2	3.5 x 2.5	~50%	Minimal	Light	3
3	2.5 x 2	~80%	Mild	Minimal	2
4	2 x 1.5	>90%	~40%	Minimal	1–2
5	1.2 x 1	>90%	>70%	None	1
6	~0.5 x 0.5	Complete	>90%	None	0

This case highlights the multifactorial nature of wound healing, especially in patients with comorbidities like diabetes and venous insufficiency. Proper wound bed preparation, control of underlying conditions, and compression therapy are key to effective healing. The patient's outcome was favorable due to multidisciplinary care, although long-term success depends on lifestyle changes and glycemic control.

CONCLUSION

Case studies demonstrate the potential of herbal wound compositions and demonstrate how well they work to promote healing, particularly when contrasted with traditional therapies. Multiple medicinal plants combined in polyherbal formulations frequently show synergistic wound healing action, resulting in quicker healing and better results. These formulations, which provide accessible and natural wound care solutions, can be especially helpful for burns and chronic wounds. Ancient wound healing is still a difficult clinical problem to effectively manage. Several cell types are involved in wound healing, including the extracellular matrix and the function of soluble mediators like as cytokines and growth factors. Numerous studies have focused on wound care, particularly on novel therapeutic approaches and the development of Ayurvedic (herbal) acute and chronic wound treatment procedures. Researchers are looking at new formulations, dressings, and medicinal plant compositions to provide a stable, sustainable, economical, and effective delivery system for wound care. New materials and the development of nanotechnology have made wound care more efficient and patient-centered. More recent technologies, such as 3D printing, are also offering beneficial alternatives for creating various drug delivery systems for wound care. Tissue engineering and regenerative medicines are the futuristic view of technologies for developing wound healing systems. New research avenues in wound care treatment will be made possible by improved quality control methods for the identification, screening, and measurement of herbal components as well as carefully planned pre-clinical and clinical trials.

REFERENCES

Al-Obaidi, J. R., Halabi, M. F., AlKhalifah, N. S., Asanar, S., Al-Soqeer, A. A., & Attia, M. F. (2017). A review on plant importance, biotechnological aspects, and cultivation challenges of jojoba plant. *Biological Research, 50*(1), 25. DOI: 10.1186/s40659-017-0131-x PMID: 28838321

Albahri, G., Badran, A., Hijazi, A., Daou, A., Baydoun, E., Nasser, M., & Merah, O. (2023). The therapeutic wound healing bioactivities of various medicinal plants. *Life (Chicago, Ill.), 13*(2), 317. DOI: 10.3390/life13020317 PMID: 36836674

Apel, L., Lorenz, P., Urban, S., Sauer, S., Spring, O., Stintzing, F. C., & Kammerer, D. R. (2021). Phytochemical characterization of different yarrow species (*Achillea* sp.) and investigations into their antimicrobial activity. *Zeitschrift für Naturforschung C, 76*(1–2), 55–65. DOI: 10.1515/znc-2020-0067 PMID: 32897872

Asif, A., Kakub, G., Mehmood, S., Khunum, R., & Gulfraz, M. (2007). Wound healing activity of root extracts of *Berberis lyceum* Royle in rats. *Phytotherapy Research, 21*(6), 589–591. DOI: 10.1002/ptr.2110 PMID: 17295382

Ayoobi, F., Shamsizadeh, A., Fatemi, I., Vakilian, A., Allahtavakoli, M., Hassanshahi, G., & Moghadam-Ahmadi, A. (2017). Bio-effectiveness of the main flavonoids of *Achillea millefolium* in the pathophysiology of neurodegenerative disorders—A review. *Iranian Journal of Basic Medical Sciences., 20*(6), 604–612. DOI: 10.22038/IJBMS.2017.8826 PMID: 28868116

Brandão, M. L., Reis, P. R., Araújo, L. A., Araújo, A. C., Santos, M. H., & Miguel, M. P. (2016). Evaluation of wound healing treated with latex derived from rubber trees and *Aloe vera* extract in rats. *Acta Cirurgica Brasileira, 31*(9), 570–577. DOI: 10.1590/S0102-865020160090000003 PMID: 27737341

Budovsky, A., Yarmolinsky, L., & Ben-Shabat, S. (2015). Effect of medicinal plants on wound healing. *Wound Repair and Regeneration, 23*(2), 171–183. DOI: 10.1111/wrr.12274 PMID: 25703533

Burusapat, C., Supawan, M., Pruksapong, C., Pitiseree, A., & Suwantemee, C. (2018). Topical *Aloe vera* gel for accelerated wound healing of split-thickness skin graft donor sites: A double-blind, randomized, controlled trial and systematic review. *Plastic and Reconstructive Surgery, 142*(1), 217–226. DOI: 10.1097/PRS.0000000000004510 PMID: 29649056

Cauich-Kumul, R., & Campos, M. R. (2019). Bee propolis: Properties, chemical composition, applications, and potential health effects. In *Bioactive Compounds* (pp. 227–243). Woodhead Publishing., DOI: 10.1016/B978-0-12-814774-0.00011-0

Chaudhary, G., Goyal, S., & Poonia, P. (2010). *Lawsonia inermis* Linnaeus: A phytopharmacological review. *International Journal of Pharmaceutical Sciences and Drug Research*, *2*(2), 91–98.

Cruceriu, D., Balacescu, O., & Rakosy, E. (2018). *Calendula officinalis*: Potential roles in cancer treatment and palliative care. *Integrative Cancer Therapies*, *17*(4), 1068–1078. DOI: 10.1177/1534735418803766 PMID: 30289008

Dubey, S., & Dixit, A. K. (2023). Preclinical evidence of polyherbal formulations on wound healing: A systematic review on research trends and perspectives. *Journal of Ayurveda and Integrative Medicine*, *14*(2), 100688. DOI: 10.1016/j.jaim.2022.100688 PMID: 36841194

Garcia-Orue, I., Gainza, G., Gutierrez, F. B., Aguirre, J. J., Evora, C., Pedraz, J. L., Hernandez, R. M., Delgado, A., & Igartua, M. (2017). Novel nanofibrous dressings containing rhEGF and *Aloe vera* for wound healing applications. *International Journal of Pharmaceutics*, *523*(2), 556–566. DOI: 10.1016/j.ijpharm.2016.11.006 PMID: 27825864

Gendrisch, F., Haarhaus, B., Krieger, N., Quirin, K. W., Schempp, C. M., & Wölfle, U. (2021). The effect of herbal medicinal products on psoriasis-like keratinocytes. *Biomolecules*, *11*(3), 371. DOI: 10.3390/biom11030371 PMID: 33801280

Gopinath, D., Ahmed, M. R., Gomathi, K., Chitra, K., Sehgal, P. K., & Jayakumar, R. (2004). Dermal wound healing processes with curcumin incorporated collagen films. *Biomaterials*, *25*(10), 1911–1917. DOI: 10.1016/j.biomaterials.2003.08.015 PMID: 14738855

Gunasekaran, S., Nayagam, A. A., & Natarajan, R. (2020). Wound healing potentials of herbal ointment containing *Calendula officinalis* Linn. on the alteration of immunological markers and biochemical parameters in excision wounded animals. *Clinical Phytoscience*, *6*(1), 77. DOI: 10.1186/s40816-020-00223-7

Gupta, S. C., Patchva, S., & Aggarwal, B. B. (2013). Therapeutic roles of curcumin: Lessons learned from clinical trials. *The AAPS Journal*, *15*(1), 195–218. DOI: 10.1208/s12248-012-9432-8 PMID: 23143785

Hamid, A. A., & Soliman, M. F. (2015). Effect of topical *Aloe vera* on the process of healing of full-thickness skin burn: A histological and immunohistochemical study. *Journal of Histology & Histopathology*, *2*(1), 3. DOI: 10.7243/2055-091X-2-3

Hekmatpou, D., Mehrabi, F., Rahzani, K., & Aminiyan, A. (2019). The effect of *Aloe vera* clinical trials on prevention and healing of skin wound: A systematic review. *Iranian Journal of Medical Sciences*, *44*(1), 1–9. PMID: 30666070

Hormozi, M., & Baharvand, P. (2024). Investigating the influence of natural compounds on the healing process of wounds. *The Open Biochemistry Journal, 18*(1). Advance online publication. DOI: 10.2174/1874091X-v18-e240219-2023-17

Huemer, M., Mairpady Shambat, S., Brugger, S. D., & Zinkernagel, A. S. (2020). Antibiotic resistance and persistence—Implications for human health and treatment perspectives. *EMBO Reports, 21*(12), e51034. DOI: 10.15252/embr.202051034 PMID: 33400359

Jain, S., Jain, N., Tiwari, A., Balekar, N., & Jain, D. K. (n.d.). *Simple evaluation of wound healing activity of polyherbal formulation of roots of Ageratum conyzoides.* Linn. [Unpublished manuscript]

Krishnan, P. (2006). The scientific study of herbal wound healing therapies: Current state of play. *Current Anaesthesia and Critical Care, 17*(1–2), 21–27. DOI: 10.1016/j.cacc.2006.03.002

Leitgeb, M., Kupnik, K., Knez, Ž., & Primožič, M. (2021). Enzymatic and antimicrobial activity of biologically active samples from *Aloe arborescens* and *Aloe barbadensis. Biology (Basel), 10*(8), 765. DOI: 10.3390/biology10080765 PMID: 34439997

Li, J., Chen, J., & Kirsner, R. (2007). Pathophysiology of acute wound healing. *Clinics in Dermatology, 25*(1), 9–18. DOI: 10.1016/j.clindermatol.2006.09.007 PMID: 17276196

Lone, A. H., Ahmad, T., Anwar, M., & Sofi, G. (2012). Clinical efficacy and safety of a pharmacopial polyherbal Unani formulation in pityriasis versicolor: A comparative randomized single-blind study. *Journal of Alternative and Complementary Medicine (New York, N.Y.), 18*(10), 978–982. DOI: 10.1089/acm.2011.0298 PMID: 22871048

Mukherjee, P. K., Mukherjee, K., Rajesh Kumar, M., Pal, M., & Saha, B. P. (2003). Evaluation of wound healing activity of some herbal formulations. *Phytotherapy Research, 17*(3), 265–268. DOI: 10.1002/ptr.1130 PMID: 12672158

Mulyaningsih, S., Sporer, F., Zimmermann, S., Reichling, J., & Wink, M. (2010). Synergistic properties of the terpenoids aromadendrene and 1,8-cineole from the essential oil of *Eucalyptus globulus* against antibiotic-susceptible and antibiotic-resistant pathogens. *Phytomedicine, 17*(13), 1061–1066. DOI: 10.1016/j.phymed.2010.06.018 PMID: 20727725

Mumtaz, R., Zubair, M., Khan, M. A., Muzammil, S., & Siddique, M. H. (2022). Extracts of *Eucalyptus alba* promote diabetic wound healing by inhibiting α-glucosidase and stimulating cell proliferation. *Evidence-Based Complementary and Alternative Medicine: eCAM*, *2022*, 4953105. Advance online publication. DOI: 10.1155/2022/4953105 PMID: 35463094

Nagoba, B., & Davane, M. (2019). Studies on wound healing potential of topical herbal formulations—Do we need to strengthen study protocol? *Journal of Ayurveda and Integrative Medicine*, *10*(4), 316–318. DOI: 10.1016/j.jaim.2018.06.009 PMID: 31685309

Olisova, O. Y., Snarskaya, E. S., Gladko, V. V., & Burova, E. P. (2018). Russian traditional medicine in dermatology. *Clinics in Dermatology*, *36*(3), 325–337. DOI: 10.1016/j.clindermatol.2018.03.006 PMID: 29908575

Saberianpour, S., Heidarzadeh, M., Geranmayeh, M. H., Hosseinkhani, H., Rahbarghazi, R., & Nouri, M. (2018). Tissue engineering strategies for the induction of angiogenesis using biomaterials. *Journal of Biological Engineering*, *12*(1), 36. DOI: 10.1186/s13036-018-0129-5 PMID: 30603044

. Saraswathy, N., Rohit, R., Shanmugam, K., Sozheeswari, S. C., & Ramalingam, P. (n.d.). A preliminary investigation of turmeric-agar composite film as bioactive wound dressing material on excision wound in rat model. [Unpublished manuscript].

Sharma, Y., Jeyabalan, G., & Singh, R. (2013). Potential wound healing agents from medicinal plants: A review. *Pharmacologia*, *4*(5), 349–358. DOI: 10.5567/pharmacologia.2013.349.358

Vollono, L., Falconi, M., Gaziano, R., Iacovelli, F., Dika, E., Terracciano, C., Bianchi, L., & Campione, E. (2019). Potential of curcumin in skin disorders. *Nutrients*, *11*(9), 2169. DOI: 10.3390/nu11092169 PMID: 31509968

Vuong, Q. V., Chalmers, A. C., Jyoti Bhuyan, D., Bowyer, M. C., & Scarlett, C. J. (2015). Botanical, phytochemical, and anticancer properties of the *Eucalyptus* species. *Chemistry & Biodiversity*, *12*(6), 907–924. DOI: 10.1002/cbdv.201400327 PMID: 26080737

Wahedi, H. M., Jeong, M., Chae, J. K., Do, S. G., Yoon, H., & Kim, S. Y. (2017). Aloesin from *Aloe vera* accelerates skin wound healing by modulating MAPK/Rho and Smad signaling pathways in vitro and in vivo. *Phytomedicine*, *28*, 19–26. DOI: 10.1016/j.phymed.2017.02.004 PMID: 28478809

Xiong, Y., Chen, L., Man, J., Hu, Y., & Cui, X. (2019). Chemical and bioactive comparison of *Panax notoginseng* root and rhizome in raw and steamed forms. *Journal of Ginseng Research*, *43*(3), 385–393. DOI: 10.1016/j.jgr.2017.11.004 PMID: 31308810

Chapter 13
Precautions in the Use of Herbal Polymers

Vaibhav Rajoriya
https://orcid.org/0000-0002-1064-4673
Vedic Institute of Pharmaceutical Education and Research, Sagar, India

Ravikant Gupta
Oriental University, India

Vibha Rajoriya
Vedic Pharmacy College, Sagar, India

Surbhi Chourasiya
Vedic Institute of Pharmaceutical Education and Research, Sagar, India

Kamlesh Patel
Gyanveer College of Pharmacy, Sagar, India

Prince Yadav
Vedic Institute of Pharmaceutical Education and Research, Sagar, India

ABSTRACT

Herbal polymers, derived from plant-based sources have become integral components in the development of advanced pharmaceutical and biomedical formulations. Their appeal lies in their biodegradability, non-toxic nature, renewability, and inherent therapeutic properties, which make them attractive alternatives to synthetic excipients. However, despite their natural origin, the assumption that herbal polymers are inherently safe is misleading and potentially hazardous. This chapter critically examines the precautionary principles necessary when incorporating herbal polymers into drug delivery systems, wound healing applications, and cosmeceutical products. Regulatory frameworks ranging from WHO guidelines to pharmacopeial standards are also discussed, with emphasis on the need for harmonization and transparency in herbal polymer governance. By integrating traditional ethnobotanical wisdom with cutting-edge scientific validation, the chapter advocates a balanced, evidence-based approach to unlocking the potential of herbal polymers without compromising patient safety.

DOI: 10.4018/979-8-3373-3977-1.ch013

INTRODUCTION

The increasing reliance on herbal polymers in wound healing reflects a global shift toward natural, sustainable, and biocompatible therapeutic materials. These polymers, derived from plant sources, offer distinct advantages including low toxicity, immune-compatibility, cost-effectiveness, and diverse functional properties such as muco-adhesion, film-forming ability, and intrinsic antimicrobial or anti-inflammatory effects (Anjum *et al.*, 2016). Consequently, they have been widely explored as excipients in modern wound care formulations—from gels and films to hydrocolloids and scaffolds. Despite their appeal, the assumption that natural equates to safe can be misleading. Herbal polymers are complex photochemical entities subject to significant variability due to environmental, botanical, and processing factors. As such, the safe and effective application of these biomaterials requires careful attention to their sourcing, characterization, formulation behavior, and biological interactions. Moreover, regulatory frameworks for herbal excipients are often fragmented or less stringent than their synthetic counterparts, further necessitating vigilance in their clinical and commercial use. This chapter provides a comprehensive analysis of the critical precautions that must be observed when utilizing herbal polymers in wound healing applications. It underscores the importance of scientific rigor, quality control, and risk mitigation strategies to ensure therapeutic consistency, patient safety, and translational viability.

Rise of Herbal Polymers in Modern Therapies

The resurgence of interest in plant-derived materials within the pharmaceutical sciences has catalyzed the development of herbal polymers as viable candidates for modern therapeutic systems. Their integration into drug delivery platforms, especially in wound healing, reflects a convergence of traditional knowledge and modern biotechnological innovation. Herbal polymers such as guar gum, xanthan gum, tragacanth, pectin, and mucilage from various medicinal plants have demonstrated a wide array of functional attributes—ranging from gelling and thickening to controlled drug release and biocompatibility. The growing interest in herbal polymers for wound care and biomedical applications is driven by several key factors. Their biological affinity to extracellular matrix components enhances cell adhesion, proliferation, and tissue regeneration. Many plant-based polymers also offer therapeutic synergy, acting as both excipients and bioactive agents due to their antimicrobial, anti-inflammatory, and antioxidant properties (Sindhu *et al.*, 2022). Environmentally, these polymers are sourced from renewable plants, making them biodegradable and aligned with global sustainability goals. Their use has now extended beyond traditional systems to sophisticated applications including nanogels, biofilms, wound dressings, transdermal patches, and 3D-bioprinted scaffolds. As their biomedical applications expand, understanding the underlying challenges and implementing appropriate precautions become paramount to ensure patient safety, formulation stability, and therapeutic efficacy (Ahmed *et al.*, 2023).

Misconceptions About Natural Safety

The phrase naturally derived is often misinterpreted as a blanket assurance of safety, efficacy, and compatibility. This misconception stems from the historical and cultural association of natural products with traditional medicine and the perception that plant-based materials are inherently benign. However, such assumptions can be dangerously misleading when translated into clinical or pharmaceutical contexts especially in the case of herbal polymers used in wound care. Several misconceptions persist around herbal polymers in wound care. First, the belief that natural equals non-toxic overlooks the fact that many plant-derived compounds can cause irritation, hypersensitivity, or systemic toxicity if not properly processed or dosed. Second, traditional use is often mistaken for scientific reliability; while valuable, empirical knowledge must be validated through rigorous pharmacological and toxicological studies (Mazzocchi, 2006).

SOURCES AND CLASSIFICATION OF HERBAL POLYMERS

Herbal polymers are high-molecular-weight biomolecules extracted from plant sources, valued for their physicochemical versatility, bio-acceptability, and therapeutic potential in wound management. Their origin and structural diversity form the basis for their functional classification, which aids in their selection for specific pharmaceutical applications. The classification of natural polymer presented in Table 1.

Table 1. Classification based on physicochemical properties

Category	Polymers	Functional roles in wound healing
Hydrocolloids	Guar gum, Xanthan gum, Pectin	Moisture retention, gel formation, exudate control (Saha and Bhattacharya, 2010)
Mucilage	Isabgol, Hibiscus mucilage	Soothing, hydration, bio-adhesion (Tosif *et al.*, 2021)
Gums and Resins	Acacia, Karaya, Tragacanth	Film-forming, thickening, stabilization (Murthy, 2022)

continued on following page

Table 1. Continued

Category	Polymers	Functional roles in wound healing
Starches and Dextrin	Potato starch, Arrowroot, Corn starch	Absorbency, mild astringency, biodegradability (Sarka *et al.*, 2023)
Cellulose derivatives	Herbal Microcrystalline Cellulose	Viscosity modifier, drug release control (Viera-Herrera *et al.*, 2020)

Plant-Based Polymers

Plant-based polymers are naturally derived macromolecules obtained from renewable botanical sources. They've become increasingly important in pharmaceutical, biomedical, and packaging industries due to their biodegradability, biocompatibility, and sustainability. Table 2, represent Plant-Based polymers with their sources. Herbal polymers are sourced from a diverse range of botanical origins, each offering unique functional benefits for wound care and biomedical applications and these sources collectively support the development of eco-friendly, bioactive, and multifunctional wound care systems.

Table 2. Plant-based polymers with their sources

Polymer	Source	Applications
Pectin, Alginate	Citrus peels, apple pomace	Gelling agent, wound dressings, drug delivery (Aderibigbe, 2018)
Guar gum	*Cyamopsis tetragonoloba* seeds	Thickener, binder, controlled-release formulations
Xanthan gum	Fermentation of plant sugars	Stabilizer, bioadhesive, hydrogel component
Starch	Corn, potato, arrowroot	Film-forming, absorbent, biodegradable packaging
Cellulose	Cotton, wood pulp	Matrix former, scaffold material, tablet binder
Gum arabic	*Acacia senegal* exudate	Emulsifier, stabilizer, wound healing formulations
Tragacanth gum	*Astragalus* species	Suspending agent, mucoadhesive, wound protectant

(Benalaya *et al.*, 2024, Zhang et al., 2021)

Structural and Functional Variability

Herbal polymers, being naturally derived macromolecules, exhibit significant structural and functional variability due to a multitude of intrinsic and extrinsic factors. Unlike synthetic polymers with uniform composition, plant-based polymers are heterogeneous systems composed of polysaccharides, glycoproteins, tannins, and other phytoconstituents. This variability poses both opportunities and challenges in their pharmaceutical application.

Factors Contributing to Structural Variability

Several factors influence the consistency and performance of herbal polymers in wound care applications. Botanical source variability, including differences in species, subspecies, and plant maturity, affects the molecular structure and branching of biopolymers. Environmental and seasonal conditions such as climate, soil quality, and harvest timing—impact yield, composition, and molecular weight distribution. Post-harvest handling, including drying, grinding, and extraction, can modify polymer conformation, solubility, and purity. Additionally, phytochemical complexity, with co-existing compounds like flavonoids, alkaloids, and essential oils, may alter polymer behavior or introduce bioactivity, influencing therapeutic outcomes (Kumar *et al.*, 2023).

Functional Implications in Wound Healing

Variability in herbal polymers can significantly influence their performance in wound care. Differences in branching and polymer chain length affect viscosity and muco-adhesion, impacting spreadability and surface adherence. Drug release dynamics may be altered by inconsistent gel strength or swelling behavior, potentially affecting therapeutic efficacy. Hydration and barrier formation can vary due to heterogeneous moisture retention, influencing exudate control and wound protection. Additionally, biological activity may fluctuate between batches depending on the presence of co-extracted bioactive, leading to inconsistent antimicrobial or anti-inflammatory effects. Standardization is key to ensuring reliable outcomes.

Analytical Strategies to Address Variability

Ensuring consistency in herbal polymer-based wound care formulations requires robust analytical and functional evaluation. Structural characterization using FTIR, NMR, and X-ray diffraction reveals polymer composition and crystalline structure. Batch profiling through HPLC and GPC enables molecular fingerprinting and determination of molecular weight distribution. Functional testing, including rheological and bio-adhesion studies, confirms application performance and patient experience. To achieve reproducibility and scalability, a quality-by-design (QbD) approach—anchored in thorough characterization and standardization—is essential for minimizing batch-to-batch variability and ensuring reliable therapeutic outcomes (Yu *et al.*, 2014).

POTENTIAL RISKS AND ASSOCIATED PRECAUTIONS

Herbal polymers, while promising in wound healing, carry potential risks due to their natural origin and inherent variability. One major concern is microbial contamination, as many herbal polysaccharides and mucilage are hygroscopic and susceptible to microbial growth during collection, storage, or processing. This necessitates stringent sterilization using validated methods such as gamma irradiation or autoclaving, along with humidity-controlled storage and regular microbial testing. Batch-to-batch variability is another critical issue, as inconsistencies in viscosity, swelling index, or bioactivity can compromise formulation performance. To mitigate this, robust quality control protocols, standard operating procedures (SOPs), and advanced analytical techniques like HPLC or FTIR should be employed to ensure consistency. Additionally, residual phytochemicals may trigger allergic or hypersensitivity reactions in certain patients, highlighting the importance of comprehensive dermal toxicity and sensitization testing.

Herbal polymers may also interact unfavorably with active pharmaceutical ingredients (APIs), affecting drug release or stability. Compatibility studies using tools such as differential scanning calorimetry (DSC) and formulation optimization are therefore essential. Regulatory challenges also arise due to varying global standards and documentation requirements; thus, maintaining traceability from botanical source to final product and adhering to GMP and pharmacopoeia guidelines are vital. Furthermore, the sustainability of herbal raw material sourcing must be addressed, as overharvesting or ecological disruption could jeopardize both supply chain integrity and environmental balance. Overall, a comprehensive, risk-mitigated formulation approach grounded in scientific validation and regulatory compliance is indispensable to unlock the full potential of herbal polymers in clinical wound care (Balian *et al.*, 2010).

Allergenic Responses

Although herbal polymers are often perceived as safe due to their natural origin, they can pose significant allergenic risks when incorporated into wound healing formulations. These responses may range from mild skin irritation and contact dermatitis to severe hypersensitivity reactions, depending on the patient's immunological profile and the nature of the herbal excipient used. Allergenic potential arises primarily from residual phytoconstituents—such as flavonoids, alkaloids, and proteins—that may not be completely removed during extraction and purification. Additionally, naturally occurring allergens within certain plant families (e.g., Asteraceae or Leguminosae) can trigger IgE-mediated or delayed-type hypersensitivity reactions upon topical application. Factors such as prolonged exposure time, high polymer concentration, and compromised skin barriers (common in chronic wounds) may amplify these risks. Precautionary strategies include rigorous screening through preclinical skin irritation and sensitization studies (e.g., Draize test, Local Lymph Node Assay) and, where possible, usage of purified or chemically modified polymers with reduced allergenic potential (Daniel *et al.*, 2018).

Microbial and Fungal Contamination

Herbal polymers are prone to microbial contamination throughout their lifecycle due to their organic, hygroscopic nature. Common threats include bacteria like *Staphylococcus aureus* and *Pseudomonas aeruginosa*, and fungi such as *Aspergillus* and *Candida*, often introduced via soil, water, or poor handling. Polysaccharide-rich excipients are especially vulnerable in warm, humid conditions. To ensure safety, materials must undergo microbial testing and validated decontamination methods like gamma irradiation or steam sterilization. Good Agricultural and Collection Practices (GACP) and hygienic post-harvest handling are essential to reduce bioburden. Formulations must also be evaluated for microbiological stability, especially when designed for prolonged use or storage. Incorporation of antimicrobial preservatives if compatible or terminal sterilization may be warranted for sterile or wound-contact applications.

Batch-to-Batch Variability

One of the major challenges in utilizing herbal polymers for pharmaceutical and wound healing applications is their inherent batch-to-batch variability. Unlike synthetic polymers, which offer consistent chemical and physical properties, herbal polymers are influenced by biological origin and environmental factors such as climate, soil composition, and harvesting conditions. These variations can significantly affect key functional attributes like viscosity, gel strength, swelling index, molecular weight distribution, and drug interaction behavior, potentially compromising formulation stability and therapeutic efficacy. Differences in plant species, subspecies, and regional cultivation practices further contribute to inconsistencies in polymer composition and secondary metabolite content. Furthermore, adopting a Quality by Design (QbD) framework allows for systematic identification of critical material attributes (CMAs) and process parameters that influence product quality. This strategy enhances product consistency, reduces risk of formulation failure, and supports regulatory compliance. Addressing batch-to-batch variability is imperative not only for ensuring therapeutic reliability, but also for scaling up herbal polymer-based wound care systems to industrial production levels. Achieving uniformity through scientific standardization will be a key determinant of their long-term clinical and commercial success (Yu *et al.*, 2014).

Chemical Residues and Toxins

The use of herbal polymers in pharmaceutical and wound healing formulations may inadvertently introduce chemical residues and toxins that compromise product safety and therapeutic efficacy. These contaminants can originate from various sources, including the use of agrochemicals during cultivation, solvent residues from extraction processes, or byproducts formed during polymer modification and storage. Pesticide and herbicide residues are among the most prevalent concerns. Plants cultivated without proper adherence to good agricultural practices (GAP) may accumulate hazardous levels of organophosphates, chlorinated compounds, or heavy metals such as lead, arsenic, and cadmium. These substances are known for their cytotoxic, genotoxic, and carcinogenic effects, making their presence in wound-contact formulations particularly dangerous.

In addition, residual solvents used during extraction or purification—especially non-pharmaceutical-grade solvents like methanol, benzene, or dichloromethane—can remain entrapped within polymer matrices. Such solvents may cause local irritation, systemic toxicity, or interfere with drug-polymer interactions. Pharmacopeial guidelines such as ICH Q3C provide strict thresholds for acceptable residual solvent levels that must be adhered to in formulation development. Furthermore, naturally occurring plant toxins such as pyrrolizidine alkaloids, oxalates, or saponins may persist in inadequately purified herbal polymers. These compounds can produce dermal irritation, allergic reactions, or long-term adverse effects upon repeated exposure. Oxidative degradation of phytoconstituents or improper storage may also generate harmful byproducts that alter the safety profile of the polymer (DeBenedictis *et al.*, 2023). Table 3, represent some examples of Chemical Residues and Toxins in Herbal Polymers.

Table 3. Examples of chemical residues and toxins in herbal polymers

Contaminant Type	Example	Source	Potential Risk
Pesticide Residues	Chlorpyrifos, Carbendazim, Bifenthrin	Agricultural use during plant cultivation	Neurotoxicity, endocrine disruption, skin irritation
Heavy Metals	Lead, Arsenic, Cadmium, Mercury	Soil contamination, irrigation water, industrial pollution	Nephrotoxicity, carcinogenicity, delayed wound healing
Residual Solvents	Methanol, Dichloromethane, Benzene	Improper extraction or purification processes	Systemic toxicity, local irritation, regulatory noncompliance
Mycotoxins	Aflatoxins, Ochratoxin A	Fungal contamination during storage (e.g., *Aspergillus* spp.)	Hepatotoxicity, immunosuppression, carcinogenicity
Plant-Derived Toxins	Pyrrolizidine alkaloids, Saponins, Oxalates	Naturally occurring in certain plant species	Hepatotoxicity, dermal irritation, allergic reactions
Unauthorized Additives	Sudan dyes (I–IV), synthetic colorants	Adulteration for visual appeal or product enhancement	Mutagenicity, regulatory violations

(Opuni *et al.*, 2023)

To mitigate these risks, comprehensive screening using validated analytical methods—including gas chromatography (GC), inductively coupled plasma mass spectrometry (ICP-MS), and liquid chromatography–mass spectrometry (LC-MS)—is essential. Establishing a contaminant profile and ensuring compliance with pharmacopeial specifications (e.g., USP, Ph. Eur., AYUSH guidelines) forms a critical component of the quality control strategy. Equally important is sourcing raw materials from certified organic or pesticide-controlled farms and enforcing stringent traceability throughout the supply chain. By proactively identifying and controlling chemical residues and toxins, formulators can uphold the safety standards required for clinical application, ensuring that the therapeutic benefits of herbal polymers are not undermined by hidden toxicological risks (Opuni *et al.*, 2023).

Drug–Excipient Interactions

Drug–excipient interactions are a pivotal yet often overlooked factor in the formulation of wound healing systems using herbal polymers. These polymers, while serving as carriers, gelling agents, or film formers, possess complex phytochemical profiles and reactive functional groups that can physically or chemically interact with active pharmaceutical ingredients (APIs). Such interactions may alter drug release kinetics, stability, bioavailability, and overall therapeutic efficacy. Physicochemical mechanisms—like hydrogen bonding, ionic interactions, or complexation—can affect drug solubility and crystallinity. For example, negatively charged polysaccharides such as pectin or gum karaya may form electrostatic complexes with basic drugs, resulting in delayed or reduced release. Chemical interactions, including oxidative degradation, hydrolysis, or Maillard-type reactions, are also possible, especially when excipients contain residual sugars or reactive metabolites.

Additionally, the inherent bioactivity of herbal polymers may synergize or antagonize the drug's pharmacological effects, influencing dose-response outcomes. To mitigate these risks, pre-formulation studies are essential. Techniques like differential scanning calorimetry (DSC), Fourier-transform infrared spectroscopy (FTIR), and high-performance liquid chromatography (HPLC) are used to assess compatibility, while rheological and in vitro release studies help evaluate formulation behavior. Stability testing under accelerated conditions is also critical to detect time-dependent degradation. Regulatory frameworks such as ICH Q8 and Q9 emphasize the need for thorough risk assessment of excipient interactions. Ultimately, a systematic evaluation of herbal polymer–API compatibility is vital to ensure formulation robustness, product quality, and clinical safety in wound care applications (Yang *et al.*, 2025).

REGULATORY AND QUALITY CONSIDERATIONS

The clinical translation and commercialization of herbal polymer-based wound healing products require adherence to stringent regulatory and quality standards. Unlike synthetic excipients, herbal polymers pose unique regulatory challenges due to their biological origin, complex composition, and potential variability. This chapter outlines the framework for ensuring regulatory compliance, product safety, and quality assurance in the development and application of herbal excipients and polymers

Regulatory Frameworks

Herbal polymers used in pharmaceutical formulations fall under the jurisdiction of various global and regional regulatory authorities.

- United States Food and Drug Administration (FDA): Herbal excipients must comply with guidelines on botanical drug development, which emphasize identity, purity, and consistency. The FDA regulates herbal polymers under its Botanical Drug Development framework, demanding rigorous testing, source verification, and stability data, especially for therapeutic claims (Rojas *et al.*, 2022).

- European Medicines Agency (EMA): Botanical substances are regulated under Traditional Herbal Medicinal Products Directive (2004/24/EC), requiring safety and quality data. The EMA focuses on quality, consistency, and safety, requiring detailed documentation and contaminant control for herbal medicines (Gatt *et al.*, 2024).
- AYUSH (India): Herbal formulations and excipients must adhere to guidelines set by the Ministry of AYUSH, which include pharmacopoeia standards and certification processes. AYUSH, supports the traditional use of herbal polymers in India, promoting innovations like graft copolymerization to improve stability and drug delivery, while ensuring adherence to pharmacopoeia standards and sustainable sourcing. Together, these agencies aim to balance tradition with scientific rigor (Kumar *et al.*, 2023).
- International Council for Harmonisation (ICH): Guidelines such as ICH Q6A (specifications), Q8 (pharmaceutical development), and Q9 (quality risk management) apply to herbal polymers.
- In China, the use of herbal polymers especially those found in traditional Chinese medicine—is carefully regulated to ensure safety and quality. The National Medical Products Administration (NMPA), previously known as the CFDA, has put strong emphasis on Good Agricultural Practice (GAP). This means that everything from how herbs are grown and harvested to how they're processed and packaged must meet strict standards.
- Australia, the Therapeutic Goods Administration (TGA) takes a slightly different but equally thorough approach. The TGA also requires specific warning labels for certain herbs. For example, *Andrographis paniculata* must carry a notice about possible taste disturbances, and artemisinin-based ingredients need pregnancy warnings. Other herbs like chelidonium, chaparral, and valerian have updated safety alerts due to recent findings (Ghosh *et al.*, 2006). Each agency requires documentation of source materials, manufacturing processes, contamination control, and stability data. These guidelines reflect a strong commitment to consumer safety while still allowing room for innovation in herbal medicine. The EMA, FDA, TGA, NMPA and AYUSH each offer distinct guidelines for the safe use of herbal polymers.

Quality Assurance and Control (QA/QC)

A robust QA/QC system is essential to ensure the consistency, safety, and performance of herbal polymer-based formulations. This begins with raw material standardization through botanical authentication, microscopic analysis, and DNA barcoding where applicable. Phytochemical profiling using techniques like HPLC, LC-MS/MS, and TLC helps identify and quantify bioactive constituents. Contaminant control is critical, involving screening for microbial load, heavy metals, pesticide residues, mycotoxins, and solvent traces in accordance with pharmacopeial standards such as USP and Functional testing—including viscosity, swelling index, film-forming ability, and drug-excipient compatibility—ensures reliable application and therapeutic performance. Maintaining validated analytical methods, standard operating procedures (SOPs), and traceable batch records throughout the product lifecycle is key to achieving reproducibility and regulatory compliance (Griffith, 2016).

Good Manufacturing Practice (GMP) and Documentation

Compliance with GMP principles is essential for herbal polymers used in pharmaceutical applications. This includes, controlled environmental conditions and equipment calibration, Validation of cleaning, sterilization, and extraction processes, Personnel training and hygiene monitoring and comprehensive batch manufacturing records and deviation handling. Electronic documentation systems and audit trails improve traceability and regulatory readiness

Stability and Shelf-Life Testing

Stability studies under ICH guidelines (e.g., ICH Q1A) must be conducted to determine the shelf-life of herbal polymer-based products. These studies evaluate (a) Physical changes (e.g., viscosity, phase separation), (b) Chemical degradation of active constituents, (c) Microbial proliferation and (d) Packaging-material compatibility. Accelerated and real-time stability testing ensures product performance throughout its labeled shelf-life.

Labeling, Traceability, and Post-Marketing Surveillance

Product labels should clearly state the botanical source, extraction method, potential allergens, and intended use. Traceability systems must document the journey of each raw material from field to finished product. Post-marketing surveillance (PMS) and pharmacovigilance mechanisms are vital for detecting delayed adverse events, especially in chronic wound applications or immunocompromised patients. A proactive regulatory and quality strategy not only protects patient safety but also facilitates global market access and long-term product success. Herbal polymers, when governed by rigorous scientific and compliance frameworks, hold great promise for safe and effective integration into modern wound care systems (Ghosh *et al.*, 2006).

Standards and Pharmacopeial Requirements

Ensuring the quality, safety, and efficacy of herbal polymers used in wound healing formulations necessitates conformity to established pharmacopeial standards and monographs. Major pharmacopoeias such as the United States Pharmacopeia (USP), the European Pharmacopoeia (Ph. Eur.), the British Pharmacopoeia (BP), and the Ayurvedic Pharmacopoeia of India (API) provide standardized specifications for several plant-based excipients. Quality specifications for herbal polymers typically include several critical parameters to ensure safety, consistency, and regulatory compliance. These begin with botanical identity verification through macroscopic, microscopic, and chromatographic analyses to confirm authenticity. Physicochemical assessments such as loss on drying, pH, solubility, viscosity, and swelling index help define material performance. Microbial limit tests, along with screening for heavy metals, pesticide residues, and aflatoxins, ensure bioburden remains within pharmacopeial limits. Lastly, residual solvent analysis must comply with ICH Q3C guidelines to prevent toxic exposure. Together, these controls form the foundation of a reliable herbal excipient profile. Where monographs for specific herbal polymers are lacking, supplementary standards—such as those published by the WHO or ISO may be adopted. In India, herbal excipients must conform to the AYUSH Good Manufacturing Practices (GMP) and relevant monographs in the Ayurvedic Pharmacopoeia, which increasingly include guidance on quality control and storage conditions for plant-based gums, mucilage, and starches (Rojas *et al.*, 2022).

Toxicological Evaluation and Documentation

A comprehensive toxicological evaluation is imperative for ensuring the safety and regulatory acceptance of herbal polymers used in pharmaceutical and wound healing applications. Despite their natural origin, these biopolymers may pose risks such as dermal irritation, systemic toxicity, mutagenicity, or allergic responses—especially if contaminated, improperly processed, or derived from toxic botanical sources. Toxicological assessments must align with international guidelines such as those set by the Organization for Economic Co-operation and Development (OECD), the U.S. FDA, CFDA/NMPA in China, TGA in Australia and the European Medicines Agency (EMA). Safety evaluation of herbal polymers involves a tiered approach to assess potential risks, especially for topical wound care applications. Key studies include acute toxicity (e.g., LD_{50}), skin and eye irritation tests, dermal sensitization assays like LLNA, and genotoxicity/mutagenicity assessments such as the Ames and micronucleus tests. Sub-chronic and chronic toxicity studies are conducted based on exposure duration and dosage. Comprehensive documentation is essential, including detailed protocols, NOAEL data, batch-specific certificates of analysis, raw vs. purified comparisons, and validated analytical methods. This ensures regulatory compliance and supports safe, reproducible product development (Soni *et al.*, 2018).

Good Manufacturing Practice (GMP) Guidelines

GMP forms the cornerstone of pharmaceutical quality assurance, ensuring that products are consistently produced and controlled according to predefined quality standards. For herbal polymers—given their biological origin and variability—adhering to GMP is especially critical to safeguard formulation integrity, patient safety, and regulatory compliance in wound care applications.

Core Principles of GMP for Herbal Polymers

Ensuring the quality and safety of herbal polymer-based formulations requires rigorous adherence to Good Manufacturing Practices (GMP). This begins with hygienic raw material handling, where environmental controls during harvesting, drying, and storage prevent contamination and degradation, and materials are authenticated and sourced from certified suppliers. Validated manufacturing processes, governed by SOPs, ensure consistency across extraction, purification, drying, and milling stages. Facility and equipment standards, including cleanrooms, stainless-steel machinery, HEPA filtration, and proper waste disposal, are essential for maintaining aseptic conditions and preventing cross-contamination. Finally, personnel training and documentation are critical—staff must be well-versed in GMP for botanical substances, with ongoing assessments and real-time recording of all procedures in master and batch records to ensure traceability and compliance.

Quality Control Integration within GMP

Effective quality control of herbal polymer-based formulations relies on three key pillars. In-process and finished product testing ensures compliance with pharmacopeial standards through routine checks of pH, viscosity, microbial load, heavy metals, and residual solvents. Stability testing, guided by ICH Q1A protocols, determines shelf life and optimal storage conditions. Finally, traceability and record keeping are vital tracking raw materials from source to final product and maintaining detailed documentation for audits, inspections, and post-market surveillance. Together, these practices uphold product integrity and regulatory readiness.

GMP Challenges Unique to Herbal Polymers

Herbal polymers present unique formulation challenges due to their natural variability and sensitivity. Batch-to-batch variation in polymer characteristics necessitates tight control over critical process parameters (CPPs) and the use of QbD strategies to ensure consistency. Sterilization and decontamination methods must be effective yet gentle enough to retain key functional properties like muco-adhesion and bioactivity. Additionally, storage and packaging require careful consideration—moisture-sensitive polymers often need specialized materials such as desiccants or barrier films, along with controlled humidity and temperature conditions. By adopting comprehensive GMP practices tailored to these complexities, manufacturers can ensure safe integration into pharmaceutical systems, streamline regulatory approval, and maintain consistent product quality throughout the lifecycle (Yu *et al.*, 2014).

ANALYTICAL AND SCREENING TECHNIQUES

The inherent complexity and variability of herbal polymers demand a robust suite of analytical and screening techniques to ensure their identity, purity, functionality, and safety. Standardized methods are essential not only for regulatory compliance but also for ensuring batch-to-batch consistency and therapeutic efficacy in pharmaceutical formulations. This chapter outlines the key analytical tools used across various stages of development—ranging from raw material authentication to finished product validation.

Phytochemical and Identity Profiling

Authentication of herbal polymers relies on a multi-tiered approach to ensure botanical integrity and prevent adulteration. Macroscopic and microscopic evaluation serves as the first line of screening, examining morphological traits and anatomical markers to verify plant identity. Thin Layer Chromatography (TLC) offers a rapid, cost-effective method for generating phytochemical fingerprint profiles. For more precise analysis, High-Performance Liquid Chromatography (HPLC) is employed to quantify marker compounds, detect adulterants, and assess extract quality. Complementing these techniques, DNA barcoding and molecular taxonomy provide advanced genomic validation, confirming species authenticity and identifying any botanical substitutions or contamination. Together, these methods form a robust framework for quality assurance in herbal polymer sourcing (Miralles *et al.*, 2024).

Physicochemical Characterization

Characterization of herbal polymers involves a suite of analytical techniques to ensure functional integrity and formulation performance. Fourier-Transform Infrared Spectroscopy (FTIR) helps identify functional groups and chemical interactions within polymer matrices. X-Ray Diffraction (XRD) assesses crystallinity, which influences drug-polymer compatibility and release kinetics. Differential Scanning Calorimetry (DSC) and Thermogravimetric Analysis (TGA) provide insights into thermal transitions, decomposition behavior, and overall polymer stability. Meanwhile, viscometry and rheological studies evaluate viscosity, shear-thinning properties, and flow dynamics critical for topical applications and controlled drug delivery. Together, these tools form the backbone of physicochemical profiling in herbal polymer research.

Contaminant and Residue Analysis

Advanced analytical techniques are crucial for ensuring the safety and purity of herbal polymers. Gas Chromatography–Mass Spectrometry (GC-MS) is employed to detect residual solvents, volatile impurities, and select pesticide residues. Inductively Coupled Plasma Mass Spectrometry (ICP-MS) enables trace-level quantification of toxic heavy metals like lead, cadmium, and arsenic. Liquid Chromatography Tandem Mass Spectrometry (LC-MS/MS) offers high sensitivity for profiling a wide range of contaminants and active phytochemicals. Additionally, aflatoxin and mycotoxin assays are vital for identifying fungal toxins, especially in mucilage-rich polymers prone to contamination under humid storage conditions. These tools collectively support rigorous quality control and regulatory compliance (Chatterjee *et al.*, 2023).

Microbial and Toxicological Screening

Safety assessment of herbal polymer-based formulations involves a comprehensive set of biological and toxicological evaluations. Total Viable Count and pathogen testing are essential to quantify microbial contamination, targeting organisms like *E. coli*, *Staphylococcus aureus*, and *Pseudomonas aeruginosa*. For topical applications, Draize tests and Local Lymph Node Assays (LLNA) help determine potential for skin irritation and allergic sensitization. Genotoxicity and mutagenicity are assessed using the Ames test and micronucleus assay, ensuring the absence of DNA-damaging effects. Finally, cytotoxicity assays such as MTT or Trypan Blue evaluate cell viability after exposure to polymer extracts, which is especially critical for scaffolds and wound films. These layered studies ensure both patient safety and regulatory compliance (Miralles *et al.*, 2024).

Functional Performance Testing

Functional evaluation of herbal polymer-based wound care systems involves several critical assessments. Swelling index and muco-adhesion studies help determine hydration capacity, film integrity, and how long the formulation remains at the wound site. In-vitro drug release and permeation assays simulate wound conditions to monitor drug diffusion and ensure therapeutic levels are maintained. Texture analysis and tensile testing provide quantitative data on mechanical strength, elasticity, and application properties, which are essential for the usability and durability of hydrogels and films. Together, these tests ensure that the formulation performs effectively in real-world clinical settings.

Chemometric and Multivariate Data Analysis

Advanced analytical techniques in herbal polymer research often yield multidimensional datasets that require robust statistical modeling for meaningful interpretation. Principal Component Analysis (PCA) simplifies complex data by identifying key variables, allowing classification of polymers based on physicochemical or bioactivity traits. Hierarchical Cluster Analysis (HCA) further organizes samples into groups with shared functional or contamination profiles, aiding in quality assessment and source tracking. Design of Experiments (DoE) plays a pivotal role in optimizing formulation parameters, systematically evaluating the impact of multiple variables while accounting for inherent natural variability. Together, these tools enhance data-driven decision-making and support reproducible, high-quality product development.

Chemical and Structural Characterization

The chemical and structural characterization of herbal polymers is a foundational step in ensuring their identity, purity, functionality, and reproducibility in pharmaceutical applications. Given their biological complexity and environmental variability, herbal polymers must undergo detailed analytical assessment to elucidate their molecular composition, structural features, and potential interactions with other formulation components (Thakur *et al.*, 2011).

Chemical Characterization

Chemical profiling focuses on identifying and quantifying the primary constituents of the polymer matrix, including monosaccharide units, functional groups, and residual phytochemicals. Key analytical tools play a vital role in characterizing herbal polymers and ensuring formulation integrity. Fourier-Transform Infrared

Spectroscopy (FTIR) identifies functional groups such as –OH, –COOH, and $-NH_2$, revealing chemical modifications or interactions with drugs and excipients. Nuclear Magnetic Resonance (NMR) Spectroscopy, particularly 1H and 13C NMR, helps elucidate monomer linkages and branching in polysaccharide chains. Ultraviolet–Visible (UV–Vis) Spectroscopy detects chromophore impurities and residual phytoconstituents, aiding in purity assessment. Elemental analysis quantifies carbon, hydrogen, nitrogen, and sulfur, supporting empirical formula estimation and verifying sample composition. Together, these tools provide a comprehensive understanding of polymer structure and quality.

Structural Characterization

Structural characterization plays a pivotal role in optimizing herbal polymer performance for wound healing applications. At the molecular level, X-ray Diffraction (XRD) distinguishes between crystalline and amorphous regions, which directly affect solubility and swelling behavior key factors in drug release and wound hydration. Differential Scanning Calorimetry (DSC) identifies thermal transitions like glass transition temperature (Tg) and melting point, offering insights into polymer stability and compatibility with active ingredients. Thermogravimetric Analysis (TGA) evaluates thermal degradation and residual moisture, crucial for shelf-life and formulation robustness. On the macroscopic front, Scanning Electron Microscopy (SEM) reveals surface morphology, porosity, and uniformity, which influence film formation and adherence to wound sites. Finally, Gel Permeation Chromatography (GPC) provides molecular weight distribution data, essential for predicting viscosity, muco-adhesion, and controlled drug release. Together, these techniques ensure that structural attributes align with therapeutic functionality.

Interpretive Considerations

Combined interpretation of chemical and structural data enables Fingerprinting and identity confirmation of botanical source, Batch-to-batch comparison for quality control, predictive modeling of drug-polymer interaction and release kinetics, optimization of processing parameters for film casting, hydrogel preparation, or scaffold fabrication. An integrated analytical approach not only ensures regulatory compliance but also supports the rational design of herbal polymer-based wound healing systems with consistent performance and safety.

Microbial Testing

Microbial testing plays a critical role in ensuring the safety and microbiological quality of herbal polymers intended for wound healing and pharmaceutical use. Due to their natural origin and hygroscopic properties, these polymers are especially prone to microbial contamination throughout cultivation, harvesting, processing, and storage. Effective microbial testing not only safeguards patient health but also ensures compliance with pharmacopoeia and regulatory standards (Sharma *et al.*, 2023).

Objectives of Microbial Testing

Microbial safety is a critical aspect of herbal polymer-based wound care formulations. First, assessing total viable aerobic count helps ensure that the overall bioburden of bacteria and fungi remains within pharmacopeial limits. Second, targeted pathogen detection—including *Escherichia coli*, *Salmonella spp.*, *Staphylococcus aureus*, and *Pseudomonas aeruginosa*—is essential, particularly for products applied to broken or compromised skin. Finally, maintaining low microbial counts or sterility is vital to prevent post-application infections, safeguarding patient health and ensuring therapeutic efficacy. These measures form the foundation of microbiological quality control in topical herbal formulations (Chuysinuan *et al.*, 2023).

Standard Test Methods

Microbial testing of herbal polymers is essential to ensure safety, especially in wound care applications. It typically involves Total Viable Count using nutrient agar and Sabouraud dextrose agar to quantify bacterial and fungal colonies. Pathogen-specific detection targets objectionable organisms: *E. coli* and *Salmonella* are identified using selective enrichment broths and differential media, while *Staphylococcus aureus* and *Pseudomonas aeruginosa* are detected via mannitol salt agar and cetrimide agar, respectively. Additionally, yeast and mold counts are crucial for mucilage-rich or hydrogel-forming polymers, which are particularly susceptible to fungal contamination under humid conditions. These tests help maintain microbial quality within pharmacopeial limits and prevent infection risks (Bhunia *et al.*, 2022).

Regulatory Standards

Best Practices for Sample Handling are use aseptic techniques and validated sterilized equipment, store test materials in sterile, airtight containers and employ neutralizers to counteract antimicrobial interference from the herbal matrix. Table 4 represent acceptable microbial limits are defined in various pharmacopoeia.

Table 4. Acceptable microbial limits are defined in various pharmacopoeia

Formulation Type	Total Aerobic Microbial Count	Total Yeast & Mold Count	Pathogen Absence
Topical products (non-sterile)	$\leq 10^3$ CFU/g or mL	$\leq 10^2$ CFU/g or mL	*E. coli, S. aureus, P. aeruginosa*
Herbal extracts/excipients (raw materials)	Specified based on intended application	Specified by pharmacopoeia	Pathogen-free as required

(USP 61, 62; Ph. Eur. 2.6.12, 2.6.13)

Complementary Testing Approaches

Microbial and contaminant control is a cornerstone of quality assurance for herbal polymers, especially in wound healing applications. Endotoxin testing, such as the Limulus Amebocyte Lysate (LAL) assay, is crucial for injectable formulations to prevent pyrogenic reactions. For multi-dose or extended-use systems, antimicrobial preservative effectiveness testing ensures sustained microbial protection. Rapid microbial detection methods, including PCR-based assays, enable efficient screening in high-throughput or time-sensitive contexts. Beyond microbial safety, herbal polymers due to their natural origin and complex processing are susceptible to a range of contaminants like pesticides, heavy metals, mycotoxins, residual solvents, and plant-derived toxins. Rigorous testing and control of these impurities not only safeguard therapeutic efficacy but also support GMP compliance and accurate shelf-life determination, ensuring that safety is built into every stage of the formulation lifecycle.

Common Contaminants and Their Sources

Herbal polymers, while promising for wound care, are susceptible to a range of chemical contaminants that can compromise safety and efficacy. Pesticide and herbicide residues, such as organophosphates and carbamates, may persist from agricultural practices. Heavy metals like lead, cadmium, arsenic, and mercury can accumulate from soil, irrigation water, or equipment contact. Mycotoxins, particularly aflatoxins from *Aspergillus* species, pose a risk under humid storage conditions. Residual solvents used during extraction such as methanol or dichloromethane must be carefully removed to avoid toxicity. Additionally, natural plant toxins like oxalates, saponins, and pyrrolizidine alkaloids may be present in unrefined materials, necessitating thorough purification and testing. Rigorous contaminant screening is essential to ensure the safety of herbal polymers in therapeutic applications.

Analytical Techniques for Detection

Each technique must be validated according to International Conference on Harmonisation (ICH) guidelines to ensure sensitivity, specificity, and reproducibility. Table 5, represent type of contamination and analytical method for their detection.

Table 5. Contaminant type and analytical methods

Contaminant Type	Analytical Methods
Pesticide Residues	Gas Chromatography–Mass Spectrometry (GC-MS), LC-MS/MS
Heavy Metals	Atomic Absorption Spectroscopy (AAS), ICP-MS
Mycotoxins	Enzyme-Linked Immunosorbent Assay (ELISA), LC-MS
Residual Solvents	Headspace GC or GC-FID (per ICH Q3C guidelines)
Natural Plant Toxins	TLC, HPLC, or spectrophotometric assays (compound-specific)

(Kadadou *et al.*, 2024)

Regulatory Requirements and Acceptance Limits

Pharmacopoeias and regulatory bodies (e.g., USP, EMA, WHO, AYUSH) provide limits for these contaminants based on route of administration and daily exposure thresholds i.e., Lead, ≤10 ppm for herbal raw materials, Methanol (Class 2 solvent) ≤3000 ppm, and Aflatoxins ≤20 µg/kg for raw herbal materials. Heavy metal limits in food, water, and soil, represent in Table 6. Meeting these limits is mandatory for product approval, especially in sensitive applications like chronic wound management or pediatric care. Regular screening for these contaminants ensures patient safety, supports regulatory compliance, and strengthens the scientific credibility of herbal polymer-based formulations (Baylor et al., 2020).

Table 6. Heavy metal limits in food, water, and soil

Metal	Food (ppm)	Drinking Water (ppm)	Soil (ppm)
Arsenic	0.1–0.2	0.01	20–40
Cadmium	0.05–2	0.003–0.005	0.9–3
Mercury	0.5–1	0.001–0.002	0.03–2
Lead	0.01–3	0.01–0.015	30–50

(FSSAI Regulations)

In-vivo and *In-vitro* Safety Models

The safety assessment of herbal polymers intended for wound healing applications necessitates a combination of *in-vitro* and *in-vivo* models to establish biocompatibility, cytotoxicity, and potential adverse biological interactions. These models provide a structured, ethical, and evidence-based approach to ensure that the polymer does not induce immunological, toxicological, or mutagenic effects before progressing to clinical use.

In-vitro Models

In-vitro assays are commonly employed as initial screening tools due to their cost-effectiveness, reproducibility, and minimal ethical concern. Safety evaluation of herbal polymers for wound healing involves a series of specialized biological assays to ensure biocompatibility and minimize adverse effects. Cytotoxicity tests such as MTT, Neutral Red Uptake, and Trypan Blue exclusion assess cell viability using fibroblast and keratinocyte cell lines like HaCaT and L929. Skin irritation and sensitization potential are evaluated using reconstructed human epidermis models like EpiDerm™ and SkinEthic™, following OECD guidelines. For dressings that contact blood, hemocompatibility assays measure hemolysis, platelet activation, and coagulation time. Additionally, oxidative stress and inflammation markers, including ELISA and ROS assays, help detect sub-toxic cellular responses by quantifying cytokines like IL-6 and TNF-α. Together, these assays provide a comprehensive safety profile essential for regulatory approval and clinical application (Menzel *et al.*, 2021).

In-vivo Models

In-vivo studies are conducted to confirm biocompatibility and safety in a physiological setting, particularly when the product is intended for prolonged contact or systemic absorption. In vivo safety assessment of herbal polymers involves a range of standardized animal studies to evaluate biocompatibility and systemic effects. Dermal toxicity studies (OECD TG 404) are conducted on rodents or rabbits to monitor skin irritation, erythema, and edema over short- and medium-term exposure. Sensitization and hypersensitivity tests, such as the Local Lymph Node Assay (LLNA) and Guinea Pig Maximization Test, help identify allergic responses. Wound healing models, using full-thickness excision or incision in rats or mice, assess not only repair efficacy but also potential adverse effects like infection or delayed healing (Palkhade *et al.*, 2025). For formulations intended for prolonged use, sub-chronic and repeated dose toxicity studies evaluate organ histopathology, hematology, and serum biochemistry. Additionally, systemic toxicity and behavioral observations track changes in weight, feeding, locomotion, and grooming to detect subtle signs of distress or dysfunction. Together, these studies provide a comprehensive safety profile essential for clinical translation and regulatory approval.

Integration into Regulatory Submissions

Both in-vitro and in-vivo studies should follow Good Laboratory Practice and align with regulatory guidelines. Data generated contributes to Risk assessment dossiers, safety margins and NOAEL estimation and Justification for clinical trials or human use. A balanced safety evaluation approach beginning with high-throughput in-vitro screens and supported by confirmatory in-vivo models—ensures that herbal polymers meet the stringent safety requirements for topical pharmaceutical products.

CASE STUDIES AND REPORTED INCIDENTS

The increasing incorporation of herbal polymers in wound care formulations has led to a growing body of observational data, post-marketing surveillance reports, and peer-reviewed case studies. These provide valuable insight into both the therapeutic promise and safety concerns associated with naturally derived excipients. Documenting such events not only reinforces the need for rigorous quality control but also illustrates potential pitfalls in formulation design, sourcing, and processing.

Case Report: Allergic Dermatitis from Aloe-Based Topical Gel

A 54-year-old diabetic patient developed erythema and pruritus after applying an over-the-counter aloe vera-based gel to a non-healing foot ulcer. Patch testing revealed hypersensitivity to aloin and anthraquinone residues components commonly found in unpurified aloe extracts. The product label failed to mention specific fractions used, and no standardized testing had been conducted on the extract. The reaction subsided upon discontinuation, emphasizing the need for allergen-screened herbal polymer components and transparent labeling (Edwards, 2025).

Regulatory Alert: Heavy Metal Contamination in Herbal Wound Powder (India, 2018)

The Central Drugs Standard Control Organization (CDSCO) issued a safety notice after finding elevated levels of lead and arsenic in a commercially marketed herbal wound dressing powder composed of *Curcuma longa* and starch derivatives.

Investigations attributed the contamination to poor soil quality and unregulated sourcing of botanical raw materials. This incident led to a temporary product ban and spurred initiatives for standardized Good Agricultural and Collection Practices (GACP) in Ayurvedic excipient manufacturing (Dashawant *et al.*, 2025).

Stability Failure: Gum-Based Hydrogel Showing Phase Separation

In a stability study conducted at 40°C/75% RH, a gum tragacanth-based wound healing hydrogel displayed significant phase separation after three months. Analytical data indicated microbial proliferation and hydrolytic degradation of polymer chains, suggesting inadequate preservative concentration and lack of sterility assurance testing. Reformulation with improved pH buffering and gamma sterilization yielded a stable and sterile product highlighting the importance of compatibility testing during formulation development (Tapia-Guerrero *et al.*, 2020).

In-vitro Safety Evaluation: Guar Gum Scaffold Exhibiting Cytotoxicity

A research group in Southeast Asia evaluated a guar gum-based wound scaffold and observed >30% cell death in L929 fibroblast cultures using MTT assay. Subsequent analysis revealed that the raw gum had not been properly deproteinized and contained residual alkaloids. After purification and retesting, cytotoxicity levels fell within acceptable limits—reinforcing the necessity of full compositional screening and preclinical safety testing for herbal excipients. These case studies illustrate that while herbal polymers hold great potential, lapses in standardization, purification, and documentation can compromise safety and undermine clinical trust. Ongoing surveillance, transparent reporting, and integration of quality-by-design approaches are essential to mitigate such risks in real-world applications (Dallabrida *et al.*, 2024).

FORMULATION CHALLENGES

Despite their therapeutic promise, herbal polymers face significant formulation challenges when translated into pharmaceutical-grade wound healing products. Their natural complexity and variability driven by environmental, botanical, and processing factors lead to batch-to-batch inconsistencies in key properties like viscosity, swelling capacity, and drug compatibility. This affects reproducibility in bio-adhesion, gel formation, and drug release kinetics. Stability is another concern, as hydrophilic polymers are prone to microbial growth and hydrolytic degradation, especially under humid conditions. Ensuring shelf-life requires optimized preservatives, drying techniques, packaging, and ICH-compliant stability testing. Solubility and pH sensitivity further limit formulation flexibility, with some polymers forming unstable gels outside narrow pH ranges. Additionally, scale-up is hindered by seasonal raw material availability and regional sourcing inconsistencies. Adopting Quality by Design (QbD) and modular processing platforms can help overcome these barriers. A multidisciplinary strategy combining polymer science, analytical rigor, and process innovation is essential to ensure safety, performance, and regulatory compliance in clinical wound care applications (Ambrogio *et al.*, 2022).

Clinical Observations

Clinical observations are essential for translating the promise of herbal polymer-based wound healing systems into therapeutic reality. While traditional use and experimental data support their efficacy, real-world studies provide critical insights into patient tolerability and formulation performance. Pilot trials—such as those using guar gum–Centella asiatica hydrogels or gum acacia–turmeric gels—have shown accelerated healing and minimal adverse effects. Observational designs like cohort and case-control studies help assess outcomes when randomized trials are impractical, and systematic reviews guided by frameworks like MOOSE and the Cochrane Handbook ensure evidence quality. Despite growing interest in herbal polymers for their biocompatibility, regulatory challenges remain due to inconsistent quality standards. Overall, clinical data affirm their potential but underscore the need for tailored formulations, rigorous monitoring, and future large-scale trials to establish long-term safety and efficacy (Song *et al.*, 2010).

Best Practices and Recommendations

The successful integration of herbal polymers into wound healing systems hinges on a well-defined framework of scientific, regulatory, and operational best practices. Given the natural origin and inherent variability of these materials, formulating safe, effective, and commercially viable products requires careful planning, multidisciplinary coordination, and continuous quality oversight. The following recommendations provide a roadmap for researchers, manufacturers, and clinicians working with herbal polymer-based formulations:

Raw Material Selection and Standardization

Raw material selection and standardization are foundational to the quality and safety of herbal polymer-based formulations. Polymers should be sourced from certified organic and traceable suppliers who adhere to Good Agricultural and Collection Practices (GACP), ensuring minimal contamination and ethical harvesting. Botanical identity must be rigorously verified using macroscopic and microscopic evaluations, supported by molecular techniques like DNA barcoding to confirm species authenticity. To ensure consistency across batches, validated chromatographic methods such as HPLC and TLC are employed to establish reliable phytochemical profiles. These profiles are then used to create a reference fingerprinting system, which serves as a benchmark for quality control and regulatory compliance throughout the formulation lifecycle (Chandra *et al.*, 2019).

Quality Control and Analytical Rigor

Ensuring the safety and consistency of herbal polymer-based formulations demands rigorous quality control across every batch. This includes comprehensive physicochemical, microbiological, and toxicological screening to detect impurities and confirm compliance with pharmacopeial standards. A suite of advanced analytical tools FTIR, NMR, XRD, TGA, and SEM is employed to characterize molecular structure, thermal stability, crystallinity, and surface morphology. Defined specifications for critical quality attributes such as viscosity, swelling index, and pH range are established to ensure reproducibility and therapeutic performance. This analytical rigor forms the backbone of GMP compliance and product reliability.

Safety and Toxicity Evaluation

Product development for herbal polymer-based wound care systems should begin with in-vitro screening, such as MTT assays for cytotoxicity and dermal irritation models to assess biocompatibility. These early tests help identify potential safety concerns before advancing to in-vivo studies, which evaluate toxicity, sensitization, and long-term stability—especially critical for high-risk or chronic-use applications. All studies must be conducted under Good Laboratory Practice (GLP) and aligned with OECD/FDA guidelines to ensure scientific validity and facilitate regulatory approval. This structured approach ensures both patient safety and compliance with global standards (Jena *et al.*, 2017).

GMP-Compliant Formulation and Manufacturing

Formulating herbal polymers for wound healing demands strict adherence to Good Manufacturing Practices (GMP). Sterilization methods such as gamma irradiation or low-temperature drying must be validated to ensure microbial safety without compromising polymer integrity. Manufacturing facilities should incorporate aseptic zones, controlled process flows, and trained personnel to minimize contamination risks and ensure safe handling of biological materials. A Quality-by-Design (QbD) framework is essential to proactively identify and control critical material attributes and process variables, ensuring consistent product performance and regulatory compliance throughout the production lifecycle (Yu *et al.*, 2014).

Patient-Centric Formulation Design

Effective wound care begins with tailoring the polymer type and form such as gels, films, or scaffolds to match the wound's location, severity, and moisture level. Ensuring biocompatibility, non-irritant behavior, and ease of removal enhances patient comfort and compliance, especially in chronic or sensitive cases. To further safeguard users, formulations must include clear labeling, precise usage instructions, and allergen disclosures, minimizing the risk of misuse and adverse reactions. This patient-focused approach bridges therapeutic efficacy with real-world usability.

REGULATORY DOCUMENTATION AND LIFECYCLE MANAGEMENT

To ensure safety and market readiness of herbal polymer-based wound care products, full traceability from source to final product is essential, supported by batch records and certificates of analysis. Regular updates to safety dossiers, pharmacovigilance reports, and post-marketing data strengthen oversight. Regulatory alignment with FDA, EMA, CDSCO, AYUSH, and ICH frameworks ensures global compliance. A proactive, science-driven approach from seed to scaffold advances innovation while maintaining reproducibility and patient safety (Makrani *et al.*, 2025).

Source Selection and Traceability

Ensuring the safety, efficacy, and reproducibility of herbal polymer-based formulations begins with meticulous source selection and transparent traceability. Due to the natural variability of botanical raw materials, a robust sourcing framework is essential for maintaining batch consistency and meeting regulatory standards. Priority should be given to materials cultivated under Good Agricultural and Collection Practices (GACP), with added assurance from certified organic farms or biodiversity-protected zones to minimize contamination and promote ecological sustainability. Selection criteria must also consider species authenticity, chemotype stability, harvest timing, and local processing traditions, all of which influence the polymer's functional properties. Traceability systems document the full lifecycle of raw materials from field to final formulation using tools like Certificates of Origin, harvest records, and Certificates of Analysis (CoA). Advanced methods such as blockchain-based documentation and DNA barcoding enhance transparency, support provenance verification, and streamline regulatory audits. These protocols help prevent adulteration, reduce ecological impact, and ensure therapeutic consistency. Ultimately, strong sourcing and traceability practices reinforce supply chain integrity, enable effective pharmacovigilance, and foster consumer confidence in herbal wound care products (Centobelli *et al.*, 2022).

Sterilization and Preservation

Sterilization and preservation strategies are essential to ensuring the microbial safety, physicochemical integrity, and therapeutic reliability of herbal polymer-based formulations. Due to their hygroscopic and bioactive nature, herbal polymers are particularly prone to microbial contamination and degradation—necessitating tailored approaches that balance microbial control with structural preservation.

Sterilization Approaches

Herbal polymers in topical wound care must be sterile or have low microbial counts to prevent infections, but sterilization methods must be carefully chosen to preserve functionality. Gamma irradiation (≤25 kGy) is effective with minimal impact but requires validation to avoid degradation. Autoclaving suits heat-stable gels but may reduce viscosity in sensitive polysaccharides. Ethylene oxide works for dry materials but poses toxicity risks due to residue. Dry heat and UV are generally inadequate for viscous or opaque formulations. Sterilization should align with the polymer's stability, dosage form, and regulatory standards (Atlanta, 2022).

Preservation Strategies

For non-sterile or multi-use herbal wound care products, preservatives are essential to prevent microbial growth. Natural options like neem oil, clove oil, and honey derivatives offer antimicrobial benefits with botanical compatibility. Synthetic preservatives such as parabens and phenoxyethanol are effective but must meet safety and regulatory standards. Preservative efficacy depends on formulation factors like pH, water activity, and polymer concentration. Techniques like buffering and sealed packaging enhance protection. Preservative efficacy testing is crucial. A tailored strategy combining sterilization validation, preservative compatibility, and stability testing ensures safety and performance.

Training, Labeling, and End-User Awareness

Effective implementation of herbal polymer-based wound care products extends beyond scientific formulation—it requires proper training, clear product labeling, and heightened awareness among end users, including healthcare professionals and patients. These elements are critical to ensure safe handling, correct usage, and improved therapeutic outcomes, while minimizing risks related to misuse, allergen exposure, or misinterpretation of product attributes.

Training and Professional Education

To ensure the safe and effective use of herbal polymers in healthcare, it is crucial that providers, pharmacists, and manufacturing personnel are equipped with accurate, up-to-date knowledge of their formulation behavior and associated risks. This can be achieved through structured workshops and continuing education programs that focus on herbal excipients, botanical pharmacology, and patient-specific wound care strategies. The implementation of standardized protocols for handling, reconstitution, and application particularly in primary care settings helps maintain consistency and safety across practices. Additionally, the provision of comprehensive Technical Data Sheets outlining compatibility, stability, and contraindications supports informed clinical decision-making. Ongoing training not only enhances professional competence but also builds confidence in recommending and managing these products, especially when caring for sensitive populations such as children, the elderly, or immunocompromised individuals (Thakur *et al.*, 2011).

Labeling and Consumer Guidance

Clear, accurate, and compliant labeling plays a vital role in ensuring transparency and safeguarding consumer health. Labels should clearly specify the botanical source and extraction method, including details about the plant part used and whether the extract is purified or crude. Disclosure of preservatives and allergens is equally important, as it helps users identify known sensitizers and anticipate potential interactions. Comprehensive instructions for use—covering frequency, application technique, duration of therapy, and storage conditions—empower consumers to use products safely and effectively. Additionally, regulatory certifications and shelf-life information enhance consumer trust and help prevent the use of expired or unstable formulations. Any claims such as natural, chemical-free, or organic must be substantiated with proper documentation to avoid misleading users or creating a false sense of safety.

End-User Awareness and Education

Engaging patients and caregivers through simple, accessible communication is essential to promote the appropriate use of healthcare products, especially in wound management. One effective strategy is the use of Patient Information Leaflets (PILs), which should be provided in local languages and include visual aids to accommodate varying literacy levels. Digital tools such as QR codes and user-friendly interfaces can link individuals to video demonstrations and detailed product FAQs, enhancing understanding and confidence in product use. Additionally, offering allergy and sensitivity checklists at the point of sale or during initial application helps identify potential adverse reactions early, ensuring safer outcomes. Raising awareness about critical practices like patch testing, correct dosing, and proper storage not only prevents complications but also empowers users to take an active role in their care (Sustersic *et al.*, 2017).

CONCLUSION

The integration of herbal polymers into wound healing formulations represents a promising convergence of traditional botanical wisdom and modern pharmaceutical innovation. Their unique properties—biocompatibility, biodegradability and intrinsic bioactivity—position them as compelling alternatives to synthetic excipients in both acute and chronic wound care applications. However, as evidenced throughout this monograph, their successful development and clinical translation are contingent upon rigorous standardization, safety profiling, and regulatory alignment. Challenges such as microbial contamination, batch-to-batch variability, allergenicity, and potential drug–excipient interactions underscore the importance of comprehensive analytical evaluation and controlled manufacturing practices. Regulatory frameworks and standards must be diligently followed to ensure consistency, traceability, and patient safety. In addition, real-world case studies and clinical observations highlight both the therapeutic benefits and potential pitfalls of herbal polymer use, reinforcing the need for robust toxicological assessment, vigilant post-marketing surveillance, and enhanced end-user education. Best practices in sourcing, sterilization, labeling, and training are not just operational necessities—they are integral to fostering trust and ensuring product success. As the field of natural-origin biomaterials continues to evolve, interdisciplinary collaboration, scientific rigor, and regulatory foresight will be essential in unlocking the full therapeutic potential of herbal polymers. By adhering to a framework of quality, transparency, and patient-centered design, these materials can play a transformative role in advancing safe, effective, and sustainable wound healing technologies.

REFERENCES

Aderibigbe, B. A. (2018). Alginate in wound dressings. *Pharmaceuticals, 11*(2), 42. DOI: 10.3390/ph11020042 PMID: 29735913

Ahmed, S., Ikram, S., & Yousaf, M. (2023). Biopolymer-based wound dressings: Recent advances and future perspectives. *Carbohydrate Polymers, 312*, 120789. DOI: 10.1016/j.carbpol.2022.120789

Ambrogio, G., Filice, L., Longo, F., & Padovano, A. (2022). Workforce and supply chain disruption as a digital and technological innovation opportunity for resilient manufacturing systems in the COVID-19 pandemic. *Computers & Industrial Engineering, 169*, 108158. DOI: 10.1016/j.cie.2022.108158 PMID: 35431410

Anjum, S., Arora, A., Alam, M. S., & Gupta, B. (2016). Development of antimicrobial and scar preventive chitosan hydrogel wound dressings. *International Journal of Pharmaceutics, 508*(1–2), 92–101. DOI: 10.1016/j.ijpharm.2016.05.014 PMID: 27163526

Balian, J. D., Wherry, J. C., Malhotra, R., & Perentesis, V. (2010). Roadmap to risk evaluation and mitigation strategies (REMS) success. *Therapeutic Advances in Drug Safety, 1*(1), 21–38. DOI: 10.1177/2042098610381419 PMID: 25083193

Baylor, N. W., & Tillman, D.-B. (2020). Regulatory approval and compliances for biotechnology products. In Shimasaki, C. (Ed.), *Biotechnology entrepreneurship* (2nd ed., pp. 429–446). Academic Press., DOI: 10.1016/B978-0-12-815585-1.00030-9

Benalaya, I., Alves, G., Lopes, J., & Silva, L. R. (2024). A Review of Natural Polysaccharides: Sources, Characteristics, Properties, Food, and Pharmaceutical Applications. *International Journal of Molecular Sciences, 25*(2), 1322. DOI: 10.3390/ijms25021322 PMID: 38279323

Bhunia, A. K., Singh, A. K., Parker, K., & Applegate, B. M. (2022). Petri-plate, bacteria, and laser optical scattering sensor. *Frontiers in Cellular and Infection Microbiology, 12*, 1087074. DOI: 10.3389/fcimb.2022.1087074 PMID: 36619754

Centobelli, P., Cerchione, R., Del Vecchio, P., Oropallo, E., & Secundo, G. (2022). Blockchain technology for bridging trust, traceability and transparency in circular supply chain. *Information & Management, 59*(7), 103508. DOI: 10.1016/j.im.2021.103508

Chandra, S., Stanford, D., Fletcher, E., & Walker, L. A. (2019). Raw Materials Production and Manufacturing Process Control Strategies. In Sasisekharan, R., Lee, S., Rosenberg, A., & Walker, L. (Eds.), *The Science and Regulations of Naturally Derived Complex Drugs. AAPS Advances in the Pharmaceutical Sciences Series* (Vol. 32). Springer., DOI: 10.1007/978-3-030-11751-1_10

Chatterjee, S., Dhole, A., Krishnan, A. A., & Banerjee, K. (2023). Mycotoxin Monitoring, Regulation and Analysis in India: A Success Story. *Foods (Basel, Switzerland), 12*(4), 705. DOI: 10.3390/foods12040705 PMID: 36832780

Chuysinuan, P., Pengsuk, C., Lirdprapamongkol, K., Thanyacharoen, T., Techasakul, S., Svasti, J., & Nooeaid, P. (2023). Turmeric Herb Extract-Incorporated Biopolymer Dressings with Beneficial Antibacterial, Antioxidant and Anti-Inflammatory Properties for Wound Healing. *Polymers, 15*(5), 1090. DOI: 10.3390/polym15051090 PMID: 36904331

Dallabrida, K. G., Braz, W. C., Marchiori, C., Alves, T. M., Cruz, L. S., Trindade, G. A. M., Machado, P., da Rosa, L. S., Khalil, N. M., Rego, F. G. M., Fajardo, A. R., Ferreira, L. M., Sari, M. H. M., & Reolon, J. B. (2024). Exploring Cationic Guar Gum: Innovative Hydrogels and Films for Enhanced Wound Healing. *Pharmaceutics, 16*(9), 1233. DOI: 10.3390/pharmaceutics16091233 PMID: 39339269

Daniel, A. B., Strickland, J., Allen, D., Casati, S., Zuang, V., Barroso, J., Whelan, M., Régimbald-Krnel, M. J., Kojima, H., Nishikawa, A., Park, H. K., Lee, J. K., Kim, T. S., Delgado, I., Rios, L., Yang, Y., Wang, G., & Kleinstreuer, N. (2018). International regulatory requirements for skin sensitization testing. Regulatory toxicology and pharmacology. *RTP, 95*, 52–65. DOI: 10.1016/j.yrtph.2018.03.003 PMID: 29518484

Dashawant, A., Khadke, R., Shete, A., & Gaikwad, V. (2025). CDSCO alerts: A retrospective dosage form–wise analysis of quality control alerts issued to pharmaceutical companies from 2018 to 2023. *Regulatory Toxicology and Pharmacology, 156*, 105775. DOI: 10.1016/j.yrtph.2025.105775 PMID: 39892642

DeBenedictis, J. N., de Kok, T. M., & van Breda, S. G. (2023). Impact of Processing Method and Storage Time on Phytochemical Concentrations in an Antioxidant-Rich Food Mixture. *Antioxidants (Basel, Switzerland), 12*(6), 1252. DOI: 10.3390/antiox12061252 PMID: 37371982

Edwards, E., & Yosipovitch, G. (2025). Skin Manifestations of Diabetes Mellitus. (Updated 2025 Mar 21). In: Feingold KR, Ahmed SF, Anawalt B, *et al.*, editors. Endotext (Internet). South Dartmouth (MA): MDText.com, Inc.; 2000-. Available from: https://www.ncbi.nlm.nih.gov/books/NBK481900/

Eur, Ph. 2.6.12, 2.6.13. http://www.uspbpep.com/ep60/2.6.13.%20microbiological%20examination%20of%20non-sterile%20products-%20test%20for%20specified%20micro-organisms%2020613e.pdf

Gatt, A. R., Vella Bonanno, P., & Zammit, R. (2024). Ethical considerations in the regulation and use of herbal medicines in the European Union. *Frontiers in Medical Technology*, *6*, 1358956. DOI: 10.3389/fmedt.2024.1358956 PMID: 38948354

Ghosh, D., Skinner, M., & Ferguson, L. R. (2006). The role of the Therapeutic Goods Administration and the Medicine and Medical Devices Safety Authority in evaluating complementary and alternative medicines in Australia and New Zealand. *Toxicology*, *221*(1), 88–94. DOI: 10.1016/j.tox.2005.12.023 PMID: 16481089

Griffith, C. (2016). Surface Sampling and the Detection of Contamination. Handbook of Hygiene Control in the Food Industry, 673–696. https://doi.org/DOI: 10.1016/B978-0-08-100155-4.00044-3

Jena, G. B., & Chavan, S. (2017). Implementation of Good Laboratory Practices (GLP) in basic scientific research: Translating the concept beyond regulatory compliance. *Regulatory Toxicology and Pharmacology*, *89*, 20–25. DOI: 10.1016/j.yrtph.2017.07.010 PMID: 28713068

Kadadou, D., Tizani, L., Alsafar, H., & Hasan, S. W. (2024). Analytical methods for determining environmental contaminants of concern in water and wastewater. *MethodsX*, *12*, 102582. DOI: 10.1016/j.mex.2024.102582 PMID: 38357632

Kumar, A. P. N., Kumar, M., Jose, A., Tomer, V., Oz, E., Proestos, C., Zeng, M., Elobeid, T. K. S., & Oz, F. (2023). Major Phytochemicals: Recent Advances in Health Benefits and Extraction Method. *Molecules (Basel, Switzerland)*, *28*(2), 887. DOI: 10.3390/molecules28020887 PMID: 36677944

Kumar, S., Gopal, K. M., Choudhary, A., Soman, A., & Namburi, U. R. S. (2023). Advancing the one health approach through integration of Ayush systems: Opportunities and way forward. *Journal of Family Medicine and Primary Care*, *12*(9), 1764–1770. DOI: 10.4103/jfmpc.jfmpc_192_23 PMID: 38024885

Makrani, M. F., Goyal, A., & Sayeed, S. Y. (2025). A comparative overview of global regulatory authorities: Ensuring quality, safety, and efficacy in medicines. International Research Journal of Pharmacy and Medical Sciences, 8(2), 93–99. http://irjpms.com/wp-content/uploads/2025/03/IRJPMS-V8N2P150Y25.pdf

Mazzocchi, F. (2006). Western science and traditional knowledge. Despite their variations, different forms of knowledge can learn from each other. *EMBO Reports*, *7*(5), 463–466. DOI: 10.1038/sj.embor.7400693 PMID: 16670675

Menzel, A., Samouda, H., Dohet, F., Loap, S., Ellulu, M. S., & Bohn, T. (2021). Common and Novel Markers for Measuring Inflammation and Oxidative Stress Ex Vivo in Research and Clinical Practice-Which to Use Regarding Disease Outcomes? *Antioxidants (Basel, Switzerland), 10*(3), 414. DOI: 10.3390/antiox10030414 PMID: 33803155

Miralles, A., Puillandre, N., & Vences, M. (2024). DNA Barcoding in Species Delimitation: From Genetic Distances to Integrative Taxonomy. *Methods in Molecular Biology (Clifton, N.J.), 2744*, 77–104. DOI: 10.1007/978-1-0716-3581-0_4 PMID: 38683312

Murthy, H. N. (2022). Chemical Constituents and Applications of Gums, Resins, and Latexes of Plant Origin. In Murthy, H. N. (Ed.), *Gums, Resins and Latexes of Plant Origin. Reference Series in Phytochemistry*. Springer., DOI: 10.1007/978-3-030-91378-6_1

Opuni, K. F. M., Kretchy, J. P., Agyabeng, K., Boadu, J. A., Adanu, T., Ankamah, S., Appiah, A., Amoah, G. B., Baidoo, M., & Kretchy, I. A. (2023). Contamination of herbal medicinal products in low-and-middle-income countries: A systematic review. *Heliyon, 9*(9), e19370. DOI: 10.1016/j.heliyon.2023.e19370 PMID: 37674839

Palkhade, R., Sammal, D., Parmar, J., & Chavhan, S. (2025). Methodological limitations and confounders in dermal toxicity evaluation of aqueous test substance by OECD technical guidelines 402, 410: Our experience of testing ethanol-based hand sanitizer. *Annals of Medicine, 57*(1). Advance online publication. DOI: 10.1080/07853890.2025.2491664 PMID: 40242887

Rojas, P., Jung-Cook, H., Ruiz-Sánchez, E., Rojas-Tomé, I. S., Rojas, C., López-Ramírez, A. M., & Reséndiz-Albor, A. A. (2022). Historical Aspects of Herbal Use and Comparison of Current Regulations of Herbal Products between Mexico, Canada and the United States of America. *International Journal of Environmental Research and Public Health, 19*(23), 15690. DOI: 10.3390/ijerph192315690 PMID: 36497761

Saha, D., & Bhattacharya, S. (2010). Hydrocolloids as thickening and gelling agents in food: A critical review. *Journal of Food Science and Technology, 47*(6), 587–597. DOI: 10.1007/s13197-010-0162-6 PMID: 23572691

Sharma, A., Sharma, N., & Luthra, G. (2023). The Crucial Role of Microbiological Testing in Ensuring Safety and Efficacy of Medical Devices: An Overview. *Journal of Pharmaceutical Research International, 35*, 47–55. DOI: 10.9734/jpri/2023/v35i127364

Sindhu, R. K., Gupta, R., Wadhera, G., & Kumar, P. (2022). Modern Herbal Nanogels: Formulation, Delivery Methods, and Applications. *Gels (Basel, Switzerland)*, *8*(2), 97. DOI: 10.3390/gels8020097 PMID: 35200478

Song, J. W., & Chung, K. C. (2010). Observational studies: Cohort and case-control studies. *Plastic and Reconstructive Surgery*, *126*(6), 2234–2242. DOI: 10.1097/PRS.0b013e3181f44abc PMID: 20697313

Soni, V., Jain, P., Haider, T., Pandey, V., & Tekade, R. K. (2018). Documentation protocol in product development including clinical records. In Tekade, R. K. (Ed.), *Advances in pharmaceutical product development and research: Dosage form design parameters* (pp. 403–440). Academic Press., DOI: 10.1016/B978-0-12-814421-3.00012-9

Sustersic, M., Gauchet, A., Foote, A., & Bosson, J. L. (2017). How best to use and evaluate Patient Information Leaflets given during a consultation: A systematic review of literature reviews. *Health Expectations*, *20*(4), 531–542. DOI: 10.1111/hex.12487 PMID: 27669682

Tapia-Guerrero, Y. S., Del Prado-Audelo, M. L., Borbolla-Jiménez, F. V., Gomez, D. M. G., García-Aguirre, I., Colín-Castro, C. A., Morales-González, J. A., Leyva-Gómez, G., & Magaña, J. J. (2020). Effect of UV and Gamma Irradiation Sterilization Processes in the Properties of Different Polymeric Nanoparticles for Biomedical Applications. *Materials (Basel, Switzerland)*, *13*(5), 1090. DOI: 10.3390/ma13051090 PMID: 32121529

Thakur, L., Ghodasra, U., Patel, N., & Dabhi, M. (2011). Novel approaches for stability improvement in natural medicines. *Pharmacognosy Reviews*, *5*(9), 48–54. DOI: 10.4103/0973-7847.79099 PMID: 22096318

Tosif, M. M., Najda, A., Bains, A., Kaushik, R., Dhull, S. B., Chawla, P., & Walasek-Janusz, M. (2021). A Comprehensive Review on Plant-Derived Mucilage: Characterization, Functional Properties, Applications, and Its Utilization for Nanocarrier Fabrication. *Polymers*, *13*(7), 1066. DOI: 10.3390/polym13071066 PMID: 33800613

USP 61. https://www.usp.org/harmonization-standards/pdg/general-methods/microbial-enumeration

USP 62. http://www.uspbpep.com/usp31/v31261/usp31nf26s1_c62.asp

Viera-Herrera, C., Santamaría-Aguirre, J., Vizuete, K., Debut, A., Whitehead, D. C., & Alexis, F. (2020). Microcrystalline Cellulose Extracted from Native Plants as an Excipient for Solid Dosage Formulations in Drug Delivery. *Nanomaterials (Basel, Switzerland)*, *10*(5), 975. DOI: 10.3390/nano10050975 PMID: 32438544

Yang, S., Hu, X., Zhu, J., Zheng, B., Bi, W., Wang, X., Wu, J., Mi, Z., & Wu, Y. (2025). Aspects and Implementation of Pharmaceutical Quality by Design from Conceptual Frameworks to Industrial Applications. *Pharmaceutics*, *17*(5), 623. DOI: 10.3390/pharmaceutics17050623 PMID: 40430914

Yu, L. X., Amidon, G., Khan, M. A., Hoag, S. W., Polli, J., Raju, G. K., & Woodcock, J. (2014). Understanding pharmaceutical quality by design. *The AAPS Journal*, *16*(4), 771–783. DOI: 10.1208/s12248-014-9598-3 PMID: 24854893

Zhang, S., Hu, J., Sun, Y., Tan, H., Yin, J., Geng, F., & Nie, S. (2021). Review of structure and bioactivity of the Plantago (Plantaginaceae) polysaccharides. *Food Chemistry: X*, *12*, 100158. DOI: 10.1016/j.fochx.2021.100158 PMID: 34825168

Chapter 14

Regulatory and Ethical Perspective on Herbal Polymers and Excipients

Kavyashree Shetty
Shobhaben Pratapbhai Patel School of Pharmacy and Technology Management, SVKM's NMIMS, India

Namita Juvale
https://orcid.org/0000-0001-7004-5675
Shobhaben Pratapbhai Patel School of Pharmacy and Technology Management, SVKM's NMIMS, India

ABSTRACT

Herbal excipients and natural polymers have gained significant attention in the field of wound healing due to their biocompatibility, biodegradability, antimicrobial properties, and cost-effectiveness. Biopolymers such as chitosan, cellulose, and hyaluronic acid, often combined with herbal bioactive like curcumin, aloe vera, and centella Asiatica, have shown significant potential for wound repair. Despite their therapeutic potential, the regulatory and ethical framework for herbal excipients is complex when compared to synthetic excipients. This involves challenges like lack of standardization and quality control due to natural variability in herbal raw materials, lack of pharmacopeial recognition, etc. Agencies such as the US FDA, EMA, and WHO have provided general frameworks for botanical products, but harmonized product-specific regulations for herbal excipients and polymers are still evolving. This chapter highlights the need for standardized regulatory framework for the development and approval of novel polymers.

DOI: 10.4018/979-8-3373-3977-1.ch014

1. INTRODUCTION

Wound healing is a complex and dynamic biological process involving a cascade of cellular and molecular events which restores the integrity and function of damaged tissue. Over the years, a growing interest has emerged in the use of herbal-based materials for wound care, to get a safer, biocompatible, and cost-effective alternatives to synthetic compounds, (Schultz et al., 2011). Among these, herbal polymers and excipients have emerged as promising agents in wound healing formulations due to their biocompatibility, biodegradability, and therapeutic potential, (Oliveira et al., 2023). Natural gums such as guar gum and xanthan gum contribute to improved swelling index and enhanced patient comfort in hydrogel wound dressings, whereas glycerin, a well-established moisturizing excipient in dermatological creams and cosmeceuticals, facilitates skin hydration and supports barrier repair, (Mohammadinejad et al., 2020). They are derived from natural plant sources like gums, mucilages and polysaccharides, which are biocompatible, non-toxic, cost-effective and widely available in addition to improving drug delivery, stability, and viscosity, (Prajapati et al., 2013).

The pharmaceutical and cosmeceutical industries are increasingly incorporating herbal polymers and excipients into wound dressings, hydrogels, films, and ointments. Despite their growing use, there are significant regulatory and ethical challenges, which include the lack of standardized pharmacopeial monographs for many herbal excipients, the risk of contamination with heavy metals, pesticides, or microbes, and concerns about ethical sourcing, (Prajapati et al., 2022). Although their traditional use is well documented in various systems of medicine such as Ayurveda, Traditional Chinese Medicine (TCM), and Unani, a systematic framework of scientific validation, safety assessment, quality control, and ethical sourcing is necessary for integrating this historical knowledge into regulated pharmaceutical products, (Patwardhan et al., 2005).

While synthetic excipients have established monographs and detailed specifications in global pharmacopeias such as the United States Pharmacopeia (USP), European Pharmacopeia (Ph. Eur), many herbal polymers lack official standards. Regulatory authorities such as the European Medicines Agency (EMA) have established guidelines to ensure the quality, safety, and efficacy of herbal medicinal products and their excipients, (European Directorate for the Quality of Medicines & HealthCare, 2025). These guidelines emphasize the need for standardized production practices, such as Good Agricultural and Collection Practice (GACP) for herbal starting materials, and require comprehensive specifications for herbal substances, including details on the name, quantity, and technological purpose of excipients, (World Health Organization, 2023). The United States Food and Drug Administration (US FDA) has not established specific monographs or formal guidelines solely dedicated to herbal excipients. The herbal excipients used in drug products must either be included in the US FDA's Inactive Ingredient Database (IID) or be supported by sufficient toxicological data to demonstrate their safety, (Center for Drug Evaluation and Research, 2019). In India, the regulation of herbal excipients is primarily governed by the Drugs and Cosmetics Act, 1940 and its associated Rules, which apply to allopathic, Ayurvedic, and homeopathic drugs. For an excipient to be used in pharmaceutical products, it must have a precedence of use, either in India or internationally, and supporting data from reputable sources like Martindale or the Handbook of Pharmaceutical Excipients can be submitted for approval, (Central Drugs Standard Control Organization, 1940).

The general quality principles as per the ICH guidelines emphasizes that pharmaceutical development must involve detailed evaluation of all excipients' functionality, compatibility, stability, and safety, (International Council for Harmonisation, 2025). Along with the regulatory concerns, there is a growing need to address ethical considerations associated with the use of herbal polymers. Many of these natural substances are derived from biodiversity-rich regions and have been historically used by indigenous and local communities for traditional healing practices such as the use of neem (*Azadirachta indica*) in India or ginseng (*Panax ginseng*) in East Asia. Companies and researchers utilizing such polymers must ensure fair and equitable benefit-sharing, proper acknowledgment of traditional knowledge. Thus, for the effective integration of herbal polymers into a medicinal product, a comprehensive knowledge of the legal frameworks, ethical issues, and scientific validation criteria is essential (Gupta et al., 2005).

Regulation of herbal excipients is necessary to ensure the safety, quality, and efficacy of the final formulation. Herbal excipients play a crucial roles in drug formulations by affecting stability, bioavailability, and patient acceptance, but their natural origin has challenges such as variability in composition, potential contamination with heavy metals or pesticides, and batch-to-batch inconsistency. The growing demand for natural and eco-friendly products has led to an increase in the use of herbal excipients, which makes it even more important to have robust standards for the sourcing, processing, and quality control. Harmonized regulations facilitate international trade, prevent the distribution of substandard products, and support the sustainable growth of the herbal excipient industry. Regulatory oversight helps to establish uniform standards for sourcing, processing, testing, and labelling. This minimizes risks to patients and ensures ethical and scientific accountability in drug development.

The use of herbal excipients in drug formulations especially for sensitive populations like wound healing in pediatric, or geriatric patients will require stringent regulations and scientific validation.

2. GLOBAL REGULATORY LANDSCAPE

The World Health Organization (WHO) recognizes the growing significance of herbal excipients in pharmaceutical formulations. WHO has developed various guidelines to ensure quality throughout the lifecycle of herbal substances. These include the Good Agricultural and Collection Practices (GACP), Good Herbal Processing Practices (GHPP), and Good Manufacturing Practices (GMP) for herbal medicines. GACP ensures that plants are correctly identified and harvested at optimal maturity, while GHPP and GMP guide the processing of plant extracts to control microbial contamination and heavy metal levels. Traceability systems track these materials from farm to finished product, and quality control tests verify identity, microbial load, and pesticide residues. These measures benefit herbal excipients by ensuring consistent quality, safety, and efficacy across batches, reducing the risk of contamination or adulteration. WHO guidelines related to herbal excipients are discussed ahead.

2.1 Good Agricultural and Collection Practices (GACP)

This guideline consists of the framework to ensure the quality, safety, and consistency of raw herbal materials. The guideline covers every stage of the herbal excipient supply chain, from plant selection to post-harvest storage with the goal of minimizing contamination, adulteration, and variability within natural products. It emphasizes on the accurate botanical identification and authentication of plant species, requiring taxonomical precision to avoid the use of incorrect or potentially harmful substitutes. During cultivation and collection, it highlights the need for appropriate site selection, optimal soil quality, and consideration of ecological factors to support the healthy growth of medicinal plants. The post-harvest phase is equally critical, requiring that inspection, sorting, and primary processing such as cutting and drying are conducted under controlled and hygienic conditions to minimize the risk of microbial or chemical contamination. It also addresses the packing and storage of the herbal materials along with clear labelling to ensure traceability. Transportation processes must also safeguard the integrity and quality of the herbal excipients by avoiding exposure to adverse environmental conditions (World Health Organization, 2023).

2.2 Good Herbal Processing Practices (GHPP)

This guideline standardizes the processing of herbs from post-harvesting stage. It supplements existing GACP and GMP by focusing specifically on the critical steps involved after harvesting, including inspection, sorting, washing, primary processing and advanced techniques like distillation, extraction, and concentration. It emphasizes the need for in-process quality control, proper documentation, and adherence to national and international standards throughout all processing stages. The GHPP also addresses technical aspects such as facility requirements, equipment maintenance, packaging, labelling, storage, and transportation, ensuring that all processed herbal products are free from contaminants (World Health Organization, 2018).

2.3 Good Manufacturing Practices (GMP) for herbal medicines

This guideline provides a regulatory framework to ensure that herbal products, including herbal excipients, are consistently produced and controlled to meet quality standards appropriate for their intended use. This guideline covers all stages of manufacturing, including raw material handling, processing, quality control, packaging, labeling, and storage. Critical aspects include facility sanitation to prevent microbial contamination, validation of extraction and processing methods to ensure batch consistency, and controlled storage conditions to preserve stability. It requires that manufacturing facilities maintain a clean and controlled environment, use qualified equipment, and employ trained personnel to minimize risks such as contamination, cross-contamination. It emphasizes the development and adherence to Standard Operating Procedures (SOPs), documentation of every manufacturing step, and implementation of quality assurance systems, such as in-process checks and final product testing. It also requires manufacturers to establish a robust quality management system, ensuring traceability of all the activities (World Health Organization, 2007).

2.4 Quality Control methods for herbal materials

This guideline highlights the importance of establishing internationally recognized standards and testing procedures to ensure the quality, safety, and efficacy of herbal medicines and raw plant materials. It provides a comprehensive set of analytical methods for the identification, sampling, and examination of herbal materials, including both macroscopic and microscopic analysis, chemical profiling, and quantitative determinations like ash, extractable matter, water content, volatile oils, and specific indices like bitterness, tannins, and foaming. It emphasizes on the detection and quantification of potential contaminants such as pesticide residues, toxic metals like arsenic, microorganisms, aflatoxins, and radioactive contamination. The guideline is intended to support national drug quality control laboratories, particularly in developing countries, by providing model procedures that can be adapted to local regulatory needs and market conditions, (World Health Organization, 2011).

3. COUNTRY SPECIFIC REGULATIONS RELATED TO HERBAL EXCIPIENTS

3.1. United States of America (USA)

The US FDA is responsible for the regulation related to herbal excipients. The US FDA defines new excipients as any inactive ingredients that are intentionally added to therapeutic and diagnostic products, but that:

(a) are not intended to exert therapeutic effects at the intended dosage, although they may act to improve product delivery
(b) are not fully qualified by existing safety data with respect to the currently proposed level of exposure, duration of exposure, or route of administration, (The United States Pharmacopeial Convention, 2020).

3.1.1. Review and Approval Process of Novel Herbal Excipients

Herbal excipients undergo a similar regulatory pathway like other synthetic excipients. Herbal excipients do not have a direct regulatory pathway and are assessed with the submission of NDA, ANDA. The manufacturer must submit a Type IV Drug Master File (DMF) to the US FDA, which includes detailed information on the excipients's manufacturing process, specifications, analytical and toxicological data, and non-clinical safety studies. The DMF holder must also provide a Letter of Authorization (LOA), allowing the US FDA to access the DMF for another applicant's submission without disclosing proprietary details. The US FDA then reviews the polymer's safety data and may request additional information before making a decision. Once approved, the polymer is listed in the Inactive Ingredient Database (IID), (Center for Drug Evaluation and Research, 2019).

3.1.2. Safety Evaluation of Herbal Excipients

Non-Clinical studies must be conducted if the excipient is novel and has no previous history of safety data. New excipients require a risk-benefit assessment and submission of relevant toxicological data. Safety evaluations should follow ICH S7A guidelines, including pharmacological activity assessments. Based on intended clinical use duration, toxicology studies are categorized into short-term (≤14 days), intermediate (2 weeks–3 months), and long-term (>3 months). Depending on the clinical use, the US FDA recommends the studies like acute toxicity and reproductive toxicity evaluations to chronic toxicology and carcinogenicity studies. Additionally, the US FDA may request further data such as pharmacokinetic profiles or drug-excipient interaction studies if existing information is inadequate, (Center for Drug Evaluation and Research, 2005).

Chronic and carcinogenicity studies are recommended for herbal wound dressings with agents like honey and polysaccharides to ensure long-term safety, (Arslan et al., 2024). The US FDA may require toxicity studies for aloe vera gel and guar gum if their safety profile for topical or systemic use is not well-established, (Chakraborty et al., 2021). Guar gum is generally recognized as safe (GRAS) by the US FDA for food use, but studies on chronic toxicity and ingredient quality are still ongoing, (EFSA Panel on Food Additives and Nutrient Sources Added to Food, 2017).

3.1.3. Inactive Ingredient Database

The Inactive Ingredient Database (IID) maintained by the US FDA provides a list of excipients used in the approved drug product. It also includes information on herbal excipients along with the excipient name, route of administration, dosage form, and the maximum potency used in approved formulations (Center for Drug Evaluation and Research, 2019). The Table 1 below provides the list of herbal excipients used in the market formulations for wound healing.

Table 1. Herbal excipients listed in the IID used in the marketed formulations for wound healing

Sr	Name of the Herbal excipient	Source	Route of Administration	Dosage form	Marketed Formulations for Wound Healing
1.	Guar Gum	Endosperm of seeds of Cyamopsis tetragonoloba (guar plant)	Topical	Lotion	Regenerex Xcellderma™ (Regenerex Pharma Inc., 2025)
2.	Starch	Extracted from cereals/tubers like Zea mays (corn), Solanum tuberosum (potato), Oryza sativa (rice)	Topical	Cream, Powder	Iodosorb Ointment (Smith-Nephew, 2025)
3.	Carrageenan	Extracted from red seaweeds, especially Chondrus crispus (Irish moss), Kappaphycus alvarezii, and Eucheuma species	Topical	Lotion	Garamycin Cream (Padagis Isreal Pharmaceuticals Ltd., 2024)
4.	Glycerin	Derived from fats and oils (animal or vegetable) by hydrolysis, transesterification, or fermentation	Topical	Aerosol, Cream, Gel, Lotion, Ointment	Elasto-Gel™ Hydrogel Sheets (Stout & McKessor, 2012)
5.	Lactose	Commercially derived from whey	Topical	Ointment	LAC-HYDRIN Cream (Bristol Myers Squibb Company, 2001)

3.1.4. GRAS (Generally Regarded as Safe) Notification Process

Herbal excipients used as taste-masking agents or flavorants in drug formulations may undergo the GRAS notification process to establish their safety for use after approval. Companies can submit a GRAS notification to the US FDA by providing comprehensive evidence of safety through scientific data or a history of safe use. The submission must include detailed information about the substance's identity, manufacturing process, specifications, and safety profile. After reviewing the notification, the US FDA may issue one of three types of responses which includes "No Question letter", "Insufficient Basis Letter" and "Cease to Evaluate Letter" (Food and Drug Administration, 2025).

Curcumin, derived from the turmeric plant (*Curcuma longa*) has undergone the GRAS Notification process. In 2017, a GRAS notice (No. 000686) was submitted to the US FDA for curcumin's use as a food ingredient. The notification included comprehensive safety data, including toxicological studies and human consumption history, to support its safe use in food products US FDA. While this GRAS notification pertains to curcumin's use in food, its established safety profile has enabled its incorporation into various pharmaceutical and cosmetic formulations (Department of Health and Human Services, 2017).

3.1.5. Pilot Program for Review of Innovation and modernization of excipients (PRIME)

In the Year 2021, the US FDA has launched the Pilot Program for Review of Innovation and modernization of excipients (PRIME) to help excipient manufacturers to overcome challenges in their development and market authorization. This voluntary program is intended to provide manufacturers of excipients with an opportunity to obtain US FDA evaluations of novel excipients prior to their use in drug formulations. PRIME targets excipients that have not been used in US FDA-approved drug products and the excipients which are not used in food. This process allows for the early identification of any concerns such as formulation issues, safety risks, or limitations, so that manufacturers can address them before proceeding with expensive and time-consuming clinical trials, (United States Pharmacopeia, 2024). The Figure 1 explains the review and approval process of herbal excipients in the USA.

Figure 1. Approval process of herbal excipients by US FDA

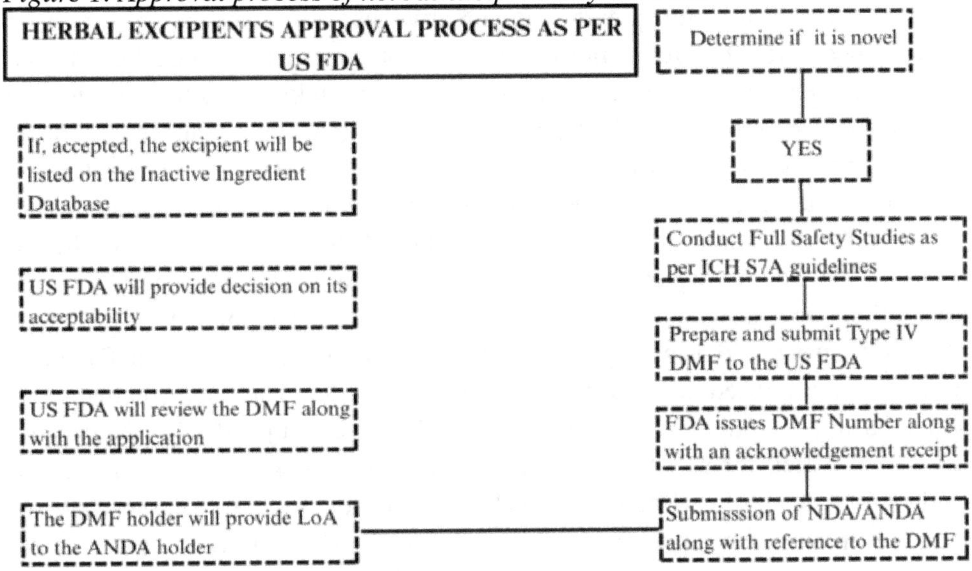

3.2. European Union (EU)

The primary regulatory authority for herbal medicinal products and excipients in the European Union (EU) is the EMA. Within the EMA, the Committee on Herbal Medicinal Products (HMPC) is responsible for issuing scientific opinions and providing guidance on the safe and effective use of herbal substances and preparations. National competent authorities (NCAs) of EU member states are involved in decentralized and national procedures. European Directorate for the Quality of Medicines & HealthCare (EDQM) maintains the Ph. Eur. and sets quality standards, (European Medicines Agency, 2025).

3.2.1. Regulations related to herbal excipients

Directive 2001/83/EC provides the legal framework for medicinal products in the European Union and includes specific provisions relevant to herbal excipients. The Directive defines key terms such as "herbal substances," "herbal preparations," and "herbal medicinal products," clarifying that herbal substances can include whole, fragmented, or cut plants, algae, fungi, or lichen, and that herbal preparations are obtained by processes like extraction, distillation, or fermentation. The Directive mandates that all ingredients, including herbal excipients, must be clearly identified and their quality, safety, and traceability must be ensured. The manufacturers must comply with Good Manufacturing Practice (GMP) standards for both the manufacture and distribution of excipients. The Directive also addresses the prevention of falsified medicines. The authenticity and quality of excipients must be documented throughout the supply chain, and that any excipient with known action or effect be properly labeled and included in the product information, (European Union, 2001).

EU Directive 2004/24/EC amends Directive 2001/83/EC and addresses the regulation of traditional herbal medicinal products along with the excipients used in these products. Traditional herbal medicinal products are defined as "Medicinal products whose active ingredients consist exclusively of herbal substances or herbal preparations, such as whole plants, plant parts, or processed plant materials, and are intended for use based on a long-standing tradition of medicinal use" The Directive introduces a simplified registration procedure for traditional herbal medicinal products requiring that all ingredients must be clearly listed and justified in the product dossier submitted for registration. The Directive mandates that the Summary of Product Characteristics (SmPC) for each product must include a comprehensive list of excipients, their quantities, and any relevant safety information or special warnings. Furthermore, excipients used in traditional herbal medicinal products must comply with established quality standards, such as those outlined in the Ph. Eur. and must be manufactured in accordance with Good Manufacturing Practice (GMP). The Directive also requires that any excipient with known action or effect be appropriately labeled and that its safety profile is assessed as part of the overall product evaluation, (European Union, 2004).

3.2.2. Guidelines related to herbal excipients

Guideline on quality of herbal medicinal products/traditional herbal medicinal products (EMA/CPMP/QWP/2819/00 Rev. 2) provides requirements related to herbal excipients. The excipients must be fully described in the product dossier along with their name and quantity. Any substance added during manufacture for purposes like stabilisation, preservation, or as a technological aid must be listed as an "excipient" and not as part of the active substance, and comprehensive details on production and control must be provided in the dossier. Safety is supported by documented long-term use and must be supplemented by toxicological data for any excipient if not listed in Ph. Eur., (European Medicines Agency, 2022).

Guideline on specifications: test procedures and acceptance criteria for herbal substances, herbal preparations and herbal medicinal products/traditional herbal medicinal products. This guideline provides requirements for establishing comprehensive specifications, including test procedures and acceptance criteria, for all components of herbal medicinal products. It also provides that the specifications for excipients cover quality attributes such as identity, purity, and content, and that appropriate test methods are applied to ensure batch-to-batch consistency and safety. For standardised herbal preparations, the guideline allows the addition of suitable inert excipients to achieve a defined content of active constituents, but for quantified or "other" herbal preparations, excipients can only be included for technological purposes, with their use and range, (European Medicines Agency, 2022).

Annexure to the European Commission guideline on 'Excipients in the labelling and package leaflet of medicinal products for human use' provides a comprehensive list of excipients with known actions or effects that must be clearly declared on the labelling and in the package leaflet of all medicinal products in the EU. The Annex specifies the exact information, warning statements, and safety details for each listed excipient that must be included in the package leaflet to ensure safe use by patients and healthcare professionals, (European Medicines Agency, 2018).

The Table 2 highlights the list of herbal excipients along with the patient information note as provided in the European Commission's Guideline.

Table 2. List of herbal excipiemt with patient information note as per the European Commission's guideline

Sr No.	Name of the Herbal Excipient	Route of Administration	Patient Information Note
1.	Arachis oil (peanut oil)	All	May cause allergic reactions in individuals allergic to peanuts.
2.	Balsam of Peru	Topical	May cause skin reactions.
3.	Bergamot oil	Topical	May increase sensitivity to UV light (natural photosensitiser)
4.	Latex (Natural Rubber)	All	Warning for allergy due to container contact
5.	Macrogolglycerol ricinoleate	Parentral	Macrogolglycerol ricinoleate
6.	Soya oil	All	Contraindicated in peanut or soya allergy

(European Medicines Agency, 2018)

EU GMP Annex 7: Manufacture of Herbal Medicinal Products. The annex emphasizes the critical importance of controlling starting materials including the herbal active substances and herbal excipients used in the formulation. It requires detailed documentation and traceability for all plant-derived materials along with the scientific (binomial) name, plant part used, source, cultivation and harvesting conditions, and any treatments or processing steps must be recorded for both actives and excipients. The annex mandates that any excipient of herbal origin must meet the same rigorous standards for quality, storage, and contamination control as active herbal substances, including tests for identity, purity, microbial and pesticide contamination, and potential adulterants or toxic metal, (ECA Academy, 2008).

3.2.3. Review and Approval process of Herbal Excipients

Figure 2. Herbal excipient approval pathway in EU

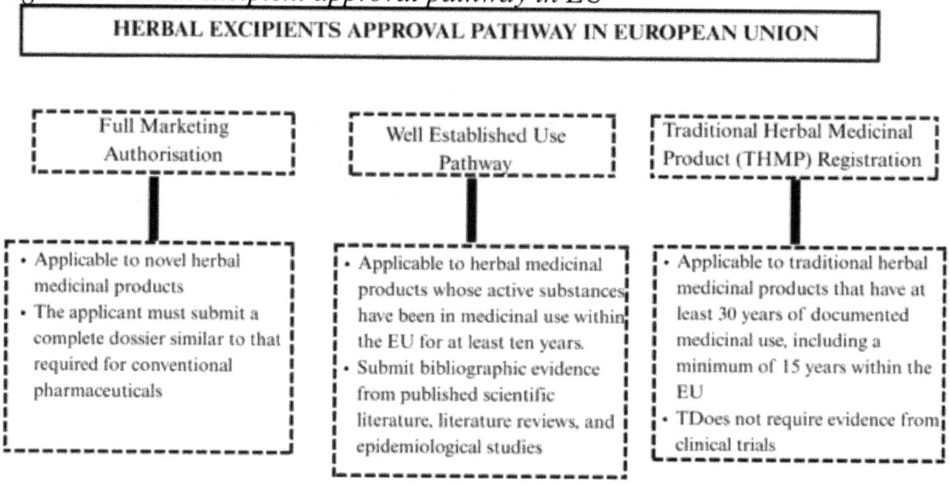

Herbal excipients do not have a direct regulatory pathway. They are submitted along with the finished product. Herbal medicinal products are regulated through national procedures overseen by each EU Member State's national competent authority. There are 3 main regulatory pathways available:

Full Marketing Authorisation pathway is required for novel herbal medicinal products that do not qualify for simplified or traditional use procedures. Under this route, the applicant must submit a complete dossier similar to that required for conventional pharmaceuticals. This dossier must include detailed data on the product's quality, safety, and efficacy, supported by results from pharmaceutical studies such as composition, manufacturing process and stability. Non-clinical studies including toxicology and pharmacology and clinical studies demonstrating efficacy and safety in humans is also required. The dossier must provide information about excipients related to their quality, safety, toxicological data and justification for their use. This pathway is typically used for new herbal products or those with novel combinations or novel indications, (European Medicines Agency, 2025).

The Well-Established Use pathway is intended for herbal medicinal products whose active substances have been in medicinal use within the EU for at least ten years, with recognized efficacy and acceptable safety. Instead of requiring new clinical trials, this route allows applicants to submit bibliographic evidence from published scientific literature, literature reviews, and epidemiological studies that collectively demonstrate the product's safety and efficacy. This approach is suitable for products where the active herbal ingredients and their effects are documented with well-established clinical safety and scientific research. Excipients used in these products must also be justified and shown to be safe, with supporting bibliographic or scientific evidence as necessary, (European Medicines Agency, 2009).

Traditional Herbal Medicinal Product (THMP) Registration procedure is for traditional herbal medicinal products that have at least 30 years of documented medicinal use, including a minimum of 15 years within the EU. Unlike the other pathways, THMP registration does not require evidence from clinical trials. The efficacy is established based on bibliographic or expert evidence of traditional use and experience. Applicants must submit a bibliographic review of safety data, as well as comprehensive information on quality, manufacturing, and stability. These products are intended for use without the supervision of a medical practitioner and cannot be administered by injection. All ingredients along with the excipients must be clearly listed, justified, and shown to be safe based on traditional use and available safety data. This pathway facilitates the availability of traditional herbal remedies while maintaining standards of safety and quality, (European Medicines Agency, 2009). The Figure 2 explains the approval process of herbal excipients in the European Union.

3.3. India

The primary regulatory authority for herbal excipients in India is the Central Drugs Standard Control Organization (CDSCO). Along with it, the Department of AYUSH (Ayurveda, Yoga & Naturopathy, Unani, Siddha, and Homoeopathy), which operates under the Ministry of Health and Family Welfare, is responsible for overseeing the manufacturing, marketing, and quality control of herbal medicines, (Central Drugs Standard Control Organization, 2025). Both CDSCO and AYUSH dont have an independent pathways for approval of herbal excipients. However, annually CDSCO publishes a list of Ayurvedic Products whose Certificate of Pharmaceutical Product (COPP) is granted by CDSCO as per WHO-GMP Certification Scheme, (Central Drugs Standard Control Organization, 2025).

3.3.1. Regulations/Guidelines

Herbal excipients used in Ayurvedic, Siddha, and Unani (ASU) medicines are regulated under the Drugs and Cosmetics Act, 1940 and Rules, 1945. Schedule T of the Act specifies GMP for herbal medicines. The Indian Pharmacopoeia (IP) and other official pharmacopoeias provide quality standards for excipients. There are no specific regulations for excipients. Instead, the excipients must comply with IP or other recognized international compendia.

3.3.2. Review and Approval Process

In India, the review and approval process for herbal excipients depends on whether the excipient is already recognized or is being newly introduced, (Zugle, 2021).

For Excipients Listed in Pharmacopoeia, a herbal excipient must either be listed in the IP or another recognized international compendium such as the USP, Ph. Eur., or have documented precedence of safe use in India or abroad. If the excipient is graded as IP, it will be regulated by the State Food and Drug Administration (State FDA). For example, curcumin is already recognized in the IP for its various medicinal properties, so it meets the initial requirement of being a compendial herbal excipient. Since it's an IP-grade substance, its use and regulation fall under the purview of the State FDA. The State FDA conducts pre-licensing inspections of the site to ensure it adheres to Good Manufacturing Practices (GMP). Once the site is approved and the manufacturing license is granted, the company can begin the manufacturing process. The license is renewable, and the State FDA conducts periodic inspections to ensure continued compliance with GMP.

For Formulations under AYUSH systems, The Pharmacopeial Laboratory for Indian Medicine (PLIM) or associated research councils evaluate the herbal excipient as per traditional medicine protocols. Additionally, the applicant is expected to submit a Certificate of Analysis (CoA), stability data, and demonstrate compliance with GMP to ensure product consistency and safety.

The Table 3 provides a comparison summarizing the review and approval process for herbal excipients in USA, EU and India.

Table 3. Comparison summarizing the review and approval process for herbal excipients in USA, EU and India

Aspect	USA	European Union	India
Regulatory Authorities	United States Food and Drug Administration (US FDA)	European Medicines Agency (EMA), Committee on Herbal Medicinal Products (HMPC), National Competent Authorities	Central Drugs Standard Control Organization, Department of AYUSH (Ayurveda, Yoga & Naturopathy, Unani, Siddha, and Homoeopathy)
Applicable Framework	US FDA Guidelines, IPEC America Guidelines	Directive 2001/83/EC, 2004/24/EC, Quality and safety Guidelines	Drugs and Cosmetics Act (1940), Schedule T
Submission Pathway	Type IV DMF, Reviewed along with NDA/ANDA	Submitted with final product dossier (Full MA, Well-Established Use, or THMP)	Requires precedence of use or recognized pharmacopoeial listing
Independent Approval Pathway for Novel Excipients	Assessed by PRIME Program for early US FDA Feedback	No independent approval pathway	No independent approval pathway
Safety and Quality	Requires toxicological data, pharmacokinetics, interactions, risk-benefit evaluation per ICH	GMP (Annex 7), EMA guidelines require full traceability, quality data, and toxicological support	GMP per Schedule T, documentation of traditional use
Traditional Use Consideration	Limited	THMP route allows 30+ years of documented use	Traditional knowledge (AYUSH systems) accepted with documentation
Regulatory database	Inactive Ingredient Database (IID) includes list of excipients used in approved formulations	A database is maintained by the European Commission providing information of the safety details of excipient in approved formulations.	No database specifically for excipients

4. REGULATORY APPROACHES IN BIODIVERSITY-RICH DEVELOPING COUNTRIES

The most biodiversity-rich countries which is often called "megadiverse countries" include Brazil, Indonesia, Colombia, China, Mexico, Peru, India, Australia,

Ecuador, the United States, South Africa, Democratic Republic of Congo, Venezuela, the Philippines, Papua New Guinea, Malaysia, and Madagascar, (Pariona, 2025). Biodiversity-rich developing countries have adopted multifaceted regulatory approaches which include national legislation, international conventions, and innovative financing strategies. They work together internationally through the Convention on Biological Diversity (CBD) which encourages countries in enforcing national laws and policies to protect habitats and species through in-situ and ex-situ conservation, environmental impact assessments, and regulation of genetic resource access, (Convenion on Biological Diversity, 2025). Legislations for enforcement of green supply chain management hold paramount importance, (Hariyani et al., 2024).

Countries such as India and Indonesia have established protected area networks, community-led sacred groves, and biodiversity monitoring schemes. In Africa, countries like Botswana, South Africa, Rwanda, Egypt, and Uganda utilize biodiversity offset banking, wildlife certification. These countries increasingly leverage modern regulatory tools, including national biodiversity finance plans in Egypt, ecological fiscal transfers in Uganda and integration of nature-related financial disclosures in South Africa. International collaborations and donor-supported frameworks provide technical and financial assistance, which enables robust enforcement and innovative conservation programs, (Kigonya et al., 2024).

5. CLINICAL DATA, CASE STUDIES, AND REAL-WORLD APPLICATIONS OF HERBAL EXCIPIENTS

Aloe vera gel is rich in polysaccharides such as acemannan, has shown significant wound healing benefits. Randomized controlled trials in patients with partial-thickness burns revealed that Aloe vera gel dressings accelerated epithelialization, reduced healing time by nearly one-third compared to silver sulfadiazine, and improved pain management. These findings highlight the dual role of Aloe vera as both a therapeutic agent and a natural excipient in topical formulations, (Hekmatpou et al., 2019). Similarly, chitosan which is a natural polymer derived from chitin has been evaluated in surgical wound management and chronic ulcer care, where clinical trials demonstrated its hemostatic, antimicrobial, and bioadhesive properties, supporting its utility as a stabilizing excipient in wound dressings and hydrogels. Curcumin-loaded gels formulated with guar gum have also shown promise in diabetic wound healing by reducing inflammation and enhancing collagen deposition, (Hekmatpou et al., 2019).

In the United States, excipients such as xanthan gum, tragacanth, and carrageenan are included in the US FDA'S IID and are widely employed in approved topical gels, creams, and suspensions. In the European Union, soya oil and arachis oil are listed as excipients in licensed medicinal products which requires safety labeling to address allergenicity.

6. ETHICAL CONSIDERATIONS AND CHALLENGES RELATED TO THE DEVELOPMENT AND APPROVAL OF HERBAL EXCIPIENTS

Ethical considerations in the use of herbal excipients ensures patient safety, product efficacy, and respect for individual and cultural values. Regulatory authorities and manufacturers must prioritize transparency, honesty, and fairness by providing accurate information about quality, safety, and efficacy, and by ensuring that products are scientifically validated.

The WHO guidelines on GACP for medicinal plants emphasize that all activities related to the cultivation, collection, and post-harvest processing of medicinal plant materials must adhere to both legal and ethical standards established at national and international levels. Legally, this includes compliance with environmental regulations, intellectual property rights, and international treaties such as the Convention on Biological Diversity (CBD) and the Convention on International Trade in Endangered Species of Wild Fauna and Flora (CITES). The includes any collection of medicinal plants from the wild or those listed as threatened or endangered, must be conducted only with the appropriate permissions and in accordance with relevant laws. Export permits, phytosanitary certificates, and CITES documentation are mandatory for international trade in such species, ensuring that the sourcing of plant materials does not contribute to the depletion of biodiversity or the illegal trade of protected species (8).

It also provides the importance of respecting the rights and interests of local communities and indigenous peoples who are often the traditional custodians of medicinal plant knowledge and resources. Prior to the collection or cultivation of medicinal plants, agreements regarding the sharing of benefits and compensation for the use of source materials must be negotiated and documented.

This approach is designed to ensure fair and equitable benefit-sharing, recognizing the contributions of local communities and upholding the principles of the CBD. It also highlights the need to avoid negative social impacts on local livelihoods, advocating for practices that support community welfare. Additionally, ethical concerns regarding the conservation of medicinal plant resources, promoting sustainable use to prevent over-harvesting and environmental degradation must be taken into consideration. The guidelines encourage the establishment of national and regional inventories of medicinal plants, which helps in the identification of endangered species, support conservation efforts, and address intellectual property rights issues, (World Health Organization, 2023).

Technical issues such as contamination with pesticides, heavy metals, or microbial agents can affect product safety. Additionally, inadequate standardization and lack of rigorous quality control during extraction, concentration, and formulation processes can result in batch-to-batch variability, affecting the efficacy and safety of the final product. The complexity of herbal mixtures, which often contain numerous active and inactive compounds, further complicates the development of reliable analytical methods for quality assurance, (World Health Organization, 2018).

One of the most cited cases is the biopiracy of Neem, where the European Patent Office granted a patent to W.R. Grace and the U.S. Department of Agriculture for neem-based pesticidal applications despite the plant's centuries-long traditional use in India. Indian scientists and NGOs challenged the patent and it was eventually revoked in 2000, reinforcing the principle that traditional knowledge cannot be misappropriated without recognition or consent (48). Similarly, the Turmeric (*Curcuma longa*) case involved a U.S. patent for its wound-healing applications, which was successfully revoked after India's Council of Scientific and Industrial Research (CSIR) demonstrated prior use in Ayurveda, making it a classic example of biopiracy in herbal medicine, (Fredriksson, 2023).

Herbal excipients requires rigorous ethical and regulatory oversight through comprehensive clinical evaluations and transparent labelling Ensuring patient safety with herbal excipients requires rigorous ethical and regulatory oversight, particularly through clinical evaluations and transparent labeling. Clinical evaluations are essential to identify potential adverse effects, interactions with other medications, and to ensure that herbal excipients are both safe and effective for their intended use. Labeling must provide clear information about the contents, proper usage, possible side effects, contraindications, and storage instructions, enabling patients and healthcare providers to make informed decisions. Clinical evaluations are essential to identify potential adverse effects, interactions with other medications, and to ensure that herbal excipients are both safe and effective for their intended use. The need for rigorous safety testing in herbs with known toxicities must also be considered to prevent adverse health outcomes, (World Health Organization, 2018).

6.1. Ethical Considerations

6.1.1. Authenticity and Accurate Botanical Identification

Accurate botanical identification of herbal excipients is required to ensure patient safety and maintain scientific integrity. Misidentification can lead to the inclusion of the wrong species, potentially resulting in reduced efficacy or serious adverse effects. Ethical sourcing demands that manufacturers use validated methods such as macroscopic, microscopic, and chromatographic techniques to confirm plant identity. Proper taxonomic classification along with standardized nomenclature, helps prevent substitution or adulteration. Ethically, it is also important to document the plant's origin, part used and its processing history to ensure transparency and traceability, (Gatt, Vella Bonanno, & Zammit, 2024). A 2021 study in India found that nearly 30% of Echinacea supplements were adulterated or contained incorrect species due to improper identification. To ensure species authenticity and avoid these issues, manufacturers are urged to use macroscopic and microscopic evaluations, DNA barcoding, and High-Performance Liquid Chromatography (HPLC), (Ferrer, 2025).

6.1.2. Sustainability and Environmental Impact

Ethical considerations must be taken to ensure that the plants must be harvested sustainably from cultivated sources as per protocols that allow for regeneration. Environmental responsibility also includes minimizing the carbon footprint in transportation, reducing water usage, and managing waste from extraction and processing. Ethical sourcing should align with international conventions such as the Convention on Biological Diversity (CBD), emphasizing the need for conservation and fair benefit-sharing with communities that rely on these natural resources, (Gatt, Vella Bonanno, & Zammit, 2024). In 2023, the Aloe vera industry in India was valued at 1,200 crore (approximately USD 190 million), with the country being the world's largest producer. This growth is attributed to the increasing demand for natural and organic products, leading to the establishment of sustainable cultivation practices. Farmers in drought-prone regions like Satara, Maharashtra, have adopted water-efficient irrigation techniques and organic farming methods to cultivate Aloe vera, ensuring environmental responsibility and economic viability, (Warak, 2025).

6.1.3. Scientific Validity and Evidence based Use

Many herbal products enter the market without sufficient evidence supporting their pharmacological activity or safety profile. This lack of scientific validation raises concerns about misleading patients. Ethical standards necessitate that herbal excipients must have stringent regulations to ensure their reliability,(Gatt, Vella Bonanno, & Zammit, 2024). In a study published in 2018, 28.8% of herbal preparations were found to be contaminated with heavy metals, and 7% were adulterated with conventional drugs to enhance efficacy. These findings underscore the need for stringent regulations to ensure the safety and efficacy of herbal products. A 2023 study assessed the safety documentation submitted for herbal medicines in Tanzania, revealing that many products lacked adequate safety data in their marketing authorization dossiers. This highlights the necessity for comprehensive safety evaluations before market approval, (Luo et al., 2021).

6.1.4. Transparency in Labeling and Marketing

Accurate labeling and marketing are essential to ensure that consumers and healthcare professionals are fully informed about the contents and properties of herbal excipients. Mislabeling or deleting information about potential allergens, contaminants, or the true concentration of active components can lead to misuse of the product. Excipient manufacturers must provide clear information on product labels and in advertising to support informed decision-making, (Pick, 2025). A 2025 bulletin from the American Botanical Council highlighted widespread mislabeling of Echinacea products. The report indicated that many products labeled as containing Echinacea roots or herbs were found to be adulterated with other plant materials, leading to discrepancies between labeled and actual contents. Such mislabeling undermines consumer trust and poses risks to individuals relying on these products for their purported health benefits, (Ferrer, 2025).

6.1.5. Fair Trade and Indigenous Knowledge Rights

Many herbal excipients are derived from traditional knowledge by indigenous or local communities. Ethical practice requires that companies and researchers obtain prior informed consent and enter into benefit-sharing agreements. Exploiting traditional knowledge without proper acknowledgment or compensation is considered as biopiracy. Ethical obligations include ensuring that these communities receive fair economic benefits and capacity-building support from commercialization, (Alum, 2024). The development of Jeevani, an anti-fatigue drug derived from *Trichopus zeylanicus*, was based on the traditional knowledge of the Kani tribe in Kerala, India. The Tropical Botanic Garden and Research Institute (TBGRI) implemented a pioneering benefit-sharing model that allocated a portion of the profits to a trust for the welfare of the Kani community, setting a precedent under the Convention on Biological Diversity (CBD), (World Intellectual Property Organization, 2010). The case of the Rosy Periwinkle (*Catharanthus roseus*) from Madagascar led to the discovery of the anticancer agents vincristine and vinblastine. Despite the immense global impact of these drugs, the communities and country of origin received no financial compensation or recognition, (Kerketta & Kumari, 2024).

6.2. Recent Developments to Combat Biopiracy

There have been recent developments related to biopiracy, particularly concerning the protection of traditional knowledge and the rights of indigenous communities. In May 2024, the World Intellectual Property Organization (WIPO) adopted the GRATK Treaty, a significant international legal action aimed at combating biopiracy. This treaty mandates that patent applicants disclose the origin of genetic resources and associated traditional knowledge used in their inventions. It also emphasizes the need for prior informed consent and equitable benefit-sharing with indigenous communities. The treaty has been signed by 30 countries, including India, and is expected to enter into force once 15 countries accept it, (World Intellectual Property Organization, 2025).

7. CERTIFICATION BODIES AND COUNCILS RELATED TO HERBAL EXCIPIENTS

7.1 International Pharmaceutical Excipient Council Federation (IPEC Federation)

The International Pharmaceutical Excipient Council Federation (IPEC Federation) is a global organization representing excipient suppliers, distributors, and pharmaceutical manufacturers. IPEC's primary mission is to develop, implement, and promote voluntary guidance for excipients, including herbal excipients, to ensure their quality and safety. The council encourages the adoption of regulatory and compendial standards and works collaboratively to advance public health. It provides updates for the excipient industry on global issues, monitors regulatory developments, and provides mechanisms for consensus-building across regions. Its members include IPEC-Americas, IPEC Europe, IPEC Japan, and IPEC China, with associate members in Brazil and India. The council is also involved in harmonizing standards through collaboration with major pharmacopoeias and promotes supply chain management through risk assessment and third-party GMP certification, (IPEC Federation, 2025).

7.2 International Regulatory Cooperation for Herbal Medicines (IRCH)

The International Regulatory Cooperation for Herbal Medicines (IRCH) is a global network established by the WHO in 2006. Its membership comprises national and regional regulatory authorities responsible for the regulation of herbal medicines. IRCH's mission is promote collaboration and provide best practices among its members to improve the regulation and safe use of herbal medicines along with the inactive ingredients. The council also assists WHO in developing recommendations for member states and raising awareness about the safety and efficacy of herbal products. As of January 2025, IRCH has 49 member authorities from around the world. The network facilitates the exchange of regulatory information, supports harmonization efforts, and addresses emerging challenges in the herbal sector, (World Health Organization, 2025).

7.3 American Herbal Products Association (AHPA)

AHPA is a US based trade association that develops industry standards and guidance documents for the responsible commerce of herbal products and excipients. It provides specific standards for identity, manufacturing, labeling, and usage of herbal ingredients. It is referred for the basis for quality management systems and reliable trade conduct for herbal products and excipients thereby encouraging suppliers and formulators globally, (American Herbal Products Association, 2025).

7.4 Pharmacopoeial Discussion Group (PDG)

The PDG is a collaboration between the United States Pharmacopeia (USP), European Pharmacopoeia (Ph. Eur.), and Japanese Pharmacopoeia (JP). It aims to harmonize pharmacopoeial standards for excipients. Harmonization of monographs and general chapters through PDG ensures that excipient specifications meet regulatory requirements across major markets, (The United States Pharmacopeial Convention, 2018).

7.5 International Organization for Standardization (ISO) – Technical Committee ISO/TC 249 (Traditional Chinese Medicine)

ISO/TC 249 provide standardization of traditional medicines which also includes herbal products and excipients. It provides international standards for raw herbal materials, processing methods, safety testing, and labeling. These ISO standards are globally recognized and assist in harmonizing quality control measures, (Secretariat Standardization Administration of China, 2009).

7.6 National Science Foundation (NSF)

NSF International is a globally recognized, independent organization that develops public health standards and certification programs to ensure the safety and quality of food, water, and consumer products, including dietary supplements and herbal ingredients. For herbal excipients, NSF provide Good Manufacturing Practices (GMP) certification. NSF also certifies raw materials, including herbal excipients, for purity, contamination risk like heavy metals, microbes, and pesticides and identity verification through rigorous analytical testing and audits. In addition to GMP, NSF's NSF/ANSI 173 standard provides criteria for ingredient testing in dietary supplements, which often include herbal excipients, (NSF-National Science Foundation, 2025.

8. FUTURE PROSPECTS

The use of herbal excipients in drug formulations is driven by the global shift toward natural, sustainable, and biocompatible ingredients in pharmaceutical formulations. The organic pharmaceutical excipients market, which includes herbal excipients, is projected to grow robustly from \$12.33 billion in 2025 to \$17.59 billion by 2029 with a annual growth rate (CAGR) of 9.3%, (Research and Markets, 2025). Additionally, the overall global excipients market including both synthetic and natural types is expected to reach \$13.06 billion by 2030, growing at a CAGR of 4.1% from 2024, (American Pharmaceutical Review, 2025). The integration of AI and in-silico modeling in excipient characterization and standardization can enhance the development of herbal excipients. AI and machine learning are increasingly applied in excipient evaluation, offering predictive insights into excipient–drug compatibility, stability, and toxicity. These in silico tools reduce lengthy trial- and enable the design of optimized formulations, (Vora et al., 2023). A 2025 study published in Pharmaceuticals reviewed AI models and tools designed to assess interactions between herbal medicines and conventional drugs. These models utilize machine learning and deep learning techniques to predict potential adverse interactions. Similarly, blockchain technology is emerging as a enabler of supply chain transparency, (Hilal et al., 2024). In 2021, the HerBChain platform was introduced as a blockchain-based system to record and verify the six critical processes in herbal product manufacturing and marketing. This platform ensures transparency and traceability, addressing challenges related to authenticity, adulteration, and ethical sourcing of herbal excipients, (Yik et al., 2021). Green technologies and sustainable processing methods are redefining the production landscape for natural excipients. Techniques such as supercritical fluid extraction, microwave-assisted extraction, and enzymatic processing are being adopted to reduce solvent use, minimize waste, and lower the environmental footprint of excipient manufacturing, (Usman, Nakagaway, & Cheng, 2023). Despite these advances, industry barriers remain significant. Challenges such as complex regulatory requirements, variability in plant material quality, financial constraints, and limited market access hinder the large-scale commercialization of herbal excipients, (Jadhav et al., 2025). The integration of herbal excipients into personalized medicine is likely to expand with natural polymers due to their multifunctional properties. The multifunctional nature of herbal excipients will help in advancing patient-tailored therapies.

9. CONCLUSION

The use of herbal excipients into wound healing formulations provides various advantages due to their biocompatibility, biodegradability. Regulatory agencies such as the WHO, US FDA, and EMA have established guidelines for ensuring the quality, safety, and efficacy of herbal excipients, but there is a need for harmonized, product-specific regulations. The EMA's 2024 annual report emphasizes the importance of scientific opinions on herbal substances and preparations, providing clear reference points for marketing authorization or registration in EU Member States. Similarly, the US FDA's 2024 roundup includes approvals for novel drugs, some of which incorporate botanical ingredients, reflecting the agency's recognition of the therapeutic potential of herbal excipients. Ethical considerations such as sustainable sourcing, benefit-sharing with indigenous communities, and transparent clinical research are equally critical to ensure innovation. The sustainable incorporation of herbal excipients into wound healing products requires a holistic approach combining scientific validation, AI-driven in silico modeling, regulatory harmonization, and ethical sourcing.

REFERENCES

Alum, E. U. (2024). The role of indigenous knowledge in advancing the therapeutic use of medicinal plants: Challenges and opportunities. *Plant Signaling & Behavior, 19*(1), 2439255. Advance online publication. DOI: 10.1080/15592324.2024.2439255 PMID: 39652401

American Herbal Products Association. (2025). *About AHPA*. https://www.ahpa.org/

American Pharmaceutical Review. (2025). The future of pharmaceutical excipients: A $14 billion market driven by global demand. *American Pharmaceutical Review, Interphex 2025 Supplement*, 25–27. https://www.americanpharmaceuticalreview.com/Featured-Articles/618347-The-Future-of-Pharmaceutical-Excipients-A-14-Billion-Market-Driven-by-Global-Demand/

Arslan, N. P., Orak, T., Ozdemir, A., Altun, R., Esim, N., Eroglu, E., Karaagac, S. I., Aktas, C., & Taskin, M. (2024). Polysaccharides and peptides with wound healing activity from bacteria and fungi. *Journal of Basic Microbiology, 64*(9), e2400510. Advance online publication. DOI: 10.1002/jobm.202400510 PMID: 39410821

Bristol Myers Squibb Company. (2001). *Drug approval package: Lac-Hydrin (ammonium lactate) cream* (NDA #20-508/S005). U.S. Food and Drug Administration. https://www.accessdata.fda.gov/drugsatfda_docs/nda/2000/20508S005_Lac-Hydrin.cfm

Center for Drug Evaluation and Research. (2005). *Nonclinical studies for the safety evaluation of pharmaceutical excipients*. U.S. Food and Drug Administration. https://www.fda.gov/regulatory-information/search-fda-guidance-documents/nonclinical-studies-safety-evaluation-pharmaceutical-excipients

Center for Drug Evaluation and Research. (2019). *Inactive ingredients in approved drug products search: Frequently asked questions*. U.S. Food and Drug Administration. https://www.fda.gov/drugs/drug-approvals-and-databases/inactive-ingredients-approved-drug-products-search-frequently-asked-questions

Center for Drug Evaluation and Research. (2019). *Drug master files guidance for industry (draft)*. U.S. Food and Drug Administration. https://www.fda.gov/drugs/forms-submission-requirements/drug-master-files-dmfs

Central Drugs Standard Control Organization. (1940). *Drugs and Cosmetics Act 1940*. https://cdsco.gov.in/opencms/opencms/en/Acts-and-rules/Drugs-and-Cosmetics-Act/

Central Drugs Standard Control Organization. (2025). *Home*. https://cdsco.gov.in/opencms/opencms/en/Home/

Central Drugs Standard Control Organization. (2025). *Ayush*. https://cdsco.gov.in/opencms/opencms/en/Aayush/

Chakraborty, T., Gupta, S., Nair, A., Chauhan, S., & Saini, V. (2021). Wound healing potential of insulin-loaded nanoemulsion with aloe vera gel in diabetic rats. *Journal of Drug Delivery Science and Technology*, *64*, 102601. Advance online publication. DOI: 10.1016/j.jddst.2021.102601

Convention on Biological Diversity. (2025). *Home*. https://www.cbd.int/

Department of Health and Human Services. (2017). *GRAS notice (GRN) No. 686: Curcumin from turmeric (Curcuma longa L.)*. U.S. Food and Drug Administration. https://www.fda.gov/files/food/published/GRAS-Notice-000686---Curcumin-from-turmeric-%28Curcuma-longa-L.%29.pdf

ECA Academy. (2008). *EU GMP Annex 7: Manufacture of herbal medicinal products*. https://www.gmp-compliance.org/guidelines/gmp-guideline/eu-gmp-annex-7-manufacture-of-herbal-medicinal-products

EFSA Panel on Food Additives and Nutrient Sources added to Food, Mortensen, A., Aguilar, F., Crebelli, R., Di Domenico, A., Frutos, M. J., … & Younes, M. (2017). Re-evaluation of guar gum (E 412) as a food additive. *EFSA Journal, 15*(2), Article e04669. https://doi.org/DOI: 10.2903/j.efsa.2017.4669

European Directorate for the Quality of Medicines & HealthCare. (2025). *Harmonisation status for excipient monographs (PDG)*. https://www.edqm.eu/en/harmonisation-status-for-excipient-monographs-pdg-

European Medicines Agency. (2009). *Herbal medicinal products*. https://www.ema.europa.eu/en/human-regulatory-overview/herbal-medicinal-products

European Medicines Agency. (2018). *Annex to the European Commission guideline on "Excipients in the labelling and package leaflet of medicinal products for human use"*. https://www.ema.europa.eu/en/annex-european-commission-guideline-excipients-labelling-package-leaflet-medicinal-products-human-use

European Medicines Agency. (2022). *Guideline on quality of herbal medicinal products/traditional herbal medicinal products* (Revision 3). https://www.ema.europa.eu/en/documents/scientific-guideline/guideline-quality-herbal-medicinal-productstraditional-herbal-medicinal-products-revision-3_en.pdf

European Medicines Agency. (2022). *Guideline on specifications: Test procedures and acceptance criteria for herbal substances, herbal preparations and herbal medicinal products/traditional herbal medicinal products* (Revision 3). https://www.ema.europa.eu/en/documents/scientific-guideline/guideline-specifications-test-procedures-and-acceptance-criteria-herbal-substances-herbal-preparations-and-herbal-medicinal-productstraditional-herbal-medicinal-products-revision-3_en.pdf

European Medicines Agency. (2025). *Herbal medicinal products*. https://www.ema.europa.eu/en/human-regulatory-overview/herbal-medicinal-products

European Medicines Agency. (2025). *Herbal medicinal products: Scientific guidelines*. https://www.ema.europa.eu/en/human-regulatory-overview/research-development/scientific-guidelines/multidisciplinary-guidelines/herbal-medicinal-products-scientific-guidelines

European Union. (2001). *Directive 2001/83/EC of the European Parliament and of the Council of 6 November 2001 on the Community code relating to medicinal products for human use. Official Journal of the European Union, L 311*, 67–128. https://eur-lex.europa.eu/eli/dir/2001/83/oj/eng

European Union. (2004). *Directive 2004/24/EC of the European Parliament and of the Council of 31 March 2004 amending, as regards traditional herbal medicinal products, Directive 2001/83/EC. Official Journal of the European Union, L 136*, 85–90. https://eur-lex.europa.eu/eli/dir/2004/24/oj/eng

Ferrer, B. (2025). *Echinacea under scrutiny: New report exposes adulteration and mislabelling*. Nutrition Insight. https://www.clearprint.com/role-of-accurate-labeling-in-consumer-safety/

Food and Drug Administration. (2025). *Generally recognized as safe (GRAS)*. https://www.fda.gov/food/food-ingredients-packaging/generally-recognized-safe-gras

Fredriksson, M. (2023). India's traditional knowledge digital library and the politics of patent classifications. *Law and Critique*, *34*(1), 1–19. DOI: 10.1007/s10978-022-09327-7 PMID: 36915708

Gatt, A. R., Vella Bonanno, P., & Zammit, R. (2024). Ethical considerations in the regulation and use of herbal medicines in the European Union. *Frontiers in Medical Technology*, *6*, 1358956. Advance online publication. DOI: 10.3389/fmedt.2024.1358956 PMID: 38948354

Gupta, R., Gabrielsen, B., & Ferguson, S. M. (2005). Nature's medicines: Traditional knowledge and intellectual property management. Case studies from the National Institutes of Health (NIH), USA. *Current Drug Discovery Technologies*, *2*(4), 203–219. DOI: 10.2174/157016305775202937 PMID: 16475917

Hariyani, D., Hariyani, P., Mishra, S., & Sharma, M. K. (2024). A literature review on green supply chain management for sustainable sourcing and distribution. *Waste Management Bulletin*, *2*(4), 231–248. DOI: 10.1016/j.wmb.2024.07.008

Hekmatpou, D., Mehrabi, F., Rahzani, K., & Aminiyan, A. (2019). The effect of aloe vera clinical trials on prevention and healing of skin wound: A systematic review. *Iranian Journal of Medical Sciences*, *44*(1), 1–9. https://pubmed.ncbi.nlm.nih.gov/30666070/ PMID: 30666070

Hilal, P. J., Harish, P., Harshita, C., Ashishkumar, P., Rashmi, D., & Prashant, K. (2024). Advancements and challenges in the integration of artificial intelligence with herbal medicine research. *IJPS Journal*, *2*(4), 973–984.

International Council for Harmonisation. (2025). *Mission - Harmonisation for better health*. https://www.ich.org/page/quality-guidelines

IPEC Federation. (2025). *Guidelines*. https://ipec-federation.org/home/guidelines/

Jadhav, R., Das, J., Rajyaguru, S., Kyada, S., Kale, V., Teja, P. K., & Bhatt, P. (2025). Regulations, current development, and future prospects of phytopharmaceuticals, a new class of herbal medicines in India. *Discover Pharma Sciences*, *1*(6). Advance online publication. DOI: 10.1007/s44338-024-00002-5

Kerketta, G. S., & Kumari, P. (2024). Overview on Madagascar periwinkle. *World Journal of Pharmaceutical Research*, *13*(4), 264–278. DOI: 10.20959/wjpr20244-30636

Kigonya, R., Byakagaba, P., Ssenyonjo, E., & Jjunju, C. N. (2024). Biodiversity offsetting in Uganda's protected areas: A pathway to restoration of forest biodiversity? *Environmental Management*, *73*(6), 1134–1149. DOI: 10.1007/s00267-023-01918-7 PMID: 38730130

Luo, L., Wang, B., Jiang, J., Fitzgerald, M., Huang, Q., & Yu, L. (2021). Heavy metal contaminations in herbal medicines: Determination, comprehensive risk assessments, and solutions. *Frontiers in Pharmacology*, *11*, 595335. Advance online publication. DOI: 10.3389/fphar.2020.595335 PMID: 33597875

Mohammadinejad, R., Kumar, A., Ranjbar-Mohammadi, M., Ashrafizadeh, M., Han, S. S., Khang, G., & Roveimiab, Z. (2020). Recent advances in natural gum-based biomaterials for tissue engineering and regenerative medicine: A review. *Polymers*, *12*(1), 176. Advance online publication. DOI: 10.3390/polym12010176 PMID: 31936590

NSF - National Science Foundation. (2025). *The importance of NSF/ANSI 173 certification for dietary supplement products*. https://www.nsf.gov/

Oliveira, C., Sousa, D., Teixeira, J. A., Ferreira-Santos, P., & Botelho, C. M. (2023). Polymeric biomaterials for wound healing. *Frontiers in Bioengineering and Biotechnology*, *11*, 1136077. Advance online publication. DOI: 10.3389/fbioe.2023.1136077 PMID: 37576995

Pariona, A. (2025). *The world's 17 megadiverse countries*. WorldAtlas. https://www.worldatlas.com/articles/ecologically-megadiverse-countries-of-the-world.html

Patwardhan, B., Warude, D., Pushpangadan, P., & Bhatt, N. (2005). Ayurveda and traditional Chinese medicine: A comparative overview. *Evidence-Based Complementary and Alternative Medicine: eCAM*, *2*(4), 465–473. DOI: 10.1093/ecam/neh140 PMID: 16322803

Pick, G. (2025). *The role of accurate labeling for consumer safety*. Clear Print. https://www.clearprint.com/role-of-accurate-labeling-in-consumer-safety/

Prajapati, V., Desai, S., Gandhi, S., & Roy, S. (2022). Pharmaceutical applications of various natural gums and mucilages. In Murthy, H. N. (Ed.), *Gums, resins and latexes of plant origin* (pp. 1–34). Springer., DOI: 10.1007/978-3-030-91378-6_1

Prajapati, V. D., Jani, G. K., Moradiya, N. G., & Randeria, N. P. (2013). Pharmaceutical applications of various natural gums, mucilages and their modified forms. *Carbohydrate Polymers*, *92*(2), 1685–1699. DOI: 10.1016/j.carbpol.2012.11.021 PMID: 23399207

Research and Markets. (2025). *Organic pharmaceutical excipients market report 2025*. https://www.researchandmarkets.com/reports/5865933/organic-pharmaceutical-excipients-market-report

Schultz, G. S., Chin, G. A., Moldawer, L., & Diegelmann, R. F. (2011). Principles of wound healing. In Fitridge, R., & Thompson, M. (Eds.), *Mechanisms of vascular disease: A reference book for vascular specialists* (pp. 423–451). University of Adelaide Press., https://www.ncbi.nlm.nih.gov/books/NBK534261/

Secretariat Standardization Administration of China. (2009). *ISO/TC 249 - Traditional medicine*. International Organization for Standardization. https://www.iso.org/committee/598435.html

Smith+Nephew. (2025). *IODOSORB Cadexomer iodine range*. https://www.smith-nephew.com/en/health-care-professionals/products/advanced-wound-management/iodosorb-global

Stout, E. I., & McKessor, A. (2012). Glycerin-based hydrogel for infection control. *Advances in Wound Care*, *1*(1), 48–51. DOI: 10.1089/wound.2011.0288 PMID: 24527279

The United States Pharmacopeial Convention. (2018). *Pharmacopeial Discussion Group (PDG)*. https://www.usp.org/harmonized-standards/pdg

The United States Pharmacopeial Convention. (2020). *Novel excipients: New hope for therapeutic innovations*. https://qualitymatters.usp.org/novel-excipients-new-hope-therapeutic-innovations

United States Pharmacopeia. (2024). *Fostering the use of novel excipients in drug products*. https://www.usp.org/sites/default/files/usp/document/public-policy/USP%20Global%20Policy%20Position_NovelExcipients_Paper_2024.pdf

Usman, M., Nakagawa, M., & Cheng, S. (2023). Emerging trends in green extraction techniques for bioactive natural products. *Processes (Basel, Switzerland)*, *11*(12), 3444. Advance online publication. DOI: 10.3390/pr11123444

Vora, L. K., Gholap, A. D., Jetha, K., Thakur, R. R. S., Solanki, H. K., & Donnelly, R. F. (2023). Artificial intelligence in pharmaceutical technology and drug delivery design. *Pharmaceutics*, *15*(7), 1916. Advance online publication. DOI: 10.3390/pharmaceutics15071916 PMID: 37514102

Warak, A. (2025). *Aloe vera farming in India*. Tractor Karvan. https://tractorkarvan.com/blog/aloe-vera-farming-in-india

World Health Organization. (2007). *WHO guidelines on good manufacturing practices (GMP) for herbal medicines*. https://www.who.int/publications/i/item/9789241547161

World Health Organization. (2011). *Quality control methods for herbal materials*. https://www.who.int/publications/i/item/9789241500739

World Health Organization. (2018). *WHO guidelines on good herbal processing practices for herbal medicines* (Annex 1). In *WHO Expert Committee on Specifications for Pharmaceutical Preparations: Fifty-second report* (WHO Technical Report Series, No. 1010, pp. 81–152). https://www.gmp-compliance.org/guidelines/gmp-guideline/who-guidelines-on-good-herbal-processing-practices-for-herbal-medicines

World Health Organization. (2023). *WHO guidelines on good agricultural and collection practices for medicinal plants.* https://www.who.int/publications/i/item/9241546271

World Health Organization. (2025). *International Regulatory Cooperation for Herbal Medicines (IRCH).* https://www.who.int/initiatives/international-regulatory-cooperation-for-herbal-medicines

World Intellectual Property Organization. (2010). *Using traditional knowledge to revive the body and a community.* IP Advantage. https://www.wipo.int/en/web/ip-advantage/w/stories/using-traditional-knowledge-to-revive-the-body-and-a-community

World Intellectual Property Organization. (2025). *WIPO treaty on intellectual property, genetic resources and associated traditional knowledge.* https://www.wipo.int/treaties/en/ip/gratk

Yik, M. H., Wong, V. C. T., Wong, T., & Shaw, P. (2021). HerBChain, a blockchain-based informative platform for quality assurance and quality control of herbal products. *Journal of Traditional and Complementary Medicine*, *11*(6), 598–600. DOI: 10.1016/j.jtcme.2021.06.005 PMID: 34765524

Zugle, D. (2021). Regulation of the use of pharmaceutical excipients in India. *Journal of Current Research in Medicine*, 2(5), 2709–8125.

Chapter 15

Wound Healing With Herbal Excipients: Navigating Regulatory and Ethical Landscapes

Vivek Pazhamalai
https://orcid.org/0000-0003-2088-7545
Department of Bioengineering, Vels Institute of Science, Technology, and Advanced Studies, India

M. Suriya
https://orcid.org/0009-0008-5398-0221
Department of Bioengineering, Vels Institute of Science, Technology, and Advanced Studies, India

V. Aarthi
https://orcid.org/0009-0004-0177-7716
Department of Bioengineering, Vels Institute of Science, Technology, and Advanced Studies, India

S. Ivo Romauld
https://orcid.org/0000-0003-0610-0646
Department of Bioengineering, Vels Institute of Science, Technology, and Advanced Studies, India

S. S. Meenambiga
https://orcid.org/0000-0002-5445-525X
Department of Bioengineering, Vels Institute of Science, Technology, and Advanced Studies, India

R. Chandrasekaran
Department of Biomedical Engineering, Vels Institute of Science, Technology, and Advanced Studies, India

Anbarasu Mariyappillai
https://orcid.org/0000-0001-7970-4454
Department of Agronomy, School of Agriculture, Vels Institute of Science, Technology, and Advanced Studies, India

DOI: 10.4018/979-8-3373-3977-1.ch015

ABSTRACT

The combination of herbal excipients and polymers, as alternatives to conventional medicines, offers the potential for a novel and effective wound healing therapeutic approach with biocompatibility, sustainability, and improved outcomes for patients. The use of herbal components derived from medicinal plants, which have anti-inflammatory, antimicrobial, and regenerative properties, combined with polymers, both natural and synthetic, as they can also affect the encapsulation of various types of therapies and create a controlled drug release system while mimicking the extra cellular matrix /wound site, heralds a new era of Herbo-polymeric technologies in wound care. Although the advancements in wound care technologies are substantial, the adoption of Herbo-polymeric technologies is hindered by a fragmented regulatory space, inconsistency in standards, and complicated ethical issues. The chapter outlines an integrated approach to explore the interdisciplinary science, formulation, as well as an analysis of the regulatory and ethical category associated with herbal and polymeric systems.

INTRODUCTION

Wound healing is a complicated physiological process (hemostasis, inflammation, proliferation and remodeling) that requires real advancement in the development of effective therapies. (Boateng & Catanzano, 2015) There has been a trend towards the use of herbal excipients, and polymers in modern medicine. These materials have biocompatibility, biodegradability and provide therapeutics for patients. (Dhivya et al., 2015) Herbal excipients (plant derived) have been found to promote wound healing, by enhancing wound repair through modulating inflammation and tissue regeneration. Polymers (natural and synthetic) are used as scaffolds and delivery systems for advanced wound care systems. (Chattopadhyay & Banerjee, 2022) While these products have great potential for wound healing, quality standards and regulatory pathways differ considerably and limit the application to clinical practices. Furthermore, there are ethical considerations with respect to using information from traditional knowledge and natural resources, including informed consent, intellectual property rights and sustainability. (Patwardhan et al., 2005) Because these products are often located in the overlap of pharmaceuticals and traditional medicine, we see the need for clear regulatory and ethical frameworks. We do intend for this review to delve into these important aspects, evaluate what currently is being done, and what that might look like to move forward.

Background on Wound Healing and Modern Therapeutics

Wound healing is an elaborate and dynamic biological process that is comprised of four overlapping phases; hemostasis, inflammation, proliferation, and tissue remodeling. (Guo & DiPietro 2010) Each of the wound healing phases must be timed precisely and coordinated with each cellular and molecular component in order to restore the skin to its previous state of integrity and function. Most acute wounds heal in a predictable time frame, whereas chronic wounds (e.g. diabetic ulcers, pressure sores, venous ulcers) often remain in a pathological- inflammatory phase of healing and thus delayed or incomplete healing. (Brem & Tomic- Canic 2007) Common treatment modalities for wounds include debridement, infection control, and moist wound dressings.

Collectively, these methods have developed to follow traditional care paths (e.g. debridement, etc.) and now use advanced therapeutic technologies (e.g. stem cells, growth factor therapies) and have improved and evolved through introducing bio-engineered skin substitutes. (Velnar et al 2009) In addition, the development of advanced wound dressings (e.g. bio-absorbable polymers, nanoparticles, antimicrobials and bioactive products) has increased treatment opportunities. Nevertheless, the cost or limited accessibility of these treatments has drawn interest in other forms of treatment that are affordable and include herbs and polymeric products/systems, even when they resemble established methods.

Phases of Wound Healing

Healing a wound is an intricate multi-stage biological process aimed at restoring damaged dermis and underlying tissue to its original state. The wound healing process includes four separate biological stages: hemostasis, inflammation, proliferation and tissue remodeling. Hemostasis happens immediately following the injury, and is the prevention of blood loss via blood vessel constriction, and clotting (Jayakumar et al., 2011). After the hemostasis phase, inflammatory phase follows and consists of the activation and recruitment of immune cells such as neutrophils and macrophages, to eliminate pathogens and debris. Inflammatory phase is followed by the proliferative healing phase in which tissue regeneration is renewed via the following processes: activation of fibroblasts, deposition of extracellular matrix, (ECM), angiogenesis, and re-epithelialization (Falanga, 2005). The final phase of tissue remodeling reinforces the repaired tissue by reorganization of the new collagen fibers, which increases tensile strength to the newly repaired skin. An organized coordination of the above four processes is critical for a well-timed and efficient healing process. Disruption of the above processes can result in chronic or non-healing wounds.

Acute vs. Chronic Wounds

Acute wounds typically adhere to a predictable and timely healing process by cycling through the phases of hemostasis, inflammation, proliferation, and remodeling without significant interruption (Frykberg & Banks, 2015). These wounds can be related to surgical cuts or small injuries, usually heal within weeks, and follow the general plan with few negative issues when managed appropriately. Chronic wounds such as diabetic foot ulcers, pressure ulcers, and venous leg ulcers, have not been able to progress through the normal stages of healing, and are likely in a prolonged inflammatory phase (Mustoe et al., 2006). This prolonged inflammatory phase is caused by underlying conditions such as infection, ischemia, neuropathy, and systemic conditions such as diabetes, resulting in tissue break down and lack of re-epithelization. Chronic wounds are also entailed in a considerable burden on the healthcare system and on the patients due to their length of time heal, high rate of recurrence, and increased likelihood of complications. (Boateng et al, 2008). A comparative summary of these characteristics is displayed in **Table 1,** while **Figure 1** compares the healing processes of both acute and chronic wounds both to help with clinical-to-clinical reasoning.

Table 1. Comparison of acute and chronic wound healing phases

Feature	Acute Wounds	Chronic Wounds
Onset and Duration	Develops suddenly; heals within predetermined timeframe	Extended healing; lasts longer than 4-6 weeks.
Inflammatory Response	Transient inflammatory response; controlled inflammation	Continuous inflammatory response; uncontrolled inflammation
Infection Risk	Low risk with appropriate management	High risk; colonization and/or infected
Healing Outcome	Complete tissue repair and regeneration	Partial/incomplete healing
Underlying Causes	Trauma, surgery	Diabetes, ischemia and/or reperfusion; pressure; ischemia; vascular insufficiency
Histological Features	Structured phases of tissue regeneration	Nonviable material, biofilm; excessive protease activity
Clinical Management	Standard dressings and/or antiseptic	Advanced therapy methods such as debridement and/or antimicrobials.

(Winter, 1962)

Figure 1. Structural differences in healing dynamics of acute vs chronic wounds

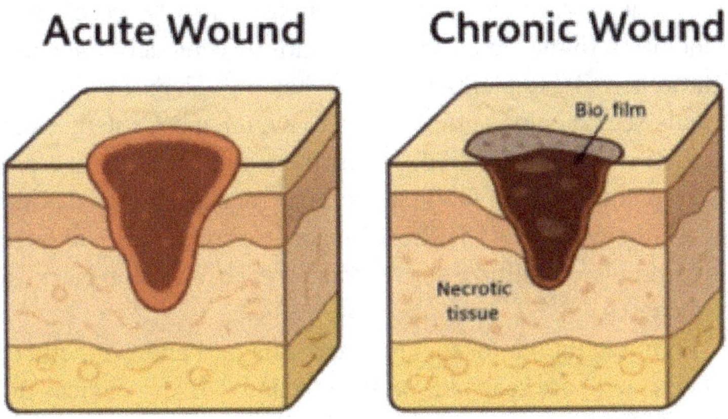

Traditional Therapeutic Approaches

Conventional wound care methods form the cornerstone of clinical wound management and include essential practices such as debridement, infection control, and the application of moist wound dressings. Debridement the removal of necrotic or infected tissue promotes the formation of healthy granulation tissue and reduces microbial load at the wound site. The individuals who conduct infection control measures with topical antiseptics and systemic antibiotics on chronic wounds are attempting to prevent or handle microbial colonization, which could slow healing. The process of healing consists of various phases and phases of healing that are sometime exclusive to acute wounds. Dressings that retain moisture (hydrocolloid, hydrogel, and alginate) will protect the wound while allowing full cover to eliminate contamination. Moist dressings provide a good moisture balance, and research established that epithelialization occurs more rapidly in moist environments, and scarring is minimized. (Sen, 2009) This coupled with the folk antibiotic and antifungal remedies for wounds that acute acid and other wound care interventions have not only advanced positive outcomes for acute wounds, they have blazed the pathways for modern wound care approaches including bioactive dressings, and tissue engineered products characterized by pharmacological and biological principles or protein dynamics in order to facilitate the improved or enhanced healing. (Shukla et al., 1999)

Role of Herbal Excipients and Polymers in Tissue Regeneration

Herbal excipients and polymers have been shown to be excellent facilitators of tissue regeneration to the superior biocompatibility, bioactivity, and multifunctionality of these herbal excipients in wound healing. Herbal excipients of plant-derived materials such as aloe vera, curcumin, neem, and Centella asiatica, select the anti-inflammatory, antimicrobial, antioxidant, and proliferative properties of these herbal excipients that can facilitate cellular regeneration and components of angiogenesis. (Hamedi et al., 2015) These bioactive compounds will facilitate faster wound closure and also minimize scar formation and infection risks, suitable for regenerative purposes.

Polymers, both natural (chitosan, alginate, collagen) and synthetic (polycaprolactone, polylactic acid) are scaffolds and controlled delivery devices that enable a sustained release of therapeutic agents in adhesion, and tissue remodeling. (Ekor, 2014) Polymers complement herbal excipients by improving stability and solubility and improving bioavailability to phytoconstituents. The combination of herbal excipients with polymers gives rise to next gen wound care platforms like hydrogel dressings, nanofibers, and films that mimic the extracellular matrix which provides functional tissue recovery. Overall, utilizing herbal excipients and polymers in wound healing formulations offers an attractive avenue towards natural, effective, and patient-friendly regenerative therapies.

The Need for Regulatory and Ethical Oversight

The incorporation of herbal excipients and polymers to contemporary wound care can introduce significant regulatory and ethical implications to safeguard the public from harm, inefficacy, and lack of trust as with herbal product use. Herbal-based therapies used in wound care do not face the same obligations as pharmaceuticals. Herbal products often face challenges involving consistency, quality, standardization with extraction and problems with the bioactive content's consistency, due to numerous differences in cultivation, harvesting, processing (Tilburt & Kaptchuk, 2008). Statistically variability of herbal products raise issues of product accuracy, probable adverse effects, or therapeutic disposition. As a result of these shortcomings, regulatory frameworks must be more defined.

Ethically the use and sourcing of herbal materials bring about unresolvable questions regarding sustainability, equitable benefit-sharing and protection of indigenous knowledge systems. Moreover, clinical exploration of herbal and polymer interventions must still ensure informed consent, data rigour, and responsible modelling practices using animals or alternatives (Eming et al., 2014). Without definable intervention oversight there is room of exploitation, misinformation and more harm to marginalized communities. Thus, establishing standardized regulatory practices and ethical guidelines are paramount with respect to preventing harm to patients, promoting innovative practices and ensuring international acceptance of innovations in wound care management.

Aim and Scope of the Review

This review will discuss regulatory and ethical contexts surrounding the use of herbal excipients and polymers utilized in wound healing. It is essential to contextualize their biomedical relevance, given the rising global interest pertaining to naturally derived and biocompatible materials - including herbal items - which interact with evolving regulations and ethics. (Houghton & Mukherjee, 2020) The review will document the types, sources, functions, challenges related to formulation, quality, and transition to clinical use of herbal excipients and polymers. Regulatory contexts will be focused primarily on the guidelines set out by regulatory agencies such as the U.S. Food and Drug Administration (FDA), European Medicines Agency (EMA), Central Drugs Standard Control Organization (CDSCO), and India's Minister of AYUSH. Relevant ethical aspects in regard to traditional knowledge, sustainability, informed consent, and fair access will also be reviewed (Javed et al., 2021). By considering all three dimensions - scientific, regulatory, and ethical - this review is intended to help researchers, clinicians, and policymakers make further progress on developing safe, effective, and ethically defensible wound care.

HERBAL EXCIPIENTS AND POLYMERS IN WOUND HEALING

The use of herbal excipients and polymers has drawn attention in wound healing because of their natural biocompatibility and bioactivity with low toxicity. Herbal excipients are extracted from plants that were traditionally used in wound care formulations as multi-functional stabilizers, gelling agents, permeation enhancers, and antimicrobial agents. Compounds that were formulated from herbal extracts such are mucilages, gums, and tannins didn't only help to improve the mechanical properties of wound dressings but possessed bioactive properties to facilitate healing by acting on inflammation, angiogenesis, and tissue regeneration. (Nayak & Pinto Pereira, 2006). The effectiveness of herbal-based wound products has also been enhanced with the use of natural and semi-synthetic polymers including chitosan, alginate and cellulose derivatives, through the use of controlled drug release, moisture retention and 3-D structural support (Venkatesan et al., 2017). The synergistic power of herbal bioactive and biocompatible polymers can allow for the development of the next generation of sustainable and effective wound healing systems.

Classification and Sources of Herbal Excipients

Herbal excipients are naturally derived components that originate from plant sources and are incorporated into pharmaceutical and nutraceutical formulations to provide stability, bioavailability, and therapeutic benefit without therapeutic effect. The excipients can be classified depending on their physicochemical properties and functions as binders, disintegrants, emulsifiers, thickeners, film formers, and stabilizers. Each excipient class (with few exceptions) is affixed to a specific part of a plant - seeds, leaves, bark, or roots that provide a source of gum, mucilage, starch, and resin. (Kulkarni et al., 2012) For example, gums, including gum acacia, come from exudates of trees; mucilages can come from seeds of plants, such as Plantago ovata or Hibiscus esculentus. Other important examples include starch from Zea mays and cellulose derivatives from Bombax ceiba. (Pandey et al., 2016)

A detailed overview of these classes, along with their botanical sources and plant parts used, is provided in **Table 2.** This classification helps in selecting appropriate excipients tailored for specific wound healing formulations, as the physicochemical characteristics of these substances significantly influence the product's mechanical properties, moisture retention, and drug-release behavior.

Table 2. Classification and sources of herbal excipients

Class	Example	Source Plant	Plant Part
Binder	Gum Acacia	*Acacia senegal*	Exudate (gum)
Disintegrant	Mucilage	*Plantago ovata*	Seed
Emulsifier	Lecithin	*Glycine max* (soybean)	Seed
Thickener	Pectin	*Citrus sinensis*	Peel
Film-forming agent	Starch	*Zea mays* (maize)	Kernel
Stabilizer	Cellulose	*Bombax ceiba*	Bark/wood

(Deshmukh et al., 2014)

Functional Classification of Herbal Excipients

Herbal excipients have functional classifications based on their intended functions when used in pharmaceutical formulations. There are many functional classes, with some common classes of excipients listed as binders (such as acacia gum), disintegrants (e.g., isabgol husk mucilage), emulsifiers (e.g., lecithin), thickeners (e.g., pectin), film formers (e.g., starch), and stabilizers (e.g., cellulose). The functionality of herbal excipients likely relates to their complex polysaccharide content, glycoproteins, or proteins which provide structure for adhesion for swelling, when used in wound dressings and in topical formulations. (Mali et al., 2010)

Botanical Sources and Plant Parts Used

Herbal excipients can be sourced from a large number of plant species, and can also be harvested from many areas of the plant. For example, Astragalus species yield gums such as gum tragacanth, mucilages are produced from Hibiscus and Plantago, starches can be sourced from maize and potato, and cellulose can be harvested from cotton and fibrous wood plants. Each area of strain provides differing amounts of chemical and/or structural content, and these will impact the effectiveness of the excipient in a formulation. (Shaikh et al., 2011).

Advantages Over Synthetic Excipients

Herbal excipients are biodegradable, environmentally friendly, cost-effective compared to synthetic excipients, and generally well tolerated. Their natural origin means that they are more biocompatible and will show lower incidence of adverse reactions, which is important in wound healing when there is sustained skin-contact. In addition, some herb-based excipients exhibit inherent antimicrobial, anti-inflammatory, and antioxidant action that help produce a healing environment (Jani et al., 2012).

Considerations in Selection and Processing

The selection of herbal excipients needs to consider prophylactic qualities of the herbal excipient and combinations of formulations, as well as their own physicochemical properties, compatibility to active ingredients, and stability in formulating conditions. Processing methods and techniques (drying, making powder, purification) are important to keep their functionality and limit microorganisms. Standardization is a challenge as variables arise from the plant source, harvest season, and geographical source, putting quality control at forefront of regulatory context. (Ravikumar et al., 2013)

Natural and Synthetic Polymers: Biocompatibility and Use

Polymers, including both biological (natural) and synthetic types, play important roles in wound healing because they provide hydrogels, films, and scaffolds that assist with tissue regeneration. Biological polymers include chitosan, alginate, gelatin, hyaluronic acid, and cellulose. These polymers, derived from biological origins, have excellent biocompatibility, biodegradability, and low antigenicity. (Ahmed, 2015), Additionally, the structural similarities of biological polymers with the extracellular matrix (ECM) allows cells to adhere, proliferate, and migrate which all are necessary processes in wound repair. There are many examples of biological polymers that assist in wound repair, and part of those processes is their nature. For instance, chitosan from crustacean shells has antimicrobial uses and supports hemostasis. Alginate from brown seaweed forms gels that are ionically cross-linked, which also provide a moist wound environment and take exudate.

Synthetic polymers are also important for their role in tissue repair and include poly (lactic acid) (PLA), poly (glycolic acid) (PGA), and polyvinyl alcohol (PVA). Synthetic polymers are different than biological polymers and offer some advantages such as mechanical robustness, structural integrity, and have defined degradation rates (Ullah et al., 2015). These types of polymers can also be fabricated at the level of the molecule which allows for degrees of freedom to meet specific physicochemical and pharmacokinetic requirements. Tempted not to, but not forgot to mention, synthetic polymers do not have biological activity and proper respects of not calling them biological. Regardless synthetic polymers are frequently utilized with bioactive compounds or natural polymers and other things to achieve a therapeutic result and reduce cytotoxicity.

The decision between natural and synthetic polymers is dependent on the application, desired healing dynamics, and prescription factors specific to the patient. A combination of both polymer types working synergistically is increasingly found in next-generation wound dressings and drug delivery systems.

Mechanisms of Action in Wound Healing

Wound healing is dynamic and multimodal. Wound healing occurs in four overlapping transition phases of: hemostasis, inflammation, proliferation, and remodeling. Each phase is characterized by unique cellular and molecular events which can be supported or augmented, by both the natural and synthetic polymers used in a variety of wound care technologies. (Balaji et al., 2016)

Hemostasis

Having an injury, blood vessels tighten up and platelets quickly join forces to form a clot that will last just a short time. As a result, the clot seals the wound and creates a place where cells can travel. As illustrated in **Figure 2,** during this stage both red blood cells and platelets are present, as are some bacteria. This process is enhanced by natural polymers such as chitosan which facilitate platelet attachment, change their activity, improve the rate of forming blood clots and add defense against bacteria. Because of polymer use, barricades form inside the wound, protecting it from outside germs. (Chen & Abatangelo, 1999).

Inflammation

The inflammatory phase of healing is characterized by the influx of white blood cells, together with macrophages to help debride and remove debris and pathogenic agents, as well as releasing cytokines for repair. Natural polymers such as hyaluronic acid modulate inflammation through regulating leukocyte migration and cytokine expression. Additionally, polymer-based systems could be employed as a delivery mechanism for anti-inflammatory agents, whether owned vehicles that could possibly target the inflammatory site in an effort to reduce the duration of inflammation (Gurtner et al., 2008).

Proliferation

In this phase, the wound bed is restocked with fibroblasts, myofibroblasts, and endothelial cells, facilitating angiogenesis, ECM deposition, or re-epithelialization. Figure 1 shows cellular activity at this phase is continuous and abetted by the provisional matrix. Hydrogels from polymers such as alginate and gelatin retain a moist wound environment that is necessary for cell migration and proliferation. Synthetic scaffolds mimic the ECM and allow for the cells to anchor and grow in addition to has the ability to allow for controlled release of growth factors to increase granulation tissue (Zhao et al., 2017).

Remodeling

In conclusion, collagen is reorganized, the new tissue matures, and scar tissue forms at this final stage of repair to restore the original function of the tissue. As shown in Figure 1, the outcome of wound healing and repair is an intact wound through vascular and epidermal remodeling. Analogs like PLA and PGA will be made to reabsorb to match tissue regeneration; they provide support only as long as needed A (Middleton & Tipton, 2000).

Figure 2. Sequential cellular and molecular events in the four phases of wound healing

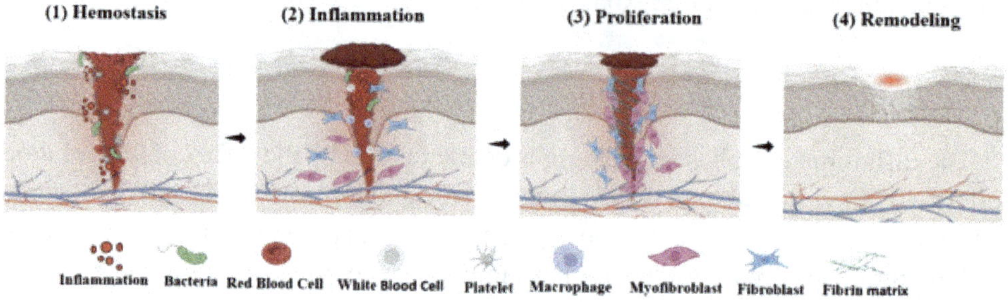

Recent Advances and Formulations

New technologies in wound healing have focused on the development of multifunctional and responsive formulations that incorporate the healing properties of natural and synthetic polymers with herbal bio actives, nanotechnology, and complex drug delivery systems to improve healing times, limit infection, and decrease scar tissue in a biocompatible and cost-efficient manner.

Polymeric Nanocomposites and Nanofibers

Electrospun nanofiber scaffolds have become the most promising wound dressings because they are built of polymers that mimic the structure of the body's native extracellular matrix, and they are designed to allow for a controlled delivery of herbal therapeutics. Commonly, natural polymers such as gelatin, chitosan, and cellulose derivatives are then blended with synthetic polymers like polycaprolactone (PCL) or polylactic acid (PLA) to develop hybrid nanofibers. For example, effective herbal agents may include curcumin or neem extract, as well as centella asiatica or aloe vera, and functional creativities include antimicrobial, anti-inflammatory, and antioxidant activities. (Mogo anu & Grumezescu, 2014)

Stimuli-Responsive Hydrogels

Recent advances in responsive smart hydrogels that can be activated electrochemically, pH, temperature, or enzymatically, could allow the hydrogel to respond to bioactive compound delivery in a wound-specific manner. A pH-responsive hydrogel that has either quercetin or curcuminoids from turmeric altered the rate release of bioactive compounds between infected and non-infected environments (to increase the therapeutic specificity of the plant extracts) such as quercetin. These active hydrogels typically utilize modified hyaluronic acid, poly(N-isopropylacrylamide) or carboxymethyl cellulose as the polymer base materials (Liu et al., 2017).

Herbal-Polymer Hybrid Films and Membranes

Film-forming polymers containing herbal extracts are used in the way of semi-occlusive dressings that can create moisture and provide NATURAL antimicrobial activity through herbal loading. Chitosan-based films load Calendula officinalis, Azadirachta indica (neem), or tea tree oil and have significant activity against common wound pathogens, such as S. aureus and P. aeruginosa, and also provide epithelialization and angiogenesis support (Iordache et al., 2022).

Injectable and Sprayable Formulations

Injectables hydrogels and spray on polymers are becoming more common for irregular/deep wounds. The majority of these systems can quickly form an in-situ matrix to cover the wound, promote tissue growth and deliver a drug dose intermittently. Alginate based injectable gels containing plant polyphenols or bioflavonoids are in active development given their anti-inflammatory and pro-healing function.

3D-Bioprinted Skin Substitutes

Moreover, new 3D-bioprinting allow for researchers to create skin constructs from bioinks based on natural polymers (gelatin, collagen and fibrin) and herbal induced growth enhancers. Engineered skin grafts show great potential especially towards full-thickness wounds and burns, with broader surface area and better integration and vascularization.

Challenges in Formulation and Standardization

Polymeric wound healing systems provide an important opportunity for therapy, in particular, when combined with herbal excipients, but much work is still needed to optimize formulation and reproducibility, safety and regulatory issues prior to being able to take these from a laboratory to a clinically approved product.

Phytochemical Variability and Standardization Issues

One major challenge faced when formulating polymeric herbal wound dressings is the wide variability in the composition of herbal excipients. The phytochemistry of herbal excipients can be affected by several ecological factors, such as plant species, soil, climate, and cropping time. Even the extraction method and solvent system can influence the concentration of the bioactive constituents of the herbal excipients. The wide variability in phytochemistry presents an obstacle to batch-to-batch consistency and reproducibility of therapeutic effects. (Kunle, Egharevba, & Ahmadu, 2012). Unquestionably, it is difficult to standardize herbal products in polymer matrices, but the multicomponent nature of herbs complicates standardization even more. These inconsistencies create significant hurdles for quality control and regulatory approval.

Formulation Compatibility and Technical Limitations

When paired with polymeric carriers, there are many obstacles to formulate a product containing herbal extracts because of chemical incompatibilities. Many of the phytochemicals derive from herbal materials, are sensitive to heat, light, and/or pH, and consequently can lose their therapeutic action during processing. The challenges in achieving optimal stability and sustained release when using hydrogels, films, or nanofibers is often complicated. The poor solubility and bioavailability of herbal actives diminishes therapeutic action. While still retaining the integrity of structures and functional properties is essential; scaling up production remains a significant barrier. These limitations create obstacles for formulation development as well as the translation to industry. (Boddupalli & Kataria, 2021)

Regulatory, Manufacturing, and Clinical Barriers

The regulatory ambiguity of herbo-polymeric wound care products as drugs, devices or combination products creates difficulty in the market place, and this ambiguity occurs at multiple levels. The lack of harmonization of herbal and polymer regulations adds another layer of complexity. Manufacturers also face challenges in regulatory consistency, compliance with GMP regulations, strong quality control standards, and limited clinical validation, there are few formal, well-designed clinical studies documenting product effectiveness. All of these issues affect both the broader acceptance by health organizations and its economic attractiveness to marketplace access. For the successful commercialization of herbo-polymeric products, it is imperative that these challenges are identified and addressed (Patel & Patel, 2021).

REGULATORY PERSPECTIVES

Herbo-polymeric wound care products are subjected to regulatory ambiguity, existing somewhere in the distinction of drugs, devices, or cosmetics, by their dual nature when offering care. The lack of harmonized global guidelines complicates approval, especially with herbal regulations and polymer technology not being aligned. Validation against GMP processes, quality control, and clinical validation are essential yet remain a barrier achieving the level of expectation related to commercializing such products. Regulatory pathways that are harmonized with respect to specific products are an opportunity to overcome barriers to global commercialization. (Langwick, 2011)

The different national frameworks for the regulatory approval of Herbo-polymeric wound care products reflects differences in the complexities of classification and the absence of harmonized international guidelines.

In the US, the Food and Drug Administration (FDA) divides products by the primary mode of action. Herbo-polymeric formulations can be regulated as a drug, device or combination product under 21 CFR part 3. Investigational New Drug (IND) and New Drug Application (NDA) filings will be required for herbal actives that have therapeutic claims, while the polymers used solely as 'carriers' will need to show safety and biocompatibility. The FDA's Guidance for Industry: Botanical Drug Development discusses the clinical and quality data necessary to support the herbal components. (FDA, 2020)

In the European Union (EU) herbal medicines and herbal medicinal products are governed by the Committee on Herbal Medicinal Products (HMPC) at the European Medicines Agency (EMA) via the Traditional Herbal Medicinal Products Directive (2004/24/EC). This framework creates pathways for registering traditionally used herbal products; however, there is presently no guidance on polymeric based systems. In the event polymeric systems come to fruition, the possibilities under Advanced Therapy Medicinal Products (ATMP) or Medical Device Regulation (MDR) regulations would likely apply based on the mechanism of action and intended use. (EMA, 2004)

A two-structured regulatory framework for India is existing. CDSCO (Central Drugs Standard Control Organization) regulates modern drugs and delivery systems under the Drugs and Cosmetics Act, 1940, while AYUSH regulates traditional systems of Ayurveda, Unani and Siddha. Herbo-polymeric products are caught in a regulatory grey area where the active herbal ingredient is covered by AYUSH and the polymer component is regulated by CDSCO, necessitating cooperation between the two regulators (Ministry of AYUSH, 2021).

In a broad sense, the absence of coherent regulatory principles between CDSCO and Ministry of AYUSH imposes considerable barriers to global commercialization. Developers of Herbo-polymeric products are faced with two sets of overlapping compliance obligations and administration that takes longer- and allows for different definitions of quality standards for herbal extracts, safety for polymers, and methods of compliance in product labelling (Parasuraman, 2012).

Regulatory Classification: Drug, Device, or Combination Product

Given their hybrid nature, it can be difficult to classify Herbo-polymeric wound healing products under regulations. These systems can consist of a bioactive herbal extract combined with a polymeric carrier or vehicles (hydrogels, nanofibers or films) – both of which can be used therapeutically or as a physical structure.

The classification in the United States will come from the FDA based on the primary mode of action (PMOA). If a product produces a therapeutic effect from the herb, it would be classified as a drug. If the effect is physical (for example barrier or scaffold), the product would be classified as a medical device. If both components independently contribute to the therapeutic effects of the product, the product includes drug and device components, making the product a combination product (21 CFR Part 3). The classification ultimately determines the route of regulation, as it is critical in pre-market submissions (for example, IND, NDA, or Premarket Approval (PMA)) depending on the classification.

A similar framework is present in the EU. The classification under the Medicinal Product Directive (2001/83/EC) or Medical Device Regulations (EU 2017/745) depends on the intended purposes and mode of action of the product. Combination product is assessed on ad-hoc basis, and uncertainty remains where herbal ingredients are added within polymeric carriers, without a well-defined pharmacological mode of action amongst the ingredients.

In India, there is no regulatory authority definition on combination products. Herbal actives may be dealt with under an AYUSH jurisdiction, while the polymeric carrier may be reviewed via CDSCO. The presence of two authorities creates and generates delay often resulting in inconsistencies in terms of regulatory arrangements, notably on new formulations in wound care that are outside the normal description usage indication bounds.

This ambiguity in classification has implications beyond regulatory route - i.e. requirements for clinical evaluation, labelling, safety testing and GMP will all be influenced. The absence of clear global standards for these hybrid systems prevents innovation and delays product development.

Quality Control and Standardization Requirements

Quality assurance and standardization of Herbo-polymeric wound care systems, or hybrid products, represent a formidable regulatory and formulation challenge. On the herbal side, extractable compounds vary due to the phytochemical nature of plants and their respective genotypes, environmental factors, harvesting and processing conditions. As such, validated chromatographic and spectroscopic methods (e.g., HPLC, NMR, LC-MS) must be used consistently to standardize bioactive constituents and reproduce an identifiable product. (Mukherjee et al., 2011)

On the polymeric front, carriers frequently must meet demanding mechanical, physicochemical and release profile specifications. For example, parameters such as porosity, swelling index, degradation rate and encapsulation efficiency must factor into evaluating performance and safety. (Patil et al., 2009) Ideally, where herbal and polymeric components interact, both components should be considered in compatibility and accelerated stability studies to ensure stability and therapeutic efficacy, to ICH specification.

Regardless of advances in analytical techniques - the absence of harmonized global standards for hybrid products remains a debilitating bottleneck. Quality benchmarks will differ according to regulatory agency requirements; furthermore, regulatory agency specifications most often focus on either herbal or polymeric components and not both in unison. This gap increases the burden on manufacturers to develop in-house validation protocols and ensure robust, GMP compliant fulfilment of processes.

Clinical Trial Regulations for Herbal and Polymer-Based Therapies

Regulatory considerations impede the clinical assessment of Herbo-polymeric wound care products in an inconsistent and rapidly changing regulatory climate. Herbal medicines were all assessed by ethnomedical use in the past, and now are being asked to provide evidence through RCTs and pharmacovigilance data. Designing an RCT for an herbal product is difficult since the composition can vary from product to product, there are not regulated or standard doses, and blinding or introducing a placebo is challenging (Goyal & Singh, 2019).

When combined with polymeric delivery systems like hydrogels, films or scaffolds used to deliver the herbal components, the regulatory issues become more complicated due to the combination device status. The majority of carriers are made from synthetic or biocompatible polymers, but all systems must adhere to Good Laboratory Practice (GLP) and Good Clinical practice (GCP) guidelines regardless. Toxicological and safety data must be provided before clinical applications. All systems require either device or drug specific approval protocols determined by a regulatory body like the FDA or EMA.

The challenge is compounded in countries like India where regulatory frameworks for AYUSH and herbal products require registrants to provide a clinical trial registry with the Clinical Trials Registry India (CTRI) and require PMT for Ayurvedic or herbal product registrations. There is currently no comprehensive regulatory framework for combination systems such as a Herbo-polymeric product incorporating herbal bio actives incorporated in a polymer matrix (Patwardhan et al., 2015). There is little clarity for registrants about the pathways on timelines or documentation to assess combination systems involving herbal bioactive embedded in polymer matrices.

Post-Market Surveillance and Compliance Challenges

The role of post-market surveillance (PMS) is fundamental to assuring the long-term safety and efficacy of Herbo-polymeric wound care products. These systems can fall into regulatory categories that overlap herbal, medical device or combination product, associated PMS protocols can be inconsistent and fragmented. Unlike mainstream pharmaceuticals, herbal products are inherently less stable due to batch variability and brand contamination that may not come to light until they are available for consumers. As such, strong pharmacovigilance should include ongoing monitoring of reported adverse events and product quality as products fall into various states of distribution (Barnes 2003).

Many countries do not have organized systems in place for ongoing monitoring of herbal or combination therapies after approval. Although some systems do exist, such as the AYUSH pharmacovigilance centers in India, and FDA MedWatch program in the USA, under-reporting of adverse events continues because of factors such as under-recognition of side effects, the poor understanding of therapeutic range, and lack of awareness among users and practitioners. After approval, establishing a commitment to maintain compliance with Good Manufacturing Practices (GMP) may also present challenges for manufacturers, particularly for those using seasonal plant materials or employing more artisanal production.

Further complexity is added by inconsistencies or instability in the supply chain that can introduce badly sourced build material or changes to formulations that culminate in products being non-conforming to the safety and regulatory requirements of the original manufacturer and the product approval. Without the benefit of continuous Quality audits, real-world data collection, and increased education stakeholders, it will be difficult to fill this gap with consumer understanding and confidence.

ETHICAL CONSIDERATIONS

There are some ethical issues associated with Herbo-polymeric wound management, which include ensuring an informed consent process, particularly in clinical trials in traditional remedies and traditional practices where participants may not fully appreciate the inherent risks. There is also the potential to undermine public confidence from misleading claims of efficacy when there is no sound clinical evidence to support those claims. Participants are entitled to fair benefit-sharing with indigenous communities, per the Nagoya Protocol, but that may not be strongly considered by researchers. Sustainability in harvesting any herbal sources is implicated by ethical obligations with respect to the environment. Ensuring there is transparency in labelling and marketing is part of the ethical obligation to protect consumers. Ethically, the oversight of this work must be investigated by multidisciplinary review boards and committees. The regulatory framework will need to adapt or draft regulations to these emerging bioethical areas. (Cohen et al., 2011)

Importance of Informed Consent

Informed consent is vitally important for respecting participants' autonomy in clinical research. In Herbal-based research, there often may be a tendency that products are safe because of their use over time and may lead participants to make assumptions. Many of these herbal products have not been subjected to questioning and clinical trials and invariably ethical oversights can occur when researchers have not taken the time to describe in detail the investigational status of the intervention. (Bhatt, 2010)

Unique Challenges with Herbal and Polymeric Formulations

Herbal extracts vary in composition depending on the source plant, season, and extraction method, increasing the unpredictability of drug delivery and efficacy when considering starting with polymer systems such as nanogels or films. Participants should also be made aware of the potential for new drug–carrier interactions and the limited available history of the same. (Sahoo, Parveen, & Panda, 2008) It is critical to highlight the increased potential for complications in consent from these interactions, an additional layer of complexity in ensuring clear communication during the consent process.

Support for Comprehension with Diverse Populations

Having a legal form of informed consent is one thing, but a thorough, comprehensive consent process must also incorporate culturally appropriate strategies. For participants from areas where herbal medicine is a cultural norm, they may never have been exposed to a clinical study protocol or may demonstrate skepticism of a biomedical framework. Use of vernacular languages, images, and the support of community leaders will aid in participants ensuring their understanding and voluntary participation. (Srinivas, Anand, & Nath, 2019)

Continuous Consent and Ethical Oversight

Consent is a feature of ethical responsibility that must be maintained. During the conduct of trials, researchers may find new adverse effects or product interactions which mean they must obtain new consent from the participants. Ethics review boards must maintain ongoing scrutiny of consent procedures, especially in cases involving new technologies and old remedies. (Langat, 2005) Such conversations foster trust from participants and are crucial to the credibility of the study.

Ethical Use of Traditional and Indigenous Knowledge

Application of traditional and indigenous knowledge (TIK) when designing Herbo-polymeric technologies for wound care offers astonishing possibilities while simultaneously creating complicated ethical issues. Communities have for many years preserved intricate and valuable medicinal knowledge, but their sponsors or contributions remain largely unrecognized or utilized for unfair exploitative practices during studies and commercial use. Creating respectful relations, obtaining prior informed consent, and designing fair benefit-sharing agreements are vital to protecting the dignity and rights of the holders of knowledge. In the case of TIK, some international documents like the Convention on Biological Diversity and Nagoya Protocol make it easy to apply them ethically in modern biomedical practices. (Bannister, 2014)

Respecting Cultural Heritage and Intellectual Property

The integration of indigenous and traditional knowledge into modern Herbo-polymeric wound care must be carried out with the most respect for the cultural tradition from which such knowledge originates. This implies recognition of traditional healers and communities as legitimate holders of knowledge and a refusal to appropriate their knowledge without their consent or acknowledgment. Ethical guidelines should provide that knowledge is not desorbed from its context or utilized in a manner that breaches cultural protocols. (Posey & Dutfield, 1996)

Benefit-Sharing and Community Consent

Ethical bioprospecting is mandated by prior informed consent (PIC) from traditional communities and equitable access and benefit-sharing (ABS) regimes. These are provided in the Nagoya Protocol, where benefits derived from the commercial or scientific use of traditional knowledge must be shared equitably. These benefits include monetary benefits, capacity development, and participation in the research process. (Morgera et al., 2012)

Avoiding Exploitation in Commercialization

Commercialization of herbal products derived from indigenous knowledge without community involvement or recognition is considered unethical exploitation. Many companies in the past have profited from such knowledge without bringing back any value for the source communities. To avoid the exploitation of communities and ensure that innovation is sustainable, transparent agreements must be in place, with legal protection of community intellectual property and ethical review mechanisms. (Shiva, 2001)

Sustainability and Environmental Ethics in Sourcing

Sustainable sourcing practices for raw materials great biodiversity and long-term existence of medicinal plants upon which Herbo-polymeric wound care products depend are imperative. Exorbitant harvesting, habitat obliteration, and non-sustainable agricultural methods are threats to the survival of agents that are valuable, including ecological upliftment and training for livelihood to human communities. Ethical sourcing entails adherence to environmental ethics with conservation and responsible harvesting and further support for regenerative cultivation methods. Supply chain transparency along with respect for international environmental agreements are also critical to lessening negative impacts and augmenting social equity among indigenous and local communities dependent on these natural resources. (Smith & Berkes, 2018)

Conservation of Medicinal Plant Biodiversity

The extensive demand for natural wound care ingredients has caused severe strains on medicinal plants through excessive harvesting which endangers biodiversity and places endangered species at risk. The protection of plants requires methods that support sustainable harvesting along with endangered species cultivation and natural habitat conservation. These methods support the creation of durable plant populations for upcoming times without disrupting ecosystem equilibrium. (Ticktin, 2004)

Responsible Harvesting and Supply Chain Transparency

The ethical standard for sourcing herbal materials depends on the disclosure of both collection methods and the specific origin of plant materials. The practice of responsible harvesting involves limiting the overall collection volume and stopping harmful extraction practices and following natural growing seasons. Product accountability and the ability to develop consumer trust in genuine sustainable products need systems that provide tracking and certification. (Marshall et al., 2006)

Supporting Indigenous and Local Communities

Environmental ethics expand their study area from ecological systems to address the social fairness needs of communities who depend on growing medicinal plants. Through benefit-sharing programs and fair-trade operations and capacity-building activities indigenous and rural communities develop improved resource management practices which support their economic growth and environmental sustainability. The implementation of collaborative stewardship models leads to industry stakeholders and traditional knowledge holders developing relationships based on mutual respect. (Berkes, 2009)

Compliance with International Environmental Frameworks

The fulfillment of international treaties including the Convention on Biological Diversity (CBD) and the Nagoya Protocol stands as a critical requirement for establishing sustainable and fair plant genetic resource utilization. The frameworks establish regulations to protect resources while supporting sustainable usage and fair benefit distribution thus developing a legal and ethical foundation for herbal-polymeric wound care product development. (Convention on Biological Diversity Secretariat, 2011)

Animal Ethics and Alternatives in Preclinical Testing

The advancement of Herbo-polymeric wound care products demands preclinical evaluations which confirm their effectiveness along with safety for human trials. In the past the research community relied on animal models to investigate biological reactions during this developmental stage. The scientific testing limitations combined with ethical animal welfare concerns have motivated researchers to discover alternative evaluation methods. Scientists dedicate their research efforts to establish non-animal models that improve ethical requirements while making their predictions better through the 3Rs guidelines of Replacement, Reduction, and Refinement. The field of preclinical research faces a major obstacle when researchers need to comply with regulations while maintaining ethical standards.

Ethical Concerns in Animal Testing

The standard preclinical test method uses animal models to evaluate Herbo-polymeric wound care products throughout their safety, efficacy, and biocompatibility assessments. Research testing follows ethical principles that mandate researchers use the least number of animals possible while controlling animal discomfort to reach scientifically valid results. The Institutional Animal Care and Use Committees (IACUCs) create regulations to maintain humane treatment practices while reducing the number of animals used for experimentation. (Steneck, 2006)

The 3Rs Principle: Replacement, Reduction, Refinement

The 3Rs Principle establishes standards that guide ethical animal research practices. Ethical animal research moves forward under the 3Rs framework by:

- **Replacement:** Researchers should prioritize non-animal testing methods which include in vitro assays along with computer simulations and organ-on-chip systems.
- **Reduction:** Conducting studies which require the smallest number of animals.
- **Refinement:** Researchers improve their protocols to decrease both pain and distress levels. (Morton & Griffiths, 1985)

Emerging Alternatives in Preclinical Testing

Biotechnology progress has created three promising substitute methods to test products that do not involve animal research. The implementation of these methods handles ethical problems and generates more human-relevant data which leads to enhanced predictability for herbal-polymeric formulations. (Russell & Burch, 1959)

Regulatory Acceptance and Challenges

The acceptance of substitute methods continues to face regulatory agency requirements for using animal data in approval processes. The process of linking these two elements requires both new proof for alternative models and adjustments to regulatory standards to include scientific and moral advancements. The adoption of animal-free testing strategies requires researchers and industry leaders to work alongside regulatory agencies through collaborative efforts. (Hartung, 2008)

Data Integrity, Transparency, and Equitable Access

The development of Herbo-polymeric wound care products depends on maintaining data integrity across the research and development lifecycle to establish trust and drive product innovation. Reliable and openly accessible data enable scientific rigor while supporting regulatory compliance and informed clinical decision-making. These innovations must provide equitable access to all individuals to prevent exclusive benefits from reaching underprivileged communities worldwide. The fulfillment of these ethical responsibilities leads to better public health outcomes through both accountability and social justice development for therapeutic innovations.

Importance of Data Integrity

The study shows that preserving data integrity serves as essential for developing herbo-polymeric wound care products. Scientific validity together with regulatory approval depends on the foundation of accurate and complete and reliable data. Trust erosion and market exposure of unsafe products occur when data undergoes manipulation or selective reporting or falsification. Researchers need to maintain strict data collection and storage and analysis protocols that guarantee both reproducibility and accountability. (Balls et al., 2012)

Transparency in Research and Publication

The research community demonstrates transparency through the public availability of research protocols and datasets and results which anyone can verify to develop scientific knowledge. Publication bias decreases while stakeholders like clinicians and regulators gain informed decision-making capabilities through transparent reporting. Research transparency improves through open-access platforms and clinical trial preregistration which becomes vital when herbal medicine research encounters difficulty in validating real efficacy because of conflicting data and undisclosed proprietary formulations. (Nosek et al., 2015)

Equitable Access to Innovations

Equitable access means that Herbo-polymeric wound care developments reach people from all walks of life especially those in underprivileged and underfunded areas. The system requires equal pricing structures and available products in low-income areas alongside culturally relevant product designs. Health equity throughout the world will improve through the progress of new products that combine traditional knowledge with modern innovations while avoiding the deepening of current disparities. (Peters et al., 2019)

Intellectual Property and Sharing of Benefits

The protection of intellectual property rights requires a delicate balance with the moral obligation to distribute advantages. Patents act as a catalyst for innovation, while at the same time restricting and raising costs. Ethical principles advocate for negotiated licensing and patent pools and engaged licensing through public-private partnerships, which would allow widespread availability of products, while still protecting the rights of every inventor. (Tobin & Lewison, 2011)

Role of Regulatory and Funding Bodies

The combination of regulatory agencies and funding institutions functions as the cornerstone to safeguard data reliability and transparency and equal access through the enforcement of standards and data sharing requirements and provision of support for underserved population programs. Their oversight enables commercial interests to harmonize with public health targets which leads to the translation of innovation into practical benefits. (Ioannidis et al., 2014)

CURRENT CHALLENGES AND FUTURE PROSPECTS

The use of herbal therapeutics through polymer-based delivery systems has great potential for integrating into a future advanced wound care process; however, there are numerous challenges for developing and commercializing Herbo-polymeric wound care products. These challenges include specific technical difficulties related to stabilizing the formulation, ensuring bioavailability, and regulatory obstacles, as well as ethical issues related to sustainability and traditional knowledge of herbs. However, present trends in material science, biotechnology, and regulation, together with increased awareness of and involvement in integrative medicine and local cooperation, provide the scope to push ahead in our present limitations. (Gatt et al., 2024) Therefore, there is a scope for transformational development in the sector, to encourage the advancement of more efficient, secure, ethical, accessible, and effective wound healing therapy.

Gaps in Global Harmonization of Herbal Product Regulations

Due to differences in culture, law, practice, and science, regulation of herbal products really varies all over the world. This lack of universal standardization poses problems for the Herbo-polymeric products trying to obtain regulatory approval and commercialize in different markets. Differences in classification, supervision of clinical trials, quality control practices, and surveillance of the market after a product's release create obstacles to reliable testing of the safety and efficacy of a product. **Table 3** presents major regulatory variations between leading regions, focusing on these variances in terms of classification, quality standards, clinical evidence, and pharmacovigilance. Harmonization of these regulatory elements is vital to support global trade, safeguard consumers, and foster innovation in herbal therapeutics. (Zhang & Li, 2022)

Table 3. Summary of key regulatory differences in major regions

Regulatory Aspect	USA (FDA)	EU (EMA)	India (AYUSH)	China (NMPA)
Division of Tasks	Diet Supplement or Drug	Drug Traditional Herbal Medicinal Medicine or Drug	Traditional Medicine	Traditional Chinese Medicine
Quality Assurance	Good Manufacturing Practices, Standards of USP-to-USP documents	UA Monographs Self passports	AYUSH Pharmacopoeia standards	Chinese Pharmacopoeia
Research of Clinical Practices	Multi-lateral reproducible tests with "Clinically Controlled Test" defined as RCT for drug removed	Rigorous Constraining supporting traditional use	Relies heavily on empirical evidence	Combination of traditional usage and clinical evidence
Surveillance of the Market after Its Launch Types and Techniques	Active EU Pharmacovigilance System	Regularly Check required Active Restriction	Passive surveillance	Frontline emerging recent years

Diverse Regulatory Classifications

Across the world, herbal products are gone through different stages of their regulatory classifications. In some countries, these products are treated as dietary supplements, which results in a more relaxed distribution, while in other countries, they are regarded as traditional treatments, pharmaceutical goods or even cosmetics. This regulates how much attention is paid to the product's safety, efficacy, and marketing claims. This fragmentation of classification poses complex challenges in the product development and approval processes for manufacturers, as a formulation that is compliant with one country's regional regulations may need drastic changes to meet another's. In addition, vague capturing definitions or boundaries, such as combination products containing herbal materials and polymers, add to pre-existing regulatory uncertainty concerning claim substantiation, increasing the cost and time for market entry. (Chan & Leung, 2021)

Inconsistent Quality Control and Standardization

Quality control for herbal products is a major concern worldwide, primarily because there aren't any standardized guidelines in place. When it comes to sourcing raw materials, several factors come into play, such as the challenges of identifying different plant species, their geographic origins, and the conditions under which they're harvested. It's important to note that there can be quite a bit of variation in the phytochemical profiles and potency of these substances. The extraction methods can differ significantly, which in turn impacts the content and qualities of the active ingredients. Regarding the evaluation of purity, the analytical techniques and tests may vary considerably between different pharmacopeias or government agencies. Such inconsistency in the monographs or standards of the majority of herbal products becomes a challenge for manufacturers attempting to address varied regulatory quality standards. Such inconsistencies may risk product safety and efficacy, make consistency assurance across batches more cumbersome, and complicate the regulation submission process. (Goyal & Bhattacharya, 2022)

Varied Clinical Evidence Requirements

Different countries have different requirements for clinical evidence when registering herbal products. Some regulatory bodies require RCTs, pharmacokinetic studies, and extensive clinical trials, while others impose stringent requirements similar to those for proprietary medicines and rely on well-documented ethnobotanical evidence and traditionally used evidence as proof of safety and efficacy. Such differences pose considerable time and financial challenges for manufacturers that need multi-regional registration. The fact that clinical trial standards for Herbo-polymeric products are also lacking contributes to the difficulty in study design and comparability. This heterogeneity thus prevents immediate patient access to new herbal medicines and inhibits their further incorporation into mainstream medicine. (Martinez et al., 2020)

Post-Market Surveillance and Pharmacovigilance

Systems to keep an eye on herbal products after they hit the market aren't well-developed and differ from country to country. To watch out for safety, we need reliable ways to follow identify, and tell others about side effects or quality issues once a product is on the shelves. In many places, there's no need to monitor products after they're sold, or the ways to report problems are all over the place. This means fewer people speak up about issues, and it takes longer to find out when something's not safe. This has sometimes led to product recalls or punishments from regulators after harmful effects come to light. Also, the complex nature of herbal mixes often with many ingredients, makes it hard to pinpoint the cause in side effect investigations. To make sure products stay safe keep public trust, and help regulators make choices, we need to beef up PMS and align safety monitoring across the board. (Singh & Gupta 2023)

Ethical Oversight in Developing Nations

This is to ensure that the research and development of herbal as well polymer based wound care products are conducted in a manner that met both international ethical standards has to be accompanied by appropriate oversight from an ethical standpoint in developing nations. Limited governance of course infrastructure, resource constrains and sociocultural disadvantages are what hit the best hardest. Closing these ethical gaps is necessary to safeguard participant rights and transparency as well as equitable benefit-sharing.

Risk of Exploitation and Inadequate Informed Consent

Critical deficiencies in developing nations are the lack of Institutional Ethics Committees (IECs)/Research Ethics Committees (RECs) which prevents meaningful ethical oversight on clinical research. In some areas, these are under-staffed committees that compromise availability of skilled personnel and are not well supported in operation. In many cases this results in delayed reviews and inadequate oversight of study designs. Also, the potential for conflicts of interests and questionable decision-making without true legislative independence is noted. Those failings ramp up the likelihood that human subject research will be done improperly. The absence of well-functioning IEC systems may leave participant rights and safety unsecured. This is essential to achieve compliance with international norms, ethics infrastructure strengthening. (Nyika et al., 2009)

Lack of Regulatory Harmonization and Legal Frameworks

No country will have unified legal/ regulatory frameworks for the research with herbal medicine and traditional knowledge in low- and middle-income countries. This results into Research Participant protection inconsistent with the welfare protection of Ethnic communities. The absence of cohesive policies can be confusing and diffuse ethical oversight. This cause traditional knowledge holders to not be fairly acknowledged or rewarded. It is critical to expand and democratize regulation (Homedes & Ugalde, 2005)

Inadequate Community Engagement and Benefit-Sharing

Ethical oversight in peer-reviewed research of developing nations often confines local communities at every stage as passive subjects of studies. Traditional healers and native knowledge holders are often left out of consultations as well decisions. This lack of engagement does not engender trust and reciprocity. Ethical issues arise around exploitation as benefit-sharing is almost never on the agenda. As this undermines community support and long-term collaboration generated from such practices. Engagement pathways need to be inclusive and transparent. (Tindana et al., 2007)

Technological Advancements in Regulatory Monitoring

Technological innovations are reshaping the landscape and practice of regulatory monitoring in healthcare, pharma, herbal/ polymer wound care products. Digitalization: fresh transparency on pre and post market surveillance for compliance. This is particularly useful in low-resource settings were regulatory bodies often battle lack of infrastructure, and workforce. Point subtopics: Technical interventions for Regulatory Oversight.

Digital Platforms for Regulatory Submissions

E-submission processes help to automate the approval process by submitting required documents electronically and providing centralized data access via digital platforms. Such systems mean less paper, less human error and quicker regulatory clearance. In terms of accountability and efficiency, real-time updates also increase transparency. Investors' better coordination can be achieved by the improved communication between stakeholders. This is to modernize the ever-evolving regulatory practices globally. (WHO, 2021)

AI and Machine Learning in Pharmacovigilance

Artificial intelligence (AI) and machine learning (ML) are currently transforming pharmacovigilance with faster detection of safety signals. They enable these tools to sift through massive adverse event data with a great degree of accuracy. Used to highlight the drug-herb interactions that could be possibly missed by manual review. AI systems are used in predictive modeling for the early signal of potential occurring risks. It makes the regulatory response mechanisms more effective. As a result, these technologies enhance the safety of natural and synthetic drugs. (De Freitas et al., 2020)

Blockchain for Supply Chain Integrity

Supply chain transparency and traceability can be considerably enhanced in the field of herbal products due to the extensive use of Blockchain technology. Cryptography secures a public, immutable and scalable ledger to register every transaction done on it and store that data cannot be changed or tampered. This assist is authentic product verification throughout production and warehousing. Similar to herbal markets, blockchain is also essential for fraud intervention and anti-counterfeiting. With that, only the identified and ethically sourced ingredients are being used. Proves Compliance with regulatory and sustainability standards that manufacturers can Share Blockchain overall helps safer herbal delivery. (Kumar et al., 2021)

Mobile and Cloud-Based Monitoring Systems

Mobile and cloud-based systems make it easier to keep an eye on clinical trials and post-market activities in real-time. Healthcare workers and the public can quickly report problems, even from remote areas. This boosts safety checks and makes regulations run smoother. With cloud storage, accessing data is both simple and secure. Overall, these tools update the way we do monitoring. (Danzon & Keuffel, 2019)

Recommendations for Policymakers and Researchers

For developing Herbo-polymer wound care products ethically and effectively, it's key for policymakers and researchers to team up. We need to get regulatory rules to line up worldwide to make approvals easier. It's really important to boost research resources, especially in developing areas, so we can build strong clinical evidence. We should focus on ethically sourcing materials and sharing the benefits with local communities. Backing sustainable farming and fair trade is really important for keeping our environment safe. When we come together and combine old farming practices with new science, we can help ensure that everyone can easily get the treatment they need.

Promote Global Regulatory Harmonization

Policymakers need to work on aligning herbal product regulations across different countries. Right now, the varying classification systems and rules make it tough to trade and innovate globally. Creating common standards for quality, safety, and testing is really important. Groups like the International Council for Harmonization can help with this. Having one set of rules would cut down on duplication and help get products to market faster, which would also increase safety and build consumer trust. (Van den Berg et al., 2020)

Strengthen Research Capacity in Developing Regions

Improving research skills in developing areas is crucial for advancing Herbo-polymeric wound care. A lot of low- and middle-income countries deal with issues like poor infrastructure, not enough skilled workers, and limited research funding. Putting money into training, lab tools, and clinical trial networks can really help improve the quality of research. Teaming up with international groups can share knowledge and inspire fresh ideas. Sticking to standard research methods makes it simpler to compare data and get regulatory approval. These steps can lead to better healthcare solutions for everyone. (Chaturvedi et al., 2019)

Encourage Ethical and Sustainable Sourcing

Promoting ethical and sustainable sourcing is essential for biodiversity conservation and respect for the indigenous knowledge systems. There should also be some fair-trade covers in higher levels of government and the industries as a means to control overexploitation of medicinal plants. The Nagoya Protocol provides a system for fair benefit-sharing and the protection of community rights. Ethical sourcing can also help in maintaining traceability and product integrity." These methods help to identify trust with local communities and guide long-term ecological stewardship. (Ten Kate & Laird, 2018)

Foster Interdisciplinary Collaboration

The development of Herbo-polymeric products for injured skin depends greatly on close cooperation across multiple fields. Input from researchers, traditional practitioners, government bodies and others in the field can improve both making and studying health products. Using the knowledge of traditional practitioners makes traditions meaningful and encourages everyone to act ethically. Early regulations guide researchers so the products comply with approval standards. Working together encourages more people to trust and use the new technology. Shared problem-solving platforms can speed up the process of bringing discoveries into actual products. They help close the divide between scientific medicine and older medical practices. Joining forces inclusively leads to safer and more fair healthcare. (Canigueral et al., 2021)

Future Scope for Integrative Ethical-Regulatory Models

Increased complexity of Herbo-polymeric wound care systems underscores the imperative for synergistic ethical and regulatory frameworks. Emerging models need to harmonize scientific progress with sensitivity towards traditional knowledge, cultural values, and environmental stewardship. An integrated, patient-oriented system that harmonizes bioethics, regulatory science, and priorities in public health has the potential to bridge existing gaps among traditional and contemporary healthcare systems. Digital technologies such as blockchain and AI are able to facilitate transparency, informed consent, and compliance monitoring. Additionally, harmonized international policy is able to facilitate cross-border collaboration with accountability, equitable access, and safety. (Bodeker & Ong, 2020) Integration of such multi-dimensional systems holds the key to a promising future of global wound care improvement.

Integration of Traditional Knowledge into Regulatory Science

Upcoming regulatory frameworks should proactively incorporate tested traditional knowledge to close the gap between timeless practice and contemporary science. This entails constructing transparent guidelines for assessing traditional evidence in a manner that is sensitive to cultural context. Acknowledgment of the skill of traditional healers and participation of the same in research and policy-making is imperative. This builds confidence, safeguards indigenous knowledge, and optimizes the applicability of regulatory decisions. This integration eventually fosters more holistic and culturally more responsive health solutions. (WHO, 2013)

Development of Unified Global Ethical Guidelines

Harmonizing global bioethical norms is important to enable ethical development and commercialization of Herbo-polymeric items. Harmonized guidelines would provide uniform safeguards for vulnerable groups in various parts of the world. Such guidelines would also harmonize informed consent practices, ensuring transparency and participant self-determination. Moreover, such guidelines must impose fair benefit-sharing consistent with international policies like the Nagoya Protocol. Such harmonization induces trust, accountability, and ethical consistency in research and industrial practices. (United Nations, 2011) It finally advocates for equitable and prudent progress in herbal-based treatments.

Use of Digital Infrastructure for Compliance and Transparency

New digital technologies such as blockchain, mobile health platforms, and artificial intelligence are strong assets to enhance compliance and transparency in regulation of Herbo-polymeric products. Blockchain offers secure, tamper-evident history of clinical trials and supply chains to provide data integrity. Mobile platforms can enable real-time monitoring and reporting, enhancing informed consent processes and follow-up on adverse events. AI enables analysis of large datasets to identify safety signals and make more effective regulatory decisions. collectively, these technologies encourage stronger ethical regulation and foster trust for the stakeholders who are involved in the production of herbal medicine. (Sharma & Singh, 2021)

Capacity Building and Education Initiatives

Investing in capacity development through focused education programs becomes crucial to enhance ethical and regulatory competence in the arena of Herbo-polymeric products. Creating specialized curricula and ethics courses designed for researchers, traditional practitioners, and regulatory staff promotes detailed awareness of compliance needs and cultural barriers. Interdisciplinary exchange programs foster collaboration and sharing of knowledge among various sectors. These initiatives together make a more educated, ethically aware workforce better qualified to promote safe and efficacious herbal treatment throughout the world.

Multistakeholder Collaboration Platforms

Building multistakeholder cooperation frameworks that bring together governments, academia, industry, NGOs, and indigenous peoples is paramount to foster inclusive policy-making. These platforms create channels for free dialogue and building trust among diverse stakeholders. By engendering collective decision-making, such avenues allow for the co-creation of rules and moral values achievable, which respect cultural and scientific values. These platforms allow for early awareness of arising challenges, which facilitates responsible innovation and sustainable development in Herbo-polymeric products.

CONCLUSION

The discovery of herbal excipients and polymers for wound healing opens up exciting therapeutic possibilities, blending the age-old traditions of herbal medicine with modern polymer science to create novel wound healing solutions. Herbal excipients rich in bioactive molecules like flavonoids, tannins, and essential oils play a vital role in wound healing by facilitating tissue regeneration, displaying anti-inflammatory, antimicrobial, and antioxidant activities. Natural and synthetic polymers are important scaffolds used to impart structural strength, ensure a moist wound bed, and allow the controlled delivery of active ingredients, thus improving the action of herbal-based products.

Herbo-polymeric systems provide distinct benefits compared with traditional wound dressings, such as biodegradability, biocompatibility, and the ability to release therapeutic agents in a targeted and sustained fashion. These combined systems can promote the rate of wound closure, minimize the risk of infection, and reduce scarring, ultimately enhancing patient outcomes. While these novel characteristics are promising, their translation from the laboratory bench to clinical use remains problematic.

Chief among such challenges are the regulatory and ethical ones that now impede commercialization and extensive clinical acceptance. Harmonized global regulatory systems for herbal excipients and polymer-based wound dressings are lacking, which leads to uneven standards of quality and safety evaluations. Inconsistency in herbal sources, extraction processes, and polymer characterization only adds to batch-to-batch variability, making it hard for quality control as well as regulatory approval. Moreover, sparse preclinical and clinical data limit setting of solid safety and efficacy profiles that are required to gain regulatory approval.

Ethical issues must also be taken into account with caution. Intellectual property rights over traditional knowledge, fair benefit-sharing with traditionally using indigenous communities and anti-biopiracy are some of the major issues which need to be addressed so that social justice and ethical accountability are not violated.

For herbal excipients and polymers to be most effective in wound healing, different experts must cooperate. All stakeholders, including regulators, scientists, industry experts and ethicists, must come together to set up quiet, clear ways to test, describe and identify materials from ethical sources. Using this method will support new ideas, enhance safety during treatments, ensure products work well and make treatments fair for all.

Generally, combined plant medicine and polymer science has great potential to restructure how wounds are being treated. If challenges related to regulations and ethics are addressed together, Herbo-polymeric wound healing systems will be valuable, lasting and successful for patients everywhere.

REFERENCES

Ahmed, E. M. (2015). Hydrogel: Preparation, characterization, and applications: A review. *Journal of Advanced Research*, *6*(2), 105–121. PMID: 25750745

Balaji, S., Wang, X., King, A., Le, L. D., Bhattacharya, S. S., Moles, C. M., & Crombleholme, T. M. (2016). Interleukin-10–mediated regenerative postnatal tissue repair is dependent on regulation of hyaluronan metabolism via fibroblast-specific STAT3 signaling. *The FASEB Journal*, *31*(1), 212–219. PMID: 27903619

Balls, M., Combes, R., Fentem, J. H., Festing, M. F., Goldberg, A. M., Holzhütter, H. G., & Whelan, M. C. (2012). The principles of humane experimental technique: Reflections on 50 years of the 3Rs. *Alternatives to Laboratory Animals*, *40*(2), 93–102.

Bannister, K. (2014). Ethical challenges of traditional knowledge protection in the age of biotechnology. *Journal of Medical Ethics and History of Medicine*, *7*(1), 8.

Barnes, J. (2003). Quality, efficacy and safety of complementary medicines: fashions, facts and the future. Part II: Efficacy and safety. *British Journal of Clinical Pharmacology*, *55*(4), 331–340. PMID: 12680880

Berkes, F. (2009). Community conserved areas: Policy issues in historic and contemporary context. *Conservation Letters*, *2*(1), 20–25.

Bhatt, A. (2010). Evolution of clinical research: A history before and beyond James Lind. *Perspectives in Clinical Research*, *1*(1), 6–10. PMID: 21829774

Boateng, J., & Catanzano, O. (2015). Advanced therapeutic dressings for effective wound healing—A review. *Journal of Pharmaceutical Sciences*, *104*(11), 3653–3680. PMID: 26308473

Boateng, J. S., Matthews, K. H., Stevens, H. N., & Eccleston, G. M. (2008). Wound healing dressings and drug delivery systems: A review. *Journal of Pharmaceutical Sciences*, *97*(8), 2892–2923. PMID: 17963217

Boddupalli, S., & Kataria, M. (2021). Herbal drug-polymer conjugates: A promising approach for novel drug delivery system. *Pharmaceutical Nanotechnology*, *9*(3), 207–220.

Bodeker, G., & Ong, C. K. (2020). *WHO global report on traditional and complementary medicine 2019*. World Health Organization.

Brem, H., & Tomic-Canic, M. (2007). Cellular and molecular basis of wound healing in diabetes. *The Journal of Clinical Investigation*, *117*(5), 1219–1222. PMID: 17476353

Canigueral, S., Vila, R., & Alvarenga, N. (2021). Bridging traditional knowledge and scientific research in herbal medicine development. *Journal of Ethnopharmacology, 278*, 114309.

Chan, K., & Leung, K. W. (2021). Regulatory challenges in global herbal product development: A comparative analysis. *Phytomedicine, 80*, 153398.

Chattopadhyay, S., & Banerjee, G. (2022). Biopolymers and their applications in wound healing: Current and emerging trends. *International Journal of Biological Macromolecules, 200*, 414–430.

Chaturvedi, S., Kumar, S., & Dey, S. (2019). Strengthening research in developing countries: Strategies for capacity building. *Global Health Research and Policy, 4*(1), 1–8.

Chen, W. Y. J., & Abatangelo, G. (1999). Functions of hyaluronan in wound repair. *Wound Repair and Regeneration, 7*(2), 79–89. PMID: 10231509

Cohen, M. M., Penman, S., Pirotta, M., & Da Costa, C. (2011). Ethics and regulation of clinical research in complementary and alternative medicine. *Evidence-Based Complementary and Alternative Medicine: eCAM, 2011*, 1–9.

. Convention on Biological Diversity Secretariat. (2011). *Nagoya Protocol on Access and Benefit-sharing*.

Danzon, P. M., & Keuffel, E. L. (2019). *Regulation of pharmaceuticals: A review of global experiences*. Oxford Research Encyclopedia of Economics and Finance.

De Freitas, R. M., Dos Santos, F. C. A., & Santos, F. J. (2020). Artificial intelligence in pharmacovigilance: Current applications and future perspectives. *Therapeutic Advances in Drug Safety, 11*, 2042098620940936.

Deshmukh, P. T., Naik, S. R., & Magdum, C. S. (2014). Plant-based natural gums and mucilages as excipients in drug delivery: A review. *Research Journal of Pharmaceutical, Biological and Chemical Sciences, 5*(6), 1178–1189.

Dhivya, S., Padma, V. V., & Santhini, E. (2015). Wound dressings—A review. *Biomedicine (Taipei), 5*(4), 22. PMID: 26615539

Ekor, M. (2014). The growing use of herbal medicines: Issues relating to adverse reactions and challenges in monitoring safety. *Frontiers in Pharmacology, 4*, 177. PMID: 24454289

EMA. (2004). *Directive 2004/24/EC of the European Parliament and of the Council*.

Eming, S. A., Martin, P., & Tomic-Canic, M. (2014). Wound repair and regeneration: Mechanisms, signaling, and translation. *Science Translational Medicine*, *6*(265), 265sr6. PMID: 25473038

Falanga, V. (2005). Wound healing and its impairment in the diabetic foot. *Lancet*, *366*(9498), 1736–1743. PMID: 16291068

FDA. (2020). *Guidance for Industry: Botanical Drug Development*. U.S. Food and Drug Administration.

Frykberg, R. G., & Banks, J. (2015). Challenges in the treatment of chronic wounds. *Advances in Wound Care*, *4*(9), 560–582. PMID: 26339534

Gatt, A. R., Vella Bonanno, P., & Zammit, R. (2024). Ethical considerations in the regulation and use of herbal medicines in the European Union. *Frontiers in Medical Technology*, *4*, 1358956. PMID: 38948354

Goyal, A., & Bhattacharya, S. (2022). Clinical evidence requirements for herbal products: Bridging traditional use and modern regulatory frameworks. *Journal of Ethnopharmacology*, *292*, 115205.

Goyal, R. K., & Singh, J. (2019). Regulatory requirements for clinical trials of herbal products: Challenges and current status. *Journal of Ayurveda and Integrative Medicine*, *10*(4), 243–247.

Guo, S., & DiPietro, L. A. (2010). Factors affecting wound healing. *Journal of Dental Research*, *89*(3), 219–229. PMID: 20139336

Gurtner, G. C., Werner, S., Barrandon, Y., & Longaker, M. T. (2008). Wound repair and regeneration. *Nature*, *453*(7193), 314–321. PMID: 18480812

Hamedi, S., Mohagheghzadeh, A., & Rivaz, S. (2015). The role of medicinal plants in the treatment of wound healing: A review on historical perspectives. *Journal of Dermatology & Cosmetic*, *6*(2), 67–83.

Hartung, T. (2008). Toxicology for the twenty-first century. *Nature*, *460*(7252), 208–212. PMID: 19587762

Homedes, N., & Ugalde, A. (2005). Clinical trial ethics in Latin America: The continuing debate over standards of care. *Journal of Medical Ethics*, *31*(4), 231–235. PMID: 15800365

Houghton, P., & Mukherjee, P. K. (2020). Regulatory and quality aspects of herbal medicines: Global scenario. *Pharmaceutical Biology*, *58*(1), 61–72.

Ioannidis, J. P., Fanelli, D., Dunne, D. D., & Goodman, S. N. (2014). Meta-research: Evaluation and improvement of research methods and practices. *PLoS Biology, 12*(10), e1001747. PMID: 26431313

Iordache, F., Ditu, L. M., Popa, M. I., Ditu, S. T., & Vasilescu, A. (2022). Natural extract-based antimicrobial polymer films for wound healing. *Polymers, 14*(4), 743. PMID: 35215664

Jani, G. K., Shah, D. P., Prajapati, V. D., & Jain, V. C. (2012). Gums and mucilages: Versatile excipients for pharmaceutical formulations. *Asian Journal of Pharmaceutical Sciences, 7*(5), 309–323.

Javed, Z., Sadia, H., Raza, S., Iqbal, M. J., Sathyapalan, T., & Hashmi, M. F. (2021). Herbal medicine use and regulation in developing countries: A review of policy and ethics. *Complementary Therapies in Clinical Practice, 43*, 101393.

Jayakumar, R., Prabaharan, M., Sudheesh Kumar, P. T., Nair, S. V., & Tamura, H. (2011). Biomaterials based on chitin and chitosan in wound dressing applications. *Biotechnology Advances, 29*(3), 322–337. PMID: 21262336

Kulkarni, G. T., Gowthamarajan, K., & Dhobale, S. (2012). Natural polymers—A comprehensive review. *International Journal of Research in Pharmaceutical and Biomedical Sciences, 3*(4), 1597–1613.

Kumar, N., Mallick, P. K., & Tripathy, B. K. (2021). Blockchain for the healthcare supply chain: Challenges and opportunities. *Materials Today: Proceedings, 49*, 2848–2854.

Kunle, O. F., Egharevba, H. O., & Ahmadu, P. O. (2012). Standardization of herbal medicines – A review. *International Journal of Biodeversity and Conservation, 4*(3), 101–112.

Langat, S. K. (2005). Ethical challenges in advance of conducting herbal clinical trials: The need for internationally acceptable guidelines. *Acta Tropica, 95*(2), 178–184.

Langwick, S. A. (2011). *Bodies, politics, and African healing: The matter of maladies in Tanzania*. Indiana University Press.

Liu, M., Zeng, X., Ma, C., Yi, H., Ali, Z., Mou, X., Li, S., Deng, Y., & He, N. (2017). Injectable hydrogels for cartilage and bone tissue engineering. *Bone Research, 5*, 17014. PMID: 28584674

Mali, G. R., Bathe, R. S., & Bhalekar, M. R. (2010). Herbal excipients: A review. *International Journal of Pharmaceutical Sciences Review and Research, 5*(3), 104–112.

Marshall, E., Newton, A. C., & Schreckenberg, K. (2006). Commercialization of non-timber forest products: First steps in analyzing the factors influencing success. *International Forestry Review*, *8*(1), 34–43.

Martinez, L., Rodrigues, A. M., & Silva, D. (2020). Quality control challenges in herbal medicine: Global perspectives. *Pharmaceutical Biology*, *58*(1), 400–410. PMID: 32420784

Middleton, J. C., & Tipton, A. J. (2000). Synthetic biodegradable polymers as orthopedic devices. *Biomaterials*, *21*(23), 2335–2346. PMID: 11055281

Ministry of AYUSH. (2021). *Guidelines for Development of Ayurveda Formulations*. Government of India.

Mogo anu, G. D., & Grumezescu, A. M. (2014). Natural and synthetic polymers for wounds and burns dressing. *International Journal of Pharmaceutics*, *463*(2), 127–136. PMID: 24368109

Morgera, E., Tsioumani, E., & Buck, M. (2012). *Unraveling the Nagoya Protocol: A commentary on the Nagoya Protocol on Access and Benefit-sharing to the Convention on Biological Diversity*. Brill Nijhoff.

Morton, D. B., & Griffiths, P. H. M. (1985). Guidelines on the recognition of pain, distress and discomfort in experimental animals and an hypothesis for assessment. *The Veterinary Record*, *116*(16), 431–436. PMID: 3923690

Mukherjee, P. K., Nema, N. K., Maity, N., & Mukherjee, D. (2011). *Standardized extracts of herbs and their significance in clinical practice. Herbal Medicine: Biomolecular and Clinical Aspects* (2nd ed.). CRC Press.

Mustoe, T. A., O'Shaughnessy, K., & Kloeters, O. (2006). Chronic wound pathogenesis and current treatment strategies: A unifying hypothesis. *Plastic and Reconstructive Surgery*, *117*(7S), 35S–41S. PMID: 16799373

Nayak, B. S., & Pinto Pereira, L. M. (2006). Catharanthus roseus flower extract has wound-healing activity in Sprague Dawley rats. *BMC Complementary and Alternative Medicine*, *6*, 41. PMID: 17184528

Nosek, B. A., Ebersole, C. R., DeHaven, A. C., & Mellor, D. T. (2015). The preregistration revolution. *Proceedings of the National Academy of Sciences of the United States of America*, *115*(11), 2600–2606. PMID: 29531091

Nyika, A., Kilama, W., Chilengi, R., & Tangwa, G. B. (2009). Composition, training needs and independence of ethics review committees across Africa: Are the gate-keepers rising to the emerging challenges? *Journal of Medical Ethics*, *35*(3), 189–193. PMID: 19251972

Pandey, R., Bhatt, G., & Johri, A. (2016). Herbal excipients in novel drug delivery systems. *International Journal of Pharmaceutical Sciences Review and Research*, *36*(1), 192–199.

Parasuraman, S. (2012). Herbal drug development: Current status and the future. *Asian Journal of Pharmaceutical and Clinical Research*, *5*(Suppl 2), 8–12.

Patel, M., & Patel, N. (2021). Regulatory challenges and approaches in herbal drug development. *Journal of Herbal Medicine*, *26*, 100406.

Patil, J. S., Kamalapur, M. V., Marapur, S. C., & Kadam, D. V. (2009). Formulation and evaluation of sustained release microparticles of aceclofenac using natural polymer. *Research Journal of Pharmacy and Technology*, *2*(5), 331–334.

Patwardhan, B., Chandran, U., & Joshi, K. (2015). Ayurveda and natural products drug discovery. *Current Science*, *109*(9), 1579–1583.

Patwardhan, B., Warude, D., Pushpangadan, P., & Bhatt, N. (2005). Ayurveda and traditional Chinese medicine: A comparative overview. *Evidence-Based Complementary and Alternative Medicine: eCAM*, *2*(4), 465–473. PMID: 16322803

Peters, M. A., Jayne, M., & Murphy, T. (2019). Global health equity and access: Towards sustainable universal health coverage. *Health Policy and Planning*, *34*(3), 195–197.

Posey, D. A., & Dutfield, G. (1996). *Beyond intellectual property: Toward traditional resource rights for indigenous peoples and local communities*. International Development Research Centre.

Ravikumar, P., Krishna, V., & Manjunath, K. (2013). Herbal excipients in novel drug delivery systems. *International Journal of Pharma and Bio Sciences*, *4*(2), 334–345.

Russell, W. M. S., & Burch, R. L. (1959). *The principles of humane experimental technique*. Methuen.

Sahoo, S. K., Parveen, S., & Panda, J. J. (2008). The present and future of nanotechnology in human health care. *Nanomedicine; Nanotechnology, Biology, and Medicine*, *3*(1), 20–31. PMID: 17379166

Sen, C. K. (2009). Wound healing essentials: Let there be oxygen. *Wound Repair and Regeneration*, *17*(1), 1–18. PMID: 19152646

Shaikh, T., Ali, J., & Baboota, S. (2011). Herbal excipients in novel drug delivery systems. *Pharmacognosy Reviews*, *5*(9), 46–52.

Sharma, S., & Singh, S. (2021). Blockchain technology for enhancing transparency and traceability in herbal medicine supply chains. *Journal of Ethnopharmacology*, *268*, 113605.

Shiva, V. (2001). *Protect or plunder? Understanding intellectual property rights*. Zed Books.

Shukla, A., Rasik, A. M., Jain, G. K., Shankar, R., Kulshrestha, D. K., & Dhawan, B. N. (1999). In vitro and in vivo wound healing activity of asiaticoside isolated from *Centella asiatica. Journal of Ethnopharmacology*, *65*(1), 1–11. PMID: 10350364

Singh, R., & Gupta, N. (2023). Pharmacovigilance in herbal medicine: Current status and future directions. *Regulatory Toxicology and Pharmacology*, *135*, 105276.

Smith, J., & Berkes, F. (2018). Sustainability and indigenous knowledge: Implications for environmental ethics in natural resource management. *Environmental Ethics*, *40*(1), 1–15.

Srinivas, K., Anand, A. R., & Nath, R. K. (2019). Informed consent in clinical research: Revisiting its history, current challenges, and future prospects. *Journal of Clinical and Diagnostic Research: JCDR*, *13*(4), JE01–JE04.

Steneck, N. H. (2006). Fostering integrity in research: Definitions, current knowledge, and future directions. *Science and Engineering Ethics*, *12*(1), 53–74. PMID: 16501647

Ten Kate, K., & Laird, S. A. (2018). *The commercial use of biodiversity: Access to genetic resources and benefit-sharing*. Earthscan.

Ticktin, T. (2004). The ecological implications of harvesting non-timber forest products. *Journal of Applied Ecology*, *41*(1), 11–21.

Tilburt, J. C., & Kaptchuk, T. J. (2008). Herbal medicine research and global health: An ethical analysis. *Bulletin of the World Health Organization*, *86*(8), 594–599. PMID: 18797616

Tindana, P. O., Kass, N., & Akweongo, P. (2007). The informed consent process in a rural African setting: A case study of the Kassena-Nankana District of northern Ghana. *IRB*, *29*(3), 1–6. PMID: 17847635

Tobin, J., & Lewison, G. (2011). Global trends in patents and intellectual property rights. *Scientometrics*, *89*(1), 1–14.

Ullah, F., Othman, M. B. H., Javed, F., Ahmad, Z., & Akil, H. M. (2015). Classification, processing and application of hydrogels: A review. *Materials Science and Engineering C, 57*, 414–433. PMID: 26354282

. United Nations. (2011). *Nagoya Protocol on Access to Genetic Resources and the Fair and Equitable Sharing of Benefits Arising from their Utilization to the Convention on Biological Diversity.*

Van den Berg, M. J., de Vries, H., & Peek, N. (2020). Harmonizing regulations for herbal medicines: An international perspective. *Regulatory Toxicology and Pharmacology, 117*, 104770.

Velnar, T., Bailey, T., & Smrkolj, V. (2009). The wound healing process: An overview of the cellular and molecular mechanisms. *The Journal of International Medical Research, 37*(5), 1528–1542. PMID: 19930861

Venkatesan, J., Bhatnagar, I., Manivasagan, P., Kang, K. H., & Kim, S. K. (2017). Alginate composites for wound healing: A review. *International Journal of Biological Macromolecules, 104*, 1388–1400.

Winter, G. D. (1962). Formation of the scab and the rate of epithelialization of superficial wounds in the skin of the young domestic pig. *Nature, 193*, 293–294. PMID: 14007593

World Health Organization. (2013). *WHO traditional medicine strategy 2014–2023.* World Health Organization.

. World Health Organization. (2021). *Good regulatory practices: guidelines for national regulatory authorities for medical products.*

Zhang, Y., & Li, X. (2022). Challenges and opportunities in the global regulation of herbal medicines: Towards harmonization. *International Journal of Regulatory Science, 7*(2), 45–57.

Zhao, X., Wu, H., Guo, B., Dong, R., Qiu, Y., & Ma, P. X. (2017). Antibacterial anti-oxidant electroactive injectable hydrogels for wound healing. *Acta Biomaterialia, 68*, 67–79.

Chapter 16
Challenges and Opportunities in Herbal Wound Care

Nidhi Bais
https://orcid.org/0009-0008-6333-7977
Oriental University, India

Ravikant Gupta
https://orcid.org/0009-0003-8349-8739
Oriental University, India

Sachin K. Jain
Oriental University, India

Sudha Vengurlekar
Oriental University, India

ABSTRACT

Healthcare wound healing has attracted a lot of attention. Biological wound healing is accurate and highly programmed by stages of hemostasis, Inflammation, proliferation and conversion. . This includes the use of antibacterial active ingredients, healing conveyors, herbs and natural products. However, there is no efficient evidencebased treatment available for specific chronic wounds that may lead to final clinical outcomes. Under general conditions, chronicity faces many challenges. With the increasing use of complementary and alternative drugs (CAMs) in healthcare, wound management applications remain diamonds in ore. The main focus is the application and limitation of currently available treatment options for nonhealing

DOI: 10.4018/979-8-3373-3977-1.ch016

wounds and the best possible alternatives. This information generates broader knowledge about chronic wound healing and can be addressed further using inter-disciplinary approaches and combination therapy.

INTRODUCTION

Use of herbal medication and ideas for recovery of one of the fundamental principles of conventional medication. Despite the fact that majority of them aren't in mainstream due to lack of evidences, some of them have efficaciously entered medical application after gaining significance in special ranges of research for infection, most cancers and different chronic illnesses. that is particularly due to specific capability of natural molecules to engage with distinct bio-molecules. Consequently, each know-how the essential cell components altered for the duration of wound and progressions of wound as well as molecules to opposite/repair those changes are critical. in this course, there's a large capacity for development of safe, sustainable and powerful remedy module the usage of trade medication from plant or different herbal sources. this could help to scientifically promote numerous conventional drug treatments for recovery special class of wounds.

HEALING OF WOUND

The process of healing is complex and time-consuming, involving the restoration of cell structure and tissue layers. It can occur through two methods:

A) Regeneration, where a like tissue replaces the extinct one, or repair, where the damaged tissue is replaced by a different type of tissue.

B) Repair – it's the process of replacing the damaged tissue with new granulation tissue. This type of tissue completely develops to create the scar tissue. The process of wound healing involves several stages: the first is haemostasis, followed by the inflammatory phase, then the proliferation or granulation phase, and finally, the remodelling and scar formation phase, (Schilling, 1968).

CLINICAL PRESENTATION AND CHALLENGES IN CHRONIC WOUND

Chronic wounds pose a significant healthcare burden, both financially and in terms of morbidity, and have a profound impact on individuals' well-being. In India, public healthcare funding has been reported at 5% of the annual gross domestic product, with over 80% of healthcare costs covered through out-of-pocket payments, (Allaman, 1988). These do not capture the economic loss, frustration, and compromised quality of life endured by individuals with chronic wounds. As a result, they pose a significant clinical challenge in long-term care, affecting the quality of life for patients and increasing healthcare expenses, (Allaman, 1988; Ruedrich et al., 2013).

Chronic wounds are often characterized by pathological reactions that lead to fibrosis and non-healing chronic ulcers.

This clinical condition is the result of a non-diagnosed or untreated wound. The most important clinical signs and symptoms in patients with chronic wounds are pullolence with pain, erythema, edema, fever, and wounds, (Stotts & Hunt, 1997). Furthermore, the symptoms and symptoms specific to secondary wounds observed in proliferative phase are as follows.

(1) Wound degradation (2) Simultaneous inflammation, (3) Foul odor, (3) Base (4) Granulation tissue (6) Delayed tissue (6) Delayed him (6) Delayed him (6) Sight (3) Base (3) Base (4) However, these signs and symptoms should be further validated for effective chronic wound management and treatment, (Gardner, Frantz, & Doebbeling, 2001).

To verify the clinical symptoms of chronic wounds, the signs showed signs specific to secondary wounds. These signs and symptoms may correlate with diseases that represent the physiological environment of the disease. This means that chronic wounds in a challenging environment are exposed to the wounds that lead to non-healing states. It is very necessary to have a detailed understanding of the underlying mechanisms in its pathological conditions. This is possible by identifying clinically relevant biological markers. This is a critical chronic factor in wounds. Therefore, the identification of a biomarker and a biomarker may address the prognosis, diagnosis, or treatment of the biomarker, (Gardner, Frantz, & Doebbeling, 2001).

Chronic wounds, often characterized by infection/biofilms, increase the production of inflammatory and inflammatory cytokines, leading to the production of matrix metalloproteases and reduced inhibitors. Extended inflammation leads to the disruption of extracellular matrix and fibroblast production. Inhibition of fibroblast production produces little collagen fiber required for wound redesign. Chronic wound-associated fibroblasts indicate senescence of fibroblasts. Chronic wound environment affects the position of angiogenesis and epithelialization. These properties represent chronic wound environments where healing is delayed.

It was estimated that ¼1% of the population develop leg ulcers during their lifespan, (Martin, 2001; Strausberg et al., 2007). An Indian study on the epidemiology of chronic wounds estimated the prevalence at a rate of 4.5/1,000 population, (Shukla, Ansari, & Gupta, 2005). Untreated or insufficient acute traumatic wounds are the common cause of these chronic wounds. Wounds associated with chronic diseases such as diabetes and cancer are a greater challenge for treatment and treatment, primarily due to molecular complexity, (Brem, Sheehan, & Boulton, 2004). Furthermore, chronic nonsymptomatic pressure ulcers are serious, often indicating the development of (such as spinal cord injuries) among immobilized and weakened patients. Based on this information, understanding wound healing activities at the molecular level is essential to identify factors that cause delayed wound repair. Current research into the treatment of chronic wounds focuses on understanding the underlying molecular mechanisms at clinically different wounds and at different stages of their progression and healing, (Brem, Sheehan, & Boulton, 2004).

HERBAL MEDICINE

Herbal medicine or plant medicine refers to herbs (including leaves, seeds, roots, bark, etc.), herbal ingredients (fresh juice, essential oils, etc.), herbal preparations (extracts, tinctures, fatty oils) and finished herbal products. This is a complex mixture of components of different chemical classes, whose biological activity produces effects caused by the complex action of independent components. As a result, the drugs taken into consideration are complex mixtures that produce specific effects, both chemically and in terms of bioactivity. The latest synthetic drugs are potentially dangerous and recurred after symptoms and very expensive. However, herbs are generally claimed to be non-toxic as they come from natural sources and have been used since civilization began.

Types of Herbal Medicine Systems: Herbal medicines have been produced in a variety of cultures and can be divided into three groups.

- Western herbal medicine
- Chinese herbal medicine
- Traditional Indian medicine (Ayurveda, Siddha, Unani).

Western Herbal Medicine

Western herbal medicine was a major type of medicine before the 20th century but has since been shaded by orthodox or inorganic medicine based on scientific medical models. However, in recent years, public opinion outside of traditional medicine has changed. By the 17th century, European herbs were based on humor that touched Hippocrates.

Chinese Herbal Medicine

Yellow Kaiser Huntty (2697-2597 V. Most Chinese herb enthusiasts use the main herbs in combinations of, because both are advantageous. They are performed in the same way, in the same way. Herbal support offers a variety of functions and benefits. One herb lead, and the other herb serves as a catalyst support. Frighteners Rede Reduce the risk of injury by reducing the strength and violence of plants in the mixture. Cancelling herbs such as laxative and string agent combinations to minimize herbs, minimizing the constipation produced by the latter is used to eliminate unwanted side effects.

Traditional Indian Medicine (Ayurveda, Siddha, Unani).

Ayurvedic Medicine is a traditional Indian public health system. Until 1400 BC, BC had developed Ayurveda or life science into a health system based on education and health promotion. This medical method is based on the biological humor of Vata (Air), Pitta (Tue), and Kapha (Wed). These Toridoshas exist in all people, but the elements govern the dominant constitution. Constitutional strength and weaknesses are defined by key elements. VATA is characterized by lack of strength and durability, shortness of breath, indigestion, flatulence and circulation problems. Pitta tends to be susceptible to rage and is a hot constitution with purple skin. They have decent digestive and circulatory health but are susceptible to inflammatory and viral disorders. Kapa has white, moist skin, and is sensitive and romantic. Different category. 7 Greasy, sticky and sweet foods should have the nature of tamasian. H. Heavy and dull for the system. Sattvic Foods are objects that calm and nourish the body, such as vegetables, fruits, nuts, and daily life, (Huffman, 2003; Dwivedi & Dwivedi, 2007).

Table 1. Role of phytoconstituent in wound healing studies (12,13,14,15,16)

Name of Phytocompound	Type of formulation	Uses and applications in wound healing	Possible mechanism of action	Outcome
Vitamin A	Topical and systemic	Anti-inflammatory property; Necessary for growth, differentiation, and maintenance of epithelial tissues	Influences morphogenesis, epithelial cell proliferation and differentiation in time and dose dependent manner	Prevents and treats infectious as well as inflammatory skin diseases
Vitamin E	Oral and topical	Used for resurfacing of the skin Modulate	cellular signaling, gene expression	Increased wound contraction
Vitamin C	Plant extract	Modulators of angiogenesis & collagen production; critically important for tensile strength of a wound	Act through induction of protein-kinase-Cdependent pathway that activates protein-1 DNA binding activity; hydroxylation of lysine and proline during the synthesis of collage	Stimulated growth of keratinocytes
Alkaloids effects	Topical	Anti-inflammatory	Stimulate the growth of colonies from fibroblast precursors	Promotes early phases of wound healing (≤7 days) in a dose-dependent manner
Flavonoids	Pure Phytocompound/ extract	Antioxidant, anti-allergic, anti-carcinogenic, anti-viral and anti-inflammatory agents	Involve hydrogen bonding and hydrophobic interactions	Collagen fibers treated with catechin are stable

CHALLENGES OF HERBAL FORMULATIONS

Herbal medications present a number of obstacles that must be addressed, such as the task of:

- Over the course of the extraction procedure, herbal Substances need special care and safeguarding. It is important to maintain ideal drying conditions. Unintentional adulteration may arise from inadequate drying. Glycosides break down by enzymatic hydrolysis, for instance, when digitalis leaves are dried above 65°.

- There is no good method to ascertain whether ingredients can be used, to what degree, and to what standards because there is no single standard that will apply to herbal formulations.
- Only a few numbers of natural ingredients can be used in the creation of herbal medicines. The challenge of creating a mixture with fewer ingredients could lead to the creation of a product that is less effective than ones based on synthetic chemicals.
- Clinical research including herbal preparations may encounter challenges.
- There are issues with pharmacological and toxicological evaluation in herbal preparations.
- Challenges with technique development, absorption site research, finding many animal models for toxicity and safety assessment, and legal and regulatory issues with herbal medicines, among other factors, (Balap & Gaikwad, 2021).

Comparison Between Synthetic and Herbal Medicine

Traditional medicine is defined as the culmination of all knowledge and practices derived from indigenous cultural conceptions and experiences, whether or not they can be explained. It is used to prevent, diagnose, and treat physical and mental illnesses as well as to maintain health. The WHO estimated in 1983 that traditional and herbal medicines represent the main source of healthcare for the majority of people in poor nations. Global interest in herbal medicines and traditional medical practices has grown within the last ten years. The acceptability of traditional and herbal medicine is impressive worldwide, particularly in third-world countries where access to modern medical technology is limited. In addition, many people in rich countries also accept herbal remedies, (World Health Organization, 2000; Bannerman, Burton, & Chen, 1983; Fong, 2002).

Numerous pieces of evidence demonstrate how much attention has been paid to the growing popularity of complementary and alternative medicine, or CAM. According to a survey by Eisenberg et al. in the USA, the percentage of adults using CAM rose from 34% in 1990 to 42% in 1997. Additionally, the survey revealed that $27 billion was spent by American consumers. on complementary therapies, and an estimated $5.1 billion on herbal remedies in 1997; in contrast, the global herbal medicine business was valued at about $20 billion, (Eisenberg et al., 1998; Dev, 1997; Dev, 2001).

A new era known as “integrative medicine” has emerged as a result of the current surge in interest in integrative techniques and numerous medicinal modalities. The practice of medicine that carefully integrates CAM components into all-encompassing treatment programs in addition to conventional techniques of diagnosis and therapy,

(Rees & Weil, 2001). It may also refer to the integration of TRM into general health care systems, which acknowledge both conventional and traditional medical practice methods. Integrative medicine is intended to be the former in industrialized nations like the United States of America. Herbal medicine should be logically incorporated into contemporary medical procedures, such as cancer treatment, using a scientific approach that considers the interconnected concerns of efficacy, safety, and quality, (World Health Organization, 1999).

Need of Standardization

As components and medication candidates, plant extracts offer a wide range of options for the treatment of numerous chronic illnesses. Plant extracts, pure forms, and derivatives are in high demand as therapeutic goods because of their unparalleled availability and chemical diversity. It's noteworthy to note that genetic and environmental influences in plants have a significant impact on the biochemical makeup of plants; therefore, standardizing herbal medicines is required. Additionally, the quality, safety, and effectiveness of the content of one or more active ingredients and marker compounds are ensured by standardization processes. Monocultures from the source plant should be used to create genetically homogeneous plant generations; additionally, biochemical consistency should be guaranteed, and safety and effectiveness should be maximized. profiles of the plant-based products. The safety and effectiveness of pant goods are also significantly impacted by commercial production and manufacturing procedures. Thus, during analysis and manufacturing, adherence to good agriculture and collection practices, good laboratory practices, good manufacturing standards, and good plant authentication and identification practices are crucial. In the post-marketing phase following production, vendor audits in supply chains and the development of standardized multilaboratory verified analytical techniques are equally crucial. IV) Clinical verification of herbal remedies, (Garg et al., 2012; Govindaraghavan & Sucher, 2015; Govindaraghavan, 2008).

REFERENCES

Allaman, R. M. (1988). The impact of pressure ulcers on health care costs and mortality. *Advances in Wound Care, 11*(2). PMID: 9729946

Balap, A. R., & Gaikwad, A. A. (2021). Challenges, advances and opportunities of herbal medicines in wound healing: A review. *International Journal of Pharmaceutical Sciences Review and Research, 71*(1). *Article, 15*, 125–136.

. Bannerman, R. H., Burton, J., & Chen, W.-C. (1983). *Traditional medicine and health care coverage: A reader for health administrators and practitioners.*

Brem, H., Sheehan, P., & Boulton, A. J. M. (2004). Protocol for treatment of diabetic foot ulcers. *American Journal of Surgery, 187*(Suppl. 1), S1–S10. PMID: 15147985

Dev, S. (1997). Ethnotherapeutics and modern drug development: The potential of Ayurveda. *Current Science, 73*(11), 909–928.

Dev, S. (2001). Ancient-modern concordance in Ayurvedic plants: Some examples. In *Development of Plant-Based Medicines: Conservation, Efficacy, and Safety* (pp. 47-67). Springer.

Dwivedi, G., & Dwivedi, S. (2007). *History of medicine: Sushruta — the clinician-teacher par excellence. National Informatics Centre.* Government of India.

Eisenberg, D. M., Davis, R. B., Ettner, S. L., Appel, S., Wilkey, S., Van Rompay, M., & Kessler, R. C. (1998). Trends in alternative medicine use in the United States, 1990-1997: Results of a follow-up national survey. *Journal of the American Medical Association, 280*(18), 1569–1575. PMID: 9820257

Fong, H. H. S. (2002). Integration of herbal medicine into modern medical practices: Issues and prospects. *Integrative Cancer Therapies, 1*(3), 287–293. PMID: 14667286

Gardner, S. E., Frantz, R. A., & Doebbeling, B. N. (2001). The validity of the clinical signs and symptoms used to identify localized chronic wound infection. *Wound Repair and Regeneration, 9*, 178–186. PMID: 11472613

Garg, V.. (2012). Facts about standardization of herbal medicine: A review. *Journal of Chinese Integrative Medicine, 10*(10), 1077–1083. PMID: 23073189

Govindaraghavan, S. (2008). Quality assurance of herbal raw materials in supply chain: Challenges and opportunities. *Journal of Dietary Supplements, 5*(2), 176–212. PMID: 22432433

Govindaraghavan, S., & Sucher, N. J. (2015). Quality assessment of medicinal herbs and their extracts: Criteria and prerequisites for consistent safety and efficacy of herbal medicines. *Epilepsy & Behavior, 52*, 363–371. PMID: 25899015

Huffman, M. A. (2003). Animal self-medication and ethno-medicine: Exploration and exploitation of the medicinal properties of plants. *The Proceedings of the Nutrition Society, 62*(2), 371–381. PMID: 14506884

Martin, G. M. (2001). Frontiers of aging. *Science, 294*(5540), 13. PMID: 11588222

Rees, L., & Weil, A. (2001). Integrated medicine: Imbues orthodox medicine with the values of complementary medicine. *BMJ (Clinical Research Ed.), 322*(7279), 119. PMID: 11159553

Ruedrich, E. D., Henzel, M. K., Hausman, B. S., & Bogie, K. M. (2013). Reference gene identification for reverse transcription-quantitative polymerase chain reaction analysis in an ischemic wound-healing model. *Journal of Biomolecular Techniques: JBT, 24*, 181–186. DOI: 10.7171/jbt.13-2404-003 PMID: 24294111

Schilling, J. A. (1968). Wound healing. *Physiological Reviews, 48*(2-4), 374. PMID: 4231314

Shukla, V. K., Ansari, M. A., & Gupta, S. K. (2005). Wound healing research: A perspective from India. *The International Journal of Lower Extremity Wounds, 4*, 7–8. PMID: 15860447

Stotts, N. A., & Hunt, T. K. (1997). Managing bacterial colonization and infection. *Clinics in Geriatric Medicine, 13*, 565–573. DOI: 10.1016/S0749-0690(18)30160-5 PMID: 9227945

Strausberg, J., Lehmann, N., Kröger, K., Maier, I., & Schneider, H. N. W. [initials expanded as per source]. (2007). Changes in secondary care may explain increasing pressure ulcer rates in a university clinic in Germany. *Wound Management, 5*, 194–198.

World Health Organization. (1999). *Traditional and modern medicine: Harmonizing the two approaches: A report of the consultation meeting on traditional and modern medicine, 22-26 November 1999, Beijing, China*. WHO Regional Office for the Western Pacific.

World Health Organization. (2000). *General guidelines for methodologies on research and evaluation of traditional medicine*. Essential Medicines and Health Products Information Portal.

Compilation of References

Abdi, G., Jain, M., Patil, N., Tariq, M., Choudhary, S., Kumar, P., Raj, N. S., Mohsen Ali, S. S., & Uthappa, U. T. (2024). Tragacanth gum-based hydrogels for drug delivery and tissue engineering applications. *Frontiers in Materials, 11*, 1296399. DOI: 10.3389/FMATS.2024.1296399/XML/NLM

Abdou, A. G., Maraee, A. H., Al-Bara, A. M., & Diab, W. M. (2011). Immunohistochemical expression of TGF-β1 in keloids and hypertrophic scars. *The American Journal of Dermatopathology, 33*(1), 84–91. DOI: 10.1097/DAD.0b013e3181d0c3ad PMID: 20559120

Abka-Khajouei, R., Tounsi, L., Shahabi, N., Patel, A. K., Abdelkafi, S., & Michaud, P. (2022). Structures, properties and applications of alginates. *Marine Drugs, 20*(6), 364. PMID: 35736167

Abourehab, M. A. S., Rajendran, R. R., Singh, A., Pramanik, S., Shrivastav, P., Ansari, M. J., Manne, R., Amaral, L. S., & Deepak, A. (2022). Alginate as a Promising Biopolymer in Drug Delivery and Wound Healing: A Review of the State-of-the-Art. *International Journal of Molecular Sciences, 23*(16), 9035. DOI: 10.3390/ijms23169035 PMID: 36012297

Aburjai, T., Al-Janabi, R., Al-Mamoori, F., & Azzam, H. (2019). In vivo wound healing and antimicrobial activity of Alkanna strigose. *Wound Med, 25*(1), 100152.

Aderibigbe, B. A. (2018). Alginate in wound dressings. *Pharmaceuticals, 11*(2), 42. DOI: 10.3390/ph11020042 PMID: 29735913

Aderibigbe, B. A., & Buyana, B. (2018). Alginate in wound dressings. *Pharmaceutics, 10*(2), 42. PMID: 29614804

Aderibigbe, B., & Buyana, B. (2018). Alginate in Wound Dressings. *Pharmaceutics, 10*(2), 42. DOI: 10.3390/pharmaceutics10020042 PMID: 29614804

Ahmad, N. (2023). In vitro and in vivo characterization methods for evaluation of modern wound dressings. *Pharmaceutics, 15*(1), 42. DOI: 10.3390/pharmaceutics15010042 PMID: 36678671

Ahmed, E. M. (2015). Hydrogel: Preparation, characterization, and applications: A review. *Journal of Advanced Research, 6*(2), 105–121. DOI: 10.1016/j.jare.2013.07.006 PMID: 25750745

Ahmed, O. M., Mohamed, T., Moustafa, H., Hamdy, H., Ahmed, R. R., & Aboud, E. (2018). Quercetin and low level laser therapy promote wound healing process in diabetic rats via structural reorganization and modulatory effects on inflammation and oxidative stress. *Biomedicine and Pharmacotherapy, 101*, 58–73. PMID: 29477473

Ahmed, S., Ikram, S., & Yousaf, M. (2023). Biopolymer-based wound dressings: Recent advances and future perspectives. *Carbohydrate Polymers, 312*, 120789. DOI: 10.1016/j.carbpol.2022.120789

Ajayi, O. E., Yoon, S. Y., Moon, S., Kim, K. H., Kim, J. H., Chung, J.-W., Jang, K.-I., & Hyun, T. K. (2023). Variability in Phytochemical Contents and Biological Activities among *Adenophora triphylla* Genotypes. *Applied Sciences (Basel, Switzerland), 13*(20), 11184. DOI: 10.3390/app132011184

Akbik, D., Ghadiri, M., Chrzanowski, W., & Rohanizadeh, R. (2014). Curcumin as a wound healing agent. *Life Sciences, 116*(1), 1–7. DOI: 10.1016/j.lfs.2014.08.016 PMID: 25200875

Aklilu, T. E. G. E. G. N. E. (2002). *Evaluation of Local Gum of Acacia Polyacantha as a Binder in Tablet Formulations*. AAU Institutional Repository.

Alam, P., Shakeel, F., Anwer, M. K., Foudah, A. I., & Alqarni, M. H. (2018). Wound healing study of eucalyptus oil containing nanoemulsion in rat model. *Journal of Oleo Science, 67*(8), 957–968. DOI: 10.5650/jos.ess18005 PMID: 30012898

Albahri, G., Badran, A., Hijazi, A., Daou, A., Baydoun, E., Nasser, M., & Merah, O. (2023). The therapeutic wound healing bioactivities of various medicinal plants. *Life (Chicago, Ill.), 13*(2), 317. DOI: 10.3390/life13020317 PMID: 36836674

Albahri, G., Badran, A., Hijazi, A., Daou, A., Baydoun, E., Nasser, M., & Merah, O. (2023). The Therapeutic Wound Healing Bioactivities of Various Medicinal Plants. *Life (Chicago, Ill.), 13*(2), 317. DOI: 10.3390/LIFE13020317 PMID: 36836674

Alberti, T., & Coelho, S, D., Voytena, A., Pitz, H., de Pra, M., Mazzarino, L., ... & Veleirinho, B. (2017). Nanotechnology: A promising tool towards wound healing. *Current Pharmaceutical Design, 23*(24), 3515–3535. PMID: 28472915

Alengebawy, A., Abdelkhalek, S. T., Qureshi, S. R., & Wang, M. Q. (2021). Heavy metals and pesticides toxicity in agricultural soil and plants: Ecological risks and human health implications. *Toxics*, *9*(3), 42. PMID: 33668829

Al-Gharibi, K. A., Sharstha, S., & Al-Faras, M. A. (2018). Cost-Effectiveness of Wound Care: A concept analysis. *Sultan Qaboos University Medical Journal*, *18*(4), e433–e439. DOI: 10.18295/squmj.2018.18.04.002 PMID: 30988960

Aliabadi, M., Chee, B. S., Matos, M., Cortese, Y. J., Nugent, M. J. D., De Lima, T. A. M., Magalhães, W. L. E., & De Lima, G. G. (2020). Yerba Mate Extract in Microfibrillated Cellulose and Corn Starch Films as a Potential Wound Healing Bandage. *Polymers*, *12*(12), 2807. DOI: 10.3390/polym12122807 PMID: 33260883

Aliabadi, M., Chee, B. S., Matos, M., Cortese, Y. J., Nugent, M. J. D., De Lima, T. A. M., Magalhães, W. L. E., De Lima, G. G., & Firouzabadi, M. D. (2021). Microfibrillated cellulose films containing chitosan and tannic acid for wound healing applications. *Journal of Materials Science. Materials in Medicine*, *32*(6), 67. DOI: 10.1007/s10856-021-06536-4 PMID: 34117926

Ali, K. A., Mohin, S. K., Mondal, P., Goswami, S., Ghosh, S., & Choudhuri, S. (2024). Influence of artificial intelligence in modern pharmaceutical formulation and drug development. *Future Journal of Pharmaceutical Sciences*, *10*(1), 53.

Ali, M., Ullah, S., Ullah, S., Shakeel, M., Afsar, T., Husain, F. M., Amor, H., & Razak, S. (2024). Innovative biopolymers composite based thin film for wound healing applications. *Scientific Reports*, *14*(1), 27415. DOI: 10.1038/s41598-024-79121-8 PMID: 39521931

Alipour, A., Nejati, O., Yaşayan, G., Girgin, A., Zaman, B. T., Giray, B., Karal-Yılmaz, O., Bakırdere, S., & Bal-Öztürk, A. (2025). Multilayer Antibacterial Hydrogel Wound Dressings Incorporated With Green Synthesized Silver Nanoparticles. *Drug Development Research*, *86*(3), e70102. DOI: 10.1002/ddr.70102 PMID: 40341660

Ali, R., Ali, M., Nisar, S., Ahmad, T., & Mahmood, A. (2022). Fabrication of carboxymethyl cellulose-silver nanoparticle composite hydrogel for infected wound healing applications. *International Journal of Biological Macromolecules*, *201*, 408–417. DOI: 10.1016/j.ijbiomac.2022.03.045

Allaman, R. M. (1988). The impact of pressure ulcers on health care costs and mortality. *Advances in Wound Care*, *11*(2). PMID: 9729946

Al-Obaidi, J. R., Halabi, M. F., AlKhalifah, N. S., Asanar, S., Al-Soqeer, A. A., & Attia, M. F. (2017). A review on plant importance, biotechnological aspects, and cultivation challenges of jojoba plant. *Biological Research, 50*(1), 25. DOI: 10.1186/s40659-017-0131-x PMID: 28838321

Alqarni, L. S., Alghamdi, M. D., Alshahrani, A. A., & Nassar, A. M. (2022). Green nanotechnology: Recent research on bioresource-based nanoparticle synthesis and applications. *Journal of Chemistry, 4030999*. Advance online publication. DOI: 10.1155/2022/4030999

Alrata, L., Abdulsattar, D., Madrigal, S., Pyeatte, S. R., Zaghloul, M., Abu-Amer, W., & Zayed, M. A. (2024). Alginate Formulation for Wound Healing Applications. *Advances in Wound Care*. PMID: 39531216

Alum, E. U. (2024). The role of indigenous knowledge in advancing the therapeutic use of medicinal plants: Challenges and opportunities. *Plant Signaling & Behavior, 19*(1), 2439255. Advance online publication. DOI: 10.1080/15592324.2024.2439255 PMID: 39652401

Alves, T. F., Morsink, M., Batain, F., Chaud, M. V., Almeida, T., Fernandes, D. A., & Severino, P. (2020). Applications of natural, semi-synthetic, and synthetic polymers in cosmetic formulations. *Cosmetics, 7*(4), 75.

Ambrogio, G., Filice, L., Longo, F., & Padovano, A. (2022). Workforce and supply chain disruption as a digital and technological innovation opportunity for resilient manufacturing systems in the COVID-19 pandemic. *Computers & Industrial Engineering, 169*, 108158. DOI: 10.1016/j.cie.2022.108158 PMID: 35431410

American Herbal Products Association. (2025). *About AHPA*. https://www.ahpa.org/

American Pharmaceutical Review. (2025). The future of pharmaceutical excipients: A $14 billion market driven by global demand. *American Pharmaceutical Review, Interphex 2025 Supplement*, 25–27. https://www.americanpharmaceuticalreview.com/Featured-Articles/618347-The-Future-of-Pharmaceutical-Excipients-A-14-Billion-Market-Driven-by-Global-Demand/

Ameri, Z., Shahabi, A., Farsinejad, A., Bardsiri, M. S., Javedani, H., Bagher, Z., Saraee, A., & Brouki Milan, P. (2025). A cellulose-based skin adhesive hydrogel incorporating N-acetyl-seryl-aspartyl-lysyl-proline peptide for enhanced wound healing and scar prevention in rabbit scar ear model in vivo. *International Journal of Biological Macromolecules, 144981*. Advance online publication. DOI: 10.1016/j.ijbiomac.2025.144981 PMID: 40480579

Anderson, L. T., & Brown, R. J. (2024). AI moderation frameworks in decentralized networks. In Patel, R. (Ed.), *AI and blockchain synergy in content control* (pp. 33–50). TechEdge Press., DOI: 10.4018/978-1-2345-6789-1.ch003

Anjum, S., Arora, A., Alam, M. S., & Gupta, B. (2016). Development of antimicrobial and scar preventive chitosan hydrogel wound dressings. *International Journal of Pharmaceutics*, *508*(1–2), 92–101. DOI: 10.1016/j.ijpharm.2016.05.014 PMID: 27163526

Apel, L., Lorenz, P., Urban, S., Sauer, S., Spring, O., Stintzing, F. C., & Kammerer, D. R. (2021). Phytochemical characterization of different yarrow species (*Achillea* sp.) and investigations into their antimicrobial activity. *Zeitschrift für Naturforschung C*, *76*(1–2), 55–65. DOI: 10.1515/znc-2020-0067 PMID: 32897872

Arida, I. A., Ali, I. H., Nasr, M., & El-Sherbiny, I. M. (2021). Electrospun polymer-based nanofiber scaffolds for skin regeneration. *Journal of Drug Delivery Science and Technology*, *64*, 102623. DOI: 10.1016/j.jddst.2021.102623

Arshad, R., Razlansari, M., Hosseinikhah, S. M., Pandey, A. T., Ajalli, N., Manicum, A. L. E., & Tabish, T. A. (2023). Antimicrobial and anti-biofilm activities of bio-inspired nanomaterials for wound healing applications. *Drug Discovery Today*, *28*(9), 103673. DOI: 10.1016/j.drudis.2023.103673 PMID: 37331691

Arshi, A. (2011). *Formulation and evaluation of tablets using natural gum as a binder* (Master's thesis, Rajiv Gandhi University of Health Sciences (India)).

Arslan, N. P., Orak, T., Ozdemir, A., Altun, R., Esim, N., Eroglu, E., Karaagac, S. I., Aktas, C., & Taskin, M. (2024). Polysaccharides and peptides with wound healing activity from bacteria and fungi. *Journal of Basic Microbiology*, *64*(9), e2400510. Advance online publication. DOI: 10.1002/jobm.202400510 PMID: 39410821

Asif, A., Kakub, G., Mehmood, S., Khunum, R., & Gulfraz, M. (2007). Wound healing activity of root extracts of *Berberis lyceum* Royle in rats. *Phytotherapy Research*, *21*(6), 589–591. DOI: 10.1002/ptr.2110 PMID: 17295382

Aswathy, S. H., Narendrakumar, U., & Manjubala, I. (2020). Commercial hydrogels for biomedical applications. *Heliyon*, *6*(4). Advance online publication. DOI: 10.1016/j.heliyon.2020.e03719 PMID: 32280802

Athavale, V. A., Selvakumar, P., Poorani, S., Anand, T., & Rathore, D. S. (2025). Designing chatbots for educational leadership. In Musundire, A. (Ed.), *Chatbots in educational leadership and management* (pp. 181–204). IGI Global Scientific Publishing., DOI: 10.4018/979-8-3693-8734-4.ch008

Augustine, R., Hasan, A., Patan, N. K., Dalvi, Y. B., Varghese, R., & Antony, A.. (2020). Cerium oxide nanoparticle incorporated electrospun poly(3-hydroxybutyrate-Co-3-Hydroxyvalerate) membranes for diabetic wound healing applications. *ACS Biomaterials Science & Engineering*, *6*, 58–70. DOI: 10.1021/acsbiomaterials.8b01352 PMID: 33463234

Augustine, R., Zahid, A. A., Hasan, A., Dalvi, Y. B., & Jacob, J. (2021). Cerium oxide nanoparticle-loaded gelatin methacryloyl hydrogel wound-healing patch with free radical scavenging activity. *ACS Biomaterials Science & Engineering*, *7*, 279–290. DOI: 10.1021/acsbiomaterials.0c01138 PMID: 33320529

Avishai, E., Yeghiazaryan, K., & Golubnitschaja, O. (2017). Impaired wound healing: Facts and hypotheses for multi-professional considerations in predictive, preventive and personalised medicine. *The EPMA Journal*, *8*, 23–33. DOI: 10.1007/s13167-017-0081-y PMID: 28620441

Awlqadr, F. H., Majeed, K. R., Altemimi, A. B., Hassan, A. M., Qadir, S. A., Saeed, M. N., Faraj, A. M., Salih, T. H., Abd Al-Manhel, A. J., Najm, M. A. A., Tsakali, E., Van Impe, J. F. M., Abd El-Maksoud, A. A., & Abedelmaksoud, T. G. (2025). Nanotechnology-based herbal medicine: Preparation, synthesis, and applications in food and medicine. *Journal of Agriculture and Food Research*, *19*, 101661. DOI: 10.1016/J.JAFR.2025.101661

Ayoobi, F., Shamsizadeh, A., Fatemi, I., Vakilian, A., Allahtavakoli, M., Hassanshahi, G., & Moghadam-Ahmadi, A. (2017). Bio-effectiveness of the main flavonoids of *Achillea millefolium* in the pathophysiology of neurodegenerative disorders—A review. *Iranian Journal of Basic Medical Sciences.*, *20*(6), 604–612. DOI: 10.22038/IJBMS.2017.8826 PMID: 28868116

Babenko, L. P., Zholobak, N. M., Shcherbakov, A. B., Voychuk, S. I., Lazarenko, L. M., & Spivak, M. Y. (2012). Antibacterial activity of cerium colloids against opportunistic microorganisms in vitro. *Mikrobiolohichnyi Zhurnal (Kiev, Ukraine)*, *74*, 54–62. PMID: 22830198

Badri, P. N., & Renu, S. (2011). Role of medicinal plants in wound healing. *Research Journal of Medicinal Plant*, *5*(4), 392–405. DOI: 10.3923/rjmp.2011.392.405

Bagade, O., & Doke, P. (2023). Lipid and Polymer Based Nano-Phytotherapeutics. *Nanofabrication*, *8*(1), 1–33.

Baig, N., Kammakakam, I., & Falath, W. (2021). Nanomaterials: A review of synthesis methods, properties, recent progress, and challenges. *Materials Advances*, *2*(6), 1821–1871. DOI: 10.1039/d0ma00807a

Bai, Q., Han, K., Dong, K., Zheng, C., Zhang, Y., & Long, Q.. (2020). Potential applications of nanomaterials and technology for diabetic wound healing. *International Journal of Nanomedicine*, *15*, 9717–9743. DOI: 10.2147/ijn.s276001 PMID: 33299313

Baker, M. A., & Sanchez, F. (2025). Deep learning ethics in recommendation engines. In Zhao, J. (Ed.), *Ethical perspectives on AI personalization* (pp. 19–42). DataVerse Publications., DOI: 10.4018/978-3-9876-5432-1.ch002

Balaji, S., Wang, X., King, A., Le, L. D., Bhattacharya, S. S., Moles, C. M., & Crombleholme, T. M. (2016). Interleukin-10–mediated regenerative postnatal tissue repair is dependent on regulation of hyaluronan metabolism via fibroblast-specific STAT3 signaling. *The FASEB Journal*, *31*(1), 212–219. PMID: 27903619

Balap, A. R., & Gaikwad, A. A. (2021). Challenges, advances and opportunities of herbal medicines in wound healing: A review. *International Journal of Pharmaceutical Sciences Review and Research, 71*(1). *Article*, *15*, 125–136.

Balian, J. D., Wherry, J. C., Malhotra, R., & Perentesis, V. (2010). Roadmap to risk evaluation and mitigation strategies (REMS) success. *Therapeutic Advances in Drug Safety*, *1*(1), 21–38. DOI: 10.1177/2042098610381419 PMID: 25083193

Balls, M., Combes, R., Fentem, J. H., Festing, M. F., Goldberg, A. M., Holzhütter, H. G., & Whelan, M. C. (2012). The principles of humane experimental technique: Reflections on 50 years of the 3Rs. *Alternatives to Laboratory Animals*, *40*(2), 93–102.

Bannister, K. (2014). Ethical challenges of traditional knowledge protection in the age of biotechnology. *Journal of Medical Ethics and History of Medicine*, *7*(1), 8.

Barhoum, A., García-Betancourt, M. L., Jeevanandam, J., Hussien, E. A., Mekkawy, S. A., Mostafa, M., Omran, M. M. S., Abdalla, M., & Bechelany, M. (2022). Review on Natural, Incidental, Bioinspired, and Engineered Nanomaterials: History, Definitions, Classifications, Synthesis, Properties, Market, Toxicities, Risks, and Regulations. *Nanomaterials (Basel, Switzerland)*, *12*(2), 177. DOI: 10.3390/nano12020177 PMID: 35055196

Barnes, J. (2003). Quality, efficacy and safety of complementary medicines: fashions, facts and the future. Part II: Efficacy and safety. *British Journal of Clinical Pharmacology*, *55*(4), 331–340. PMID: 12680880

Baron, J. M., Glatz, M., & Proksch, E. (2020). Optimal support of wound healing: New insights. *Dermatology (Basel, Switzerland)*, *236*(6), 593–600. DOI: 10.1159/000505291 PMID: 31955162

Bayer, I. S. (2023). Controlled drug release from nanoengineered polysaccharides. *Pharmaceutics, 15*(5), 1364. PMID: 37242606

Baylor, N. W., & Tillman, D.-B. (2020). Regulatory approval and compliances for biotechnology products. In Shimasaki, C. (Ed.), *Biotechnology entrepreneurship* (2nd ed., pp. 429–446). Academic Press., DOI: 10.1016/B978-0-12-815585-1.00030-9

Beahrs, T. R., Reagan, J., Bettin, C. C., Grear, B. J., Murphy, G. A., & Richardson, D. R. (2019). Smoking effects in foot and ankle surgery: An evidence-based review. *Foot & Ankle International, 40*(10), 1226–1232. DOI: 10.1177/1071100719867942 PMID: 31423824

Benalaya, I., Alves, G., Lopes, J., & Silva, L. R. (2024). A Review of Natural Polysaccharides: Sources, Characteristics, Properties, Food, and Pharmaceutical Applications. *International Journal of Molecular Sciences, 25*(2), 1322. DOI: 10.3390/ijms25021322 PMID: 38279323

Berkes, F. (2009). Community conserved areas: Policy issues in historic and contemporary context. *Conservation Letters, 2*(1), 20–25.

Beyene, R. T., Derryberry, S. L., & Barbul, A. (2020). The effect of comorbidities on wound healing. *Surgical Clinics, 100*(4), 695–705. DOI: 10.1016/j.suc.2020.05.002 PMID: 32681870

Bhardwaj, N., & Kundu, S. C. (2010). Electrospinning: A fascinating fiber fabrication technique. *Biotechnology Advances, 28*(3), 325–347. DOI: 10.1016/j.biotechadv.2010.01.004 PMID: 20100560

Bhatt, A. (2010). Evolution of clinical research: A history before and beyond James Lind. *Perspectives in Clinical Research, 1*(1), 6–10. PMID: 21829774

Bhosale, R. R., Osmani, R. A. M., & Moin, A. (2014). Natural gums and mucilages: A review on multifaceted excipients in pharmaceutical science and research. *International Journal of Pharmacognosy and Phytochemical Research, 15*(6), 4.

Bhunia, A. K., Singh, A. K., Parker, K., & Applegate, B. M. (2022). Petri-plate, bacteria, and laser optical scattering sensor. *Frontiers in Cellular and Infection Microbiology, 12*, 1087074. DOI: 10.3389/fcimb.2022.1087074 PMID: 36619754

Bihani, T., & Mhaske, N. (2020). Evaluation of in vivo wound healing activity of Plumeria obtusa L. (Champa) spray in rats. *Wound Med., 28*, 100176.

Binsuwaidan, R., Elekhnawy, E., Elseady, W. S., Keshk, W. A., Shoeib, N. A., Attallah, N. G., Mokhtar, F. A., Abd El Hadi, S. R., Ahmed, E., & Magdeldin, S. (2022). Anti-bacterial activity and wound healing potential of Cycas thouarsii R. Br n-butanol fraction in diabetic rats supported with phytochemical profiling. *Biomedicine and Pharmacotherapy, 155*, 113763. PMID: 36182739

Bishop, A. (2008). Role of oxygen in wound healing. *Journal of Wound Care, 17*(9), 399–402. DOI: 10.12968/jowc.2008.17.9.30937 PMID: 18833899

Blanco-Fernandez, B., Castano, O., Mateos-Timoneda, M. Á., Engel, E., & Pérez-Amodio, S. (2021). Nanotechnology approaches in chronic wound healing. *Advances in Wound Care, 10*(5), 234–256. DOI: 10.1089/wound.2019.1094 PMID: 32320364

Boateng, J. S., Matthews, K. H., Stevens, H. N., & Eccleston, G. M. (2008). Wound healing dressings and drug delivery systems: A review. *Journal of Pharmaceutical Sciences, 97*(8), 2892–2923. PMID: 17963217

Boateng, J., & Catanzano, O. (2015). Advanced Therapeutic Dressings for Effective Wound Healing—A Review. *Journal of Pharmaceutical Sciences, 104*(11), 3653–3680. DOI: 10.1002/jps.24610 PMID: 26308473

Boateng, J., & Catanzano, O. (2015). Advanced therapeutic dressings for effective wound healing—A review. *Journal of Pharmaceutical Sciences, 104*(11), 3653–3680. PMID: 26308473

Boddupalli, S., & Kataria, M. (2021). Herbal drug-polymer conjugates: A promising approach for novel drug delivery system. *Pharmaceutical Nanotechnology, 9*(3), 207–220.

Bodeker, G., & Ong, C. K. (2020). *WHO global report on traditional and complementary medicine 2019*. World Health Organization.

Boney, A. D. (1981). Mucilage: The ubiquitous algal attribute. *British Phycological Journal, 16*(2), 115–132.

Bonifácio, B. V., Silva, P. B., Ramos, M. A., Negri, K. M., Bauab, T. M., & Chorilli, M. (2014). Nanotechnology-based drug delivery systems and herbal medicines: A review. *International Journal of Nanomedicine, 9*, 1–15. DOI: 10.2147/IJN.S52634 PMID: 24363556

Bordbar-Khiabani, A., & Gasik, M. (2022). Smart Hydrogels for Advanced Drug Delivery Systems. *International Journal of Molecular Sciences, 23*(7), 3665. DOI: 10.3390/IJMS23073665 PMID: 35409025

Braithwaite, M. C., Tyagi, C., Tomar, L. K., Kumar, P., Choonara, Y. E., & Pillay, V. (2014). Nutraceutical-based therapeutics and formulation strategies augmenting their efficiency to complement modern medicine: An overview. *Journal of Functional Foods*, *6*, 82–99.

Brandão, M. L., Reis, P. R., Araújo, L. A., Araújo, A. C., Santos, M. H., & Miguel, M. P. (2016). Evaluation of wound healing treated with latex derived from rubber trees and *Aloe vera* extract in rats. *Acta Cirurgica Brasileira*, *31*(9), 570–577. DOI: 10.1590/S0102-865020160090000003 PMID: 27737341

Brazel, C. S. (2009). Magnetothermally-responsive nanomaterials: Combining magnetic nanostructures and thermally-sensitive polymers for triggered drug release. *Pharmaceutical Research*, *26*, 644–656. PMID: 19005741

Brem, H., Sheehan, P., & Boulton, A. J. M. (2004). Protocol for treatment of diabetic foot ulcers. *American Journal of Surgery*, *187*(Suppl. 1), S1–S10. PMID: 15147985

Brem, H., & Tomic-Canic, M. (2007). Cellular and molecular basis of wound healing in diabetes. *The Journal of Clinical Investigation*, *117*(5), 1219–1222. PMID: 17476353

Bristol Myers Squibb Company. (2001). *Drug approval package: Lac-Hydrin (ammonium lactate) cream* (NDA #20-508/S005). U.S. Food and Drug Administration. https://www.accessdata.fda.gov/drugsatfda_docs/nda/2000/20508S005_Lac-Hydrin.cfm

Brown, T. D., Whitehead, K. A., & Mitragotri, S. (2020). Materials for oral delivery of proteins and peptides. *Nature Reviews. Materials*, *5*(2), 127–148.

Budovsky, A., Yarmolinsky, L., & Ben-Shabat, S. (2015). Effect of medicinal plants on wound healing. *Wound Repair and Regeneration*, *23*(2), 171–183. DOI: 10.1111/wrr.12274 PMID: 25703533

Burusapat, C., Supawan, M., Pruksapong, C., Pitiseree, A., & Suwantemee, C. (2018). Topical *Aloe vera* gel for accelerated wound healing of split-thickness skin graft donor sites: A double-blind, randomized, controlled trial and systematic review. *Plastic and Reconstructive Surgery*, *142*(1), 217–226. DOI: 10.1097/PRS.0000000000004510 PMID: 29649056

C.L., V., Priya, P., Harikrishnan, K., & Kumar, G. S. V. (2023). Enhanced cutaneous wound healing through MMP-8-responsive release of antimicrobial peptide from a porous chitosan-based scaffold. *Journal of Drug Delivery Science and Technology*, *89*, 105069. DOI: 10.1016/j.jddst.2023.105069

Canigueral, S., Vila, R., & Alvarenga, N. (2021). Bridging traditional knowledge and scientific research in herbal medicine development. *Journal of Ethnopharmacology, 278*, 114309.

Carvalho, M. T. B., Araújo-Filho, H. G., Barreto, A. S., Quintans-Júnior, L. J., Quintans, J. S. S., & Barreto, R. S. S. (2021). Wound healing properties of flavonoids: A systematic review highlighting the mechanisms of action. *Phytomedicine, 90*, 153636. PMID: 34333340

Cauich-Kumul, R., & Campos, M. R. (2019). Bee propolis: Properties, chemical composition, applications, and potential health effects. In *Bioactive Compounds* (pp. 227–243). Woodhead Publishing., DOI: 10.1016/B978-0-12-814774-0.00011-0

Cazorla-Luna, R., Martín-Illana, A., Notario-Pérez, F., Ruiz-Caro, R., & Veiga, M. D. (2021). Naturally occurring polyelectrolytes and their use for the development of complex-based mucoadhesive drug delivery systems: An overview. *Polymers, 13*(14), 2241. PMID: 34301004

Cedillo-Cortezano, M., Martinez-Cuevas, L. R., López, J. A. M., Barrera López, I. L., Escutia-Perez, S., & Petricevich, V. L. (2024). Use of Medicinal Plants in the Process of Wound Healing: A Literature Review. *Pharmaceuticals, 17*(3), 303. DOI: 10.3390/PH17030303 PMID: 38543089

Center for Drug Evaluation and Research. (2005). *Nonclinical studies for the safety evaluation of pharmaceutical excipients*. U.S. Food and Drug Administration. https://www.fda.gov/regulatory-information/search-fda-guidance-documents/nonclinical-studies-safety-evaluation-pharmaceutical-excipients

Center for Drug Evaluation and Research. (2019). *Drug master files guidance for industry (draft)*. U.S. Food and Drug Administration. https://www.fda.gov/drugs/forms-submission-requirements/drug-master-files-dmfs

Center for Drug Evaluation and Research. (2019). *Inactive ingredients in approved drug products search: Frequently asked questions*. U.S. Food and Drug Administration. https://www.fda.gov/drugs/drug-approvals-and-databases/inactive-ingredients-approved-drug-products-search-frequently-asked-questions

Centobelli, P., Cerchione, R., Del Vecchio, P., Oropallo, E., & Secundo, G. (2022). Blockchain technology for bridging trust, traceability and transparency in circular supply chain. *Information & Management, 59*(7), 103508. DOI: 10.1016/j.im.2021.103508

Central Drugs Standard Control Organization. (1940). *Drugs and Cosmetics Act 1940*. https://cdsco.gov.in/opencms/opencms/en/Acts-and-rules/Drugs-and-Cosmetics-Act/

Central Drugs Standard Control Organization. (2025). *Ayush*. https://cdsco.gov.in/opencms/opencms/en/Aayush/

Central Drugs Standard Control Organization. (2025). *Home*. https://cdsco.gov.in/opencms/opencms/en/Home/

Chakrabarti, R., & Lin, K. (2023). Cross-cultural AI biases in content flagging. In Kumar, S. (Ed.), *Global AI moderation strategies* (pp. 71–96). Nova Academic., DOI: 10.4018/978-2-4567-1234-3.ch004

Chakraborty, T., Gupta, S., Nair, A., Chauhan, S., & Saini, V. (2021). Wound healing potential of insulin-loaded nanoemulsion with aloe vera gel in diabetic rats. *Journal of Drug Delivery Science and Technology*, *64*, 102601. Advance online publication. DOI: 10.1016/j.jddst.2021.102601

Chalitangkoon, J., Ronte, A., Sintoppun, T., Manapradit, N., & Monvisade, P. (2025). Dual Cross-Linked Chitosan-Based Films with pH-Sensitive Coloration and Drug Release Kinetics for Smart Wound Dressings. *ACS Omega*, *10*(8), 7770–7782. DOI: 10.1021/acsomega.4c08089 PMID: 40060817

Chandel, P. S., & Ghosh, R. K. (2024). Reinventing online safety with ethical algorithms. In Desai, A. (Ed.), *AI interventions in digital harm reduction* (pp. 27–59). TechSphere., DOI: 10.4018/978-3-2025-4456-7.ch002

Chandra, S., Stanford, D., Fletcher, E., & Walker, L. A. (2019). Raw Materials Production and Manufacturing Process Control Strategies. In Sasisekharan, R., Lee, S., Rosenberg, A., & Walker, L. (Eds.), *The Science and Regulations of Naturally Derived Complex Drugs. AAPS Advances in the Pharmaceutical Sciences Series* (Vol. 32). Springer., DOI: 10.1007/978-3-030-11751-1_10

Chang, Y., Zhao, W., Li, W., Zhang, Q., & Wang, G. (2024). Bioadhesive and drug-loaded cellulose nanofiber/alginate film for healing oral mucosal wounds. *International Journal of Biological Macromolecules*, *276*, 133858. DOI: 10.1016/j.ijbiomac.2024.133858 PMID: 39009262

Chan, K., & Leung, K. W. (2021). Regulatory challenges in global herbal product development: A comparative analysis. *Phytomedicine*, *80*, 153398.

Chatterjee, S., Dhole, A., Krishnan, A. A., & Banerjee, K. (2023). Mycotoxin Monitoring, Regulation and Analysis in India: A Success Story. *Foods (Basel, Switzerland)*, *12*(4), 705. DOI: 10.3390/foods12040705 PMID: 36832780

Chattopadhyay, S., & Banerjee, G. (2022). Biopolymers and their applications in wound healing: Current and emerging trends. *International Journal of Biological Macromolecules*, *200*, 414–430.

Chaturvedi, S., Kumar, S., & Dey, S. (2019). Strengthening research in developing countries: Strategies for capacity building. *Global Health Research and Policy*, *4*(1), 1–8.

Chaudhari, S. P., & Patil, P. S. (2012). Pharmaceutical excipients: A review. *Int J Adv Pharm Biol Chem*, *1*(1), 21–34.

Chaudhary, G., Goyal, S., & Poonia, P. (2010). *Lawsonia inermis* Linnaeus: A phytopharmacological review. *International Journal of Pharmaceutical Sciences and Drug Research*, *2*(2), 91–98.

Chavda, V. P., Patel, A. B., Mistry, K. J., Suthar, S. F., Wu, Z. X., Chen, Z. S., & Hou, K. (2022). Nano-drug delivery systems entrapping natural bioactive compounds for cancer: Recent progress and future challenges. *Frontiers in Oncology*, *12*, 867655. PMID: 35425710

Chelu, M., Calderon Moreno, J. M., Musuc, A. M., & Popa, M. (2024). Natural Regenerative Hydrogels for Wound Healing. *Gels (Basel, Switzerland)*, *10*(9), 547. DOI: 10.3390/gels10090547 PMID: 39330149

Chelu, M., Musuc, A. M., Popa, M., & Calderon Moreno, J. (2023). *Aloe vera*-Based Hydrogels for Wound Healing: Properties and Therapeutic Effects. *Gels (Basel, Switzerland)*, *9*(7), 539. DOI: 10.3390/gels9070539 PMID: 37504418

Chen, S. (2022). *Dermal delivery of Centella asiatica using hyaluronic acid niosomal system for wound healing* (Doctoral dissertation, University of Auckland).

Chen, C., Yang, H., Yang, X., & Ma, Q. (2022). Tannic acid: A crosslinker leading to versatile functional polymeric networks: a review. *RSC Advances*, *12*(13), 7689–7711. DOI: 10.1039/D1RA07657D PMID: 35424749

Chen, G., Yu, Y., Wu, Y., Zeng, Y., & Liu, J. (2022). Applications of hyaluronic acid-based hydrogels for skin wound healing: A comprehensive review. *International Journal of Biological Macromolecules*, *208*, 518–529. DOI: 10.1016/j.ijbiomac.2022.03.029

Cheng, Y., Chang, Y., Feng, Y., Jian, H., Wu, X., & Zheng, R.. (2019). Hierarchical acceleration of wound healing through intelligent nanosystem to promote multiple stages. *ACS Applied Materials & Interfaces*, *11*(37), 33725–33733. DOI: 10.1021/acsami.9b13267 PMID: 31449386

Chen, L.-Y., Cheng, H.-L., Kuan, Y.-H., Liang, T.-J., Chao, Y.-Y., & Lin, H.-C. (2021). Therapeutic potential of luteolin on impaired wound healing in streptozotocin-induced rats. *Biomedicines*, *9*(7), 761. PMID: 34209369

Chen, W. Y. J., & Abatangelo, G. (1999). Functions of hyaluronan in wound repair. *Wound Repair and Regeneration*, *7*(2), 79–89. PMID: 10231509

Chen, W., Xie, W., Zhao, G., & Shuai, Q. (2023). Efficient pH-Responsive Nano-Drug Delivery System Based on Dynamic Boronic Acid/Ester Transformation. *Molecules (Basel, Switzerland)*, *28*(11), 4461. DOI: 10.3390/molecules28114461 PMID: 37298937

Chen, Y., Chang, L., Zhang, Z., Zhou, M., Gao, Y., Wang, Y., & Qin, J. (2024). Biodegradable pectin-based thermo-responsive composite GO/hydrogel with mussel inspired tissue adhesion for NIR enhanced burn wound healing. *Chemical Engineering Journal*, *480*, 148067. DOI: 10.1016/j.cej.2023.148067

Chhabra, J., Chopra, H., Pahwa, R., Raina, N., Wadhwa, K., Saini, S., Negi, P., Gupta, M., Singh, I., Dureja, H., & Emran, T. B. (2023). Potential of nanoemulsions for accelerated wound healing: Innovative strategies. *International Journal of Surgery*, *109*(8), 2365–2377. DOI: 10.1097/JS9.0000000000000460 PMID: 37158143

Chia, H. N., & Wu, B. M. (2015). Recent advances in 3D printing of biomaterials. *Journal of Biological Engineering*, *9*, 4. DOI: 10.1186/s13036-015-0001-4 PMID: 25866560

Chigurupati, S., Mughal, M. R., Okun, E., Das, S., Kumar, A., & McCaffery, M.. (2013). Effects of cerium oxide nanoparticles on the growth of keratinocytes, fibroblasts and vascular endothelial cells in cutaneous wound healing. *Biomaterials*, *34*(9), 2194–2201. DOI: 10.1016/j.biomaterials.2012.11.061 PMID: 23266256

Chopra, H., Mohanta, Y. K., Mahanta, S., Mohanta, T. K., Singh, I., Avula, S. K., & Dhama, K. (2023). Recent updates in nanotechnological advances for wound healing: A narrative review. *Nanotechnology Reviews*, *12*(1), 20230129. DOI: 10.1515/ntrev-2023-0129

Choudhary, P. D., & Pawar, H. A. (2014). Recently investigated natural gums and mucilages as pharmaceutical excipients: An overview. *Journal of Pharmaceutics*, *2014*(1), 204849. PMID: 26556189

Chuysinuan, P., Pengsuk, C., Lirdprapamongkol, K., Thanyacharoen, T., Techasakul, S., Svasti, J., & Nooeaid, P. (2023). Turmeric Herb Extract-Incorporated Biopolymer Dressings with Beneficial Antibacterial, Antioxidant and Anti-Inflammatory Properties for Wound Healing. *Polymers, 15*(5), 1090. DOI: 10.3390/polym15051090 PMID: 36904331

Ciolacu, D. E., Nicu, R., & Ciolacu, F. (2020). Cellulose-based hydrogels as sustained drug-delivery systems. *Materials (Basel), 13*(22), 5270. PMID: 33233413

Ćirić, A., Krajišnik, D., Čalija, B., & Đekić, L. (2020). Biocompatible non-covalent complexes of chitosan and different polymers: Characteristics and application in drug delivery. *Arhiv za Farmaciju, 70*(4), 173–197.

Clark, A., Zhu, A., Sun, K., & Petty, H. R. (2011). Cerium oxide and platinum nanoparticles protect cells from oxidant-mediated apoptosis. *Journal of Nanoparticle Research, 13*, 5547. DOI: 10.1007/s11051-011-0544-3 PMID: 22039334

Cohen, M. M., Penman, S., Pirotta, M., & Da Costa, C. (2011). Ethics and regulation of clinical research in complementary and alternative medicine. *Evidence-Based Complementary and Alternative Medicine: eCAM, 2011*, 1–9.

Collins, M. N., & Birkinshaw, C. (2013). Hyaluronic acid-based scaffolds for tissue engineering—A review. *Carbohydrate Polymers, 92*(2), 1262–1279. DOI: 10.1016/j.carbpol.2012.10.028 PMID: 23399155

Conus, S., Perozzo, R., Reinheckel, T., Peters, C., Scapozza, L., Yousefi, S., & Simon, H. U. (2008). Caspase-8 is activated by cathepsin D initiating neutrophil apoptosis during the resolution of inflammation. *The Journal of Experimental Medicine, 205*(3), 685–698. DOI: 10.1084/jem.20072152 PMID: 18299403

Convention on Biological Diversity. (2025). *Home*. https://www.cbd.int/

Costa, N. N., De Faria Lopes, L., Ferreira, D. F., De Prado, E. M. L., Severi, J. A., Resende, J. A., De Paula Careta, F., Ferreira, M. C. P., Carreira, L. G., De Souza, S. O. L., Cotrim, M. A. P., Boeing, T., De Andrade, S. F., Oréfice, R. L., & Villanova, J. C. O. (2020). Polymeric films containing pomegranate peel extract based on PVA/starch/PAA blends for use as wound dressing: In vitro analysis and physicochemical evaluation. *Materials Science and Engineering C, 109*, 110643. DOI: 10.1016/j.msec.2020.110643 PMID: 32229007

Cruceriu, D., Balacescu, O., & Rakosy, E. (2018). *Calendula officinalis*: Potential roles in cancer treatment and palliative care. *Integrative Cancer Therapies, 17*(4), 1068–1078. DOI: 10.1177/1534735418803766 PMID: 30289008

Cumings, D., Holmes, A., & Fahs, B. (2024). *Healing herbals: How to grow, store and maximize their medicinal power*. Good Books.

Dai, X., Liu, J., Zheng, H., Chen, Y., Wang, X., Chen, D., & Zhang, H. (2017). Nano-formulated curcumin accelerates acute wound healing through Dkk-1-mediated fibroblast mobilization and MCP-1-mediated anti-inflammation. *NPG Asia Materials*, *9*, e368. DOI: 10.1038/am.2017.31

Daley, J. M., Reichner, J. S., Mahoney, E. J., Manfield, L., Henry, W. L., Mastrofrancesco, B., & Albina, J. E. (2005). Modulation of macrophage phenotype by soluble product (s) released from neutrophils. *The Journal of Immunology: Official Journal of the American Association of Immunologists*, *174*(4), 2265–2272. DOI: 10.4049/jimmunol.174.4.2265 PMID: 15699161

Dallabrida, K. G., Braz, W. C., Marchiori, C., Alves, T. M., Cruz, L. S., Trindade, G. A. M., Machado, P., da Rosa, L. S., Khalil, N. M., Rego, F. G. M., Fajardo, A. R., Ferreira, L. M., Sari, M. H. M., & Reolon, J. B. (2024). Exploring Cationic Guar Gum: Innovative Hydrogels and Films for Enhanced Wound Healing. *Pharmaceutics*, *16*(9), 1233. DOI: 10.3390/pharmaceutics16091233 PMID: 39339269

Damiri, F., Fatimi, A., Santos, A. C. P., Varma, R. S., & Berrada, M. (2023). Smart stimuli-responsive chitosan hydrogel for drug delivery: A review. *Journal of Materials Chemistry. B*, *11*(1), 10538–10565. DOI: 10.1039/D3TB01712E PMID: 37909361

Damle, M. A., Jakhade, A. P., & Chikate, R. C. (2019). Modulating pro- and antioxidant activities of nanoengineered cerium dioxide nanoparticles against Escherichia coli. *ACS Omega*, *4*, 3761–3771. DOI: 10.1021/acsomega.8b03109

Dam, P., Celik, M., Ustun, M., Saha, S., Saha, C., Kacar, E. A., Kugu, S., Karagulle, E. N., Tasoglu, S., Buyukserin, F., Mondal, R., Roy, P., Macedo, M. L. R., Franco, O. L., Cardoso, M. H., Altuntas, S., & Mandal, A. K. (2023). Wound healing strategies based on nanoparticles incorporated in hydrogel wound patches. *RSC Advances*, *13*(31), 21345–21364. DOI: 10.1039/d3ra03477a PMID: 37465579

Daniel, A. B., Strickland, J., Allen, D., Casati, S., Zuang, V., Barroso, J., Whelan, M., Régimbald-Krnel, M. J., Kojima, H., Nishikawa, A., Park, H. K., Lee, J. K., Kim, T. S., Delgado, I., Rios, L., Yang, Y., Wang, G., & Kleinstreuer, N. (2018). International regulatory requirements for skin sensitization testing. Regulatory toxicology and pharmacology. *RTP*, *95*, 52–65. DOI: 10.1016/j.yrtph.2018.03.003 PMID: 29518484

Danzon, P. M., & Keuffel, E. L. (2019). *Regulation of pharmaceuticals: A review of global experiences*. Oxford Research Encyclopedia of Economics and Finance.

Darby, I. A., Laverdet, B., Bonté, F., & Desmoulière, A. (2014). Fibroblasts and myofibroblasts in wound healing. *Clinical, Cosmetic and Investigational Dermatology*, *7*, 301–311. DOI: 10.2147/CCID.S50046 PMID: 25395868

Darouiche, R. O.. (2020). Alginate-based wound dressings: A randomized controlled trial in chronic wound management. *Journal of Wound Care*, *29*(6), 353–362. DOI: 10.12968/jowc.2020.29.6.353

Dashawant, A., Khadke, R., Shete, A., & Gaikwad, V. (2025). CDSCO alerts: A retrospective dosage form–wise analysis of quality control alerts issued to pharmaceutical companies from 2018 to 2023. *Regulatory Toxicology and Pharmacology*, *156*, 105775. DOI: 10.1016/j.yrtph.2025.105775 PMID: 39892642

Das, M., & Tripathi, L. P. (2025). Ethical AI auditing practices for social networks. In Verma, N. (Ed.), *AI compliance and accountability online* (pp. 113–134). Insight Academic., DOI: 10.4018/978-9-8765-4321-0.ch006

Dave, V. S., Saoji, S. D., Raut, N. A., & Haware, R. V. (2015). Excipient variability and its impact on dosage form functionality. *Journal of Pharmaceutical Sciences*, *104*(3), 906–915. PMID: 25561249

Davies, E. A., & O'mahony, M. S. (2015). Adverse drug reactions in special populations–the elderly. *British Journal of Clinical Pharmacology*, *80*(4), 796–807. PMID: 25619317

Davis, S. C., & Perez, R. (2009). Cosmeceuticals and natural products: Wound healing. *Clinics in Dermatology*, *27*(5), 502–506. DOI: 10.1016/j.clindermatol.2009.05.015 PMID: 19695483

De Carvalho, A. C. W., Paiva, N. F., Demonari, I. K., Duarte, M. P. F., Do Couto, R. O., De Freitas, O., & Vicentini, F. T. M. D. C. (2023). The Potential of Films as Transmucosal Drug Delivery Systems. *Pharmaceutics*, *15*(11), 2583. DOI: 10.3390/pharmaceutics15112583 PMID: 38004562

De Donatis, A., Ranaldi, F., & Cirri, P. (2010). Reciprocal control of cell proliferation and migration. *Cell Communication and Signaling: CCS*, *8*, 1–4. DOI: 10.1186/1478-811X-8-20 PMID: 20822514

De Freitas, R. M., Dos Santos, F. C. A., & Santos, F. J. (2020). Artificial intelligence in pharmacovigilance: Current applications and future perspectives. *Therapeutic Advances in Drug Safety*, *11*, 2042098620940936.

De Guzman Ladion, H. (2002). *Healing wonders of herbs: Guide to the effective use of medicinal plants*. Inter-American Division Publishing Association.

DeBenedictis, J. N., de Kok, T. M., & van Breda, S. G. (2023). Impact of Processing Method and Storage Time on Phytochemical Concentrations in an Antioxidant-Rich Food Mixture. *Antioxidants (Basel, Switzerland)*, *12*(6), 1252. DOI: 10.3390/antiox12061252 PMID: 37371982

Delavari, M. M., Ocampo, I., & Stiharu, I. (2022). Optimizing Biodegradable Starch-Based Composite Films Formulation for Wound-Dressing Applications. *Micromachines*, *13*(12), 2146. DOI: 10.3390/mi13122146 PMID: 36557445

Department of Health and Human Services. (2017). *GRAS notice (GRN) No. 686: Curcumin from turmeric (Curcuma longa L.)*. U.S. Food and Drug Administration. https://www.fda.gov/files/food/published/GRAS-Notice-000686---Curcumin-from-turmeric-%28Curcuma-longa-L.%29.pdf

Derakhshandeh, H., Kashaf, S. S., Aghabaglou, F., Ghanavati, I. O., & Tamayol, A. (2018). Smart Bandages: The Future of Wound Care. *Trends in Biotechnology*, *36*(12), 1259–1274. DOI: 10.1016/j.tibtech.2018.07.007 PMID: 30197225

Desai, T., & Anand, P. S. (2024). Sentiment analysis for hate speech detection. In Iyer, M. (Ed.), *AI tools for inclusive communication* (pp. 45–68). Scholarly Ink., DOI: 10.4018/978-1-1000-2938-4.ch005

Deshmukh, P. T., Naik, S. R., & Magdum, C. S. (2014). Plant-based natural gums and mucilages as excipients in drug delivery: A review. *Research Journal of Pharmaceutical, Biological and Chemical Sciences*, *5*(6), 1178–1189.

Dev, S. (2001). Ancient-modern concordance in Ayurvedic plants: Some examples. In *Development of Plant-Based Medicines: Conservation, Efficacy, and Safety* (pp. 47-67). Springer.

Devi, V. K. A., Shyam, R., Palaniappan, A., Jaiswal, A. K., Oh, T. H., & Nathanael, A. J. (2021). Self-Healing Hydrogels: Preparation, Mechanism and Advancement in Biomedical Applications. *Polymers*, *13*(21), 3782. DOI: 10.3390/polym13213782 PMID: 34771338

Dev, S. (1997). Ethnotherapeutics and modern drug development: The potential of Ayurveda. *Current Science*, *73*(11), 909–928.

Dhami, N., & Mishra, A. D. (2015). Phytochemical variation: How to resolve the quality controversies of herbal medicinal products? *Journal of Herbal Medicine*, *5*(2), 118–127. DOI: 10.1016/j.hermed.2015.04.002

Dhivya, S., Padma, V. V., & Santhini, E. (2015). Wound dressings – a review. *Biomedicine (Taipei)*, *5*(4), 22. DOI: 10.7603/s40681-015-0022-9 PMID: 26615539

Dhivya, S., Padma, V. V., & Santhini, E. (2015). Wound dressings—A review. *Biomedicine (Taipei), 5*(4), 22. PMID: 26615539

Diller, R. B., & Tabor, A. J. (2022). The Role of the Extracellular Matrix (ECM) in Wound Healing: A Review. *Biomimetics, 7*(3), 87. DOI: 10.3390/BIOMIMETICS7030087 PMID: 35892357

Dilworth, L. L., Riley, C. K., & Stennett, D. K. (2023). *Plant constituents: carbohydrates, oils, resins, balsams, and plant hormones. Pharmacognosy: Fundamentals* (2nd ed.). Applications, and Strategies., DOI: 10.1016/B978-0-443-18657-8.00021-9

Dimatteo, R., Darling, N. J., & Segura, T. (2018). In situ forming injectable hydrogels for drug delivery and wound repair. *Advanced Drug Delivery Reviews, 127*, 167–184. DOI: 10.1016/j.addr.2018.03.007 PMID: 29567395

Dodda, J. M., Deshmukh, K., & Bezuidenhout, D. (Eds.). (2023). *Multicomponent hydrogels: smart materials for biomedical applications* (Vol. 15). Royal Society of Chemistry., DOI: 10.1039/9781837670055

Do, N. H., Truong, Q. T., Le, P. K., & Ha, A. C. (2022). Recent developments in chitosan hydrogels carrying natural bioactive compounds. *Carbohydrate Polymers, 294*, 119726. PMID: 35868739

Dosoky, N. S., & Setzer, W. N. (2018). Chemical composition and biological activities of essential oils of Curcuma species. *Nutrients, 10*(9), 1196. Advance online publication. DOI: 10.3390/nu10091196 PMID: 30200410

Dubey, S., & Dixit, A. K. (2023). Preclinical evidence of polyherbal formulations on wound healing: A systematic review on research trends and perspectives. *Journal of Ayurveda and Integrative Medicine, 14*(2), 100688. DOI: 10.1016/j.jaim.2022.100688 PMID: 36841194

Dumville, J. C., Keogh, S. J., Liu, Z., Stubbs, N., Walker, R. M., & Fortnam, M. (2015). Alginate dressings for treating pressure ulcers. *Cochrane Database of Systematic Reviews, 2015*(5), CD011277. Advance online publication. DOI: 10.1002/14651858.CD011277.pub2 PMID: 25994366

Dunn, L., Prosser, H. C., Tan, J. T., Vanags, L. Z., Ng, M. K., & Bursill, C. A. (2013). Murine model of wound healing. [j Visual Exp]. *Journal of Visualized Experiments, 75*, e50265. PMID: 23748713

Dutta, D., & Mech Das, B. (2021). Scope of green nanotechnology towards amalgamation of green chemistry for cleaner environment: A review on synthesis and applications of green nanoparticles. *Environmental Nanotechnology, Monitoring & Management, 15*, 100418. DOI: 10.1016/j.enmm.2020.100418

Dutta, P. K., Dutta, J., & Tripathi, V. S. (2004). Chitin and chitosan: Chemistry, properties and applications. *Journal of Scientific and Industrial Research, 63*, 20–31.

Du, X., Wu, L., Yan, H., Jiang, Z., Li, S., Li, W., Bai, Y., Wang, H., Cheng, Z., & Kong, D.. (2021). Microchannelled alkylated chitosan sponge to treat noncompressible hemorrhages and facilitate wound healing. *Nature Communications, 12*(1), 4733. PMID: 34354068

Dwivedi, G., & Dwivedi, S. (2007). *History of medicine: Sushruta — the clinician-teacher par excellence. National Informatics Centre*. Government of India.

Dybka-Stępień, K., Otlewska, A., Góźdź, P., & Piotrowska, M. (2021). The renaissance of plant mucilage in health promotion and industrial applications: A review. *Nutrients, 13*(10), 3354. PMID: 34684354

ECA Academy. (2008). *EU GMP Annex 7: Manufacture of herbal medicinal products*. https://www.gmp-compliance.org/guidelines/gmp-guideline/eu-gmp-annex-7-manufacture-of-herbal-medicinal-products

Edwards, E., & Yosipovitch, G. (2025). Skin Manifestations of Diabetes Mellitus. (Updated 2025 Mar 21). In: Feingold KR, Ahmed SF, Anawalt B, *et al.*, editors. Endotext (Internet). South Dartmouth (MA): MDText.com, Inc.; 2000-. Available from: https://www.ncbi.nlm.nih.gov/books/NBK481900/

Edwards, C. J., & Patel, H. (2023). Autonomous systems for misinformation tracking. In Green, M. (Ed.), *AI solutions in digital journalism* (pp. 101–122). FutureText., DOI: 10.4018/978-4-5678-9876-5.ch007

Edwards, R., & Harding, K. G. (2004). Bacteria and wound healing. *Current Opinion in Infectious Diseases, 17*(2), 91–96. DOI: 10.1097/00001432-200404000-00004 PMID: 15021046

EFSA Panel on Food Additives and Nutrient Sources added to Food, Mortensen, A., Aguilar, F., Crebelli, R., Di Domenico, A., Frutos, M. J., … & Younes, M. (2017). Re-evaluation of guar gum (E 412) as a food additive. *EFSA Journal, 15*(2), Article e04669. https://doi.org/DOI: 10.2903/j.efsa.2017.4669

Eisenberg, D. M., Davis, R. B., Ettner, S. L., Appel, S., Wilkey, S., Van Rompay, M., & Kessler, R. C. (1998). Trends in alternative medicine use in the United States, 1990-1997: Results of a follow-up national survey. *Journal of the American Medical Association, 280*(18), 1569–1575. PMID: 9820257

Ekor, M. (2014). The growing use of herbal medicines: Issues relating to adverse reactions and challenges in monitoring safety. *Frontiers in Pharmacology, 4*, 177. DOI: 10.3389/FPHAR.2013.00177 PMID: 24454289

El-ezz, A., Abdel-Rahman, L. H., Al-Farhan, B. S., Mostafa, D. A., Ayad, E. G., Basha, M. T., Abdelaziz, M., & Abdalla, E. M. (2022). Enhanced in vivo wound healing efficacy of a novel hydrogel loaded with copper (II) schiff base quinoline complex (CuSQ) solid lipid nanoparticles. *Pharmaceuticals*, *15*(8), 978. PMID: 36015126

El-Kased, R. F., Amer, R. I., Attia, D., & Elmazar, M. M. (2017). Honey-based hydrogel: In vitro and comparative In vivo evaluation for burn wound healing. *Scientific Reports*, *7*(1), 9692. DOI: 10.1038/s41598-017-08771-8 PMID: 28851905

Ellis, S., Lin, E. J., & Tartar, D. (2018). Immunology of wound healing. *Current Dermatology Reports*, *7*, 350–358. DOI: 10.1007/s13671-018-0234-9 PMID: 30524911

Elloumi, W., Mahmoudi, A., Ortiz, S., Boutefnouchet, S., Chamkha, M., & Sayadi, S. (2022). Wound healing potential of quercetin-3-O-rhamnoside and myricetin-3-O-rhamnoside isolated from Pistacia lentiscus distilled leaves in rats model. *Biomedicine and Pharmacotherapy*, *146*, 112574. PMID: 35062055

El-Sakhawy, M., Salama, A., & Tohamy, H. A. S. (2023). Applications of propolis-based materials in wound healing. *Archives of Dermatological Research*, *316*(1), 61. DOI: 10.1007/S00403-023-02789-X PMID: 38151671

El-Tanani, M., Satyam, S. M., Rabbani, S. A., El-Tanani, Y., Aljabali, A. A., Al Faouri, I., & Rehman, A. (2025). Revolutionizing Drug Delivery: The Impact of Advanced Materials Science and Technology on Precision Medicine. *Pharmaceutics*, *17*(3), 375. PMID: 40143038

Elumalai, P., Muninathan, N., Megalatha, S. T., Suresh, A., Kumar, K. S., Jhansi, N., Kalaivani, K., & Krishnamoorthy, G. (2022). An Insight into Anticancer Effect of Propolis and Its Constituents: A Review of Molecular Mechanisms. *Evidence-Based Complementary and Alternative Medicine: eCAM*, *2022*(1), 5901191. DOI: 10.1155/2022/5901191 PMID: 35754701

EMA. (2004). *Directive 2004/24/EC of the European Parliament and of the Council.*

Eming, S. A., Martin, P., & Tomic-Canic, M. (2014). Wound repair and regeneration: Mechanisms, signaling, and translation. *Science Translational Medicine*, *6*(265), 265sr6. PMID: 25473038

Enoch, S., & Leaper, D. J. (2008). Basic science of wound healing. *Surgery (Oxford)*, *26*(2), 31–37. DOI: 10.1016/j.mpsur.2007.11.005

Eriksson, P., Tal, A. A., Skallberg, A., Brommesson, C., Hu, Z., & Boyd, R. D.. (2018). Cerium oxide nanoparticles with antioxidant capabilities and gadolinium integration for MRI contrast enhancement. *Scientific Reports*, *8*, 6999. DOI: 10.1038/s41598-018-25390-z PMID: 29725117

Eskilson, O., Zattarin, E., Berglund, L., Oksman, K., Hanna, K., Rakar, J., Sivlér, P., Skog, M., Rinklake, I., Shamasha, R., Sotra, Z., Starkenberg, A., Odén, M., Wiman, E., Khalaf, H., Bengtsson, T., Junker, J. P. E., Selegård, R., Björk, E. M., & Aili, D. (2023). Nanocellulose composite wound dressings for real-time pH wound monitoring. *Materials Today. Bio*, *19*, 100574. DOI: 10.1016/j.mtbio.2023.100574 PMID: 36852226

Eur, Ph. 2.6.12, 2.6.13. http://www.uspbpep.com/ep60/2.6.13.%20microbiological%20examination%20of%20non-sterile%20products-%20test%20for%20specified%20micro-organisms%2020613e.pdf

European Directorate for the Quality of Medicines & HealthCare. (2025). *Harmonisation status for excipient monographs (PDG)*. https://www.edqm.eu/en/harmonisation-status-for-excipient-monographs-pdg-

European Medicines Agency. (2009). *Herbal medicinal products*. https://www.ema.europa.eu/en/human-regulatory-overview/herbal-medicinal-products

European Medicines Agency. (2018). *Annex to the European Commission guideline on "Excipients in the labelling and package leaflet of medicinal products for human use"*. https://www.ema.europa.eu/en/annex-european-commission-guideline-excipients-labelling-package-leaflet-medicinal-products-human-use

European Medicines Agency. (2022). *Guideline on quality of herbal medicinal products/traditional herbal medicinal products* (Revision 3). https://www.ema.europa.eu/en/documents/scientific-guideline/guideline-quality-herbal-medicinal-productstraditional-herbal-medicinal-products-revision-3_en.pdf

European Medicines Agency. (2022). *Guideline on specifications: Test procedures and acceptance criteria for herbal substances, herbal preparations and herbal medicinal products/traditional herbal medicinal products* (Revision 3). https://www.ema.europa.eu/en/documents/scientific-guideline/guideline-specifications-test-procedures-and-acceptance-criteria-herbal-substances-herbal-preparations-and-herbal-medicinal-productstraditional-herbal-medicinal-products-revision-3_en.pdf

European Medicines Agency. (2025). *Herbal medicinal products*. https://www.ema.europa.eu/en/human-regulatory-overview/herbal-medicinal-products

European Medicines Agency. (2025). *Herbal medicinal products: Scientific guidelines*. https://www.ema.europa.eu/en/human-regulatory-overview/research-development/scientific-guidelines/multidisciplinary-guidelines/herbal-medicinal-products-scientific-guidelines

European Union. (2001). *Directive 2001/83/EC of the European Parliament and of the Council of 6 November 2001 on the Community code relating to medicinal products for human use. Official Journal of the European Union, L 311*, 67–128. https://eur-lex.europa.eu/eli/dir/2001/83/oj/eng

European Union. (2004). *Directive 2004/24/EC of the European Parliament and of the Council of 31 March 2004 amending, as regards traditional herbal medicinal products, Directive 2001/83/EC. Official Journal of the European Union, L 136*, 85–90. https://eur-lex.europa.eu/eli/dir/2004/24/oj/eng

Falanga, V. (2005). Wound healing and its impairment in the diabetic foot. *Lancet, 366*(9498), 1736–1743. PMID: 16291068

Fang, Y., Egorov, M., Behnisch, J., & Yang, F. (2021). Hyaluronic acid in skin wound healing. *Polymers, 13*(12), 2104. DOI: 10.3390/polym13122104

Fang, Z., Lin, T., Fan, S., Qiu, X., Zhong, Z., Yang, G., Yang, J., Zhang, G., Feng, Y., Ai, F., Shi, Q., & Wan, W. (2023). Antibacterial, injectable, and adhesive hydrogel promotes skin healing. *Frontiers in Bioengineering and Biotechnology, 11*, 1180073. DOI: 10.3389/fbioe.2023.1180073 PMID: 37334269

Fan, Y., Wang, H., Wang, C., Xing, Y., Liu, S., Feng, L., Zhang, X., & Chen, J. (2024). Advances in Smart-Response Hydrogels for Skin Wound Repair. *Polymers, 16*(19), 2818. DOI: 10.3390/polym16192818 PMID: 39408528

Farrugia, C. E., Burke, E. S., Haley, M. E., Bedi, K. T., & Gandhi, M. A. (2019). The use of aloe vera in cancer radiation: An updated comprehensive review. *Complementary Therapies in Clinical Practice, 35*, 126–130. DOI: 10.1016/j.ctcp.2019.01.013 PMID: 31003648

Fathi, A. N., Sakhaie, M. H., Babaei, S., Babaei, S., Slimabad, F., & Babaei, S. (2020). Use of bromelain in cutaneous wound healing in streptozocin-induced diabetic rats: An experimental model. *Journal of Wound Care, 29*(9), 488–495. PMID: 32924815

Fatimi, A., Okoro, O. V., Podstawczyk, D., Siminska-Stanny, J., & Shavandi, A. (2022). Natural hydrogel-based bio-inks for 3D bioprinting in tissue engineering: A review. *Gels (Basel, Switzerland), 8*(3), 179. PMID: 35323292

FDA. (2020). *Guidance for Industry: Botanical Drug Development*. U.S. Food and Drug Administration.

Feng, M., Dai, X., Yang, C., Zhang, Y., Tian, Y., Qu, Q., & Shi, X. (2023). Unification of medicines and excipients: The roles of natural excipients for promoting drug delivery. *Expert Opinion on Drug Delivery*, *20*(5), 597–620. PMID: 37150753

Feng, P., Luo, Y., Ke, C., Qiu, H., Wang, W., Zhu, Y., Hou, R., Xu, L., & Wu, S. (2021). Chitosan-based functional materials for skin wound repair: Mechanisms and applications. *Frontiers in Bioengineering and Biotechnology*, *9*, 650598. DOI: 10.3389/fbioe.2021.650598 PMID: 33681176

Feng, Q., Li, Y., Yang, Y., Zhang, Z., & Xiao, B. (2019). Injectable and self-healing polysaccharide-based hydrogels for hemostasis and wound healing. *Frontiers in Bioengineering and Biotechnology*, *7*, 288. DOI: 10.3389/fbioe.2019.00288

Fernandez, J., & Zhao, L. (2024). Reinforcement learning in ethical content curation. In Li, H. (Ed.), *AI agents in dynamic environments* (pp. 87–109). MetaScholars., DOI: 10.4018/978-1-1111-2222-3.ch004

Ferrer, B. (2025). *Echinacea under scrutiny: New report exposes adulteration and mislabelling*. Nutrition Insight. https://www.clearprint.com/role-of-accurate-labeling-in-consumer-safety/

Fiorentini, F., Suarato, G., Grisoli, P., Zych, A., Bertorelli, R., & Athanassiou, A. (2021). Plant-based biocomposite films as potential antibacterial patches for skin wound healing. *European Polymer Journal*, *150*, 110414. DOI: 10.1016/j.eurpolymj.2021.110414

Fisichella, M., Berenguer, F., Steinmetz, G., Auffan, M., Rose, J., & Prat, O. (2014). Toxicity evaluation of manufactured CeO2 nanoparticles before and after alteration: Combined physicochemical and whole-genome expression analysis in Caco-2 cells. *BMC Genomics*, *15*(1), 700. DOI: 10.1186/1471-2164-15-700 PMID: 25145350

Fong, H. H. S. (2002). Integration of herbal medicine into modern medical practices: Issues and prospects. *Integrative Cancer Therapies*, *1*(3), 287–293. PMID: 14667286

Food and Drug Administration. (2025). *Generally recognized as safe (GRAS)*. https://www.fda.gov/food/food-ingredients-packaging/generally-recognized-safe-gras

Fornaguera, C., & García-Celma, M. J. (2017). Personalized Nanomedicine: A Revolution at the Nanoscale. *Journal of Personalized Medicine*, *7*(4), 12. DOI: 10.3390/jpm7040012 PMID: 29023366

Fraga-Corral, M., García-Oliveira, P., Pereira, A. G., Lourenço-Lopes, C., Jimenez-Lopez, C., Prieto, M. A., & Simal-Gandara, J. (2020). Technological application of tannin-based extracts. *Molecules (Basel, Switzerland)*, *25*(3), 614. PMID: 32019231

Fraga-Corral, M., Otero, P., Cassani, L., Echave, J., Garcia-Oliveira, P., Carpena, M., & Simal-Gandara, J. (2021). Traditional applications of tannin rich extracts supported by scientific data: Chemical composition, bioavailability and bioaccessibility. *Foods, 10*(2), 251. PMID: 33530516

Franz, M. G., Steed, D. L., & Robson, M. C. (2007). Optimizing healing of the acute wound by minimizing complications. *Current Problems in Surgery, 44*(11), 691–763. DOI: 10.1067/j.cpsurg.2007.07.001 PMID: 18036992

Fredriksson, M. (2023). India's traditional knowledge digital library and the politics of patent classifications. *Law and Critique, 34*(1), 1–19. DOI: 10.1007/s10978-022-09327-7 PMID: 36915708

Froelich, A., Jakubowska, E., Wojtyłko, M., Jadach, B., Gackowski, M., Gadziński, P., Napierała, O., Ravliv, Y., & Osmałek, T. (2023). Alginate-Based Materials Loaded with Nanoparticles in Wound Healing. *Pharmaceutics, 15*(4), 1142. DOI: 10.3390/pharmaceutics15041142 PMID: 37111628

Frykberg Robert, G. (2015). Challenges in the treatment of chronic wounds. *Advances in Wound Care (New Rochelle, N.Y.), 4*(9), 560–582. PMID: 26339534

Frykberg, R. G., & Banks, J. (2015). Challenges in the treatment of chronic wounds. *Advances in Wound Care, 4*(9), 560–582. PMID: 26339534

Futosi, K., Fodor, S., & Mócsai, A. (2013). Neutrophil cell surface receptors and their intracellular signal transduction pathways. *International Immunopharmacology, 17*, 638–650. DOI: 10.1016/j.intimp.2013.06.034 PMID: 23994464

Gabbiani, G. (2003). The myofibroblast in wound healing and fibrocontractive diseases. *The Journal of Pathology, 200*, 500–503. DOI: 10.1002/path.1427 PMID: 12845617

Gantwerker, E. A., & Hom, D. B. (2011). Skin: Histology and physiology of wound healing. *Facial Plastic Surgery Clinics of North America, 19*(3), 441. DOI: 10.1016/j.fsc.2011.06.009 PMID: 21856533

Gao, J.. (2021). Artificial intelligence in the design and optimization of biomaterials for medical applications. *Materials Science and Engineering R Reports, 145*, 100426. DOI: 10.1016/j.mser.2020.100426

Gao, Z., Golland, B., Tronci, G., & Thornton, P. D. (2021). A redox-responsive hyaluronic acid-based hydrogel for chronic wound management. *arXiv*. https://arxiv.org/abs/2101.01638

Garcia-Orue, I., Gainza, G., Gutierrez, F. B., Aguirre, J. J., Evora, C., Pedraz, J. L., Hernandez, R. M., Delgado, A., & Igartua, M. (2017). Novel nanofibrous dressings containing rhEGF and *Aloe vera* for wound healing applications. *International Journal of Pharmaceutics*, *523*(2), 556–566. DOI: 10.1016/j.ijpharm.2016.11.006 PMID: 27825864

Gardner, S. E., Frantz, R. A., & Doebbeling, B. N. (2001). The validity of the clinical signs and symptoms used to identify localized chronic wound infection. *Wound Repair and Regeneration*, *9*, 178–186. PMID: 11472613

Garg, V.. (2012). Facts about standardization of herbal medicine: A review. *Journal of Chinese Integrative Medicine*, *10*(10), 1077–1083. PMID: 23073189

Garima, Sharma, D., & Mittal, N. (2025). Greener nanomaterials for soft tissue regeneration: Diagnostic and therapeutic advances. *Journal of Drug Delivery Science and Technology*, *106*, 106747. DOI: 10.1016/j.jddst.2025.106747

Gatt, A. R., Vella Bonanno, P., & Zammit, R. (2024). Ethical considerations in the regulation and use of herbal medicines in the European Union. *Frontiers in Medical Technology*, *6*, 1358956. DOI: 10.3389/FMEDT.2024.1358956 PMID: 38948354

Gebremeskel, L., Bhoumik, D., Sibhat, G. G., & Tuem, K. B. (2018). In vivo wound healing and anti-inflammatory activities of leaf latex of aloe megalacantha baker (Xanthorrhoeaceae). *Evidence-Based Complementary and Alternative Medicine: eCAM*, *2018*, 1–7. PMID: 30057643

Gendrisch, F., Haarhaus, B., Krieger, N., Quirin, K. W., Schempp, C. M., & Wölfle, U. (2021). The effect of herbal medicinal products on psoriasis-like keratinocytes. *Biomolecules*, *11*(3), 371. DOI: 10.3390/biom11030371 PMID: 33801280

George Broughton, I. I., Janis, J. E., & Attinger, C. E. (2006). The basic science of wound healing. *Plastic and Reconstructive Surgery*, *117*(7S), 12S–34S. DOI: 10.1097/01.prs.0000225430.42531.c2 PMID: 16799372

George, A., Shah, P. A., & Shrivastav, P. S. (2019). Guar gum: Versatile natural polymer for drug delivery applications. *European Polymer Journal*, *112*, 722–735. DOI: 10.1016/J.EURPOLYMJ.2018.10.042

George, B., & Suchithra, T. V. (2019). Plant-derived bioadhesives for wound dressing and drug delivery system. *Fitoterapia*, *137*, 104241. DOI: 10.1016/j.fitote.2019.104241 PMID: 31201885

Gholamali, I. (2019). Stimuli-responsive polysaccharide hydrogels for biomedical applications: A review. *Regenerative Engineering and Translational Medicine*, *7*, 91–114. DOI: 10.1007/s40883-019-00134-1

Gholap, A. D., Uddin, M. J., Faiyazuddin, M., Omri, A., Gowri, S., & Khalid, M. (2024). Advances in artificial intelligence in drug delivery and development: A comprehensive review. *Computers in Biology and Medicine*, •••, 108702. PMID: 38878397

Ghosh, A., & Pillai, M. N. (2025). AI-driven language filters for social platforms. In Mukherjee, D. (Ed.), *Multilingual AI safety mechanisms* (pp. 61–89). Informed AI Press., DOI: 10.4018/978-5-5555-6666-6.ch005

Ghosh, A., Saha, K., Bhattacharya, T., Sarkar, S., Sengupta, D., Maiti, A., Ghoshal, D., Dey, S., & Chattopadhyay, D. (2024). Electrospun cerium oxide nanoparticle/aloe vera extract-loaded nanofibrous poly(ethylene oxide)/polyurethane mats as diabetic wound dressings. *ACS Applied Bio Materials*, *7*(8), 5268–5278. DOI: 10.1021/acsabm.4c00475 PMID: 39093691

Ghosh, D., Skinner, M., & Ferguson, L. R. (2006). The role of the Therapeutic Goods Administration and the Medicine and Medical Devices Safety Authority in evaluating complementary and alternative medicines in Australia and New Zealand. *Toxicology*, *221*(1), 88–94. DOI: 10.1016/j.tox.2005.12.023 PMID: 16481089

Ghosh, P. K., & Gaba, A. (2013). Phyto-extracts in wound healing. *Journal of Pharmacy & Pharmaceutical Sciences*, *16*(5), 760–820. PMID: 24393557

Goetz, P. (2019). Aloe vera. *Phytothérapie*, *17*(6), 352–356. DOI: 10.3166/phyto-2019-0213

Golebiewska, E. M., & Poole, A. W. (2015). Platelet secretion: From haemostasis to wound healing and beyond. *Blood Reviews*, *29*(3), 153–162. DOI: 10.1016/j.blre.2014.10.003 PMID: 25468720

Gonçalves, M. M., Carneiro, J., Justus, B., Espinoza, J. T., Budel, J. M., Farago, P. V., & Paula, J. P. D. (2020). Preparation and characterization of a novel antimicrobial film dressing for wound healing application. *Brazilian Journal of Pharmaceutical Sciences*, *56*, e18784. DOI: 10.1590/s2175-97902020000118784

Gopinath, D., Ahmed, M. R., Gomathi, K., Chitra, K., Sehgal, P. K., & Jayakumar, R. (2004). Dermal wound healing processes with curcumin incorporated collagen films. *Biomaterials*, *25*(10), 1911–1917. DOI: 10.1016/j.biomaterials.2003.08.015 PMID: 14738855

Gounden, V., & Singh, M. (2024). Hydrogels and Wound Healing: Current and Future Prospects. *Gels (Basel, Switzerland)*, *10*(1), 43. DOI: 10.3390/GELS10010043 PMID: 38247766

Govindaraghavan, S. (2008). Quality assurance of herbal raw materials in supply chain: Challenges and opportunities. *Journal of Dietary Supplements*, *5*(2), 176–212. PMID: 22432433

Govindaraghavan, S., & Sucher, N. J. (2015). Quality assessment of medicinal herbs and their extracts: Criteria and prerequisites for consistent safety and efficacy of herbal medicines. *Epilepsy & Behavior*, *52*, 363–371. PMID: 25899015

Goyal, A., & Bhattacharya, S. (2022). Clinical evidence requirements for herbal products: Bridging traditional use and modern regulatory frameworks. *Journal of Ethnopharmacology*, *292*, 115205.

Goyal, R. K., & Singh, J. (2019). Regulatory requirements for clinical trials of herbal products: Challenges and current status. *Journal of Ayurveda and Integrative Medicine*, *10*(4), 243–247.

Grattapaglia, D., & Kirst, M. (2008). Eucalyptus applied genomics: From gene sequences to breeding tools. *The New Phytologist*, *179*(4), 911–929. DOI: 10.1111/j.1469-8137.2008.02503.x PMID: 18537893

Griffith, C. (2016). Surface Sampling and the Detection of Contamination. Handbook of Hygiene Control in the Food Industry, 673–696. https://doi.org/DOI: 10.1016/B978-0-08-100155-4.00044-3

Gunasekaran, S., Nayagam, A. A., & Natarajan, R. (2020). Wound healing potentials of herbal ointment containing *Calendula officinalis* Linn. on the alteration of immunological markers and biochemical parameters in excision wounded animals. *Clinical Phytoscience*, *6*(1), 77. DOI: 10.1186/s40816-020-00223-7

Guo, S., & Dipietro, L. A. (2010). Factors affecting wound healing. *Journal of Dental Research*, *89*(3), 219–229. DOI: 10.1177/0022034509359125 PMID: 20139336

Gupta, R., & Bhatia, S. P. (2024). Digital well-being and ethical nudges. In Singh, N. (Ed.), *Behavioral AI for online harmony* (pp. 21–47). Cognitia Press., DOI: 10.4018/978-3-4444-7777-7.ch002

Gupta, R., Gabrielsen, B., & Ferguson, S. M. (2005). Nature's medicines: Traditional knowledge and intellectual property management. Case studies from the National Institutes of Health (NIH), USA. *Current Drug Discovery Technologies*, *2*(4), 203–219. DOI: 10.2174/157016305775202937 PMID: 16475917

Gupta, S. C., Patchva, S., & Aggarwal, B. B. (2013). Therapeutic roles of curcumin: Lessons learned from clinical trials. *The AAPS Journal*, *15*(1), 195–218. DOI: 10.1208/s12248-012-9432-8 PMID: 23143785

Gurtner, G. C., Werner, S., Barrandon, Y., & Longaker, M. T. (2008). Wound repair and regeneration. *Nature*, *453*(7193), 314–321. PMID: 18480812

Haalboom, M. (2018). Chronic wounds: Innovations in diagnostics and therapeutics. *Current Medicinal Chemistry*, *25*(42), 5772–5781. DOI: 10.2174/0929867324666170710120556 PMID: 28699502

Hajimiri, M., Shahverdi, A., Oryan, A., Mohammadi, A. A., & Bandegi, A. R. (2020). A review on dextran hydrogels: Synthesis, properties, and biomedical applications. *Carbohydrate Polymers*, *232*, 115800. DOI: 10.1016/j.carbpol.2019.115800

Hamdani, A. M., Wani, I. A., & Bhat, N. A. (2019). Sources, structure, properties and health benefits of plant gums: A review. *International Journal of Biological Macromolecules*, *135*, 46–61. DOI: 10.1016/J.IJBIOMAC.2019.05.103 PMID: 31121233

Hamedi, S., Mohagheghzadeh, A., & Rivaz, S. (2015). The role of medicinal plants in the treatment of wound healing: A review on historical perspectives. *Journal of Dermatology & Cosmetic*, *6*(2), 67–83.

Hamed, R., Magamseh, K. H., Al-Shalabi, E., Hammad, A., Abu-Sini, M., Abuleb-dah, D. H., Tarawneh, O., & Sunoqrot, S. (2025). Green Hydrogels Prepared from Pectin Extracted from Orange Peels as a Potential Carrier for Dermal Delivery Systems. *ACS Omega*, *10*(17), 17182–17200. DOI: 10.1021/acsomega.4c08449 PMID: 40352493

Hamed, S. H., Azooz, E. A., & Al-Mulla, E. A. J. (2023). Nanoparticles-assisted wound healing: A review. *Nano Biomedicine and Engineering*, *15*(4), 425–435. DOI: 10.26599/NBE.2023.9290039

Hamid, A. A., & Soliman, M. F. (2015). Effect of topical *Aloe vera* on the process of healing of full-thickness skin burn: A histological and immunohistochemical study. *Journal of Histology & Histopathology*, *2*(1), 3. DOI: 10.7243/2055-091X-2-3

Hamman, H., Steenekamp, J., & Hamman, J. (2015). Use of natural gums and mucilages as pharmaceutical excipients. *Current Pharmaceutical Design*, *21*(33), 4775–4797. PMID: 26290212

Hanif, W., Hardiansyah, A., Randy, A., & Asri, L. A. T. W. (2021). Physically cross-linked PVA/graphene-based materials/aloe vera hydrogel with antibacterial activity. *RSC Advances*, *11*(46), 29029–29041. DOI: 10.1039/d1ra04992e PMID: 35478571

Hansen, V. T., & Ng, C. Y. (2025). Legal frameworks for AI governance in media. In Alami, M. (Ed.), *Policy and AI in the public sphere* (pp. 109–130). Juridica Publishing., DOI: 10.4018/978-6-7654-3210-9.ch006

Haq, A., Kumar, S., Mao, Y., Berthiaume, F., & Michniak-Kohn, B. (2020). Thymoquinone-loaded polymeric films and hydrogels for bacterial disinfection and wound healing. *Biomedicines*, *8*(10), 386. PMID: 32998437

Hardman, M. J., & Ashcroft, G. S. (2008). Estrogen, not intrinsic aging, is the major regulator of delayed human wound healing in the elderly. *Genome Biology*, *9*, 1–17. DOI: 10.1186/gb-2008-9-5-r80 PMID: 18477406

Hariyani, D., Hariyani, P., Mishra, S., & Sharma, M. K. (2024). A literature review on green supply chain management for sustainable sourcing and distribution. *Waste Management Bulletin*, *2*(4), 231–248. DOI: 10.1016/j.wmb.2024.07.008

Hartung, T. (2008). Toxicology for the twenty-first century. *Nature*, *460*(7252), 208–212. PMID: 19587762

Hekmatpou, D., Mehrabi, F., Rahzani, K., & Aminiyan, A. (2019). The effect of aloe vera clinical trials on prevention and healing of skin wound: A systematic review. *Iranian Journal of Medical Sciences*, *44*(1), 1–9. https://pubmed.ncbi.nlm.nih.gov/30666070/ PMID: 30666070

Hekmatpou, D., Mehrabi, F., Rahzani, K., & Aminiyan, A. (2019). The effect of *Aloe vera* clinical trials on prevention and healing of skin wound: A systematic review. *Iranian Journal of Medical Sciences*, *44*(1), 1–9. PMID: 30666070

He, W., Ma, Z., Wang, Z., Zheng, Y., Sun, Y., & Wang, Y. (2021). A multifunctional hydrogel dressing with pH-responsive drug release, antioxidant and antibacterial activities for chronic wound healing. *Materials Science and Engineering C*, *124*, 112019. DOI: 10.1016/j.msec.2021.112019

Hilal, P. J., Harish, P., Harshita, C., Ashishkumar, P., Rashmi, D., & Prashant, K. (2024). Advancements and challenges in the integration of artificial intelligence with herbal medicine research. *IJPS Journal*, *2*(4), 973–984.

Hinz, B. (2006). Masters and servants of the force: The role of matrix adhesions in myofibroblast force perception and transmission. *European Journal of Cell Biology*, *85*(3-4), 175–181. DOI: 10.1016/j.ejcb.2005.09.004 PMID: 16546559

Hirst, S. M., Karakoti, A. S., Tyler, R. D., Sriranganathan, N., Seal, S., & Reilly, C. M. (2009). Anti-inflammatory properties of cerium oxide nanoparticles. *Small*, *5*(24), 2848–2856. DOI: 10.1002/smll.200901048 PMID: 19802857

Hoffman, A. S. (2002). Hydrogels for biomedical applications. *Advanced Drug Delivery Reviews*, *54*(1), 3–12. DOI: 10.1016/s0169-409x(01)00239-3 PMID: 11755703

Homedes, N., & Ugalde, A. (2005). Clinical trial ethics in Latin America: The continuing debate over standards of care. *Journal of Medical Ethics, 31*(4), 231–235. PMID: 15800365

Hormozi, M., & Baharvand, P. (2024). Investigating the influence of natural compounds on the healing process of wounds. *The Open Biochemistry Journal, 18*(1). Advance online publication. DOI: 10.2174/1874091X-v18-e240219-2023-17

Horn, D. B., Adams, G. L., & Monyak, D. (1995). Irradiated soft tissue and its management. *Otolaryngologic Clinics of North America, 28*(5), 1003–1019. DOI: 10.1016/S0030-6665(20)30472-2 PMID: 8559569

Horváth, A., Pandur, E., Sipos, K., Micalizzi, G., Mondello, L., Böszörményi, A., Birinyi, P., & Horváth, G. (2022). Anti-inflammatory effects of lavender and eucalyptus essential oils on the in vitro cell culture model of bladder pain syndrome using T24 cells. *BMC Complementary Medicine and Therapies, 22*(1), 119. DOI: 10.1186/S12906-022-03604-2 PMID: 35490236

Hosseini, M., Amjadi, I., Mohajeri, M., & Mozafari, M. (2020). Sol-gel synthesis, physico-chemical and biological characterization of cerium oxide/polyallylamine nanoparticles. *Polymers, 12*(7), 1444. DOI: 10.3390/polym12071444 PMID: 32605197

Ho, T. T., Tran, H. A., Doan, V. K., Maitz, J., Li, Z., Wise, S. G., Lim, K. S., & Rnjak-Kovacina, J. (2024). Natural Polymer-Based Materials for Wound Healing Applications. *Advanced NanoBiomed Research, 4*(5), 2300131. DOI: 10.1002/anbr.202300131

Houghton, P., & Mukherjee, P. K. (2020). Regulatory and quality aspects of herbal medicines: Global scenario. *Pharmaceutical Biology, 58*(1), 61–72.

Hou, Y., Xin, M., Li, Q., & Wu, X. (2021). Glycyrrhizin micelle as a genistein nanocarrier: Synergistically promoting corneal epithelial wound healing through blockage of the HMGB1 signaling pathway in diabetic mice. *Experimental Eye Research, 204*, 108454. PMID: 33497689

Huemer, M., Mairpady Shambat, S., Brugger, S. D., & Zinkernagel, A. S. (2020). Antibiotic resistance and persistence—Implications for human health and treatment perspectives. *EMBO Reports, 21*(12), e51034. DOI: 10.15252/embr.202051034 PMID: 33400359

Huffman, M. A. (2003). Animal self-medication and ethno-medicine: Exploration and exploitation of the medicinal properties of plants. *The Proceedings of the Nutrition Society, 62*(2), 371–381. PMID: 14506884

Hwang, J., Kang, Y., Park, H.-J., Kim, S., Lee, S.-H., Kim, H., Nam, S.-J., & Lim, K.-M. (2023). Skin wound healing effects of (+)-syringaresinol from ginseng berry. *Journal of Ginseng Research, 47*(5), 654–661. DOI: 10.1016/j.jgr.2023.04.003 PMID: 37720576

Ibrahim, A. A. E., Bagherani, N., Smoller, B. R., Reyes-Baron, C., & Bagherani, N. (2020). Functions of the Skin. In Smoller, B., & Bagherani, N. (Eds.), *Atlas of Dermatology, Dermatopathology and Venereology* (pp. 1–11). Springer International Publishing.

Ilina, O., & Friedl, P. (2009). Mechanisms of collective cell migration at a glance. *Journal of Cell Science, 122*, 3203–3208. DOI: 10.1242/jcs.036525 PMID: 19726629

Ilkar Erdagi, S., Asabuwa Ngwabebhoh, F., & Yildiz, U. (2020). Genipin crosslinked gelatin-diosgenin-nanocellulose hydrogels for potential wound dressing and healing applications. *International Journal of Biological Macromolecules, 149*, 651–663. DOI: 10.1016/j.ijbiomac.2020.01.279 PMID: 32006574

Iñiguez-moreno, M., Ragazzo-sánchez, J. A., & Calderón-santoyo, M. (2021). An Extensive Review of Natural Polymers Used as Coatings for Postharvest Shelf-Life Extension: Trends and Challenges. *Polymers 2021, Vol. 13, Page 3271, 13*(19), 3271. DOI: 10.3390/POLYM13193271

International Council for Harmonisation. (2025). *Mission - Harmonisation for better health.* https://www.ich.org/page/quality-guidelines

Ioannidis, J. P., Fanelli, D., Dunne, D. D., & Goodman, S. N. (2014). Meta-research: Evaluation and improvement of research methods and practices. *PLoS Biology, 12*(10), e1001747. PMID: 26431313

Iordache, F., Ditu, L. M., Popa, M. I., Ditu, S. T., & Vasilescu, A. (2022). Natural extract-based antimicrobial polymer films for wound healing. *Polymers, 14*(4), 743. PMID: 35215664

Iovene, A., Zhao, Y., Wang, S., & Amoako, K. (2021). Bioactive polymeric materials for the advancement of regenerative medicine. *Journal of Functional Biomaterials, 12*(1), 14. PMID: 33672492

IPEC Federation. (2025). *Guidelines*. https://ipec-federation.org/home/guidelines/

Iqbal, Y., Amin, F., Fatima, M., Khalid, M., Kanwal, N., Abdel Hafez, A. A., Farooq, A. S., Issa, S. A. M., Zakaly, H. M. H., & Alam, M. (2024). Chitosan-based functional materials combined with plant extract: A promising strategy in the stimulation of wound healing process. *Journal of Drug Delivery Science and Technology, 101*(Part B), 106314. https://doi.org/DOI: 10.1016/j.jddst.2024.106314

Iqbal, R., & Nair, K. J. (2024). User-centric AI ethics in platform design. In Shah, B. (Ed.), *Ethics-first AI in digital experience* (pp. 55–84). PeopleFirst Books., DOI: 10.4018/978-0-1111-9999-9.ch004

Irfan-Maqsood, M. (2016). Classification of wounds: Know before research and clinical practice. *Journal of Genes and Cells*, *4*(1), 1–4. DOI: 10.15562/gnc.61

Ishfaq, B., Khan, I. U., Khalid, S. H., & Asghar, S. (2023). Design and evaluation of sodium alginate-based hydrogel dressings containing *Betula utilis* extract for cutaneous wound healing. *Frontiers in Bioengineering and Biotechnology*, *11*, 1042077. DOI: 10.3389/fbioe.2023.1042077 PMID: 36777244

Isopencu, G. O., Covaliu-Mierlă, C.-I., & Deleanu, I.-M. (2023). From Plants to Wound Dressing and Transdermal Delivery of Bioactive Compounds. *Plants*, *12*(14), 2661. DOI: 10.3390/plants12142661 PMID: 37514275

Ivanková V, Belovičová M 2020 Consequences of chronic wounds on patient's lif. Україна Здоров'я нації. 2(3).

Jadhav, R., Das, J., Rajyaguru, S., Kyada, S., Kale, V., Teja, P. K., & Bhatt, P. (2025). Regulations, current development, and future prospects of phytopharmaceuticals, a new class of herbal medicines in India. *Discover Pharma Sciences*, *1*(6). Advance online publication. DOI: 10.1007/s44338-024-00002-5

Jahanbekam, S., Asare-Addo, K., Alipour, S., & Nokhodchi, A. (2025). Smart hydrogels and the promise of multi-responsive in-situ systems. *Journal of Drug Delivery Science and Technology*, *107*, 106758. DOI: 10.1016/J.JDDST.2025.106758

Jain, A., Radiya, P., Wadekar, R., Limaye, S., & Pawar, C. (2014). Natural excipients-an alternative to synthetic excipients: A comprehensive review. *International Journal of Pharmaceutical and Medicinal Research*, 2(4), 123–127.

Jain, R. A. (2000). The manufacturing techniques of various drug loaded biodegradable poly(lactide-co-glycolide) (PLGA) devices. *Biomaterials*, *21*(23), 2475–2490. DOI: 10.1016/S0142-9612(00)00115-0 PMID: 11055295

Jain, S., Jain, N., Tiwari, A., Balekar, N., & Jain, D. K. (n.d.). *Simple evaluation of wound healing activity of polyherbal formulation of roots of Ageratum conyzoides*. Linn. [Unpublished manuscript]

Jalili, A., Bagherifar, R., Nokhodchi, A., Conway, B., & Javadzadeh, Y. (2023). Current Advances in Nanotechnology-Mediated Delivery of Herbal and Plant-Derived Medicines. *Advanced Pharmaceutical Bulletin*, *13*(4), 712–722. DOI: 10.34172/apb.2023.087 PMID: 38022806

Jangde, R., Srivastava, S., Singh, M. R., & Singh, D. (2018). In vitro and In vivo characterization of quercetin loaded multiphase hydrogel for wound healing application. *International Journal of Biological Macromolecules, 115*, 1211–1217. PMID: 29730004

Jangid, A. K., & Sharma, S. (2025). Overview of Herbal Nanoparticles: A Patent Review. *Current Nanomedicine.*

Jangra, N., Singla, A., Puri, V., Dheer, D., Chopra, H., Malik, T., & Sharma, A. (2025). Herbal bioactive-loaded biopolymeric formulations for wound healing applications. *RSC Advances, 15*(16), 12402–12442. DOI: 10.1039/D4RA08604J PMID: 40248229

Jani, G. K., Shah, D. P., Prajapati, V. D., & Jain, V. C. (2012). Gums and mucilages: Versatile excipients for pharmaceutical formulations. *Asian Journal of Pharmaceutical Sciences, 7*(5), 309–323.

Javed, Z., Sadia, H., Raza, S., Iqbal, M. J., Sathyapalan, T., & Hashmi, M. F. (2021). Herbal medicine use and regulation in developing countries: A review of policy and ethics. *Complementary Therapies in Clinical Practice, 43*, 101393.

Jayakumar, R., Prabaharan, M., Sudheesh Kumar, P. T., Nair, S. V., & Tamura, H. (2011). Biomaterials based on chitin and chitosan in wound dressing applications. *Biotechnology Advances, 29*(3), 322–337. PMID: 21262336

Jee, J.-P., Pangeni, R., Jha, S. K., Byun, Y., & Park, J. W. (2019). Preparation and in vivo evaluation of a topical hydrogel system incorporating highly skin-permeable growth factors, quercetin, and oxygen carriers for enhanced diabetic wound-healing therapy. *International Journal of Nanomedicine, 14*, 5449. PMID: 31409998

Jena, G. B., & Chavan, S. (2017). Implementation of Good Laboratory Practices (GLP) in basic scientific research: Translating the concept beyond regulatory compliance. *Regulatory Toxicology and Pharmacology, 89*, 20–25. DOI: 10.1016/j.yrtph.2017.07.010 PMID: 28713068

Jiang, Y., Liu, Z., Guo, S., Zhang, Y., & Huang, Y. (2023). Thermosensitive chitosan-based hydrogels for controlled drug delivery and wound healing. *Carbohydrate Polymers, 301*, 120347. DOI: 10.1016/j.carbpol.2022.120347

Jirofti, N., Golandi, M., Movaffagh, J., Ahmadi, F. S., & Kalalinia, F. (2021). Improvement of the Wound-Healing Process by Curcumin-Loaded Chitosan/Collagen Blend Electrospun Nanofibers: In Vitro and In Vivo Studies. *ACS Biomaterials Science & Engineering, 7*(8), 3886–3897. DOI: 10.1021/acsbiomaterials.1c00131 PMID: 34256564

Ji, Z., Wang, X., Zhang, H., Lin, S., Meng, H., & Sun, B.. (2012). Designed synthesis of CeO2 nanorods and nanowires for studying toxicological effects of high aspect ratio nanomaterials. *ACS Nano*, *6*(6), 5366–5380. DOI: 10.1021/nn3012114 PMID: 22564147

Johnson, K. E., & Wilgus, T. A. (2014). Vascular endothelial growth factor and angiogenesis in the regulation of cutaneous wound repair. *Advances in Wound Care (New Rochelle, N.Y.)*, *3*, 647–661. DOI: 10.1089/wound.2013.0517 PMID: 25302139

Johnson, K. E., & Wilgus, T. A. (2014). Vascular Endothelial Growth Factor and Angiogenesis in the Regulation of Cutaneous Wound Repair. *Advances in Wound Care*, *3*(10), 647. DOI: 10.1089/WOUND.2013.0517 PMID: 25302139

Jones, A., & Vaughan, D. (2005). Hydrogel dressings in the management of a variety of wound types: A review. *Journal of Orthopaedic Nursing*, *9*, S1–S11. DOI: 10.1016/S1361-3111(05)80001-9

Jones, M. L. (2015). A short history of the development of wound care dressings. *British Journal of Healthcare Assistants*, *9*(10), 482–485.

Jones, V., Grey, J. E., & Harding, K. G. (2006). Wound dressings. *BMJ (Clinical Research Ed.)*, *332*(7544), 777–780. DOI: 10.1136/bmj.332.7544.777 PMID: 16575081

Joseph, T. M., Kar Mahapatra, D., Esmaeili, A., Piszczyk, Ł., Hasanin, M. S., Kattali, M., Haponiuk, J., & Thomas, S. (2023). Nanoparticles: Taking a Unique Position in Medicine. *Nanomaterials 2023, Vol. 13, Page 574*, *13*(3), 574. DOI: 10.3390/NANO13030574

Kaarniranta, K., Pawlowska, E., Szczepanska, J., Jablkowska, A., & Blasiak, J. (2019). Role of mitochondrial DNA damage in ROS-mediated pathogenesis of age-related macular degeneration (AMD). *International Journal of Molecular Sciences*, *20*, 2374. DOI: 10.3390/ijms20102374 PMID: 31091656

Kaczmarek-Szczepańska, B., Glajc, P., Chmielniak, D., Gwizdalska, K., Swiontek Brzezinska, M., Dembińska, K., Shinde, A. H., Gierszewska, M., Łukowicz, K., Basta-Kaim, A., D'Amora, U., & Zasada, L. (2025). Development and Characterization of Biocompatible Chitosan-Aloe Vera Films Functionalized with Gluconolactone and Sorbitol for Advanced Wound Healing Applications. *ACS Applied Materials & Interfaces*, *17*(10), 15196–15207. DOI: 10.1021/acsami.5c00715 PMID: 39999379

Kadadou, D., Tizani, L., Alsafar, H., & Hasan, S. W. (2024). Analytical methods for determining environmental contaminants of concern in water and wastewater. *MethodsX*, *12*, 102582. DOI: 10.1016/j.mex.2024.102582 PMID: 38357632

Kalalinia, F., Aamiri, N., Bayat, S., Movaffagh, J., & Hahsemi, M. (2021). (20211 burn wound healing effect of bromelain-loaded chitosan nanofibers. *Journal of Burn Care & Research; Official Publication of the American Burn Association, 42*(1), S192–S192.

Kalpana Manivannan, R., Sharma, N., Kumar, V., Jayaraj, I., Vimal, S., & Umesh, M. (2024). A comprehensive review on natural macromolecular biopolymers for biomedical applications: Recent advancements, current challenges, and future outlooks. *Carbohydrate Polymer Technologies and Applications, 8*, 100536. DOI: 10.1016/J.CARPTA.2024.100536

Kamalipooya, S., Fahimirad, S., Abtahi, H., Golmohammadi, M., Satari, M., & Dadashpour, M.. (2024). Diabetic wound healing function of PCL/cellulose acetate nanofiber engineered with chitosan/cerium oxide nanoparticles. *International Journal of Pharmaceutics, 653*, 123880. DOI: 10.1016/j.ijpharm.2024.123880 PMID: 38350498

Kamoun, E. A., Kenawy, E. S., & Chen, X. (2017). A review on polymeric hydrogel membranes for wound dressing applications: PVA-based hydrogel dressings. *Journal of Advanced Research, 8*(3), 217–233. DOI: 10.1016/j.jare.2017.01.005 PMID: 28239493

Kant, V., Jangir, B. L., Kumar, V., Nigam, A., & Sharma, V. (2020a). Quercetin accelerated cutaneous wound healing in rats by modulation of different cytokines and growth factors. *Growth Factors (Chur, Switzerland), 38*(2), 105–119. PMID: 32957814

Kanwar, R., Rathee, J., Salunke, D. B., & Mehta, S. K. (2019). Green nanotechnology-driven drug delivery assemblies. *ACS Omega, 4*(5), 8804–8815. DOI: 10.1021/acsomega.9b00304 PMID: 31459969

Karami, Z.. (2019). Polysaccharide-based biomaterials: Challenges in commercial production. *Biomaterials Science, 7*(12), 3856–3869. DOI: 10.1039/C9BM01194F

Karkare, P., Odijie, M. E., Ukaoha, K., & van Seters, J. (2022). Inconsistent policies or political realities. *Nigeria's trade and industrial policy imperatives (No. Discussion Paper No. 31).*

Kaur, H., Gogoi, B., Sharma, I., Das, D. K., Azad, M. A., Das Pramanik, D., & Pramanik, A. (2024). Hydrogels as a Potential Biomaterial for Multimodal Therapeutic Applications. *Molecular Pharmaceutics, 21*(10), 4827. DOI: 10.1021/ACS.MOLPHARMACEUT.4C00595 PMID: 39290162

Kaushik, A., Jayant, R. D., & Nair, M. (Eds.). (2017). *Advances in personalized nanotherapeutics* (1st ed.). Springer Cham., DOI: 10.1007/978-3-319-63633-7

Kerketta, G. S., & Kumari, P. (2024). Overview on Madagascar periwinkle. *World Journal of Pharmaceutical Research, 13*(4), 264–278. DOI: 10.20959/wjpr20244-30636

Khalid, A., Bai, D., & Abraham, A.. (2020). Electrospun nanodiamond-silk fibroin membranes: A multifunctional platform for biosensing and wound healing applications. *arXiv*. https://arxiv.org/abs/2006.00614

Khan, S. T., & Rodrigues, V. (2023). Building trust in AI content filtering. In Venkatesan, S. (Ed.), *Trustworthy AI: Models and measures* (pp. 89–112). AI Insights., DOI: 10.4018/978-2-3344-5566-2.ch005

Khayambashi, P., Iyer, J., Pillai, S., Upadhyay, A., Zhang, Y., & Tran, S. D. (2021). Hydrogel Encapsulation of Mesenchymal Stem Cells and Their Derived Exosomes for Tissue Engineering. *International Journal of Molecular Sciences, 22*(2), 684. DOI: 10.3390/ijms22020684 PMID: 33445616

Kigonya, R., Byakagaba, P., Ssenyonjo, E., & Jjunju, C. N. (2024). Biodiversity offsetting in Uganda's protected areas: A pathway to restoration of forest biodiversity? *Environmental Management, 73*(6), 1134–1149. DOI: 10.1007/s00267-023-01918-7 PMID: 38730130

Kim, J. O., Noh, J.-K., Thapa, R. K., Hasan, N., Choi, M., Kim, J. H., Lee, J.-H., Ku, S. K., & Yoo, J.-W. (2015). Nitric oxide-releasing chitosan film for enhanced antibacterial and in vivo wound-healing efficacy. *International Journal of Biological Macromolecules, 79*, 217–225. DOI: 10.1016/j.ijbiomac.2015.04.073 PMID: 25957720

Kizi, K. S. A. (2022). Pharmacological properties of Plantago major L. and its active constituents. *International Journal of Medical Science and Public Health Research, 3*(4), 9–12. DOI: 10.37547/ijmsphr/volume03issue04-03

Kocaadam, B., & Şanlier, N. (2017). Curcumin, an active component of turmeric (Curcuma longa), and its effects on health. *Critical Reviews in Food Science and Nutrition, 57*(13), 2889–2895. DOI: 10.1080/10408398.2015.1077195 PMID: 26528921

Koshy, J. T., Vasudevan, D., Sangeetha, D., & Prabu, A. A. (2023). Biopolymer Based Multifunctional Films Loaded with Anthocyanin Rich Floral Extract and ZnO Nano Particles for Smart Packaging and Wound Healing Applications. *Polymers, 15*(10), 2372. DOI: 10.3390/polym15102372 PMID: 37242946

Kozłowska, J., Skopińska-Wiśniewska, J., Kaczmarek-Szczepańska, B., Grabska-Zielińska, S., Makurat-Kasprolewicz, B., Michno, A., Ronowska, A., & Wekwejt, M. (2023). Gelatin and gelatin/starch-based films modified with sorbitol for wound healing. *Journal of the Mechanical Behavior of Biomedical Materials*, *148*, 106205. DOI: 10.1016/j.jmbbm.2023.106205 PMID: 37948920

Krausz, A. E., Adler, B. L., Cabral, V., Navati, M., Doerner, J., Charafeddine, R. A., Chandra, D., Liang, H., Gunther, L., Clendaniel, A., Harper, S., Friedman, J. M., Nosanchuk, J. D., & Friedman, A. J. (2015). Curcumin-encapsulated nanoparticles as innovative antimicrobial and wound healing agent. *Nanomedicine; Nanotechnology, Biology, and Medicine*, *11*(1), 195–206. DOI: 10.1016/j.nano.2014.09.004 PMID: 25240595

Krischak, G. D., Augat, P., Claes, L., Kinzl, L., & Beck, A. (2007). The effects of non-steroidal anti-inflammatory drug application on incisional wound healing in rats. *Journal of Wound Care*, *16*(2), 76–78. DOI: 10.12968/jowc.2007.16.2.27001 PMID: 17319622

Krishnan, P. (2006). The scientific study of herbal wound healing therapies: Current state of play. *Current Anaesthesia and Critical Care*, *17*(1–2), 21–27. DOI: 10.1016/j.cacc.2006.03.002

Küçük, K., Van Gysel, J., Del Marmol, V., & White, J. M. L. (2025). Allergic Contact Dermatitis Induced by Modern Wound Dressings: A Comprehensive Analysis of Risks and Allergenic Components. *International Wound Journal*, *22*(3), e70153. DOI: 10.1111/iwj.70153 PMID: 40069101

Kujur, A. R., & D'Souza, N. T. (2019). Comparison of Three Methods of Dressings for Split Thickness Skin Graft Donor Site-Non-Woven Dressing Impregnated with Amorphous Hydrogel, Amorphous Hydrogel with Colloidal Silver and Conventional Paraffin Gauze Dressing. *International Journal of Contemporary Medical Research*, *6*(12), 17–22.

Kulkarni, G. T., Gowthamarajan, K., & Dhobale, S. (2012). Natural polymers—A comprehensive review. *International Journal of Research in Pharmaceutical and Biomedical Sciences*, *3*(4), 1597–1613.

Kumar, A. P. N., Kumar, M., Jose, A., Tomer, V., Oz, E., Proestos, C., Zeng, M., Elobeid, T. K. S., & Oz, F. (2023). Major Phytochemicals: Recent Advances in Health Benefits and Extraction Method. *Molecules (Basel, Switzerland)*, *28*(2), 887. DOI: 10.3390/molecules28020887 PMID: 36677944

Kumar, A., Tyagi, P. K., & Tyagi, S. (2024). Integrating green nanotechnology with sustainable development goals: A pathway to sustainable innovation. *Discover Sustainability*, *5*, 364. DOI: 10.1007/s43621-024-00610-x

Kumari, A., Raina, N., Wahi, A., Goh, K. W., Sharma, P., Nagpal, R., Jain, A., Ming, L. C., & Gupta, M. (2022). Wound-Healing Effects of Curcumin and Its Nanoformulations: A Comprehensive Review. *Pharmaceutics*, *14*(11), 2288. DOI: 10.3390/pharmaceutics14112288 PMID: 36365107

Kumari, M., & Nanda, D. K. (2023). Potential of curcumin nanoemulsion as antimicrobial and wound healing agent in burn wound infection. *Burns*, *49*(5), 1003–1016. DOI: 10.1016/j.burns.2022.10.008 PMID: 36402615

Kumari, S., Goyal, A., Gürer, E. S., Yapar, E. A., Garg, M., Sood, M., & Sindhu, R. K. (2022). Bioactive Loaded Novel Nano-Formulations for Targeted Drug Delivery and Their Therapeutic Potential. *Pharmaceutics*, *14*(5), 1091. DOI: 10.3390/PHARMACEUTICS14051091 PMID: 35631677

Kumar, N., Mallick, P. K., & Tripathy, B. K. (2021). Blockchain for the healthcare supply chain: Challenges and opportunities. *Materials Today: Proceedings*, *49*, 2848–2854.

Kumar, S., Gopal, K. M., Choudhary, A., Soman, A., & Namburi, U. R. S. (2023). Advancing the one health approach through integration of Ayush systems: Opportunities and way forward. *Journal of Family Medicine and Primary Care*, *12*(9), 1764–1770. DOI: 10.4103/jfmpc.jfmpc_192_23 PMID: 38024885

Kumar, S., Kumar, A., Kumar, N., Singh, P., Singh, T. U., Singh, B. R., Gupta, P. K., & Thakur, V. K. (2022). In vivo therapeutic efficacy of Curcuma longa extract loaded ethosomes on wound healing. *Veterinary Research Communications*, *46*(4), 1033–1049. PMID: 35796857

Kumi, M., Chen, T., Zhang, Z., Wang, A., Li, G., Hou, Z., & Li, P. (2024). Integration of Hydrogels and 3D Bioprinting Technologies for Chronic Wound Healing Management. *ACS Biomaterials Science & Engineering*, *10*(10), 5995–6016. PMID: 39228365

Kunle, O. F., Egharevba, H. O., & Ahmadu, P. O. (2012). Standardization of herbal medicines – A review. *International Journal of Biodeversity and Conservation*, *4*(3), 101–112.

Kuryanova, A. S., Kardumyan, V. V., Kaplin, V. S., Aksenova, N. A., Chernyak, A. V., Timofeeva, V. A., Glagolev, N. N., Timashev, P. S., & Solovieva, A. B. (2023). Effect of amphiphilic polymers and sodium alginate on the activity of methylene blue in photogeneration of singlet oxygen^1 O_2. *Laser Physics*, *33*(9), 095601. DOI: 10.1088/1555-6611/ace70e

Kushwaha, A., Goswami, L., & Kim, B. S. (2022). Nanomaterial-based therapy for wound healing. *Nanomaterials (Basel, Switzerland)*, *12*(4), 618. DOI: 10.3390/nano12040618 PMID: 35214947

Langat, S. K. (2005). Ethical challenges in advance of conducting herbal clinical trials: The need for internationally acceptable guidelines. *Acta Tropica*, *95*(2), 178–184.

Langwick, S. A. (2011). *Bodies, politics, and African healing: The matter of maladies in Tanzania*. Indiana University Press.

LaPelusa, A., & Dave, H. D. (2023). Physiology, Hemostasis. *StatPearls*. https://www.ncbi.nlm.nih.gov/books/NBK545263/

Latos-Brozio, M., Masek, A., & Piotrowska, M. (2022). Polymeric forms of plant flavonoids obtained by enzymatic reactions. *Molecules (Basel, Switzerland)*, *27*(12), 3702. PMID: 35744827

Lee, C. H., Hsieh, M. J., Chang, S. H., Lin, Y. H., Liu, S. J., Lin, T. Y., & Juang, J. H. (2014). Enhancement of diabetic wound repair using biodegradable nanofibrous metformin-eluting membranes: In vitro and in vivo. *ACS Applied Materials & Interfaces*, *6*(6), 3979–3986. DOI: 10.1021/am405329g PMID: 24568239

Lee, C.-S., & Hwang, H. S. (2023). Starch-Based Hydrogels as a Drug Delivery System in Biomedical Applications. *Gels (Basel, Switzerland)*, *9*(12), 951. DOI: 10.3390/gels9120951 PMID: 38131937

Lee, G., Ko, Y.-G., Bae, K. H., Kurisawa, M., Kwon, O. K., & Kwon, O. H. (2022). Green tea catechin-grafted silk fibroin hydrogels with reactive oxygen species scavenging activity for wound healing applications. *Biomaterials Research*, *26*(1), 1–6. PMID: 36352485

Lee, H. M., & Chen, Y. J. (2023). Inclusive dataset strategies for fair AI. In Wong, L. (Ed.), *AI training sets and ethical representation* (pp. 33–58). DataJustice Press., DOI: 10.4018/978-8-8888-2222-2.ch003

Lee, J. H.. (2020). Efficacy of hyaluronic acid in the treatment of osteoarthritis: A systematic review and meta-analysis. *Journal of Clinical Medicine*, *9*(8), 2480. DOI: 10.3390/jcm9082480 PMID: 32748835

Lee, K. Y.. (2021). Biodegradable electronics based on polysaccharide-based materials for medical applications. *Nature Communications*, *12*, 1459. DOI: 10.1038/s41467-021-21606-0

Lee, K. Y., & Mooney, D. J. (2012). Alginate: Properties and biomedical applications. *Progress in Polymer Science*, *37*(1), 106–126. DOI: 10.1016/j.progpolymsci.2011.06.003 PMID: 22125349

Leitgeb, M., Kupnik, K., Knez, Ž., & Primožič, M. (2021). Enzymatic and antimicrobial activity of biologically active samples from *Aloe arborescens* and *Aloe barbadensis*. *Biology (Basel)*, *10*(8), 765. DOI: 10.3390/biology10080765 PMID: 34439997

Lei, X. X., Zou, C. Y., Hu, J. J., Jiang, Y. L., Zhang, X. Z., Zhao, L. M., & Xie, H. Q. (2023). Click-crosslinked in-situ hydrogel improves the therapeutic effect in wound infections through antibacterial, antioxidant and anti-inflammatory activities. *Chemical Engineering Journal*, *461*, 142092. DOI: 10.1016/j.cej.2023.142092

Leveen, H. H., Falk, G., Borek, B., Diaz, C., Lynfield, Y., Wynkoop, B. J., Mabunda, G. A., Rubricius, J. L., & Christoudias, G. C. (1973). Chemical acidification of wounds. An adjuvant to healing and the unfavorable action of alkalinity and ammonia. *Annals of Surgery*, *178*(6), 745–753. DOI: 10.1097/00000658-197312000-00011 PMID: 4759406

Li, D., Tang, G., Yao, H., Zhu, Y., Shi, C., Fu, Q., Yang, F., & Wang, X. (2022). Formulation of pH-responsive PEGylated nanoparticles with high drug loading capacity and programmable drug release for enhanced antibacterial activity. *Bioactive Materials*, *16*, 47–56. DOI: 10.1016/j.bioactmat.2022.02.018 PMID: 35386319

Li, F., Shi, Y., Liang, J., & Zhao, L. (2019). Curcumin-loaded chitosan nanoparticles promote diabetic wound healing via attenuating inflammation in a diabetic rat model. *Journal of Biomaterials Applications*, *34*(4), 476–486. DOI: 10.1177/0885328219860929 PMID: 31280635

Li, J. H., Wen, J., Li, B., Li, W., Qiao, W., & Shen, J.. (2018). Valence state manipulation of cerium oxide nanoparticles on a titanium surface for modulating cell fate and bone formation. *Advanced Science (Weinheim, Baden-Wurttemberg, Germany)*, *5*(2), 1700678. DOI: 10.1002/advs.201700678 PMID: 29610729

Li, J., Chen, J., & Kirsner, R. (2007). Pathophysiology of acute wound healing. *Clinics in Dermatology*, *25*(1), 9–18. DOI: 10.1016/j.clindermatol.2006.09.007 PMID: 17276196

Li, J., & Mooney, D. (2016). Designing hydrogels for controlled drug delivery. *Nature Reviews. Materials, 1*, 16071. DOI: 10.1038/natrevmats.2016.71 PMID: 29657852

Li, J., Wang, X., Yao, Z., Yuan, F., Liu, H., & Sun, Z.. (2023). NLRP3-Dependent crosstalk between pyroptotic macrophage and senescent cell orchestrates trauma-induced heterotopic ossification during aberrant wound healing. *Advanced Science (Weinheim, Baden-Wurttemberg, Germany), 10*(19), e2207383. DOI: 10.1002/advs.202207383 PMID: 37204068

Lin, X., Zhang, X., Wang, Y., Chen, W., Zhu, Z., & Wang, S. (2024). Hydrogels and hydrogel-based drug delivery systems for promoting refractory wound healing: Applications and prospects. *International Journal of Biological Macromolecules, 285*, 138098. DOI: 10.1016/j.ijbiomac.2024.138098 PMID: 39608543

Li, R., Song, Y., Fouladian, P., Arafat, M., Chung, R., Kohlhagen, J., & Garg, S. (2021). Three-dimensional printing of curcumin-loaded biodegradable and flexible scaffold for intracranial therapy of glioblastoma multiforme. *Pharmaceutics, 13*(4), 471. PMID: 33807243

Liu, H., Wang, C., Li, C., Qin, Y., Wang, Z., Yang, F., & Wang, J. (2018). A functional chitosan-based hydrogel as a wound dressing and drug delivery system in the treatment of wound healing. *RSC Advances, 8*(14), 7533–7549. PMID: 35539132

Liu, M., Jin, J., Zhong, X., Liu, L., Tang, C., & Cai, L. (2023). Polysaccharide hydrogels for skin wound healing. *Heliyon, 9*(3), e12999. DOI: 10.1016/j.heliyon.2023.e12999 PMID: 39144923

Liu, M., Zeng, X., Ma, C., Yi, H., Ali, Z., Mou, X., Li, S., Deng, Y., & He, N. (2017). Injectable hydrogels for cartilage and bone tissue engineering. *Bone Research, 5*, 17014. PMID: 28584674

Liu, M., Zhang, X., Yang, H., Yang, Q., & Wei, X. (2020). Dextran-based injectable hydrogels embedded with quercetin for promoting chronic wound healing. *ACS Omega, 5*(17), 9642–9649. DOI: 10.1021/acsomega.0c00374

Liu, S.. (2020). Polysaccharide-based materials for biodegradable bioelectronics: Progress and prospects. *Biomaterials, 237*, 119822. DOI: 10.1016/j.biomaterials.2020.119822

Liu, W., Xie, R., Zhu, J., Wu, J., Hui, J., Zheng, X., Huo, F., & Fan, D. (2022). A temperature responsive adhesive hydrogel for fabrication of flexible electronic sensors. *NPJ Flexible Electronics, 6*(1), 68. DOI: 10.1038/s41528-022-00193-5

Lone, A. H., Ahmad, T., Anwar, M., & Sofi, G. (2012). Clinical efficacy and safety of a pharmacopial polyherbal Unani formulation in pityriasis versicolor: A comparative randomized single-blind study. *Journal of Alternative and Complementary Medicine (New York, N.Y.)*, *18*(10), 978–982. DOI: 10.1089/acm.2011.0298 PMID: 22871048

Loo, H. L., Goh, B. H., Lee, L.-H., & Chuah, L. H. (2022). Application of chitosan-based nanoparticles in skin wound healing. *Asian Journal of Pharmaceutical Sciences*, *17*(3), 299–332. DOI: 10.1016/j.ajps.2022.04.001 PMID: 35782330

Lopes, A. I., Pintado, M. M., & Tavaria, F. K. (2024). Plant-Based Films and Hydrogels for Wound Healing. *Microorganisms*, *12*(3), 438. DOI: 10.3390/microorganisms12030438 PMID: 38543489

Lopes, P., Joaquinito, A. S. M., Ribeiro, A., Moura, N. M. M., Gomes, A. T. P., Guerreiro, S. G., Faustino, M. A. F., Almeida, A., Ferreira, P., Coimbra, M. A., Neves, M. G. P. M. S., & Gonçalves, I. (2023). Starch-based films doped with porphyrinoid photosensitizers for active skin wound healing. *Carbohydrate Polymers*, *313*, 120894. DOI: 10.1016/j.carbpol.2023.120894 PMID: 37182978

López-Estévez, A. M., Lapuhs, P., Pineiro-Alonso, L., & Alonso, M. J. (2024). Personalized cancer nanomedicine: Overcoming biological barriers for intracellular delivery of biopharmaceuticals. *Advanced Materials, 36*(n/a), 2309355. https://doi.org/DOI: 10.1002/adma.202309355

López, J. A.. (2021). Clinical trial of Hyalofill® in the treatment of venous leg ulcers: A prospective randomized study. *The Journal of Dermatological Treatment*, *32*(2), 173–181. DOI: 10.1080/09546634.2021.1870736

Lüer, S., Troller, R., & Aebi, C. (2012). Anti-bacterial and antiinflammatory kinetics of curcumin as a potential antimucositis agent in cancer patients. *Nutrition and Cancer*, *64*(7), 975–981. PMID: 22973975

Lukiswanto, B. S., Miranti, A., Sudjarwo, S. A., Primarizky, H., & Yuniarti, W. M. (2019). Evaluation of wound healing potential of pomegranate (Punica granatum) whole fruit extract on skin burn wound in rats (Rattus norvegicus). *Journal of Advanced Veterinary and Animal Research*, *6*(2), 202–207. DOI: 10.5455/javar.2019.f333 PMID: 31453192

Luo, L., Wang, B., Jiang, J., Fitzgerald, M., Huang, Q., & Yu, L. (2021). Heavy metal contaminations in herbal medicines: Determination, comprehensive risk assessments, and solutions. *Frontiers in Pharmacology*, *11*, 595335. Advance online publication. DOI: 10.3389/fphar.2020.595335 PMID: 33597875

Luong, P. T., Browning, M. B., Bixler, R. S., & Cosgriff-Hernandez, E. (2014). Drying and storage effects on poly (ethylene glycol) hydrogel mechanical properties and bioactivity. *Journal of Biomedical Materials Research. Part A, 102*(9), 3066–3076. DOI: 10.1002/jbm.a.34977 PMID: 24123725

Maan, A. A., Nazir, A., Khan, M. K. I., Ahmad, T., Zia, R., Murid, M., & Abrar, M. (2018). The therapeutic properties and applications of Aloe vera: A review. *Journal of Herbal Medicine*, *12*, 1–10. DOI: 10.1016/j.hermed.2018.01.002

Madgule, M., Vinayaka, N., Sonkhaskar, Y. M., Patel, D. R., Karthikeyan, R., & Selvakumar, P. (2023). Mechanical properties and microstructure of activated TIG welded similar joints of Inconel alloys by desirability approaches. *Materials Today: Proceedings*, *77*, 528–533.

Magangana, T. P., Makunga, N. P., Fawole, O. A., & Opara, U. L. (2020). Processing factors affecting the phytochemical and nutritional properties of pomegranate (Punica granatum L.) peel waste: A review. *Molecules (Basel, Switzerland)*, *25*(20), 4690. Advance online publication. DOI: 10.3390/molecules25204690 PMID: 33066412

Mai, B. T., Fernandes, S., Balakrishnan, P. B., & Pellegrino, T. (2018). Nanosystems based on magnetic nanoparticles and thermo- or pH-responsive polymers: An update and future perspectives. *Accounts of Chemical Research*, *51*(5), 999–1013. DOI: 10.1021/acs.accounts.7b00549 PMID: 29733199

Majtan, J., & Jesenak, M. (2018). β-Glucans: Multi-functional modulator of wound healing. *Molecules (Basel, Switzerland)*, *23*(4), 80. PMID: 29614757

Makrani, M. F., Goyal, A., & Sayeed, S. Y. (2025). A comparative overview of global regulatory authorities: Ensuring quality, safety, and efficacy in medicines. International Research Journal of Pharmacy and Medical Sciences, 8(2), 93–99. http://irjpms.com/wp-content/uploads/2025/03/IRJPMS-V8N2P150Y25.pdf

Malabadi, R. B., Kolkar, K. P., & Chalannavar, R. K. (2021). Natural plant gum exudates and mucilage: Pharmaceutical updates. *Int J Innov Sci Res Rev*, *3*(10), 1897–1912.

Malhotra, R., & Jain, I. (2024). Bias detection in social recommendation systems. In Sharma, M. (Ed.), *AI integrity in digital influence* (pp. 97–118). Equity Press., DOI: 10.4018/978-1-5555-8888-3.ch006

Mali, G. R., Bathe, R. S., & Bhalekar, M. R. (2010). Herbal excipients: A review. *International Journal of Pharmaceutical Sciences Review and Research*, *5*(3), 104–112.

Mamun, A. A., Shao, C., Geng, P., Wang, S., & Xiao, J. (2024). Recent advances in molecular mechanisms of skin wound healing and its treatments. *Frontiers in Immunology, 15*, 1395479. DOI: 10.3389/fimmu.2024.1395479 PMID: 38835782

Mandal, M. D., & Mandal, S. (2011). Honey: Its medicinal property and antibacterial activity. *Asian Pacific Journal of Tropical Biomedicine, 1*(2), 154. DOI: 10.1016/S2221-1691(11)60016-6 PMID: 23569748

Mansuri, S., Kesharwani, P., Jain, K., Tekade, R. K., & Jain, N. K. (2016). Mucoadhesion: A promising approach in drug delivery system. *Reactive & Functional Polymers, 100*, 151–172.

Marshall, E., Newton, A. C., & Schreckenberg, K. (2006). Commercialization of non-timber forest products: First steps in analyzing the factors influencing success. *International Forestry Review, 8*(1), 34–43.

Martinez, L., Rodrigues, A. M., & Silva, D. (2020). Quality control challenges in herbal medicine: Global perspectives. *Pharmaceutical Biology, 58*(1), 400–410. PMID: 32420784

Martin, G. M. (2001). Frontiers of aging. *Science, 294*(5540), 13. PMID: 11588222

Martins-Gomes, C., Nunes, F. M., & Silva, A. M. (2024). Linking Variability in Phytochemical Composition with Safety Profile of *Thymus carnosus* Boiss. Extracts: Effect of Major Compounds and Evaluation of Markers of Oxidative Stress and Cell Death. *International Journal of Molecular Sciences, 25*(10), 5343. DOI: 10.3390/ijms25105343 PMID: 38791385

Ma, X., Cheng, Y., Jian, H., Feng, Y., Chang, Y., & Zheng, R.. (2019). Hollow, rough, and nitric oxide-releasing cerium oxide nanoparticles for promoting multiple stages of wound healing. *Advanced Healthcare Materials, 8*(16), e1900256. DOI: 10.1002/adhm.201900256 PMID: 31290270

Mayrand, D., Laforce-Lavoie, A., Larochelle, S., Langlois, A., Genest, H., Roy, M., & Moulin, V. J. (2012). Angiogenic properties of myofibroblasts isolated from normal human skin wounds. *Angiogenesis, 15*, 199–212. DOI: 10.1007/s10456-012-9253-5 PMID: 22350743

Mazzocchi, F. (2006). Western science and traditional knowledge. Despite their variations, different forms of knowledge can learn from each other. *EMBO Reports, 7*(5), 463–466. DOI: 10.1038/sj.embor.7400693 PMID: 16670675

Mehta, A. K., Yashoda, L., Selvakumar, P., Mishra, B. R., Das, A., & C. T. C., M. (2025). Teaching methods: Techniques for disadvantaged learners. In S. Hai-Jew (Ed.), Mitigating learner disadvantages in teaching and learning (pp. 181–206). IGI Global Scientific Publishing. https://doi.org/DOI: 10.4018/979-8-3693-8623-1.ch007

Mekuye, B., & Abera, B. (2023). Nanomaterials: An overview of synthesis, classification, characterization, and applications. *Nano Select*, *4*(8), 486–501. DOI: 10.1002/nano.202300038

Memon, A. Q., Shah, A., Rana, N. A., & Bangash, S. A. (2025). AI for Wound Healing and Management. *Prospects*, *29*(6), 378–385.

Menzel, A., Samouda, H., Dohet, F., Loap, S., Ellulu, M. S., & Bohn, T. (2021). Common and Novel Markers for Measuring Inflammation and Oxidative Stress Ex Vivo in Research and Clinical Practice-Which to Use Regarding Disease Outcomes? *Antioxidants (Basel, Switzerland)*, *10*(3), 414. DOI: 10.3390/antiox10030414 PMID: 33803155

Metwally, W. M., El-Habashy, S. E., El-Hosseiny, L. S., Essawy, M. M., Eltaher, H. M., & El-Khordagui, L. K. (2023). Bioinspired 3D-printed scaffold embedding DDAB-nano ZnO/nanofibrous microspheres for regenerative diabetic wound healing. *Biofabrication*, *16*(1), 015001. PMID: 37751750

Middleton, J. C., & Tipton, A. J. (2000). Synthetic biodegradable polymers as orthopedic devices. *Biomaterials*, *21*(23), 2335–2346. PMID: 11055281

Ministry of AYUSH. (2021). *Guidelines for Development of Ayurveda Formulations*. Government of India.

Miralles, A., Puillandre, N., & Vences, M. (2024). DNA Barcoding in Species Delimitation: From Genetic Distances to Integrative Taxonomy. *Methods in Molecular Biology (Clifton, N.J.)*, *2744*, 77–104. DOI: 10.1007/978-1-0716-3581-0_4 PMID: 38683312

Mirhosseini, H., & Amid, B. T. (2012). A review study on chemical composition and molecular structure of newly plant gum exudates and seed gums. *Food Research International*, *46*(1), 387–398.

Mizuno, K., Yamamura, K., Yano, K., Osada, T., Saeki, S., Takimoto, N., Sakurai, T., & Nimura, Y. (2003). Effect of chitosan film containing basic fibroblast growth factor on wound healing in genetically diabetic mice. *Journal of Biomedical Materials Research. Part A*, *64A*(1), 177–181. DOI: 10.1002/jbm.a.10396 PMID: 12483711

Mo, X., Zhang, L., & Zhang, Y. (2021). Polysaccharide-based hydrogels: New insights and futuristic prospects in wound healing. *PubMed*. https://pubmed.ncbi.nlm.nih.gov/36395945/

Moghadam, A. M.. (2020). Chitosan nanoparticles for controlled delivery of antibiotics in wound infections: A clinical approach. *Pharmaceutical Development and Technology*, *25*(5), 543–552. DOI: 10.1080/10837450.2020.1751294

Mogoşanu, G. D., & Grumezescu, A. M. (2014). Natural and synthetic polymers for wounds and burns dressing. *International Journal of Pharmaceutics*, *463*(2), 127–136. DOI: 10.1016/j.ijpharm.2013.12.015 PMID: 24368109

Mohammadinejad, R., Kumar, A., Ranjbar-Mohammadi, M., Ashrafizadeh, M., Han, S. S., Khang, G., & Roveimiab, Z. (2020). Recent advances in natural gum-based biomaterials for tissue engineering and regenerative medicine: A review. *Polymers*, *12*(1), 176. Advance online publication. DOI: 10.3390/polym12010176 PMID: 31936590

Mohammad, M.. (2021). Biocompatibility and production of polysaccharide-based biomaterials for wound healing applications. *Journal of Biomaterials Science. Polymer Edition*, *32*(10), 1335–1346. DOI: 10.1080/09205063.2021.1923181

Mohan, A., Santhamoorthy, M., & Lee, Y.-C. (2024). Recent advances in the pH-responsive organic–inorganic mesoporous hybrid silica for targeted drug delivery. *European Polymer Journal*, *206*, 112783. DOI: 10.1016/j.eurpolymj.2024.112783

Molan, P. C. (2001). Potential of honey in the treatment of wounds and burns. *American Journal of Clinical Dermatology*, *2*(1), 13–19. DOI: 10.2165/00128071-200102010-00003 PMID: 11702616

Mondello, F., Fontana, S., Scaturro, M., Girolamo, A., Colone, M., Stringaro, A., Di Vito, M., & Ricci, M. L. (2022). Terpinen-4-ol, the Main Bioactive Component of Tea Tree Oil, as an Innovative Antimicrobial Agent against Legionella pneumophila. *Pathogens (Basel, Switzerland)*, *11*(6), 682. DOI: 10.3390/PATHOGENS11060682/S1 PMID: 35745536

Monika, P., Chandraprabha, M. N., Rangarajan, A., Waiker, P. V., & Chidambara Murthy, K. N. (2022). Challenges in healing wound: Role of complementary and alternative medicine. *Frontiers in Nutrition*, *8*, 791899. DOI: 10.3389/fnut.2021.791899 PMID: 35127787

Morgera, E., Tsioumani, E., & Buck, M. (2012). *Unraveling the Nagoya Protocol: A commentary on the Nagoya Protocol on Access and Benefit-sharing to the Convention on Biological Diversity*. Brill Nijhoff.

Morton, D. B., & Griffiths, P. H. M. (1985). Guidelines on the recognition of pain, distress and discomfort in experimental animals and an hypothesis for assessment. *The Veterinary Record, 116*(16), 431–436. PMID: 3923690

Mukherjee, P. K., Mukherjee, K., Rajesh Kumar, M., Pal, M., & Saha, B. P. (2003). Evaluation of wound healing activity of some herbal formulations. *Phytotherapy Research, 17*(3), 265–268. DOI: 10.1002/ptr.1130 PMID: 12672158

Mukherjee, P. K., Nema, N. K., Maity, N., & Mukherjee, D. (2011). *Standardized extracts of herbs and their significance in clinical practice. Herbal Medicine: Biomolecular and Clinical Aspects* (2nd ed.). CRC Press.

Mulyaningsih, S., Sporer, F., Zimmermann, S., Reichling, J., & Wink, M. (2010). Synergistic properties of the terpenoids aromadendrene and 1,8-cineole from the essential oil of *Eucalyptus globulus* against antibiotic-susceptible and antibiotic-resistant pathogens. *Phytomedicine, 17*(13), 1061–1066. DOI: 10.1016/j.phymed.2010.06.018 PMID: 20727725

Mumtaz, R., Zubair, M., Khan, M. A., Muzammil, S., & Siddique, M. H. (2022). Extracts of *Eucalyptus alba* promote diabetic wound healing by inhibiting α-glucosidase and stimulating cell proliferation. *Evidence-Based Complementary and Alternative Medicine: eCAM, 2022*, 4953105. Advance online publication. DOI: 10.1155/2022/4953105 PMID: 35463094

Mu, Q., Jiang, G., Chen, L., Zhou, H., Fourches, D., Tropsha, A., & Yan, B. (2014). Chemical basis of interactions between engineered nanoparticles and biological systems. *Chemical Reviews, 114*(15), 7740–7781. PMID: 24927254

Mura, S., & Couvreur, P. (2012). Nanotheranostics for personalized medicine. *Advanced Drug Delivery Reviews, 64*(13), 1394–1416. DOI: 10.1016/j.addr.2012.06.006 PMID: 22728642

Murphy, S. V., & Atala, A. (2014). 3D bioprinting of tissues and organs. *Nature Biotechnology, 32*(8), 773–785. DOI: 10.1038/nbt.2958 PMID: 25093879

Murthy, H. N. (2022). Chemical Constituents and Applications of Gums, Resins, and Latexes of Plant Origin. In Murthy, H. N. (Ed.), *Gums, Resins and Latexes of Plant Origin. Reference Series in Phytochemistry*. Springer., DOI: 10.1007/978-3-030-91378-6_1

Mushtaq, F., Raza, Z. A., Batool, S. R., Zahid, M., Onder, O. C., Rafique, A., & Nazeer, M. A. (2022). Preparation, properties, and applications of gelatin-based hydrogels (GHs) in the environmental, technological, and biomedical sectors. *International Journal of Biological Macromolecules, 218*, 601–633. PMID: 35902015

Mustoe, T. A., O'Shaughnessy, K., & Kloeters, O. (2006). Chronic wound pathogenesis and current treatment strategies: A unifying hypothesis. *Plastic and Reconstructive Surgery*, *117*(7S), 35S–41S. PMID: 16799373

Muthulakshmi, V., & Rajarajeswari, G. R. (2021). *In vivo* wound healing efficiency of curcumin-incorporated pectin-chitosan biodegradable films. *New Journal of Chemistry*, *45*(38), 17918–17929. DOI: 10.1039/D1NJ03477D

Nada, A. A., Ali, E. A., Soliman, A. A. F., Shen, J., Abou-Zeid, N. Y., & Hudson, S. M. (2020). Multi-layer dressing made of laminated electrospun nanowebs and cellulose-based adhesive for comprehensive wound care. *International Journal of Biological Macromolecules*, *162*, 629–644. DOI: 10.1016/j.ijbiomac.2020.06.184 PMID: 32574744

Nagoba, B., & Davane, M. (2019). Studies on wound healing potential of topical herbal formulations—Do we need to strengthen study protocol? *Journal of Ayurveda and Integrative Medicine*, *10*(4), 316–318. DOI: 10.1016/j.jaim.2018.06.009 PMID: 31685309

Nami, N., Feci, L., Napoliello, L., Giordano, A., Lorenzini, S., Galeazzi, M., & Fimiani, M. (2016). Crosstalk between platelets and PBMC: New evidence in wound healing. *Platelets*, *27*(2), 143–148. DOI: 10.3109/09537104.2015.1048216 PMID: 26030799

Namuga, C., Ocan, M., Kinengyere, A. A., Richard, S., Namisango, E., Muwonge, H., Kirabira, J. B., Lawrence, M., & Obuku, E. A. (2023). Efficacy of nano encapsulated herbal extracts in the treatment of induced wounds in animal models: A systematic review protocol. *Systematic Reviews*, *12*(1), 215. DOI: 10.1186/s13643-023-02370-7 PMID: 37968731

Nandhini, J., Karthikeyan, E., & Rajeshkumar, S. (2024). Nanomaterials for wound healing: Current status and futuristic frontier. *Biomedical Technology*, *6*, 26–45. DOI: 10.1016/j.bmt.2023.10.001

Nasrollahzadeh, M., Sajjadi, M., Sajadi, S. M., & Issaabadi, Z. (2019). Green nanotechnology. In Nasrollahzadeh, M., Sajadi, S. M., Sajjadi, M., Issaabadi, Z., & Atarod, M. (Eds.), *Interface science and technology* (Vol. 28, pp. 145–198). Elsevier., DOI: 10.1016/B978-0-12-813586-0.00005-5

Natarajan, V., Krithica, N., Madhan, B., & Sehgal, P. K. (2013). Preparation and properties of tannic acid cross-linked collagen scaffold and its application in wound healing. *Journal of Biomedical Materials Research. Part B, Applied Biomaterials*, *101B*(4), 560–567. DOI: 10.1002/jbm.b.32856 PMID: 23255343

Nathan, C. (2006). Neutrophils and immunity: Challenges and opportunities. *Nature Reviews. Immunology, 6*(3), 173–182. DOI: 10.1038/nri1785 PMID: 16498448

Nayak, B. S., & Pinto Pereira, L. M. (2006). Catharanthus roseus flower extract has wound-healing activity in Sprague Dawley rats. *BMC Complementary and Alternative Medicine, 6*, 41. PMID: 17184528

Nazemi, Z., Sahraro, M., Janmohammadi, M., Nourbakhsh, M. S., & Savoji, H. (2023). A review on tragacanth gum: A promising natural polysaccharide in drug delivery and cell therapy. *International Journal of Biological Macromolecules, 241*, 124343. PMID: 37054856

Nguyen Le, N.-M., Le-Vinh, B., Friedl, J. D., Jalil, A., & Kali, G. (2022). Polyaminated pullulan, a new biodegradable and cationic pullulan derivative for mucosal drug delivery. *Carbohydrate Polymers, 277*, 118848. DOI: 10.1016/j.carbpol.2021.118848

Nguyen, T. D., Nguyen, T. T., Ly, K. L., Tran, A. H., Nguyen, T. T. N., Vo, M. T., & Nguyen, T. H. (2019). In vivo study of the antibacterial chitosan/polyvinyl alcohol loaded with silver nanoparticle hydrogel for wound healing applications. *International Journal of Polymer Science, 2019*(1), 7382717. DOI: 10.1155/2019/7382717

Nguyen, T. L. C., Narayanan, M., Chinnathambi, A., Govindasamy, C., Subramani, B., Brindhadevi, K., Pimpimon, T., & Pikulkaew, S. (2022). Fabrication, characterization, anti-inflammatory, and anti-diabetic activity of silver nanoparticles synthesized from *Azadirachta indica* kernel aqueous extract. *Environmental Research, 208*, 112684. DOI: 10.1016/j.envres.2022.112684 PMID: 34995544

Nguyen, T. T. T., Tran, N. T. K., Le, T. Q., Nguyen, T. T. A., Nguyen, L. T. M., & Tran, T. V. (2023). Passion fruit peel pectin/chitosan based antibacterial films incorporated with biosynthesized silver nanoparticles for wound healing application. *Alexandria Engineering Journal, 69*, 419–430. DOI: 10.1016/j.aej.2023.01.066

Nordin, N. N., Aziz, N. K., Naharudin, I., & Anuar, N. K. (2022). Effects of Drug-Free Pectin Hydrogel Films on Thermal Burn Wounds in Streptozotocin-Induced Diabetic Rats. *Polymers, 14*(14), 2873. DOI: 10.3390/polym14142873 PMID: 35890648

Noreen, S., Hasan, S., Ghumman, S. A., Bukhari, S. N. A., Ijaz, B., Hameed, H., & Ejaz, H. (2022). pH responsive Abelmoschus esculentus mucilage and administration of methotrexate: In-vitro antitumor and in-vivo toxicity evaluation. *International Journal of Molecular Sciences, 23*(5), 2725. PMID: 35269867

Norris, K. D., & Ahmed, Z. (2024). Regulation of AI-powered political ads. In Choi, J. (Ed.), *Governance of AI in digital campaigns* (pp. 91–113). MediaEthics Press., DOI: 10.4018/978-3-764-3210-8.ch006

Nosek, B. A., Ebersole, C. R., DeHaven, A. C., & Mellor, D. T. (2015). The preregistration revolution. *Proceedings of the National Academy of Sciences of the United States of America, 115*(11), 2600–2606. PMID: 29531091

Nqoro, X., Adeyemi, S. A., & Ubanako, P.. (2024). Wound healing potential of sodium alginate-based topical gels loaded with a combination of essential oils, iron oxide nanoparticles and tranexamic acid. *Polymer Bulletin, 81*, 3459–3478. DOI: 10.1007/s00289-023-04879-2

NSF - National Science Foundation. (2025). *The importance of NSF/ANSI 173 certification for dietary supplement products*. https://www.nsf.gov/

Nyika, A., Kilama, W., Chilengi, R., & Tangwa, G. B. (2009). Composition, training needs and independence of ethics review committees across Africa: Are the gate-keepers rising to the emerging challenges? *Journal of Medical Ethics, 35*(3), 189–193. PMID: 19251972

O'Connor, B., & Dubey, R. (2025). Deepfake detection and ethical implications. In Fraser, L. (Ed.), *Truth and trust in AI-generated media* (pp. 59–84). RealMedia Academic., DOI: 10.4018/978-9-3210-7654-3.ch004

Ofridam, F., Tarhini, M., Lebaz, N., Gagnière, É., Mangin, D., & Elaissari, A. (2021). pH-sensitive polymers: Classification and some fine potential applications. *Polymers for Advanced Technologies, 32*(4), 1455–1484.

Ogaji, I. J., Nep, E. I., & Audu-Peter, J. D. (2012). Advances in natural polymers as pharmaceutical excipients. *Pharmaceutica Analytica Acta, 3*(1), 1–16.

Ogeh, P.C., E. A. B. (n.d.). Evaluation of Physico-Mechanical and Mucoadhesive Properties of Biopolymer Films From Cola Acuminata Gum. *Nigerian Journal of Pharmaceutical Research, 14*, 13.

Okan, D., Woo, K., Ayello, E. A., & Sibbald, G. (2007). The role of moisture balance in wound healing. *Advances in Skin & Wound Care, 20*(1), 39–55. DOI: 10.1097/00129334-200701000-00013 PMID: 17195786

Olisova, O. Y., Snarskaya, E. S., Gladko, V. V., & Burova, E. P. (2018). Russian traditional medicine in dermatology. *Clinics in Dermatology, 36*(3), 325–337. DOI: 10.1016/j.clindermatol.2018.03.006 PMID: 29908575

Oliveira, C., Sousa, D., Teixeira, J. A., Ferreira-Santos, P., & Botelho, C. M. (2023). Polymeric biomaterials for wound healing. *Frontiers in Bioengineering and Biotechnology, 11*, 1136077. DOI: 10.3389/fbioe.2023.1136077 PMID: 37576995

Omar, F., & Wang, L. (2023). AI in flagging extremist content: Challenges and progress. In Becker, T. (Ed.), *Machine learning in content moderation* (pp. 103–125). SafeAI Press., DOI: 10.4018/978-3-2109-8754-1.ch007

Opuni, K. F. M., Kretchy, J. P., Agyabeng, K., Boadu, J. A., Adanu, T., Ankamah, S., Appiah, A., Amoah, G. B., Baidoo, M., & Kretchy, I. A. (2023). Contamination of herbal medicinal products in low-and-middle-income countries: A systematic review. *Heliyon*, *9*(9), e19370. DOI: 10.1016/j.heliyon.2023.e19370 PMID: 37674839

Orive, G., & Desimone, M. F. (2024). Biopolymers Take Center Stage in Wound Healing Advancements. *Pharmaceutics*, *16*(6), 755. DOI: 10.3390/PHARMACEUTICS16060755 PMID: 38931877

Otranto, M., Souza-Netto, I., Aguila, M. B., & Monte-Alto-Costa, A. (2009). Male and female rats with severe protein restriction present delayed wound healing. *Applied Physiology, Nutrition, and Metabolism*, *34*(6), 1023–1031. DOI: 10.1139/H09-100 PMID: 20029510

Pagano, C., Puglia, D., Luzi, F., Michele, A. D., Scuota, S., Primavilla, S., Ceccarini, M. R., Beccari, T., Iborra, C. A. V., Ramella, D., Ricci, M., & Perioli, L. (2021). Development and Characterization of Xanthan Gum and Alginate Based Bioadhesive Film for Pycnogenol Topical Use in Wound Treatment. *Pharmaceutics*, *13*(3), 324. DOI: 10.3390/pharmaceutics13030324 PMID: 33802607

Paladini, F., & Pollini, M. (2019). Antimicrobial Silver Nanoparticles for Wound Healing Application: Progress and Future Trends. *Materials (Basel, Switzerland)*, *12*(16), 2540. DOI: 10.3390/ma12162540 PMID: 31404974

Pala, R., Mohieldin, A. M., Shamloo, K., Sherpa, R. T., Kathem, S. H., Zhou, J., Luan, Z., Zheng, J. G., Ahsan, A., & Nauli, S. M. (2019). Personalized Nanotherapy by Specifically Targeting Cell Organelles To Improve Vascular Hypertension. *Nano Letters*, *19*(2), 904–914. DOI: 10.1021/acs.nanolett.8b04138 PMID: 30582331

Palkhade, R., Sammal, D., Parmar, J., & Chavhan, S. (2025). Methodological limitations and confounders in dermal toxicity evaluation of aqueous test substance by OECD technical guidelines 402, 410: Our experience of testing ethanol-based hand sanitizer. *Annals of Medicine*, *57*(1). Advance online publication. DOI: 10.1080/07853890.2025.2491664 PMID: 40242887

Pandey, M. M., Rastogi, S., & Rawat, A. K. S. (2013). Indian Traditional Ayurvedic System of Medicine and Nutritional Supplementation. *Evidence-Based Complementary and Alternative Medicine: eCAM*, *376327*. Advance online publication. DOI: 10.1155/2013/376327 PMID: 23864888

Pandey, R., Bhatt, G., & Johri, A. (2016). Herbal excipients in novel drug delivery systems. *International Journal of Pharmaceutical Sciences Review and Research, 36*(1), 192–199.

Pang, Q., Jiang, Z., Wu, K., Hou, R., & Zhu, Y. (2023). Nanomaterials-based wound dressing for advanced management of infected wound. *Antibiotics (Basel, Switzerland), 12*(2), 351. DOI: 10.3390/antibiotics12020351 PMID: 36830262

Pang, Q., Yang, F., Jiang, Z., Wu, K., Hou, R., & Zhu, Y. (2023). Smart wound dressing for advanced wound management: Real-time monitoring and on-demand treatment. *Materials & Design, 229*, 111917. DOI: 10.1016/J.MATDES.2023.111917

Parasuraman, S. (2012). Herbal drug development: Current status and the future. *Asian Journal of Pharmaceutical and Clinical Research, 5*(Suppl 2), 8–12.

Paras, Yadav, K., Kumar, P., Teja, D. R., Chakraborty, S., Chakraborty, M., Mohapatra, S. S., Sahoo, A., Chou, M. M. C., Liang, C. T., & Hang, D. R. (2022). A Review on Low-Dimensional Nanomaterials: Nanofabrication, Characterization and Applications. *Nanomaterials (Basel, Switzerland), 13*(1), 160. DOI: 10.3390/nano13010160 PMID: 36616070

Pariona, A. (2025). *The world's 17 megadiverse countries*. WorldAtlas. https://www.worldatlas.com/articles/ecologically-megadiverse-countries-of-the-world.html

Park, D. H., Park, J. Y., Shin, M.-S., & Hwang, G. S. (2023). Wound Healing Effect of 20(*S*)-Protopanaxadiol of Ginseng Involves VEGF-ERK Pathways in HUVECs and Diabetic Mice. *Processes (Basel, Switzerland), 11*(3), 692. DOI: 10.3390/pr11030692

Park, K. S., & Park, D. H. (2019). The effect of Korean Red Ginseng on full-thickness skin wound healing in rats. *Journal of Ginseng Research, 43*(2), 226–235. DOI: 10.1016/j.jgr.2017.12.006 PMID: 30976160

Parveen, A., Kulkarni, N., Yalagatti, M., Abbaraju, V., & Deshpande, R. (2018). In vivo efficacy of biocompatible silver nanoparticles cream for empirical wound healing. *Journal of Tissue Viability, 27*(4), 257–261. PMID: 30190175

Parveen, A., Parveen, B., Parveen, R., & Ahmad, S. (2015). Challenges and guidelines for clinical trial of herbal drugs. *Journal of Pharmacy & Bioallied Sciences, 7*(4), 329–333. DOI: 10.4103/0975-7406.168035 PMID: 26681895

Patel, A.. (2022). Bioelectronics and biodegradable sensors: Future prospects of polysaccharide-based materials. *Journal of Electronic Materials, 51*(7), 3567–3584. DOI: 10.1007/s11664-022-09409-1

Patel, M., Gade, S., & Jadhav, P. (2020). Cellulose-based dressings for wound healing applications: A review. *Materials Today: Proceedings*, *33*, 2987–2993. DOI: 10.1016/j.matpr.2020.02.604

Patel, M., & Patel, N. (2021). Regulatory challenges and approaches in herbal drug development. *Journal of Herbal Medicine*, *26*, 100406.

Patil, J. S., Kamalapur, M. V., Marapur, S. C., & Kadam, D. V. (2009). Formulation and evaluation of sustained release microparticles of aceclofenac using natural polymer. *Research Journal of Pharmacy and Technology*, *2*(5), 331–334.

Patitucci, F., Motta, M. F., Dattilo, M., Malivindi, R., Leonetti, A. E., Pezzi, G., Prete, S., Mileti, O., Gabriele, D., Parisi, O. I., & Puoci, F. (2024). 3D-Printed Alginate/Pectin-Based Patches Loaded with Olive Leaf Extracts for Wound Healing Applications: Development, Characterization and In Vitro Evaluation of Biological Properties. *Pharmaceutics*, *16*(1), 99. DOI: 10.3390/pharmaceutics16010099 PMID: 38258109

Patwardhan, B., Chandran, U., & Joshi, K. (2015). Ayurveda and natural products drug discovery. *Current Science*, *109*(9), 1579–1583.

Patwardhan, B., Warude, D., Pushpangadan, P., & Bhatt, N. (2005). Ayurveda and traditional Chinese medicine: A comparative overview. *Evidence-Based Complementary and Alternative Medicine: eCAM*, *2*(4), 465–473. DOI: 10.1093/ecam/neh140 PMID: 16322803

Pawar, S. R., Patel, P., & Jain, K. (2025). Herbal Formulations: Development, Challenges, Testing, Stability, and Regulatory Guidelines. In *Advances in Pharmaceutical Product Development* (pp. 379-397). Singapore: Springer Nature Singapore. https://doi.org/DOI: 10.1007/978-981-97-9230-6_15

Pawar, S. R., Patel, P., & Jain, K. (2025). Herbal Formulations: Development, Challenges, Testing, Stability, and Regulatory Guidelines. In *Advances in Pharmaceutical Product Development* (pp. 379–397). Springer Nature Singapore.

Payne, W. G., Naidu, D. K., Wheeler, C. K., Barkoe, D., Mentis, M., Salas, R. E., & Robson, M. C. (2008). Wound healing in PatientsWith cancer. *Eplasty*, *8*, e9. PMID: 18264518

Pazyar, N., Yaghoobi, R., Rafiee, E., Mehrabian, A., & Feily, A. (2014). Skin wound healing and phytomedicine: A review. *Skin Pharmacology and Physiology*, *27*(6), 303–310. PMID: 24993834

Peppas, N. A., Bures, P., Leobandung, W. S., & Ichikawa, H. (2000). Hydrogels in pharmaceutical formulations. *European Journal of Pharmaceutics and Biopharmaceutics*, *50*(1), 27–46. DOI: 10.1016/S0939-6411(00)00090-4 PMID: 10840191

Peppas, N. A., Hilt, J. Z., Khademhosseini, A., & Langer, R. (2006). Hydrogels in biology and medicine: From molecular principles to bionanotechnology. *Advanced Materials*, *18*(11), 1345–1360. DOI: 10.1002/adma.200501612

Percival, S. L., & McCarty, S. M. (2015). Silver and Alginates: Role in Wound Healing and Biofilm Control. *Advances in Wound Care*, *4*(7), 407–414. DOI: 10.1089/wound.2014.0541 PMID: 26155383

Peters, M. A., Jayne, M., & Murphy, T. (2019). Global health equity and access: Towards sustainable universal health coverage. *Health Policy and Planning*, *34*(3), 195–197.

Petreaca, M. L., Yao, M., Liu, Y., DeFea, K., & Martins-Green, M. (2007). Transactivation of vascular endothelial growth factor receptor-2 by interleukin-8 (IL-8/CXCL8) is required for IL-8/CXCL8-induced endothelial permeability. *Molecular Biology of the Cell*, *18*(12), 5014–5023. DOI: 10.1091/mbc.e07-01-0004 PMID: 17928406

Pick, G. (2025). *The role of accurate labeling for consumer safety*. Clear Print. https://www.clearprint.com/role-of-accurate-labeling-in-consumer-safety/

Pifferi, G., & Restani, P. (2003). The safety of pharmaceutical excipients. *Il Farmaco*, *58*(8), 541–550. PMID: 12875883

Pockle, R. D., Masareddy, R. S., Patil, A. S., & Patil, P. D. (2023). A comprehensive review on pharmaceutical excipients. *Therapeutic Delivery*, *14*(7), 443–458. PMID: 37464784

Pooprommin, P., Manaspon, C., Dwivedi, A., Mazumder, A., Sangkaew, S., Wanmasae, S., Tangpong, J., Ongtanasup, T., & Eawsakul, K. (2022). Alginate/pectin dressing with niosomal mangosteen extract for enhanced wound healing: Evaluating skin irritation by structure-activity relationship. *Heliyon*, *8*(12), e12032. DOI: 10.1016/j.heliyon.2022.e12032 PMID: 36506386

Pormohammad, A., Monych, N. K., Ghosh, S., Turner, D. L., & Turner, R. J. (2021). Nanomaterials in Wound Healing and Infection Control. *Antibiotics (Basel, Switzerland)*, *10*(5), 473. DOI: 10.3390/antibiotics10050473 PMID: 33919072

Posey, D. A., & Dutfield, G. (1996). *Beyond intellectual property: Toward traditional resource rights for indigenous peoples and local communities*. International Development Research Centre.

Pradeep, E., Mukherjee, S. K., Selvakumar, P., Koppaka, A. K., Chandel, P. S., & Vats, C. (2025). Empowering social media users with ethical AI. In Chakraborty, S. (Ed.), *Ethical AI solutions for addressing social media influence and hate speech* (pp. 91–118). IGI Global Scientific Publishing., DOI: 10.4018/979-8-3693-9904-0.ch005

Prajapati, V. D., Jani, G. K., Moradiya, N. G., & Randeria, N. P. (2013). Pharmaceutical applications of various natural gums, mucilages and their modified forms. *Carbohydrate Polymers*, *92*(2), 1685–1699. DOI: 10.1016/j.carbpol.2012.11.021 PMID: 23399207

Pramanik, S., Aggarwal, A., Kadi, A., Alhomrani, M., Alamri, A. S., Alsanie, W. F., & Bellucci, S. (2024). Chitosan alchemy: Transforming tissue engineering and wound healing. *RSC Advances*, *14*(27), 19219–19256. PMID: 38887635

Prasad, N., Thombare, N., Sharma, S. C., & Kumar, S. (2022). Gum arabic–A versatile natural gum: A review on production, processing, properties and applications. *Industrial Crops and Products*, *187*, 115304.

Prasad, N., Thombare, N., Sharma, S. C., & Kumar, S. (2023). Recent development in the medical and industrial applications of gum karaya: A review. *Polymer Bulletin*, *80*(4), 3425–3447.

Priya, S., Choudhari, M., Tomar, Y., Desai, V. M., Innani, S., Dubey, S. K., & Singhvi, G. (2024). Exploring polysaccharide-based bio-adhesive topical film as a potential platform for wound dressing application: A review. *Carbohydrate Polymers*, *327*, 121655. DOI: 10.1016/j.carbpol.2023.121655 PMID: 38171676

Purohit, S. D., Singh, H., Bhaskar, R., Yadav, I., Chou, C.-F., & Gupta, M. K.. (2020). Gelatin—alginate—cerium oxide nanocomposite scaffold for bone regeneration. *Materials Science and Engineering C*, *116*, 111111. DOI: 10.1016/j.msec.2020.111111 PMID: 32806319

Qian, Y., Lin, X., Sun, Y., Wang, J., & Zhao, Y. (2022). Self-healing hydrogels with antibacterial and antioxidant activities based on dynamic Schiff base linkages for wound healing. *International Journal of Biological Macromolecules*, *213*, 321–331. DOI: 10.1016/j.ijbiomac.2022.07.153

Qiu, Y., & Park, K. (2012). Environment-sensitive hydrogels for drug delivery. *Advanced Drug Delivery Reviews*, *64*, 49–60. DOI: 10.1016/j.addr.2012.09.024 PMID: 11744175

Quave, C. L. (2018). Wound healing with botanicals: A review and future perspectives. *Current Dermatology Reports*, *7*(4), 287–295. DOI: 10.1007/s13671-018-0247-4 PMID: 31106027

Qureshi, L., & Dasgupta, T. (2024). AI fairness in targeting marginalized comunities. In Pillai, M. (Ed.), *Inclusive AI for social platforms* (pp. 29–55). Unity Press., DOI: 10.4018/978-6-1212-7777-1.ch003

Raghupathi, K. R., Koodali, R. T., & Manna, A. C. (2011). Size-dependent bacterial growth inhibition and mechanism of antibacterial activity of zinc oxide nanoparticles. *Langmuir*, *27*(7), 4020–4028. DOI: 10.1021/la104825u PMID: 21401066

Raina, R., Prawez, S., Verma, P. K., & Pankaj, N. K. (2008). Medicinal plants and their role in wound healing. *Vet Scan*, *3*(1), 24.

Raja, I. S., & Fathima, N. N. (2018). Gelatin-cerium oxide nanocomposite for enhanced excisional wound healing. *ACS Applied Bio Materials*, *1*(2), 487–495. DOI: 10.1021/acsabm.8b00208 PMID: 35016389

Rajendran, N. K., Kumar, S. S. D., Houreld, N. N., & Abrahamse, H. (2018). A review on nanoparticle based treatment for wound healing. *Journal of Drug Delivery Science and Technology*, *44*, 421–430. DOI: 10.1016/j.jddst.2018.01.009

Rajinikanth B, S., Rajkumar, D. S. R., K, K., & Vijayaragavan, V. (2024). Chitosan-Based Biomaterial in Wound Healing: A Review *Cureus*, *16*(2), e55193. DOI: 10.7759/cureus.55193

Rajkumari, N. P., Roy, P., Siddika, S., Adhikary, K., & Goswami, P. (2023). Enhancing anti-inflammatory and antibacterial activity of curcumin by nano composing with curcumin reduced copper nano for the treatment of bacterial infection. *Materials Science and Engineering B*, *292*, 116416. DOI: 10.1016/j.mseb.2023.116416

Raju, R., & Prasad, A. S., & S, R. K. (2024). Anti-inflammatory and Antioxidant Activity of Neem and Kirata-Induced Silver Nanoparticles Against Oral Biofilm: An In Vitro Study. *Cureus*, *16*(8), e67708. DOI: 10.7759/cureus.67708 PMID: 39318902

Ramakrishnan, T., Mohan Gift, M. D., Chitradevi, S., Jegan, R., & Subha Hency Jose, P. Nagaraja, Rajneesh Sharma H.N., Selvakumar P., Sintayehu Mekuria Hailegiorgis, (2022). "Study of Numerous Resins Used in Polymer Matrix Composite Materials", Advances in Materials Science and Engineering, vol. 2022, Article ID 1088926, 8 pages, 2022. https://doi.org/DOI: 10.1155/2022/1088926

Ranjbar-Mohammadi, M., & Bahrami, S. H. (2018). Alginate-based wound dressings: Recent advances and future perspectives. *Carbohydrate Polymers*, *206*, 473–488. DOI: 10.1016/j.carbpol.2018.11.035

Ranjitha, P. K., Selvakumar, P., Anute, N., Manjunath, T., Sureshkrishna, G., & Pougajendy, S. (2025). Transportation challenges in islands tourism. In Hassan, V. (Ed.), *Navigating mass tourism to island destinations: Preservation and cultural heritage challenges* (pp. 287–312). IGI Global Scientific Publishing., DOI: 10.4018/979-8-3693-9107-5.ch011

Rathod, L., Bhowmick, S., Patel, P., & Sawant, K. (2022). Calendula flower extract loaded collagen film exhibits superior wound healing potential: Preparation, evaluation, in-vitro & in-vivo wound healing study. *Journal of Drug Delivery Science and Technology*, *72*, 103363.

Ravikumar, P., Krishna, V., & Manjunath, K. (2013). Herbal excipients in novel drug delivery systems. *International Journal of Pharma and Bio Sciences*, *4*(2), 334–345.

Rees, L., & Weil, A. (2001). Integrated medicine: Imbues orthodox medicine with the values of complementary medicine. *BMJ (Clinical Research Ed.)*, *322*(7279), 119. PMID: 11159553

Ren, H., Zhang, Z., Chen, X., & He, C. (2024). Stimuli-Responsive Hydrogel Adhesives for Wound Closure and Tissue Regeneration. *Macromolecular Bioscience*, *24*(3), 2300379. DOI: 10.1002/mabi.202300379 PMID: 37827713

Research and Markets. (2025). *Organic pharmaceutical excipients market report 2025*. https://www.researchandmarkets.com/reports/5865933/organic-pharmaceutical-excipients-market-report

Rezvanian, M., Ng, S.-F., Alavi, T., & Ahmad, W. (2021). In-vivo evaluation of Alginate-Pectin hydrogel film loaded with Simvastatin for diabetic wound healing in Streptozotocin-induced diabetic rats. *International Journal of Biological Macromolecules*, *171*, 308–319. DOI: 10.1016/j.ijbiomac.2020.12.221 PMID: 33421467

Rigo, C., Ferroni, L., Tocco, I., Roman, M., Munivrana, I., Gardin, C., Cairns, W. R., Vindigni, V., Azzena, B., Barbante, C., & Zavan, B. (2013). Active silver nanoparticles for wound healing. *International Journal of Molecular Sciences*, *14*(3), 4817–4840. DOI: 10.3390/ijms14034817 PMID: 23455461

Rodrigues, M., Kosaric, N., Bonham, C. A., & Gurtner, G. C. (2019). Wound Healing: A Cellular Perspective. *Physiological Reviews*, *99*(1), 665–706. DOI: 10.1152/physrev.00067.2017 PMID: 30475656

Rodriguez, P. G., Felix, F. N., Woodley, D. T., & Shim, E. K. (2008). The role of oxygen in wound healing: A review of the literature. *Dermatologic Surgery*, *34*(9), 1159–1169. DOI: 10.1111/j.1524-4725.2008.34254.x PMID: 18513296

Rojas, P., Jung-Cook, H., Ruiz-Sánchez, E., Rojas-Tomé, I. S., Rojas, C., López-Ramírez, A. M., & Reséndiz-Albor, A. A. (2022). Historical Aspects of Herbal Use and Comparison of Current Regulations of Herbal Products between Mexico, Canada and the United States of America. *International Journal of Environmental Research and Public Health, 19*(23), 15690. DOI: 10.3390/ijerph192315690 PMID: 36497761

Rosyid, F. N. (2022). Wounds: Physiological mechanisms and factors affecting healing. *International Journal of Research in Medical Sciences, 10*(4), 1001–1006. DOI: 10.18203/2320-6012.ijrms20221000

Rousseaux, C. G. (2023). Herbal remedies. In *Haschek and Rousseaux's handbook of toxicologic pathology* (pp. 183–303). Academic Press.

Ruedrich, E. D., Henzel, M. K., Hausman, B. S., & Bogie, K. M. (2013). Reference gene identification for reverse transcription-quantitative polymerase chain reaction analysis in an ischemic wound-healing model. *Journal of Biomolecular Techniques: JBT, 24*, 181–186. DOI: 10.7171/jbt.13-2404-003 PMID: 24294111

Ruel-Gariepy, E., & Leroux, J. C. (2004). In situ-forming hydrogels—Review of temperature-sensitive systems. *European Journal of Pharmaceutics and Biopharmaceutics, 58*(2), 409–426. DOI: 10.1016/j.ejpb.2004.03.019 PMID: 15296964

Rujitanaroj, P. O., Pimpha, N., & Supaphol, P. (2008). Wound-dressing materials with antibacterial activity from electrospun gelatin fiber mats containing silver nanoparticles. *Polymer, 49*(21), 4723–4732. DOI: 10.1016/j.polymer.2008.08.021

Russell, W. M. S., & Burch, R. L. (1959). *The principles of humane experimental technique*. Methuen.

Ryu, W. H.. (2017). Clinical evaluation of chitosan-based wound dressing in diabetic foot ulcers: A randomized controlled trial. *Diabetes Research and Clinical Practice, 126*, 117–123. DOI: 10.1016/j.diabres.2017.01.027

Sabando, C., Ide, W., Rodríguez-Díaz, M., Cabrera-Barjas, G., Castaño, J., Bouza, R., Müller, N., Gutiérrez, C., Barral, L., Rojas, J., Martínez, F., & Rodríguez-Llamazares, S. (2020). A Novel Hydrocolloid Film Based on Pectin, Starch and Gunnera tinctoria and Ugni molinae Plant Extracts for Wound Dressing Applications. *Current Topics in Medicinal Chemistry, 20*(4), 280–292. DOI: 10.2174/15680266206662001241 00631 PMID: 31976835

Saberianpour, S., Heidarzadeh, M., Geranmayeh, M. H., Hosseinkhani, H., Rahbarghazi, R., & Nouri, M. (2018). Tissue engineering strategies for the induction of angiogenesis using biomaterials. *Journal of Biological Engineering, 12*(1), 36. DOI: 10.1186/s13036-018-0129-5 PMID: 30603044

Saenchoopa, A., Plaeyao, K., Talodthaisong, C., Thet Tun, W. S., Nasomjai, P., Lapmanee, S., Somsakeesit, L. O., Hutchison, J. A., & Kulchat, S. (2025). Development of Antibacterial Hydrogels Based on Biopolymer Aloe Vera/Gelatin/Sodium Alginate Composited With SM-AgNPs Loaded Curcumin-Nanoliposomes. *Macromolecular Bioscience*, *25*(4), e2400504. DOI: 10.1002/mabi.202400504 PMID: 39748596

Safta, D. A., Bogdan, C., Iurian, S., & Moldovan, M.-L. (2025). Optimization of Film-Dressings Containing Herbal Extracts for Wound Care—A Quality by Design Approach. *Gels 2025, Vol. 11, Page 322, 11*(5), 322. DOI: 10.3390/GELS11050322

Saha, D., & Bhattacharya, S. (2010). Hydrocolloids as thickening and gelling agents in food: A critical review. *Journal of Food Science and Technology*, *47*(6), 587–597. DOI: 10.1007/s13197-010-0162-6 PMID: 23572691

Sahoo, S. K., Parveen, S., & Panda, J. J. (2008). The present and future of nanotechnology in human health care. *Nanomedicine; Nanotechnology, Biology, and Medicine*, *3*(1), 20–31. PMID: 17379166

Said, N. S., Olawuyi, I. F., & Lee, W. Y. (2023). Pectin Hydrogels: Gel-Forming Behaviors, Mechanisms, and Food Applications. *Gels (Basel, Switzerland)*, *9*(9), 732. DOI: 10.3390/gels9090732 PMID: 37754413

Salehi, B., Mishra, A. P., Nigam, M., Sener, B., Kilic, M., Sharifi-Rad, M., Fokou, P. V. T., Martins, N., & Sharifi-Rad, J. (2018). Resveratrol: A Double-Edged Sword in Health Benefits. *Biomedicines*, *6*(3), 91. DOI: 10.3390/biomedicines6030091 PMID: 30205595

Salmaso, S., & Caliceti, P. (2021). Pullulan-based bioconjugates for ocular drug delivery. *European Journal of Pharmaceutical Sciences*, *158*, 105667. DOI: 10.1016/j.ejps.2021.105667

Sangnim, T., Puri, V., Dheer, D., Venkatesh, D. N., Huanbutta, K., & Sharma, A. (2024). Nanomaterials in the Wound Healing Process: New Insights and Advancements. *Pharmaceutics*, *16*(3), 300. DOI: 10.3390/pharmaceutics16030300 PMID: 38543194

Saporito, F., Sandri, G., Bonferoni, M. C., Rossi, S., Boselli, C., Cornaglia, A. I., Mannucci, B., Grisoli, P., Vigani, B., & Ferrari, F. (2017). Essential oil-loaded lipid nanoparticles for wound healing. *International Journal of Nanomedicine*, *13*, 175. DOI: 10.2147/IJN.S152529 PMID: 29343956

Satchanska, G., Davidova, S., & Petrov, P. D. (2024). Natural and Synthetic Polymers for Biomedical and Environmental Applications. *Polymers*, *16*(8), 1159. DOI: 10.3390/POLYM16081159 PMID: 38675078

Savekar, P. L., Nadaf, S. J., Killedar, S. G., Kumbar, V. M., Hoskeri, J. H., Bhagwat, D. A., & Gurav, S. S. (2024). Citric acid cross-linked pomegranate peel extract-loaded pH-responsive β-cyclodextrin/carboxymethyl tapioca starch hydrogel film for diabetic wound healing. *International Journal of Biological Macromolecules, 274*, 133366. DOI: 10.1016/j.ijbiomac.2024.133366 PMID: 38914385

Schilling, J. A. (1968). Wound healing. *Physiological Reviews, 48*(2-4), 374. PMID: 4231314

Schraufstatter, I. U., Chung, J., & Burger, M. (2001). IL-8 activates endothelial cell CXCR1 and CXCR2 through Rho and Rac signaling pathways. *American Journal of Physiology. Lung Cellular and Molecular Physiology, 280*(6), L1094–L1103. DOI: 10.1152/ajplung.2001.280.6.L1094 PMID: 11350788

Schultz, G. S., Chin, G. A., Moldawer, L., & Diegelmann, R. F. (2011). Principles of Wound Healing. *Diabetic Foot Problems*, 395–402. DOI: 10.1142/9789812791535_0028

Schultz, G. S., Chin, G. A., Moldawer, L., & Diegelmann, R. F. (2011). Principles of wound healing. In Fitridge, R., & Thompson, M. (Eds.), *Mechanisms of vascular disease: A reference book for vascular specialists* (pp. 423–451). University of Adelaide Press., https://www.ncbi.nlm.nih.gov/books/NBK534261/

Scully, D., Sfyri, P., Wilkinson, H. N., Acebes-Huerta, A., Verpoorten, S., Muñoz-Turrillas, M. C., & Matsakas, A. (2020). Optimising platelet secretomes to deliver robust tissue-specific regeneration. *Journal of Tissue Engineering and Regenerative Medicine, 14*(1), 82–98. DOI: 10.1002/term.2965 PMID: 31603629

Secretariat Standardization Administration of China. (2009). *ISO/TC 249 - Traditional medicine*. International Organization for Standardization. https://www.iso.org/committee/598435.html

Sekar, M. P., Budharaju, H., Sethuraman, S., & Sundaramurthi, D. (2023). Carboxymethyl cellulose-agarose-gelatin: A thermoresponsive triad bioink composition to fabricate volumetric soft tissue constructs. *SLAS Technology, 28*(3), 183–198. DOI: 10.1016/j.slast.2023.04.005 PMID: 37149220

Sen, C. K. (2009). Wound healing essentials: Let there be oxygen. *Wound Repair and Regeneration, 17*(1), 1–18. PMID: 19152646

Sen, C. K. (2021). Human wounds and its burden: An updated compendium of estimates. *Advances in Wound Care, 8*(2), 39–48. DOI: 10.1089/wound.2021.0026 PMID: 30809421

Serini, S., Trombino, S., Cassano, R., Marino, M., & Calviello, G. (2025). Anti-inflammatory effects of curcumin-based nanoparticles containing α-linolenic acid in a model of psoriasis in vitro. *Nutrients*, *17*(4), 692. DOI: 10.3390/nu17040692 PMID: 40005020

Serrano, D. R., Kara, A., Yuste, I., Luciano, F. C., Ongoren, B., Anaya, B. J., & Lalatsa, A. (2023). 3D printing technologies in personalized medicine, nanomedicines, and biopharmaceuticals. *Pharmaceutics*, *15*(2), 313. PMID: 36839636

Shah, J., Patel, D., Rananavare, D., Hudson, D., Tran, M., Schloss, R., Langrana, N., Berthiaume, F., & Kumar, S. (2025). Recent advancements in chitosan-based biomaterials for wound healing. *Journal of Functional Biomaterials*, *16*(2), 45. DOI: 10.3390/jfb16020045 PMID: 39997579

Shaikh, R., Singh, T. R. R., Garland, M. J., Woolfson, A. D., & Donnelly, R. F. (2011). Mucoadhesive drug delivery systems. *Journal of Pharmacy & Bioallied Sciences*, *3*(1), 89–100. PMID: 21430958

Shaikh, T., Ali, J., & Baboota, S. (2011). Herbal excipients in novel drug delivery systems. *Pharmacognosy Reviews*, *5*(9), 46–52.

Sharma, A., Puri, V., Bakshi, I. S., & Kumar, P. (2022). Herbal bioactive-incorporated scaffolds for wound healing applications. In *Herbal Bioactive-Based Drug Delivery Systems* (pp. 311–330). Academic Press.

Sharma, A., Sharma, N., & Luthra, G. (2023). The Crucial Role of Microbiological Testing in Ensuring Safety and Efficacy of Medical Devices: An Overview. *Journal of Pharmaceutical Research International*, *35*, 47–55. DOI: 10.9734/jpri/2023/v35i127364

Sharma, S., & Singh, S. (2021). Blockchain technology for enhancing transparency and traceability in herbal medicine supply chains. *Journal of Ethnopharmacology*, *268*, 113605.

Sharma, S., Sudhakara, P., Singh, J., Ilyas, R. A., Asyraf, M. R. M., & Razman, M. R. (2021). Critical review of biodegradable and bioactive polymer composites for bone tissue engineering and drug delivery applications. *Polymers*, *13*(16), 2623. PMID: 34451161

Sharma, Y., Jeyabalan, G., & Singh, R. (2013). Potential wound healing agents from medicinal plants: A review. *Pharmacologia*, *4*(5), 349–358. DOI: 10.5567/pharmacologia.2013.349.358

Shedoeva, A., Leavesley, D., Upton, Z., & Fan, C. (2019a). Wound Healing and the Use of Medicinal Plants. *Evidence-Based Complementary and Alternative Medicine: eCAM, 2684108*. Advance online publication. DOI: 10.1155/2019/2684108 PMID: 31662773

Sheokand, B., Vats, M., Kumar, A., Srivastava, C. M., Bahadur, I., & Pathak, S. R. (2023). Natural polymers used in the dressing materials for wound healing: Past, present and future. *Journal of Polymer Science*, *61*(14), 1389–1414. DOI: 10.1002/POL.20220734

Shiva, V. (2001). *Protect or plunder? Understanding intellectual property rights*. Zed Books.

Shukla, A., Rasik, A. M., Jain, G. K., Shankar, R., Kulshrestha, D. K., & Dhawan, B. N. (1999). In vitro and in vivo wound healing activity of asiaticoside isolated from *Centella asiatica. Journal of Ethnopharmacology*, *65*(1), 1–11. PMID: 10350364

Shukla, V. K., Ansari, M. A., & Gupta, S. K. (2005). Wound healing research: A perspective from India. *The International Journal of Lower Extremity Wounds*, *4*, 7–8. PMID: 15860447

Siddiqui, M. Z. (2011). Boswellia Serrata, A Potential Antiinflammatory Agent: An Overview. *Indian Journal of Pharmaceutical Sciences*, *73*(3), 255. DOI: 10.4103/0250-474X.93507 PMID: 22457547

Siefert, S. A., & Sarkar, R. (2012). Matrix metalloproteinases in vascular physiology and disease. *Vascular*, *20*(4), 210–216. DOI: 10.1258/vasc.2011.201202 PMID: 22896663

Simpson, D. M., & Ross, R. U. S. S. E. L. L. (1972). The neutrophilic leukocyte in wound repair: A study with antineutrophil serum. *The Journal of Clinical Investigation*, *51*(8), 2009–2023. DOI: 10.1172/JCI107007 PMID: 5054460

Sindhu, R. K., Gupta, R., Wadhera, G., & Kumar, P. (2022). Modern Herbal Nanogels: Formulation, Delivery Methods, and Applications. *Gels (Basel, Switzerland)*, *8*(2), 97. DOI: 10.3390/gels8020097 PMID: 35200478

Singh, R., Shitiz, K., & Singh, A. (2017). Chitin and chitosan: biopolymers for wound management. International Wound Journal, 14(6), 1276–1289. Portico. https://doi.org/DOI: 10.1111/iwj.12797

Singh, J., & Nayak, P. (2023). pH-responsive polymers for drug delivery: Trends and opportunities. *Journal of polymer science*, *61*(22), 2828–2850.

Singh, M. A., Wahi, A., Teotia, A., Thota, P., Varshney, R., & Gupta, M. (2024). *Novel phyto-pharmaceuticals used for wound healing*. CRC Press.

Singh, R., & Gupta, N. (2023). Pharmacovigilance in herbal medicine: Current status and future directions. *Regulatory Toxicology and Pharmacology*, *135*, 105276.

Singh, S.. (2022). Artificial intelligence in green chemistry: Designing sustainable polysaccharides for biomedical applications. *Green Chemistry*, *24*(2), 512–523. DOI: 10.1039/D1GC03982A

Sipponen, A., Kuokkanen, O., Tiihonen, R., Kauppinen, H., & Jokinen, J. J. (2012). Natural coniferous resin salve used to treat complicated surgical wounds: Pilot clinical trial on healing and costs. *International Journal of Dermatology*, *51*(6), 726–732. DOI: 10.1111/J.1365-4632.2011.05397.X PMID: 22607295

Sivamani, R. K., Ma, B. R., Wehrli, L. N., & Maverakis, E. (2012). Phytochemicals and naturally derived substances for wound healing. *Advances in Wound Care (New Rochelle, N.Y.)*, *1*(5), 213–217. PMID: 24527308

Smith+Nephew. (2025). *IODOSORB Cadexomer iodine range*. https://www.smith-nephew.com/en/health-care-professionals/products/advanced-wound-management/iodosorb-global

Smith, J., & Berkes, F. (2018). Sustainability and indigenous knowledge: Implications for environmental ethics in natural resource management. *Environmental Ethics*, *40*(1), 1–15.

Solovieva, A., Kopylov, A., Cherkasova, A., Shershnev, I., Kaplin, V., Timofeeva, V., Akovantseva, A., Savko, M., Gulin, A., Zarkhina, T., Aksenova, N., & Timashev, P. (2024). Methylene Blue Solid Alginate Gels for Photodynamic Therapy: The Peculiarities of Production and Controlled Release of the Dye. *Polymers*, *16*(19), 2819. DOI: 10.3390/polym16192819 PMID: 39408531

Sonawane, S. R., Gokhale, J. S., Mulla, M. Z., Kandu, V. R., & Patil, S. A. (2021). A comprehensive overview of functional and rheological properties of Aloe vera and its application in foods. *Journal of Food Science and Technology*, *58*(4), 1217–1226. DOI: 10.1007/s13197-020-04661-6 PMID: 33746250

Song, J. W., & Chung, K. C. (2010). Observational studies: Cohort and case-control studies. *Plastic and Reconstructive Surgery*, *126*(6), 2234–2242. DOI: 10.1097/PRS.0b013e3181f44abc PMID: 20697313

Soni, N. S.. (2021). Chitosan-based hydrogels in the treatment of chronic diabetic ulcers: A clinical trial. *Biomaterials Science*, *9*(4), 633–644. DOI: 10.1039/D0BM02180D

Soni, S., Namdeo, S., Agrawal, P., Haider, T., & Soni, V. (2023). Novel modalities of delivering herbal medicines for wound healing: A review. *Dermatological Reviews*, *4*(5), 194–210.

Soni, V., Jain, P., Haider, T., Pandey, V., & Tekade, R. K. (2018). Documentation protocol in product development including clinical records. In Tekade, R. K. (Ed.), *Advances in pharmaceutical product development and research: Dosage form design parameters* (pp. 403–440). Academic Press., DOI: 10.1016/B978-0-12-814421-3.00012-9

Soulaidopoulos, S., Tsiogka, A., Chrysohoou, C., Lazarou, E., Aznaouridis, K., Doundoulakis, I., Tyrovola, D., Tousoulis, D., Tsioufis, K., Vlachopoulos, C., & Lazaros, G. (2022). Overview of Chios Mastic Gum (Pistacia lentiscus) Effects on Human Health. *Nutrients*, *14*(3), 590. DOI: 10.3390/NU14030590 PMID: 35276949

Sreenivasulu, A., & Manimozhi, T. Satheesh kumar P., Selvakumar P. and Singh P.,(2022). "The Model of Smart Sensing Device For Sensitive Nanoclusters Modification in Sensing Properties," 2022 2nd International Conference on Advance Computing and Innovative Technologies in Engineering (ICACITE), Greater Noida, India, 2022, pp. 1043-1047, doi: DOI: 10.1109/ICACITE53722.2022.9823846

Srinivas, K., Anand, A. R., & Nath, R. K. (2019). Informed consent in clinical research: Revisiting its history, current challenges, and future prospects. *Journal of Clinical and Diagnostic Research: JCDR*, *13*(4), JE01–JE04.

Steinhoff, B. (2021). Challenges in the quality of herbal medicinal products with a specific focus on contaminants. *Phytochemical Analysis*, *32*(2), 117–123. PMID: 31402494

Steneck, N. H. (2006). Fostering integrity in research: Definitions, current knowledge, and future directions. *Science and Engineering Ethics*, *12*(1), 53–74. PMID: 16501647

Stotts, N. A., & Hunt, T. K. (1997). Managing bacterial colonization and infection. *Clinics in Geriatric Medicine*, *13*, 565–573. DOI: 10.1016/S0749-0690(18)30160-5 PMID: 9227945

Stout, E. I., & McKessor, A. (2012). Glycerin-based hydrogel for infection control. *Advances in Wound Care*, *1*(1), 48–51. DOI: 10.1089/wound.2011.0288 PMID: 24527279

Strausberg, J., Lehmann, N., Kröger, K., Maier, I., & Schneider, H. N. W. [initials expanded as per source]. (2007). Changes in secondary care may explain increasing pressure ulcer rates in a university clinic in Germany. *Wound Management*, *5*, 194–198.

Su, C., Chen, Y., Tian, S., Lu, C., & Lv, Q. (2022). Natural materials for 3D printing and their applications. *Gels (Basel, Switzerland)*, *8*(11), 748. PMID: 36421570

Sugumaran, K. M. D., Pandiyarajan V., Y. B S, Selvakumar P. and M. S, (2024). "Analysis of Electromyography Signals for Control of Mechanical Prosthesis using Machine Learning Techniques," 2024 2nd International Conference on Intelligent Data Communication Technologies and Internet of Things (IDCIoT), Bengaluru, India, 2024, pp. 1059-1067, doi: DOI: 10.1109/IDCIoT59759.2024.10467707

Sustersic, M., Gauchet, A., Foote, A., & Bosson, J. L. (2017). How best to use and evaluate Patient Information Leaflets given during a consultation: A systematic review of literature reviews. *Health Expectations*, *20*(4), 531–542. DOI: 10.1111/hex.12487 PMID: 27669682

Takahashi, A., Flanigan, M. E., McEwen, B. S., & Russo, S. J. (2018). Aggression, social stress, and the immune system in humans and animal models. *Frontiers in Behavioral Neuroscience*, *12*, 56. DOI: 10.3389/fnbeh.2018.00056 PMID: 29623033

Tamilarasi, G. P., Krishnan, M., Sabarees, G., Gouthaman, S., Alagarsamy, V., & Solomon, V. R. (2022). Emerging trends in curcumin embedded electrospun nanofibers for impaired diabetic wound healing. *Applied Nanoscience*, *3*(4), 202–232.

Tanaka, Y., & Velasquez, C. (2024). Multi-agent AI and online safety. In Bennett, J. (Ed.), *Distributed AI in public discourse* (pp. 119–144). GridAI Publishers., DOI: 10.4018/978-9-9999-2222-3.ch007

Tan, G., Wang, L., Pan, W., & Chen, K. (2022). Polysaccharide electrospun nanofibers for wound healing applications. *International Journal of Nanomedicine*, *17*, 3913–3931. DOI: 10.2147/IJN.S371900 PMID: 36097445

Tang, N., Zheng, Y., Jiang, X., Zhou, C., Jin, H., Jin, K., Wu, W., & Haick, H. (2021). Wearable Sensors and Systems for Wound Healing-Related pH and Temperature Detection. *Micromachines*, *12*(4), 430. DOI: 10.3390/mi12040430 PMID: 33919752

Tao, Y., Li, J., Hu, W., & Zhou, X. (2023). Advances in ionically crosslinked polysaccharide hydrogels for biomedical applications. *Gels (Basel, Switzerland)*, *9*(3), 206. DOI: 10.3390/gels9030206 PMID: 36975655

Tapia-Guerrero, Y. S., Del Prado-Audelo, M. L., Borbolla-Jiménez, F. V., Gomez, D. M. G., García-Aguirre, I., Colín-Castro, C. A., Morales-González, J. A., Leyva-Gómez, G., & Magaña, J. J. (2020). Effect of UV and Gamma Irradiation Sterilization Processes in the Properties of Different Polymeric Nanoparticles for Biomedical Applications. *Materials (Basel, Switzerland)*, *13*(5), 1090. DOI: 10.3390/ma13051090 PMID: 32121529

Tatarusanu, S. M., Lupascu, F. G., Profire, B. S., Szilagyi, A., Gardikiotis, I., Iacob, A. T., & Profire, L. (2023). Modern approaches in wounds management. *Polymers*, *15*(17), 3648. DOI: 10.3390/polym15173648 PMID: 37688274

Tejada, S., Manayi, A., Daglia, M., Nabavi, S. F., Sureda, A., Hajheydari, Z., Gortzi, O., Pazoki-Toroudi, H., & Nabavi, S. M. (2016). Wound Healing Effects of Curcumin: A Short Review. *Current Pharmaceutical Biotechnology*, *17*(11), 1002–1007. DOI: 10.2174/1389201017666160721123109 PMID: 27640646

Teja, P. K., Mithiya, J., Kate, A. S., Bairwa, K., & Chauthe, S. K. (2022). Herbal nanomedicines: Recent advancements, challenges, opportunities and regulatory overview. *Phytomedicine*, *96*, 153890. DOI: 10.1016/j.phymed.2021.153890 PMID: 35026510

Tekleyes, B., Huluka, S. A., Wondu, K., & Wondmkun, Y. T. (2021). Wound healing activity of 80% methanol leaf extract of zehneria scabra (lf) sond (cucurbitaceae) in mice. *Journal of Experimental Pharmacology*, *13*, 537. PMID: 34104005

Ten Kate, K., & Laird, S. A. (2018). *The commercial use of biodiversity: Access to genetic resources and benefit-sharing*. Earthscan.

Teodorescu, M., Bercea, M., & Morariu, S. (2018). Biomaterials of poly (vinyl alcohol) and natural polymers. *Polymer Reviews (Philadelphia, Pa.)*, *58*(2), 247–287.

Tessema, Z., & Molla, Y. (2021). Evaluation of the wound healing activity of the crude extract of root bark of Brucea antidysentrica, the leaves of Dodonaea angustifolia and Rhamnus prinoides in mice. *Heliyon*, *7*(1), e05901. PMID: 33521349

Thakkar, S., Anklam, E., Xu, A., Ulberth, F., Li, J., Li, B., & Tong, W. (2020). Regulatory landscape of dietary supplements and herbal medicines from a global perspective. *Regulatory Toxicology and Pharmacology*, *114*, 104647. PMID: 32305367

Thakur, L., Ghodasra, U., Patel, N., & Dabhi, M. (2011). Novel approaches for stability improvement in natural medicines. *Pharmacognosy Reviews*, *5*(9), 48–54. DOI: 10.4103/0973-7847.79099 PMID: 22096318

Thakur, N., Manna, P., & Das, J. (2019). Synthesis and biomedical applications of nanoceria, a redox active nanoparticle. *Journal of Nanobiotechnology*, *17*(1), 84. DOI: 10.1186/s12951-019-0516-9 PMID: 31291944

Thangapazham, R. L., Sharad, S., & Maheshwari, R. K. (2016). Phytochemicals in Wound Healing. *Advances in Wound Care*, *5*(5), 230. DOI: 10.1089/WOUND.2013.0505 PMID: 27134766

Thang, N. H., Chien, T. B., & Cuong, D. X. (2023). Polymer-Based Hydrogels Applied in Drug Delivery: An Overview. *Gels (Basel, Switzerland)*, *9*(7), 523. DOI: 10.3390/GELS9070523 PMID: 37504402

The United States Pharmacopeial Convention. (2018). *Pharmacopeial Discussion Group (PDG)*. https://www.usp.org/harmonized-standards/pdg

The United States Pharmacopeial Convention. (2020). *Novel excipients: New hope for therapeutic innovations*. https://qualitymatters.usp.org/novel-excipients-new-hope-therapeutic-innovations

Thomas, A. B., & Farooq, M. (2023). Ethical design patterns in content moderation. In Lee, R. (Ed.), *Architecting AI for human dignity* (pp. 51–76). DesignCode Press., DOI: 10.4018/978-3-2023-3030-1.ch003

Thomas, S. (1990). *Wound management and dressings*. Pharmaceutical Press.

Ticktin, T. (2004). The ecological implications of harvesting non-timber forest products. *Journal of Applied Ecology*, *41*(1), 11–21.

Tilburt, J. C., & Kaptchuk, T. J. (2008). Herbal medicine research and global health: An ethical analysis. *Bulletin of the World Health Organization*, *86*(8), 594–599. PMID: 18797616

Tindana, P. O., Kass, N., & Akweongo, P. (2007). The informed consent process in a rural African setting: A case study of the Kassena-Nankana District of northern Ghana. *IRB*, *29*(3), 1–6. PMID: 17847635

Tiwari, R., & Ochieng, J. (2024). Youth safey and AI policy on social media. In Mendez, A. (Ed.), *AI regulation for vulnerable populations* (pp. 88–112). DigitalCare Publishing., DOI: 10.4018/978-0-9876-1000-5.ch005

Tobin, J., & Lewison, G. (2011). Global trends in patents and intellectual property rights. *Scientometrics*, *89*(1), 1–14.

Tosif, M. M., Najda, A., Bains, A., Kaushik, R., Dhull, S. B., Chawla, P., & Walasek-Janusz, M. (2021). A Comprehensive Review on Plant-Derived Mucilage: Characterization, Functional Properties, Applications, and Its Utilization for Nanocarrier Fabrication. *Polymers*, *13*(7), 1066. DOI: 10.3390/polym13071066 PMID: 33800613

Tottoli, E. M.. (2020). Alginate-based dressings in chronic wound care: A review of their properties and clinical applications. *Journal of Applied Biomaterials & Functional Materials*, *18*(1), 1–10. DOI: 10.1177/2280800019900693

Tracy, L. E., Minasian, R. A., & Caterson, E. J. (2016). Extracellular matrix and dermal fibroblast function in the healing wound. *Advances in Wound Care (New Rochelle, N.Y.)*, *5*, 119–136. DOI: 10.1089/wound.2014.0561 PMID: 26989578

Trigo-Gutierrez, J. K., Vega-Chacón, Y., Soares, A. B., & Mima, E. G. O. (2021). Antimicrobial Activity of Curcumin in Nanoformulations: A Comprehensive Review. *International Journal of Molecular Sciences*, *22*(13), 7130. DOI: 10.3390/ijms22137130 PMID: 34281181

Tripathi, L. P., & Deshmukh, A. (2025). Decoding algorithmic bias in AI filters. In Bhat, R. (Ed.), *AI ethics across cultures* (pp. 42–69). InsightBridge Press., DOI: 10.4018/978-3-3333-4444-6.ch004

Tudoroiu, E.-E., Dinu-Pîrvu, C.-E., Albu Kaya, M. G., Popa, L., Anu a, V., Prisada, R. M., & Ghica, M. V. (2021). An Overview of Cellulose Derivatives-Based Dressings for Wound-Healing Management. *Pharmaceuticals*, *14*(12), 1215. DOI: 10.3390/ph14121215 PMID: 34959615

Uddin, M. N., & Jensen, T. (2024). Preventing radicalization through AI moderation. In Das, K. (Ed.), *AI in extremism prevention* (pp. 121–144). PeaceTech Academic., DOI: 10.4018/978-1-5678-9999-0.ch006

Ukaegbu, K., Allen, E., & Svoboda, K. K. H. (2025). Reactive Oxygen Species and Antioxidants in Wound Healing: Mechanisms and Therapeutic Potential. *International Wound Journal*, *22*(5), e70330. DOI: 10.1111/IWJ.70330 PMID: 40288766

Ullah, F., Othman, M. B. H., Javed, F., Ahmad, Z., & Akil, H. M. (2015). Classification, processing and application of hydrogels: A review. *Materials Science and Engineering C*, *57*, 414–433. PMID: 26354282

United States Pharmacopeia. (2024). *Fostering the use of novel excipients in drug products*. https://www.usp.org/sites/default/files/usp/document/public-policy/USP%20Global%20Policy%20Position_NovelExcipients_Paper_2024.pdf

Upadhaya, A.. (2009). *Healing herbs of India*. Satish Serial Publishing House.

Usman, M., Nakagawa, M., & Cheng, S. (2023). Emerging trends in green extraction techniques for bioactive natural products. *Processes (Basel, Switzerland)*, *11*(12), 3444. Advance online publication. DOI: 10.3390/pr11123444

Usman, S., Fawzy, K. A., Beevi, R., & Usman, A. (2019). Basis of Pharmaceutical Formulation. In *Nanoscale Networking and Communications Handbook* (pp. 281–319). CRC Press.

USP 61. https://www.usp.org/harmonization-standards/pdg/general-methods/microbial-enumeration

USP 62. http://www.uspbpep.com/usp31/v31261/usp31nf26s1_c62.asp

Vaibhavi, J., Rakesh, R., & Pankaj, K. (2010). Cinnamon: A pharmacological review. *Journal of Advanced Scientific and Engineering Research*, *1*(2), 19–23.

Valdez, A., & Krishnan, M. S. (2023). AI ethics in meme and short-form content. In Ho, C. (Ed.), *Content formats and AI challenges* (pp. 36–63). PopTech Press., DOI: 10.4018/978-6-7777-8888-8.ch003

Valle, K. Z. M., Saucedo Acuña, R. A., Ríos Arana, J. V., Lobo, N., Rodriguez, C., Cuevas-Gonzalez, J. C., & Tovar-Carrillo, K. L. (2020). Natural Film Based on Pectin and Allantoin for Wound Healing: Obtaining, Characterization, and Rat Model. *BioMed Research International*, *2020*(1), 6897497. DOI: 10.1155/2020/6897497 PMID: 33123582

Van den Berg, M. J., de Vries, H., & Peek, N. (2020). Harmonizing regulations for herbal medicines: An international perspective. *Regulatory Toxicology and Pharmacology*, *117*, 104770.

Van Den Bulcke, A. I., Bogdanov, B., De Rooze, N., Schacht, E. H., Cornelissen, M., & Berghmans, H. (2000). Structural and rheological properties of methacrylamide modified gelatin hydrogels. *Biomacromolecules*, *1*(1), 31–38. DOI: 10.1021/bm990017d PMID: 11709840

Vaz, V. M., & Kumar, L. (2021). 3D printing as a promising tool in personalized medicine. *AAPS PharmSciTech*, *22*, 1–20. PMID: 33458797

Veerapandian, M., Ramasundaram, S., Jerome, P., Chellasamy, G., Govindaraju, S., Yun, K., & Oh, T. H. (2023). Drug delivery application of functional nanomaterials synthesized using natural sources. *Journal of Functional Biomaterials*, *14*(8), 426. PMID: 37623670

Veith, A. P., Henderson, K., Spencer, A., Sligar, A. D., & Baker, A. B. (2019). Therapeutic strategies for enhancing angiogenesis in wound healing. *Advanced Drug Delivery Reviews*, *146*, 97–125. DOI: 10.1016/j.addr.2018.09.010 PMID: 30267742

Velnar, T., Bailey, T., & Smrkolj, V. (2009). The wound healing process: An overview of the cellular and molecular mechanisms. *The Journal of International Medical Research*, *37*(5), 1528–1542. DOI: 10.1177/147323000903700531 PMID: 19930861

Venkatesan, J., Bhatnagar, I., Manivasagan, P., Kang, K. H., & Kim, S. K. (2017). Alginate composites for wound healing: A review. *International Journal of Biological Macromolecules, 104*, 1388–1400.

Verma, A., Gautam, S. P., Bansal, K. K., Prabhakar, N., & Rosenholm, J. M. (2019). Green Nanotechnology: Advancement in Phytoformulation Research. *Medicines (Basel, Switzerland), 6*(1), 39. DOI: 10.3390/medicines6010039 PMID: 30875823

Viera-Herrera, C., Santamaría-Aguirre, J., Vizuete, K., Debut, A., Whitehead, D. C., & Alexis, F. (2020). Microcrystalline Cellulose Extracted from Native Plants as an Excipient for Solid Dosage Formulations in Drug Delivery. *Nanomaterials (Basel, Switzerland), 10*(5), 975. DOI: 10.3390/nano10050975 PMID: 32438544

Vijayakumar, G. (2024). Muniyandi Rajkumar, Rajiv Chandar N, Selvakumar P and Ramesh Duraisamy, (2024). Environmentally friendly TDS removal from waste water by electrochemical ion exchange batch-type recirculation (EIR) technique. *Environmental Science. Water Research & Technology, 10*, 826–835. DOI: 10.1039/D3EW00793F

Vijayakumar, G., Rajkumar, M., Chandar, N. R., Selvakumar, P., & Duraisamy, R. (2024). Environmentally friendly TDS removal from waste water by electrochemical ion exchange batch-type recirculation (EIR) technique. *Environmental Science. Water Research & Technology, 10*(4), 826–835.

Vilchez, A., Acevedo, F., Cea, M., Seeger, M., & Navia, R. (2020). Applications of electrospun nanofibers with antioxidant properties: A review. *Nanomaterials (Basel, Switzerland), 10*(1), 175. PMID: 31968539

Vinchhi, P., Wui, W. T., & Patel, M. M. (2024). Healing with herbs: An alliance with 'nano'for wound management. *Expert Opinion on Drug Delivery, 21*(7), 1115–1141. PMID: 39095934

Volenzo, T., & Odiyo, J. (2020). Integrating endemic medicinal plants into the global value chains: The ecological degradation challenges and opportunities. *Heliyon, 6*(9). PMID: 32995638

Vollono, L., Falconi, M., Gaziano, R., Iacovelli, F., Dika, E., Terracciano, C., Bianchi, L., & Campione, E. (2019). Potential of curcumin in skin disorders. *Nutrients, 11*(9), 2169. DOI: 10.3390/nu11092169 PMID: 31509968

Vora, L. K., Gholap, A. D., Jetha, K., Thakur, R. R. S., Solanki, H. K., & Donnelly, R. F. (2023). Artificial intelligence in pharmaceutical technology and drug delivery design. *Pharmaceutics, 15*(7), 1916. Advance online publication. DOI: 10.3390/pharmaceutics15071916 PMID: 37514102

Vowden, P., & Vowden, K. (2017). Wound dressings: Principles and practice. *Surgery (Oxford), 35*(9), 489–494. DOI: 10.1016/j.mpsur.2017.06.005

Vuong, Q. V., Chalmers, A. C., Jyoti Bhuyan, D., Bowyer, M. C., & Scarlett, C. J. (2015). Botanical, phytochemical, and anticancer properties of the *Eucalyptus* species. *Chemistry & Biodiversity*, *12*(6), 907–924. DOI: 10.1002/cbdv.201400327 PMID: 26080737

Wagner, L., & Kumar, A. (2024). Bridging digital divides with ethical AI access. In Foster, D. (Ed.), *Equity in AI technologies* (pp. 51–77). FutureVision Press., DOI: 10.4018/978-5-1212-6543-2.ch004

Wahedi, H. M., Jeong, M., Chae, J. K., Do, S. G., Yoon, H., & Kim, S. Y. (2017). Aloesin from *Aloe vera* accelerates skin wound healing by modulating MAPK/Rho and Smad signaling pathways in vitro and in vivo. *Phytomedicine*, *28*, 19–26. DOI: 10.1016/j.phymed.2017.02.004 PMID: 28478809

Walkey, C., Das, S., Seal, S., Erlichman, J., Heckman, K., & Ghibelli, L.. (2015). Catalytic properties and biomedical applications of cerium oxide nanoparticles. *Environmental Science. Nano*, *2*(1), 33–53. DOI: 10.1039/c4en00138a PMID: 26207185

Wallace, H. A., Basehore, B. M., & Zito, P. M. (2023). Wound Healing Phases. *StatPearls*. https://www.ncbi.nlm.nih.gov/books/NBK470443/

Wang, F., Liu, J., An, Q., Wang, Y., Yang, Y., Huo, T., Yang, S., Ju, R., & Quan, Q. (2023). Aloe Extracts Inhibit Skin Inflammatory Responses by Regulating NF-κB, ERK, and JNK Signaling Pathways in an LPS-Induced RAW264.7 Macrophages Model. *Clinical, cosmetic and investigational*

Wang, H., Chen, Y., Wang, L., Liu, Q., Yang, S., & Wang, C. (2023). Advancing herbal medicine: Enhancing product quality and safety through robust quality control practices. *Frontiers in Pharmacology*, *14*, 1265178. DOI: 10.3389/FPHAR.2023.1265178 PMID: 37818188

Wang, J., Wang, X., Yuan, X., & Zhang, W. (2021). Bioactive hyaluronic acid-based hydrogel loaded with VEGF for promoting diabetic wound healing. *Materials Science and Engineering C*, *120*, 111719. DOI: 10.1016/j.msec.2020.111719

Wang, J., Wang, X., Yuan, X., & Zhang, W. (2024). Recent advances in 3D bioprinted polysaccharide hydrogels for biomedical applications: A comprehensive review. *International Wound Journal*. Advance online publication. DOI: 10.1111/iwj.14533 PMID: 38069620

Wang, L., Ai, W., Zhai, Y., Li, H., Zhou, K., & Chen, H. (2015). Effects of nano-CeO with different nanocrystal morphologies on cytotoxicity in HepG2 cells. *International Journal of Environmental Research and Public Health, 12*(9), 10806–10819. DOI: 10.3390/ijerph120910806 PMID: 26404340

Wang, L., Hu, L., Peng, Z., Cao, H., Cao, D., Long, Y., & Zou, Z. (2022). Luteolin is an effective component of platycodon grandiflorus in promoting wound healing in rats with cutaneous scald injury. *Clinical, Cosmetic and Investigational Dermatology, 15*, 1715–1727. PMID: 36032411

Wang, L., Mu, Y., Xu, M., & Gao, J. (2021). Recent advances of chitosan-based injectable hydrogels for wound healing. *Journal of Materials Chemistry. B, 9*(15), 3279–3291. DOI: 10.1039/D0TB02785B

Wang, M., Huang, X., Zheng, H., Tang, Y., Zeng, K., Shao, L., & Li, L. (2021). Nanomaterials applied in wound healing: Mechanisms, limitations and perspectives. *Journal of Controlled Release, 337*, 236–247. DOI: 10.1016/j.jconrel.2021.07.017 PMID: 34273419

Wang, R., Chen, M., Pan, W., Chu, Y., & Chen, F. (2025). The design principle of natural polysaccharide hydrogels for promoting wound healing: A prospective review. *Journal of Materials Chemistry. B*. Advance online publication. DOI: 10.1039/D4TB02576H PMID: 40145143

Wang, Y., Zhang, X., & Wei, X. (2024). Recent advances in polysaccharide-based hydrogels for controlled delivery of therapeutic biomolecules. *ACS Biomaterials Science & Engineering, 10*(1), 1–15. DOI: 10.1021/acsbiomaterials.0c01784 PMID: 38186359

Wang, Z., & Fernandes, J. (2023). Algorithmic explainability for content decisions. In Silva, M. (Ed.), *Understanding AI in social media governance* (pp. 67–93). Clarity Publishing., DOI: 10.4018/978-0-2310-3210-0.ch003

Wang, Z., Xie, X., Wang, M., Ding, M., Gu, S., Xing, X., & Sun, X. (2023). Analysis of common and characteristic actions of *Panax ginseng* and *Panax notoginseng* in wound healing based on network pharmacology and meta-analysis. *Journal of Ginseng Research, 47*(4), 493–505. DOI: 10.1016/j.jgr.2023.02.005 PMID: 37397412

Warak, A. (2025). *Aloe vera farming in India*. Tractor Karvan. https://tractorkarvan.com/blog/aloe-vera-farming-in-india

Wayal, S. R., & Gurav, S. S. (2021). Evaluation of wound healing potential of Bhallatakadi Ghrita–cow ghee based polyherbal formulation: In-vivo excision and incision wound model. *Journal of Complementary & Integrative Medicine, 18*(3), 507–515. PMID: 33691354

White, E. T., & Raman, R. (2024). Ethical dilemmas in AI nudging. In Noor, I. (Ed.), *Digital influence and ethical AI* (pp. 34–58). EthicAI Press., DOI: 10.4018/978

Wichterle, O., & Lim, D. (1960). Hydrophilic gels for biological use. *Nature, 185*(4706), 117–118. DOI: 10.1038/185117a0

Wilkinson, H. N., & Hardman, M. J. (2020). Wound healing: Cellular mechanisms and pathological outcomes. *Open Biology, 10*(9), 200223. DOI: 10.1098/rsob.200223 PMID: 32993416

Winter, G. D. (1962). Formation of the scab and the rate of epithelialization of superficial wounds in the skin of the young domestic pig. *Nature, 193*, 293–294. PMID: 14007593

Witkowska, K., Paczkowska-Walendowska, M., Garbiec, E., & Cielecka-Piontek, J. (2024). Topical Application of Centella asiatica in Wound Healing: Recent Insights into Mechanisms and Clinical Efficacy. *Pharmaceutics, 16*(10), 1252. DOI: 10.3390/PHARMACEUTICS16101252 PMID: 39458583

World Health Organization. (1999). *Traditional and modern medicine: Harmonizing the two approaches: A report of the consultation meeting on traditional and modern medicine, 22-26 November 1999, Beijing, China*. WHO Regional Office for the Western Pacific.

World Health Organization. (2000). *General guidelines for methodologies on research and evaluation of traditional medicine*. Essential Medicines and Health Products Information Portal.

World Health Organization. (2007). *WHO guidelines on good manufacturing practices (GMP) for herbal medicines*. https://www.who.int/publications/i/item/9789241547161

World Health Organization. (2011). *Quality control methods for herbal materials*. https://www.who.int/publications/i/item/9789241500739

World Health Organization. (2013). *WHO traditional medicine strategy 2014–2023*. World Health Organization.

World Health Organization. (2018). *WHO guidelines on good herbal processing practices for herbal medicines* (Annex 1). In *WHO Expert Committee on Specifications for Pharmaceutical Preparations: Fifty-second report* (WHO Technical Report Series, No. 1010, pp. 81–152). https://www.gmp-compliance.org/guidelines/gmp-guideline/who-guidelines-on-good-herbal-processing-practices-for-herbal-medicines

World Health Organization. (2023). *WHO guidelines on good agricultural and collection practices for medicinal plants*. https://www.who.int/publications/i/item/9241546271

World Health Organization. (2025). *International Regulatory Cooperation for Herbal Medicines (IRCH)*. https://www.who.int/initiatives/international-regulatory-cooperation-for-herbal-medicines

World Intellectual Property Organization. (2010). *Using traditional knowledge to revive the body and a community*. IP Advantage. https://www.wipo.int/en/web/ip-advantage/w/stories/using-traditional-knowledge-to-revive-the-body-and-a-community

World Intellectual Property Organization. (2025). *WIPO treaty on intellectual property, genetic resources and associated traditional knowledge*. https://www.wipo.int/treaties/en/ip/gratk

Wu, Y.. (2020). 3D printing of alginate-based scaffolds for cartilage tissue engineering. *Materials Science and Engineering C*, *116*, 111198. DOI: 10.1016/j.msec.2020.111198

Xiong, Y., Chen, L., Man, J., Hu, Y., & Cui, X. (2019). Chemical and bioactive comparison of *Panax notoginseng* root and rhizome in raw and steamed forms. *Journal of Ginseng Research*, *43*(3), 385–393. DOI: 10.1016/j.jgr.2017.11.004 PMID: 31308810

Xuan, H., Du, Q., Li, R., Shen, X., Zhou, J., Li, B., & Yuan, H. (2023). Shape-memory-reduced graphene/chitosan cryogels for non-compressible wounds. *International Journal of Molecular Sciences*, *24*(2), 1389. DOI: 10.3390/ijms24021389 PMID: 36674906

Xuan, H., Wu, S., Fei, S., Li, B., Yang, Y., & Yuan, H. (2021). Injectable nanofiber-polysaccharide self-healing hydrogels for wound healing. *Materials Science and Engineering C*, *128*, 112264. DOI: 10.1016/j.msec.2021.112264 PMID: 34474823

Xue, Y., Yang, F., Wu, L., Xia, D., & Liu, Y. (2024). CeO2 nanoparticles to promote wound healing: A systematic review. *Advanced Healthcare Materials, 13*(6), e2302858. DOI: 10.1002/adhm.202302858 PMID: 37947125

Xu, N., Wang, L., Guan, J., Tang, C., He, N., Zhang, W., & Fu, S. (2018). Wound healing effects of a Curcuma zedoaria polysaccharide with platelet-rich plasma exosomes assembled on chitosan/silk hydrogel sponge in a diabetic rat model. *International Journal of Biological Macromolecules, 117*, 102–107. PMID: 29772339

Yadav, B. K., Gidwani, B., & Vyas, A. (2016). Rosin: Recent advances and potential applications in novel drug delivery system. *Journal of Bioactive and Compatible Polymers, 31*(2), 111–126.

Yamaguchi, N.. (2019). Hyaluronic acid-based hydrogel dressings for burn wound healing: A clinical evaluation. *Journal of Burn Care & Research; Official Publication of the American Burn Association, 40*(4), 512–518. DOI: 10.1093/jbcr/iry047

Yang, B. Y., Zhou, Z. Y., Liu, S. Y., Shi, M. J., Liu, X. J., & Cheng, T. M.. (2022). Porous Se@SiO2 nanoparticles enhance wound healing by ROS-PI3K/akt pathway in dermal fibroblasts and reduce scar formation. *Frontiers in Bioengineering and Biotechnology, 10*, 852482. DOI: 10.3389/fbioe.2022.852482 PMID: 35387298

Yang, D., Chen, H., Wei, H., Liu, A., Wei, D.-X., & Chen, J. (2024). Hydrogel wound dressings containing bioactive compounds originated from traditional Chinese herbs: A review. *Smart Materials in Medicine, 5*(1), 153–165. DOI: 10.1016/j.smaim.2023.10.004

Yang, G., Xiao, Z., Ren, X., Long, H., & Qian, H. (2021). Redox-responsive hydrogels for drug delivery and tissue engineering applications. *Reactive & Functional Polymers, 163*, 104895. DOI: 10.1016/j.reactfunctpolym.2021.104895

Yang, J., Pi, A., Yan, L., Li, J., Nan, S., Zhang, J., & Hao, Y. (2022). Research Progress on Therapeutic Effect and Mechanism of Propolis on Wound Healing. *Evidence-Based Complementary and Alternative Medicine: eCAM, 5798941*. Advance online publication. DOI: 10.1155/2022/5798941 PMID: 35911156

Yang, J., & Wang, S. (2023). Polysaccharide-based multifunctional hydrogel bioadhesives for wound healing: A review. *Gels (Basel, Switzerland), 9*(2), 138. DOI: 10.3390/gels9020138 PMID: 36826308

Yang, J., & Weinberg, R. A. (2008). Epithelial-mesenchymal transition: At the crossroads of development and tumor metastasis. *Developmental Cell, 14*(6), 818–829. DOI: 10.1016/j.devcel.2008.05.009 PMID: 18539112

Yang, S., Hu, X., Zhu, J., Zheng, B., Bi, W., Wang, X., Wu, J., Mi, Z., & Wu, Y. (2025). Aspects and Implementation of Pharmaceutical Quality by Design from Conceptual Frameworks to Industrial Applications. *Pharmaceutics*, *17*(5), 623. DOI: 10.3390/pharmaceutics17050623 PMID: 40430914

Yang, W., Zhang, Q., Zhou, J., Li, L., Li, Y., Zhu, L., Narain, R., Nan, K., & Chen, Y. (2024). Self-Healing Guar Gum-Based Nanocomposite Hydrogel Promotes Infected Wound Healing through Photothermal Antibacterial Therapy. *Biomacromolecules*, *25*(6), 3432–3448. DOI: 10.1021/ACS.BIOMAC.4C00080 PMID: 38771294

Yan, M., Hu, S.-Y., Wang, Z.-G., Hong, R., Peng, X., Kuzmanović, M., Yang, M., Dai, R., Wang, Y., Gou, J., Li, K., Xu, J.-Z., & Li, Z.-M. (2024). Antibacterial, fatigue-resistant, and self-healing dressing from natural-based composite hydrogels for infected wound healing. *Biomacromolecules*, *25*(4), 2438–2448. DOI: 10.1021/acs.biomac.3c01385 PMID: 38502912

Yaşayan, G. (2020). Chitosan films and chitosan/pectin polyelectrolyte complexes encapsulating silver sulfadiazine for wound healing. *İstanbul Journal of Pharmaceutics*, *50*(3). DOI: 10.26650/IstanbulJPharm.2020.0021

Yaseen, H. S., Asif, M., Saadullah, M., Asghar, S., Shams, M. U., Bazmi, R. R., Saleem, M., Yousaf, H. M., & Yaseen, M. (2020). Methanolic extract of Ephedra ciliata promotes wound healing and arrests inflammatory cascade in vivo through downregulation of TNF-α. *Inflammopharmacology*, *28*(6), 1691–1704. PMID: 32385747

Yasin, S. N. N., Said, Z., Halib, N., Rahman, Z. A., & Mokhzani, N. I. (2023). Polymer-based hydrogel loaded with honey in drug delivery system for wound healing applications. *Polymers*, *15*(14), 3085. DOI: 10.3390/polym15143085 PMID: 37514474

Yik, M. H., Wong, V. C. T., Wong, T., & Shaw, P. (2021). HerBChain, a blockchain-based informative platform for quality assurance and quality control of herbal products. *Journal of Traditional and Complementary Medicine*, *11*(6), 598–600. DOI: 10.1016/j.jtcme.2021.06.005 PMID: 34765524

Yildizbakan, L., Iqbal, N., Ganguly, P., Kumi-Barimah, E., Do, T., & Jones, E.. (2023). Fabrication and characterisation of the cytotoxic and antibacterial properties of chitosan-cerium oxide porous scaffolds. *Antibiotics (Basel, Switzerland)*, *12*(6), 1004. DOI: 10.3390/antibiotics12061004 PMID: 37370323

Yin, G., Wang, Z., Wang, Z., & Wang, X. (2018). Topical application of quercetin improves wound healing in pressure ulcer lesions. *Experimental Dermatology*, *27*(7), 779–786. PMID: 29733461

Yin, Y., Huang, J., Wang, T., Yang, R., Hu, H., Manuka, M., & Ma, B. (2023). Effect of Hydroxypropyl methyl cellulose (HPMC) on rheology and printability of the first printed layer of cement activated slag-based 3D printing concrete. *Construction & Building Materials*, *405*, 133347.

Young, A., & McNaught, C. E. (2011). The physiology of wound healing. *Surgery (Oxford)*, *29*(10), 475–479. DOI: 10.1016/s0196-0644(88)80351-2

Yu, L. X., Amidon, G., Khan, M. A., Hoag, S. W., Polli, J., Raju, G. K., & Woodcock, J. (2014). Understanding pharmaceutical quality by design. *The AAPS Journal*, *16*(4), 771–783. DOI: 10.1208/s12248-014-9598-3 PMID: 24854893

Yu, S., Sun, H., Li, Y., Wei, S., Xu, J., & Liu, J. (2022). Hydrogels as promising platforms for engineered living bacteria-mediated therapeutic systems. *Materials Today. Bio*, *16*, 100435. PMID: 36164505

Zahedi, P., Rezaeian, I., Ranaei-Siadat, S. O., Jafari, S. H., & Supaphol, P. (2010). A review on wound dressings with an emphasis on electrospun nanofibrous polymeric bandages. *Polymers for Advanced Technologies*, *21*(2), 77–95.

Zaidi, A., & Green, L. (2019). Physiology of haemostasis. *Anaesthesia and Intensive Care Medicine*, *20*(3), 152–158. DOI: 10.1016/j.mpaic.2019.01.005

Zarei, N., & Hassanzadeh-Tabrizi, S. A. (2023). Alginate/hyaluronic acid-based systems as a new generation of wound dressings: A review. *International Journal of Biological Macromolecules*, *253*(Part 6), 127249. DOI: 10.1016/j.ijbiomac.2023.127249 PMID: 37802435

Zeng, Q., Qi, X., Shi, G., Zhang, M., & Haick, H. (2022). Wound dressing: From nanomaterials to diagnostic dressings and healing evaluations. *ACS Nano*, *16*(2), 1708–1733. DOI: 10.1021/acsnano.1c0841 PMID: 35050565

Zhang, J., Hu, K., Di, L., Wang, P., Liu, Z., Zhang, J., Yue, P., Song, W., Zhang, J., Chen, T., Wang, Z., Zhang, Y., Wang, X., Zhan, C., Cheng, Y.-C., Li, X., Li, Q., Fan, J.-Y., Shen, Y., & Qiao, H. (2021). Traditional herbal medicine and nanomedicine: Converging disciplines to improve therapeutic efficacy and human health. *Advanced Drug Delivery Reviews*, *178*, 113964. DOI: 10.1016/j.addr.2021.113964 PMID: 34499982

Zhang, J., Jiang, X., Wen, X., Xu, Q., Zeng, H., Zhao, Y., & Wang, Y. (2019). Bio-responsive smart polymers and biomedical applications. *JPhys Materials*, *2*(3), 032004.

Zhang, L., Zhang, Y., & Zhang, L. (2023). Exploring the potential of polysaccharide-based hybrid hydrogel systems for their biomedical and therapeutic applications: A review. *International Journal of Biological Macromolecules, 256*, 128348. DOI: 10.1016/j.ijbiomac.2023.128348 PMID: 38007021

Zhang, S., Hu, J., Sun, Y., Tan, H., Yin, J., Geng, F., & Nie, S. (2021). Review of structure and bioactivity of the Plantago (Plantaginaceae) polysaccharides. *Food Chemistry: X, 12*, 100158. DOI: 10.1016/j.fochx.2021.100158 PMID: 34825168

Zhang, W., Hu, J., Wu, H., Lin, X., & Cai, L. (2025). Stimuli-responsive hydrogel dressing for wound healing. *APL Materials, 13*(1), 010601. DOI: 10.1063/5.0245545

Zhang, W., Liu, L., Cheng, H., Zhu, J., Li, X., Ye, S., & Li, X. (2024). Hydrogel-based dressings designed to facilitate wound healing. *Materials Advances, 5*(4), 1364–1394. DOI: 10.1039/d3ma00682d

Zhang, X., Liang, Y., Huang, S., & Guo, B. (2024). Chitosan-based self-healing hydrogel dressing for wound healing. *Advances in Colloid and Interface Science, 332*, 103267. DOI: 10.1016/j.cis.2024.103267 PMID: 39121832

Zhang, X., Zhang, Z., & Zhang, L. (2020). Rational design and latest advances of polysaccharide-based hydrogels for wound healing. *Biomaterials Science, 8*(8), 2040–2055. DOI: 10.1039/D0BM00055H PMID: 32118241

Zhang, Y., & Li, X. (2022). Challenges and opportunities in the global regulation of herbal medicines: Towards harmonization. *International Journal of Regulatory Science, 7*(2), 45–57.

Zhao, R., Zhao, C., Wan, Y., Majid, M., Abbas, S. Q., & Wang, Y. (2023). In vitro and in vivo evaluation of alginate hydrogel-based wound dressing loaded with green chemistry cerium oxide nanoparticles. *Frontiers in Chemistry, 11*, 1298808. DOI: 10.3389/fchem.2023.1298808 PMID: 38075491

Zhao, X., Wu, H., Guo, B., Dong, R., Qiu, Y., & Ma, P. X. (2017). Antibacterial anti-oxidant electroactive injectable hydrogels for wound healing. *Acta Biomaterialia, 68*, 67–79.

Zhao, Y.. (2020). Regulatory hurdles for polysaccharide-based biomaterials in wound care: Challenges and solutions. *Biomaterials, 235*, 119758. DOI: 10.1016/j.biomaterials.2020.119758

Zhou, X., Zhang, X., & Zhang, L. (2024). A review of recent advances of cellulose-based intelligent-responsive hydrogels as vehicles for controllable drug delivery system. *International Journal of Biological Macromolecules, 264*, 130525. DOI: 10.1016/j.ijbiomac.2024.130525 PMID: 38431004

Zhou, Y., Wang, M., Yan, C., Liu, H., & Yu, D. G. (2022). Advances in the application of electrospun drug-loaded nanofibers in the treatment of oral ulcers. *Biomolecules*, *12*(9), 1254. PMID: 36139093

Zhu, H., Ao, H. T., Fu, Y., Zou, C., Chen, Z., Jin, Z., Zhou, H., Sun, B., & Guo, S. (2024). Optimizing alginate dressings with allantoin and chemical modifiers to promote wound healing. *International Journal of Biological Macromolecules*, *275*(Part 1), 133524. DOI: 10.1016/j.ijbiomac.2024.133524 PMID: 38945316

Zhu, J. (2010). Bioactive modification of poly (ethylene glycol) hydrogels for tissue engineering. *Biomaterials*, *31*(17), 4639–4656. DOI: 10.1016/j.biomaterials.2010.02.044 PMID: 20303169

Zhu, J., Cheng, H., Zhang, Z., Chen, K., Zhang, Q., Zhang, C., Gao, W., & Zheng, Y. (2024). Antibacterial Hydrogels for Wound Dressing Applications: Current Status, Progress, Challenges, and Trends. *Gels (Basel, Switzerland)*, *10*(8), 495. DOI: 10.3390/gels10080495 PMID: 39195024

Zhu, J., Zhou, H., Gerhard, E. M., Zhang, S., Parra Rodríguez, F. I., Pan, T., Yang, H., Lin, Y., Yang, J., & Cheng, H. (2023). Smart bioadhesives for wound healing and closure. *Bioactive Materials*, *19*, 360–375. PMID: 35574051

Zindle, J. K., Wolinsky, E., & Bogie, K. M. (2021). A review of animal models from 2015 to 2020 for preclinical chronic wounds relevant to human health. *Journal of Tissue Viability*, *30*(3), 291–300. PMID: 34103213

Zugle, D. (2021). Regulation of the use of pharmaceutical excipients in India. *Journal of Current Research in Medicine*, *2*(5), 2709–8125.

Zulkiflee, I., & Fauzi, M. B. (2021). Gelatin-polyvinyl alcohol film for tissue engineering: A concise review. *Biomedicines*, *9*(8), 979. PMID: 34440183

About the Contributors

Sachin Jain Working as a Professor & Principal in Oriental College of Pharmacy & Research Oriental University Indore MP (India). Dr. Jain having 18 years of teaching experience. He has received best researcher award, Received Best Pharmacy Professional Award & Young talent award in various Nation and International Conferences. Dr. Jain published more 12 books in various reputed Publisher Bentham Science, Taylor and Francis, Springer Nature, Cambridge Scholar Library, Iterative International Publishers and many more. Dr. Jain is active peer reviewer in various National and International Journal with high impact factor and very good publishers. Dr. Jain Publish More than 105 research/ review articles in National and International Journals with good indexing. Dr. Jain also Publish more than 18 Book chapters in International Publishers (Bentham Science, Springer Nature, Taylor and Francis, Cambridge Scholar Library, Iterative International Publishers).

Ravikant Gupta having decade of pharmaceutical industry experience, worked in many MNCS like IPCA, Mylan, Torrent. RGPV, AFRC, PCI, AICTE, NIRF, NAAC, NABL, FDA, US FDA, TGA, EU audit experience. PhD holder, more than 50 national and international conference/seminar/webinar/ symposium attended, More than 27 research paper published in national and international journals, 08 book published, 8 chapters published & 6 chapters communicated, 5 FDP attended, registered pharmacist, health excellence award winner, research excellence award, Young scientist award, inspirational Associate professor award, Young Researcher award winner.

Sudha Vengurlekar, Dean, Faculty of Pharmacy, Oriental University, Indore, is an accomplished academician with 21 years of expertise in pharmaceutical education, research, and administration. She has in-depth knowledge of healthcare systems, workflows, and regulatory compliance related to drug design. Her research expertise includes antimicrobial drug design, herbal drug development and molecular modeling techniques, along with a strong understanding of healthcare technologies and data analysis tools. She has published 70 research articles, 15 book chapters, and 6 books in reputed journals and publications. She has secured grants from AICTE, PCI, and ICMR for conducting various events and established strong collaboration with industries. Her contributions to scientific committees, editorial boards, and industry collaborations continue to drive advancements in pharmaceutical sciences.

***

Yogita Dhurandhar Research Scholar Department of Pharmacy Guru Ghasidas Central University, Bilaspur, C.G., she served as an Assistant Professor at the Institute of Pharmaceutical Sciences, Sanjay Rungta College, Kohka, Bhilai, Chhattisgarh. She had done M. Pharm (Pharmacology) (Gold Medalist) From GLA University, Mathura. Ms. Dhurandhar has authored four peer-reviewed & 2 research articles published in indexed journals and holds two design patents, in addition to one granted and published patent.she has contributed to three scholarly book chapters. She is actively participated in various government-sponsored workshops and has attended several national and international conferences

Sandipan Jige is working as assistant professor in botany from 25 years and also five year experience in subject horticultural science in under graduate college. He has visited Dubai, Indonesia, Thailand, Singapore, Malaysia, Germany, France, Netherlands, Switzerland and Belgium attend conferences. He has published more than thirty book chapter and research paper at national and international level. Also work on different academic committees at college and university level.

Namita Juvale is a curious research scientist with a decade long experience of teaching and mentoring pharmacy aspirants. Her research interest involves development of nanotechnological formulations, polymer synthesis and herbal extractions for the anticancer activity. Her research work also includes development of delivery systems for repurposed drugs. Dr. Namita Juvale holds prominent research contributions in the areas of pharmaceutical development and their regulatory considerations for domestic and international markets.

Suriya Mohan is a B.TECH Biotechnology undergraduate student at VISTAS, Pallavaram.

T.C. Manjunath was born on 6th February 1967. He did his B.E. from RV College of Engg. in 1989 (B'lore Univ), M.E. in Robotics & Automation from Govt.'s LD College of Engg., (Gujarat Univ., Ahmedabad) in 1992 with FCD-First Rank & PhD in Systems & Control Engg. from IIT Bombay in the year 2007, got best research scholar award for the entire IITB. He is currently working as the Dean

Research (R & D) and as Professor in Dept. of Computer Science & Engg. with specialization in IoT, Cyber Security, Blockchain Technology in Rajarajeswari College of Engineering, Bengaluru, Karnataka. He has got a teaching (academic), research & administrative experience of more than 35+ years (10 years as Principal & 8 years as HoD, 1 year as Dean Research & rest as faculty) and has published more than 1500+ research papers in various national & international journals & conferences, with 175+ patents, 100+ book-chapters, 25 awards, 100s of Keynote talks and also published 25 text books in various field of science, engineering & technology, completed projects worth Rs. 9 Crores till date & guided 10 PhD scholars in VTU. He is a member of 30 Professional Society Chapters and is a fellow of IE, IETE, AMIEE, Sr. Member of IEEE and a chartered engineer.

Arya Rajesh Nambiar is a 6th-semester student of B.F.Tech (Bachelor of Fashion Technology) at the National Institute of Fashion Technology (NIFT). With a specialization in Apparel Management, Arya has a strong interest in the convergence of fashion technology, sustainability, and material innovation. Her academic work reflects a balance of technical proficiency and creative problem-solving, particularly in areas such as functional textiles and herbal-polymer applications in wellness and fashion. Arya is passionate about contributing to future-ready, eco-conscious design solutions.

Kamta Prasad Namdeo (M. Pharm, PhD, FIC) Professor (Pharmaceutical Chemistry) Department of Pharmacy Guru Ghasidas Vishwavidyalaya (A Central University) Bilaspur (CG). He is having 27 years of Research and Academic Experience. He has taught at BMCP Pilani (Raj), BRNCP Mandsaur (MP) and IOP Bundelkhand University Jhansi (UP). He has completed three research project funded by UGC, AICTE and AYUSH, published Two books, 10 book chapters, 7 Indian patent and 87 research papers in various National and International journals. He has presented more than 60 research papers invited Lectures and Chair the session in various National, International conferences. Four Ph.D and 40 M.Pharm awarded under his supervision. He is receipient of Shanti Bharti Award (1991), Prof. K.A.Thaker award (2007) and Prof. S. B. Sonwane memorial award (2013) for best paper published. He is Life member of APTI(Association of Pharmaceutical Teachers of India), Indian Phamaceutical Association and Institution of Chemists.

P. Selvakumar is currently an Associate Professor in the Department of Science and Humanities at Nehru Institute of Technology, Coimbatore, Tamil Nadu, India. Prior to joining Nehru Institute of Technology, he held positions as an Assistant Professor in the Department of Science and Humanities various engineering colleges in Coimbatore, Tamil Nadu, India, spanning from 2011 to 2023. Dr.P. Selvakumar's academic and research interests lie primarily in the field of phytochemistry. He has made significant contributions to his field, with an impressive record that includes 30 journal publications, 12 patents, and 20 conference papers. Additionally, he has organized 5 seminars and conferences, further demonstrating his commitment to academic and scientific exchange. Throughout his career, Dr. P.Selvakumar has been recognized for his dedication and excellence in teaching, having been honored with several awards, including the Best Teacher Awards. He holds a prominent position in the academic community, contributing actively to research.

Vivek Pazhamalai working as Associate Professor at Vels Institute of Science, Technology and Advanced Studies, and has teaching experience of 16 years. He has published more than 69 research articles in international and national journals to his credit.

Ayona Padhi is a 6th-semester student of B.F.Tech (Bachelor of Fashion Technology) at the National Institute of Fashion Technology (NIFT). Specializing in Apparel Management, she has a growing interest in sustainable materials and product innovation. Her academic pursuits include exploring the application of herbal excipients and polymers in modern healthcare and fashion-tech domains. Ayona combines scientific curiosity with a managerial perspective to contribute to interdisciplinary research and development.

Tarun Kumar Patel is a distinguished academician and researcher in the field of biotechnology, currently serving as an Assistant Professor and Head of the Department of Biotechnology at Sant Guru Ghasidas Government P.G. College, Kurud, Dhamtari, Chhattisgarh, India. With a robust academic background and a decade-long teaching career, Dr. Patel has made significant contributions to fungal biology, mass spectrometry, and microbial biotechnology. Educational Background and Qualifications Dr. Patel earned his M.Sc. in Biotechnology and subsequently his Ph.D. in Biotechnology from Guru Ghasidas Vishwavidyalaya, Bilaspur, with research focused on detecting and analyzing aflatoxin production in Aspergillus flavus strains using advanced mass spectrometry techniques. His academic excellence is further demonstrated by qualifying the CSIR-NET (Life Sciences) and the GATE examination. Research Contributions Dr. Patel's research encompasses a wide array of topics within biotechnology. His notable works include studies on the biosynthesis of aflatoxin B1 in Aspergillus flavus, identification of genetic relationships in Chlorophytum species, and the exploration of entomopathogenic fungi as biocontrol agents in agriculture. He has contributed to several peer-reviewed journals and book chapters, including publications in Biologia, Biotechnology and Bioprocess Engineering, and contributions to books published by Elsevier and

Springer. Professional Experience and Teaching With over ten years of teaching experience at the undergraduate level and seven years at the postgraduate level, Dr. Patel has been instrumental in shaping the academic journey of numerous students. His commitment to education is evident in his active participation in various workshops and training programs, enhancing both his knowledge and teaching methodologies. Professional Affiliations and Recognitions Dr. Patel is an active member of esteemed scientific societies, including the Asian Federation of Biotechnology (AFOB) and the Association of Microbiologists of India (AMI). His research has garnered citations and recognition within the scientific community, reflecting the impact of his work on the field of biotechnology. Dr. Tarun Kumar Patel's dedication to research and education in biotechnology has significantly contributed to advancements in fungal biology and microbial biotechnology. His work continues to inspire students and researchers alike, fostering innovation and excellence in the scientific community.

Yashvi Patel is a research scholar pursuing integrated master's degree in pharmaceutical technology and healthcare management. Her research interest involves development and evaluation of drug delivery systems and pharmaceutical formulations using herbal and allopathic medicaments. She has hands on experience of working in the pharmacovigilance department, where she honed literature screening, medical coding and documentation skills.

Jeevan Lal Prajapati is an emerging researcher and academician in pharmaceutical sciences, currently pursuing a Ph.D. at Central University Guru Ghasidas Vishwavidyalaya, Bilaspur. He holds a Master's degree in Pharmaceutical Chemistry and a Bachelor's degree in Pharmacy from Central University Indira Gandhi National Tribal University, Amarkantak. With over 2 years of research experience and 2 years of teaching experience as an Assistant Professor, he currently serves as Dean for Diploma in Pharmacy students at LCIT College of Pharmacy, Bilaspur. His research primarily focuses on the design, synthesis, and evaluation of redox-based chemical delivery systems, with specific applications in treating neurological disorders. He has authored two peer-reviewed research papers published in prestigious Scopus-indexed journals such as Expert Opinion on Drug Delivery and ACS Neuroscience, with impact factors of 7.2 and 4.4, respectively. He also holds three Indian patents related to neurological drug delivery systems. Jeevan has contributed to four book chapters with reputed publishers including Springer and Cambridge Scholars Publishing, covering topics like QSAR methodologies, sickle cell anemia, and AI in hospital management. His academic projects include work on PAMAM dendrimers for drug solubility enhancement and phytochemical investigations of tribal medicinal plants. He has participated in several national and international conferences and workshops, enhancing his expertise in drug development and delivery. His skill set includes proficiency in techniques such as FT-IR spectroscopy, UV-Vis spectroscopy, and molecular docking tools like Autodock. Driven by a passion for innovation in pharmacy and teaching, Jeevan is committed to advancing pharmaceutical education and research.

Rupayan Roy is an Assistant Professor at the National Institute of Fashion Technology (NIFT), Kannur, with a Ph.D. and M.Tech from the Indian Institute of Technology (IIT) Delhi. His academic and research pursuits span textile engineering, apparel production, and smart materials, with a strong emphasis on sustainability, ergonomics, and advanced manufacturing technologies. Dr. Roy has authored multiple book chapters and journal articles on topics such as IoT in garment manufacturing, AI in research writing, protective gear design, nonwoven materials, and polymeric energy harvesting. His recent work explores the integration of hydrothermal liquefaction (HTL) with textile waste sorting and the development of intelligent air filter media using IoT. An active contributor to curriculum development and interdisciplinary research, Dr. Roy is currently working on emerging areas like soft body armour for women, consumer behavior in circular economy models, and virtual try-on technology in retail. He is committed to bridging traditional knowledge with modern innovations to drive sustainable and inclusive growth in the textile and apparel sector.

S. Baskar completed Ph.D. in Vels Institute of Science, Technology and Advanced Studies. He completed his M.E. in Refrigeration and Air Conditioning at the College of Engineering, Anna University, Guindy, in 2012, and obtained his B.E. in Mechanical Engineering from M. Kumarasamy College of Engineering in 2010. Since 2017, he has been serving as an Assistant Professor, Assistant Director (International Affairs), and Research Supervisor at Vels Institute of Science, Technology and Advanced Studies. With over 12 years of teaching experience, he has guided numerous undergraduate and postgraduate student projects. Currently, he is supervising one full-time Ph.D. scholar. He has published more than 80 research papers in reputed journals, attended 47 workshops, and presented papers at 14 national and 26 international conferences.

S. Ivo Romauld Ph.D. in Biotechnology and currently serving as a Associate Professor at the Vels Institute of Science, Technology and Advanced Studies (VISTAS), Chennai.

Meenambiga S S, Assistant Professor completed 6 years of teaching experience and 4 years of research experience in the field of Biotechnology. Passionate about teaching and have trained many young students in the field of Mycology, Natural

Product Research, Nanoparticle synthesis, Drug Discovery from Plants and fungal sources and in-silico analysis of drug targets using modern Bio-informatics tools. Skilled in scientific writing covering the following aspects: Proposal submission, research articles suitable for national and international publications,drafting, proof reading and editing research thesis and expertise in critically reviewing the research manuscript for indexed journals. Member of Board of Studies for B.Tech Biotechnology curriculum in VISTAS. Guided more than 20 undergraduate students projects and served as Principal Investigator in the student's project funded by Tamilnadu State Council for Science and Technology. Published more than 30 research and review articles in national and international indexed journal and has volunteered as reviewer for many reputed journals. Life member of Mycological Society of India, BRSI, IARA, IAENG and many other professional organizations. Completed

Kavyashree Shetty is currently working with a pharmaceutical industry and has completed master's degree in the field of pharmaceutical regulatory affairs. She has hands on experience of working in the clinical research department, where she acquired knowledge of volunteer screening, informed consent documentation and bioequivalence studies. Her areas of interest include regulatory compliance, generic drug development, medical devices, biologics and nutraceuticals.

Aspee Singh is an emerging researcher and academician in pharmaceutical sciences, currently pursuing a Ph.D. at Central University Guru Ghasidas Vishwavidyalaya, Bilaspur. He holds a Master's degree in Pharmaceutics and a Bachelor's degree in Pharmacy from Bundelkhand University, Jhansi, U.P. With over 2 years of research experience and 6 years of teaching experience as an Assistant Professor, he is working for Shri Ramdham Mahavidyalaya (Department of Pharmacy), Mauranipur, Jhansi, U.P. His research primarily focuses on the Development of some modified chemical entities, a prodrug approach, specific drug delivery for Alzheimer's disease, with specific applications in treating neurological disorders. He has authored six peer-reviewed research papers published in prestigious Scopus-indexed journals such as Expert Opinion on Drug Delivery and ACS Neuroscience, with impact factors of 7.2 and 4.4, respectively. He also holds three Indian patents related to neurological drug delivery systems. As Pee Singh has contributed to three book chapters with reputed publishers, including Springer and Cambridge Scholars Publishing, covering topics like QSAR methodologies, sickle cell anemia, and AI in hospital management. His academic projects include work on the Formulation and evaluation of mucoadhesive buccal patches of furosemide. He has participated in several national and international conferences and workshops, enhancing his expertise in formulation development and delivery. His skill set includes proficiency in techniques such as FT-IR spectroscopy, UV-Vis spectroscopy, and molecular docking tools like Autodock. Driven by a passion for innovation in pharmacy and teaching, As Pee Singh is committed to advancing pharmaceutical education and research.

Shubham Tomar currently working as Pharmacovigilance Associate at National Coordination Centre Pharmacovigilance Programme of India, Indian Pharmacopoeia Commission (IPC). Previously he has worked as Assistant professor at Anjali College of Pharmacy, Etmadpur Agra. He has completed Master of Pharmacy in Pharmacology from GLA University, Mathura. His master's study comprises of investigation of Neuroprotection potential of a compound on Alzheimer's Disease. Currently, he has 3 peer reviewed publications in indexed journals and holds two granted and published patent to his record. He has attended and gained knowledge from various government sponsored workshops. He has also attended various national and international conferences.

Aarthi V, student of vels university studying b-tech biotechnology

Vaibhavi Bhosale is an 8th-semester student of B.F.Tech (Bachelor of Fashion Technology) at the National Institute of Fashion Technology (NIFT). With a strong foundation in apparel production and fashion management, she is particularly interested in advanced material science, sustainable manufacturing, and innovative product development. Vaibhavi combines technical knowledge with industry-oriented insights, aiming to contribute to the evolving landscape of fashion technology through research and practical application.

Index

Symbols

A

B

C

D

E

G

H

I

L

M

S

T

U

W

www.ingramcontent.com/pod-product-compliance
Lightning Source LLC
LaVergne TN
LVHW081318300926
849161LV00008B/1804